Medical Terminology, Documentation, and Coding

Giving students the strongest possible baseline in medical terminology, and explaining how and why it is used in documentation and basic coding, this is a vital text for all students taking courses in the medical arena. It allows readers to use their knowledge immediately in any medical setting (including being a patient), in their workplaces, and in the journey to future careers.

Using a body systems approach to medical terminology, this textbook supports students to:

- Recognize words by constructing medical terms based on root words, prefixes, linking forms, and suffixes.

- Define, spell, pronounce, and use medical terms, acronyms, and abbreviations in the context of patient care with appropriate documentation and coding examples.

- Identify anatomical directions, fundamental anatomical terminology, basic physiologic functions, and common pathology of all major organ systems with related medical investigation tools, procedures, and pharmaceuticals.

- Relate the use of medical language and medical record-keeping to the SOAP format, common medical reports, and coding tools, along with their impact on patient care.

Accompanied by plentiful color illustrations and activities, as well as a companion website with resources for both instructors and students, this is a fresh and readable textbook.

Anne P. Stich is a retired Physician Assistant and former Assistant Professor in the College of Arts and Science at Bellevue University, Nebraska, USA. As the program director for the BA in Health Science, Anne developed many of the courses including Medical Terminology.

Medical Terminology, Documentation, and Coding

Anne P. Stich

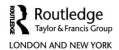

Routledge
Taylor & Francis Group

LONDON AND NEW YORK

First published 2018
by Routledge
2 Park Square, Milton Park, Abingdon, Oxon OX14 4RN

and by Routledge
711 Third Avenue, New York, NY 10017

Routledge is an imprint of the Taylor & Francis Group, an informa business

© 2018 Anne P. Stich

British Library Cataloguing-in-Publication Data
A catalogue record for this book is available from the British Library

Library of Congress Cataloging-in-Publication Data
Names: Stich, Anne P., author.
Title: Medical terminology, documentation, and coding / Anne P. Stich.
Description: Abingdon, Oxon ; New York, NY : Routledge, 2018. |
Includes bibliographical references and index.
Identifiers: LCCN 2017030227| ISBN 9780415792851 (hardback) |
ISBN 9780415792868 (pbk.) | ISBN 9781315211367 (ebook)
Subjects: | MESH: Terminology as Topic | Documentation—methods |
Clinical Coding—methods
Classification: LCC R123 | NLM W 15 | DDC 610.1/4—dc23LC
record available at https://lccn.loc.gov/2017030227

ISBN: 978-0-415-79285-1 (hbk)
ISBN: 978-0-415-79286-8 (pbk)
ISBN: 978-1-315-21136-7 (ebk)

Typeset in Bembo and Futura
by Florence Production Ltd, Stoodleigh, Devon, UK

Visit the companion website: www.routledge.com/cw/Stich

Contents

Illustrations and photographs

The majority of the illustrations and photographs are royalty free via Shutterstock as purchased by the author for use in this text and its online website. The others are from Public Domain, used with permission, or taken by the author.

Author rendered illustrations or photographs: Figures 1.2; 2.4; 2.6; 2.7; 2.8 (set); 2.9; 2.10; 2.11; 2.12; 2.17; 2.18; 2.19; 2.20; 3.5; 4.14 (set); 8.3 (set).

Public Domain: Figures 1.5; 9.2; 12.21.

Dr. Karthi Aimanan: Figure 13.16.

Karen Mayhood Art and Design: Figures 4.6; 4.19; 11.5; 11.8; 11.25; 14.3.

Coding references

The ICD-10-CM is produced and copyrighted by the World Health Organization (WHO). Its thousands of specific codes are considered public domain by virtue of extensive use for all medical care worldwide. Current codes are available in print and online. This is true for the ICD-10-PCS, HCPCS, and cpt® resource companion texts as well. These codes are available to all persons, worldwide.

IMPORTANT NOTE: The reader is notified that the examples in this book are from an online search made in 2016. The exercises utilize only a fraction of the information contained in the original resources and are not presented as a precise transcription. Do <u>not</u> use these codes for patient care episodes; look up the new ones!

Finally, the author intentionally avoided any direct quotes or statistics. This was done to illustrate that science and medicine are constantly changing; there are very few absolutes. The estimates utilized in the textbook were based on 2016 research. The statistics on cancer or sexually transmitted disease have already changed. Please do your own current research and be thankful for the many people ahead of you who produced the first books on terminology and anatomy and physiology and genetics and so much more.

Reviewers and initial review by institute

Reviewers

Susan (Sue) M. Cox, MD
Executive Vice Dean for Academics
UT Austin Dell Medical School

John Glover ScDPT
Doctor of Science in Physical Therapy

Lisa D. Hiykel IAC, BBA, RN, MSN
Retired

Karem Ralls, PT, MPT
Clinical Rehab Coordinator
Vibra Rehab and LTACH Hospital

Tammie Tabor, BSN, RN
Chief Operating Officer
Vibra Rehabilitation Hospital

Kevin Nicholson, PT
Director of Therapy Services
Vibra Rehabilitation Hospital

Heather N. Stich, OTA
Occupational Therapy Assistant

Tony Jasnowski, PhD
Professor and Writing Center Director
Bellevue University, NE

Initial review by institute

National American University, New Mexico

University of Toledo, Ohio

The Salter School, Massachusetts

Dorsey School, Michigan

Herzing University-Akron Campus, Ohio

Bristol Community College, Massachusetts

Baker College of Jackson, Michigan

Florida Technical College, Florida

Florida National University, Allied Health, Florida

New England Institute of Technology, Rhode Island

Kansas City Kansas Community College, Kansas

Stratford University, Virginia

Bryant and Stratton, Ohio

Henry Ford College, Michigan

Introduction

PRELUDE TO A TREK . . .

This textbook is for *you*! Whether you are learning medical terminology to become a medical technician and/or preparing for a professional school or as a patient who wants to understand the language, you are in the right place. The textbook is written in the context of patient care; it demonstrates how, why, and where these terms, acronyms, and abbreviations are used in a myriad of medical locations. It demonstrates why spelling, directions, numbers, and more are so vital to the delivery of quality care. Documentation review, a bit of coding, pharmacy, genetics, oncology, subspecialities, history, and even a measure of ethics is included. Why? Because how *you* use the language of medicine does tell a story.

Why this textbook? I have been learning and using the medical language since taking my first medical terminology course at age 19. When moving through several medical jobs on my way to degrees and the practice of medicine, I was struck by the interconnectivity of all the elements and how they come together to provide quality care for patients. As a patient, the language tells my story. As a provider, it is my communication tool with everyone from the ward clerk to the physician. **Medical terminology** is the glue, the interlocking network permitting our individual medical story to be told. As a teacher, I want to convey the terms, their use, and their value to the continuity of care from inception to death. Teaching the terms and word parts based on my learning of 30+ years, I aspire to reflect the amazing relationships in tracking illness and injury via documentation. **Documentation and coding** propels our research, our innovation, our preparation and response to catastrophes, patient safety initiatives, and it permits tracking, reimbursement, and so much more. No one will become a 'coder' with this textbook – however, you will know how the medical terms, spelling, and accuracy influence patient care, coding, and health informatics. This textbook endeavors to teach the old while making room for the growth and creativity of the users, YOU!

Each **unit** has much more than the terms to be learned. Explaining within context and with examples aids the student to relate the terms to the actual work of medicine. New technologies, medications, therapies, and fields of research are included to enable students to use the knowledge and skills they will learn immediately. Identifying the rationale for documentation and coding will give the learner a head start for any medical occupation in their future. This is not an 'essentials' text; it is a comprehensive medical terminology, documentation, and a coding primer.

A DIFFERENT ROAD . . .

All medical terminology textbooks cover word roots, linking forms with lots of prefixes and suffixes. This is a **working textbook**; it has a number of unique facets representing work and discovery for students and instructors alike. Making it easy for the reader to spot topics and challenges, we have recurrent icons to set these innovations apart:

Kitchen lab

The **Kitchen lab** feature is to remind all of us of a world full of science and medicine and even, medical terminology. The Kitchen lab encourages you to look around and in the mirror to find examples of your learning in your world!

The **Check it!** symbol is part of the workbook side of the text. These follow topics page to page. A quick set of questions to check understanding with the answer immediately available in the second column. A few case-related **Check it! symbols will be for discussion with the instructor.**

Word building

This construction symbol signals an opportunity to do some **Word building**. Three or four word roots with linking vowel are presented with a number of suffixes and/or prefixes to encourage word building. The instructor has the list of acceptable words. This would be a good in-class activity and will teach you to *find* and *use* a dictionary.

Did You Know **Did You Know?** is a short piece of information concerning the topic of the **unit**. It might be the source of a particular word, such as 'surgeon' or a factoid on the number of miles our nervous system covers.

Pharmacy corner

Pharmacy corner will cover medications associated with the **Unit** concept from actual medications to revealing how numbers and spelling can impact patient safety and quality care.

The **Unit worksheets** at the end of each **unit** contain a plethora of practice opportunities including the usual fill in the blanks, matching, etc. . . . *and* a case study with attached questions or essay questions. All designed to provide visuals and kinesthetics (moving a pen across the paper) to repeat, use, and understand the terms, documentation use, and coding interactions.

Online you will find any number of review activities including **practice quizzes**, **a glossary** of all the terms used in each **unit**, **flashcards**, **crossword puzzles**, **spelling challenges**, and **power point presentations** with notes. There is a full glossary and pronunciation guide online. There is more. Take the trek and find all the fun and innovative ways we have to help you learn the new language of medicine.

THE TREK, A CROSS-TRAINING PROCESS . . .

Each **unit** will illustrate the process of coming face to face with terms you already use (yes, you already know some medical terminology) and guide you to new and exciting associations with word roots, suffixes, and prefixes. Each is a 'stop and do' opportunity.

The **unit** is led off by a tree with a core word-root at its base, the root. This is the core, the root, the beginning of the trek. The words surrounding the blooming tree reveal how a simple word root with a linking vowel will become many terms and concepts on the journey.

Each **unit** begins a short list of **key word parts** to emphasize their import. The table here and at the end of the unit are color coded to reinforce the word part distinctions.

KEY WORD PARTS

Word roots with linking vowel	Prefixes	Suffixes
Anat/o > dissection	a- or an-	-al
Arteri/o > arteries	anti-	-algia

Note the COLORS of the three word parts and other elements; this visual aid is carried out throughout each **unit** to reinforce the elemental concepts. Repetition with visuals (vision), auditory (listening), and kinesthetics (movement) is crucial to memory and use.

- **Blue** is for the linking forms > word root/linking vowel > cardi/o; angi/o; oste/o; my/o . . .

- **Green** is for the prefixes > pre-; un-; supra-; hyper-; micro- . . .

- **Maroon** is for the suffixes > -ectomy; -osis; -er; -poiesis; -scope . . .

- **Magenta** is for the pronunciation guide > arteriogram > are-**tier**-ee-oh-gram

- **Red** is for **Alerts** for words or word parts which may be easily confused and potentially impact patient safety. **Alerts** may be found in any areas, look for the **RED**.

Every **unit** has **Feature boxes** to help students locate key concepts quickly. The medical terminology, directions, numbers, and definitions are found in the two column tables. The second column is numbered and may include more terms, or word parts associated with the first column. Pink is for documentation discussions. Purple is for pharmacy and yellow is for coding. The gray summary box will review the **unit**.

UNITS DELIVER . . .

1 **Word building** with the introduction of word parts and the use of suffixes making nouns and adjectives to describe and illustrate illness and disease.

2 **Systems, directions, and numbers** provides a preliminary look at the body systems these medical terms describe and enumerate. The functions and elements of the SOAP note and radiology reports are examples of where and how the anatomical position, directions, regions, cavities, and numbers are utilized day-to-day.

3 **Cells, tissue, and pathology** investigates the neighborhood of the cells and how they relate to the pathology and laboratory sciences, oncology, and genetics.

4 **Skin and soft tissues** evaluates the terms related to skin and soft tissues with their common injuries, descriptions, diagnostics, and therapies. There is a focus on burn units and ICD Injury coding.

5 **The skeleton** encompasses the pile of bones and joints and how they stand up. Injury, illnesses, diagnostics, surgery, and non-surgical therapeutics are reviewed as each term is presented.

6 **The muscles** considers a good number of the 600 muscles, tendons, and ligaments. Knowing the terms and relationships of muscle action will aid the student in recognizing the disease and injuries related to muscles as they move to their careers. There is a focus on rehabilitation medicine and the use of **cpt**®.

7 **Nervous system and psychiatry** examines the brain. A myriad of terms describe the physical and emotional context of the nervous system: central and peripheral. Diagnostics and therapies are reviewed with each appropriate term. There is a review on the ICD Table of Drugs and Chemicals.

8 **Special senses** yields many new terms covering the skin sensors, eyes, ears, nose, throat, and cranial nerves. Some of the most common reasons for an office visit are within the reach of these topics and they will be covered with diagnostics and pharmacy options. There is a short look at the ICD Tabular List of Disease.

9 **Immune and endocrine systems** brings the amazing internal survival and protection mechanisms to the student via terms, diagnostics, and the emerging therapies. Genetics is revisited here with its burgeoning testing and impact on therapies. The function of the EHR for tracking epidemics via the CDC and epidemiology provides a case study to illustrate the use of many of these terms.

10 **Blood and lymphatics** embraces a huge number of terms and interactions via the fluids of life. Students also explore the many hematological laboratory assessments and how they are coded in **cpt**® and HCPCS.

11 **Cardiovascular system** studies the terms, diagnostics, and therapeutics of the heart and blood vessels. The ICD procedural coding will illustrate cardiac and vessel procedures.

12 **Respiratory system** includes both the upper and lower respiratory systems, their terms, diagnostics, and therapies. The function of medical records during catastrophe and terrorist events will illustrate occupational respiratory diseases by tracing respiratory illness after 9/11/2001.

13 **Gastrointestinal system** is another enormous area to learn terms, diagnostics, and procedures – both to investigate and provide therapy for multiple conditions. There are some specifics for dental care and using online resources to perform basic coding from the ICD Index of Illness and Injury. There is an ethics question on the extremes of food intake: starvation and obesity.

14 **Renal system** examines the terms related to the micro- and macro-anatomy of the kidneys and urinary system, which clear waste daily. There is a brief look at documentation and the law with more use of online resources to perform basic coding from ICD Index of Illness and Injury.

15 **Reproductive systems and genetics** provides the beginning and the end of this textbook. Beginnings because without our reproductive organs, our species would cease to exit. A look at the ethical questions generated by reproductive health.

ALL THE GOODIES FOR THE TREK . . .

- Full **Glossary and pronunciation table**

- Appendix A: **Singular and plural suffix list**

- Appendix B: **Likes, opposites, and very close with spelling difference between USA and UK**

- **Unit worksheets** review all the topics with a variety of question types and exercises to check recall, ability to use the concepts, and critical thinking.

- Instructor templates, tests, practice quizzes, unit outlines, and suggested interactive learning opportunities.

- Topics for discussion boards or class: HIPAA, health agencies, government regulations, health informatics, safety initiatives, and more.

- PowerPoints with notes cover topics with new illustrations and photos to expand learning.

- Flashcards, seek and find, and crossword puzzles to provide plenty of repetition.

INDEBTED TO . . .

We are products of our environment; as children we learn from the generation who came before us. We, in turn, will teach the next child and together we develop a data-base built by literally thousands of people. My expertise is born of thousands of scientists, educators, and practitioners who came before me building the medical language you will be learning. From ancient times and faraway places the language was and is forged. It is a work in progress. I want to acknowledge all the originators who have written the dictionaries, produced the textbooks of medicine, and did the scientific research for their dedication and contributions to our collective experience and knowledge.

My deepest gratitude to my parents, Tom and Patricia, who taught me the value of education, hard work, and compassion. The guidance and love of my parents has given me the courage to write this tome. Thanks to my brothers (Marc, John, and Paul) and their families who have put up with my wandering and my incessant 'Did you know?' over the dinner table. They have each contributed with their gifts and skills as well. Respect and appreciation to my friends and colleagues who used their gifts to hone my syntax (Tony), my clarity, and my knowledge for the benefit of others.

THE AUTHOR . . .

Anne P. Stich, MMS, MPS, PA-C (retired), is a former Assistant Professor in the College of Arts and Science with Bellevue University, Nebraska. As the program director for the BA in Health Science, Anne developed many of the courses including medical terminology to give the undergraduate a strong baseline in medical fundamentals as preparation for professional studies and careers.

A medical professional, Anne was a certified physician assistant, practicing for 25 years and taught other medical professionals for 20 of those years. From the age of 19, Anne has had a broad range of experiences including operating room technician, medical records, ward clerk, emergency medical technician, medical coding, hospice care, emergency department care, and family practice. She served her country proudly in the U.S. Air Force and retired as a Lt. Colonel in 2007. She has written for and co-edited textbooks and written for the National Board of Medical Examiners. This extensive familiarity with medicine has given Anne a unique perspective on the value of all jobs within the medical arena. Learn well and share!

Unit 1

Word building

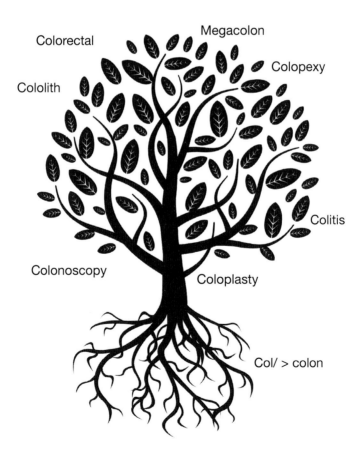

TARGETED LEARNING

1 Identify the beginnings of the language of medicine.

2 Recognize word parts and the basic assembly of medical terms.

3 Correctly construct, define, pronounce, and spell medical terms.

4 Use the understanding of word formation to pick out the fundamental components from unfamiliar terms.

5 Explain what a medical record is and its uses.

KEY WORD PARTS

Word roots with linking vowel	Prefixes	Suffixes
Anat/o > dissection	a- or an-	-al
Arteri/o > arteries	anti-	-algia
Arthr/o > joints	brady-	-ectomy
Cardi/o > heart	ec- or ecto-	-er and -or
Chondr/o > cartilage	en- and endo-	-ic
Col/o or Colon/o > colon	ex- or exo-	-ics
Cyt/o or Cellul/o > cell	in- or intra-	-ist
Dermat/o or Derm/o > skin	in-, im-, ir-, and il-	-itis
Duoden/o > duodenum	hyper-	-logy
Gastr/o > stomach	hypo-	-osis
Medic/o > medicine	pre- or pro-	-ostomy
My/o > muscle	sub-	-scopy
Oste/o > bone	tachy-	-scope
Rhin/o > nose	uni-	-tomy

IN THE BEGINNING

Once upon a time a very long time ago an ancestor burned his fingers on the fire that his next door neighbor discovered and someone took on the role of healer. Medicine was born in this healer. Perhaps a cave drawing recorded the event to warn others about the dangers of fire (Figure 1.2).

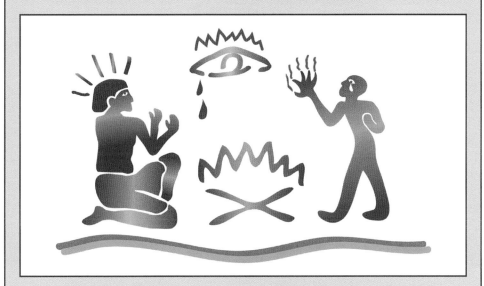

Figure 1.2

The word root with linking vowel **medic/o** is Greek for physician and over time medicine became defined as the art and science of treating disease with drugs or curative substances. In the day of Hippocrates, surgery or other procedures were not considered 'medical'. Today, the term is inclusive of all science fields which research, restore, or preserve health and wellness. Like many words there are other uses for medicine; it is the term for pharmacy drugs and topical applications (medications). The term is used to admonish someone, 'If you do that, you will have to take your medicine' meaning there are consequences to actions.

WORD ROOTS

'Word root' or 'root word' or 'primary term' are all names for the core of medical term, literally, the root of the term. It represents the meaning of the term: a thing, place, or procedure in the case of the language of medicine. It is the beginning piece for word construction. In medicine, it is often the name of an anatomical part of the body, such as the heart > cardi/o:

Cardiac (**kar**-dee-ak) > pertaining to the *heart*. -ac is 'pertaining to'

Endocarditis (**en**-doe-kar-**die**-tis) > inflammation of the inside of the *heart*. Endo- (inside) and -itis (inflammation)

Cardiologist (**kar**-dee-**ol**-oh-jist) > Specialist who studies and treats *heart* disease. -log/ist is a person who studies

Cardiomegaly (**kar**-dee-oh-**meg**-a-lee) > Enlargement of the *heart*. -megaly is enlargement

Cardiocentesis (**kar**-dee-oh-sen-**tea**-sis) > Removal of fluid from the *heart*. -centesis is removal of fluid, usually with a needle

1.1

Cardi- is the word root

Cardi/o is the linking form which is how the term is presented in most textbooks and dictionaries.

 Mrs. Rentoria has cardiopulmonary disease. The first word root in this term means?

1.2
Heart (cardi-)

 Dermatitis, dermatome, dermatologist, and dermatosis all have the word root of _____ .

1.3
Dermat- (skin)

LINKING FORMS AND ANATOMY

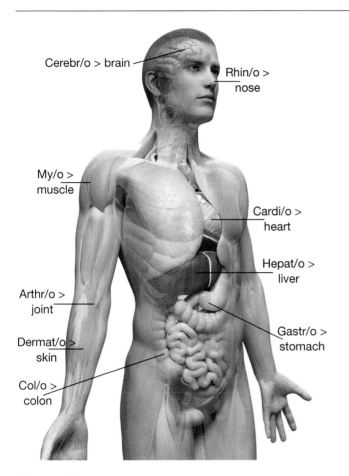

Cerebr/o > brain

Rhin/o > nose

My/o > muscle

Cardi/o > heart

Hepat/o > liver

Arthr/o > joint

Dermat/o > skin

Gastr/o > stomach

Col/o > colon

Figure 1.3

1.4
These linking forms denote body parts:

Rhin/o > Nose

Dermat/o > Skin

Oste/o > Bone

Chondr/o > Cartilage

Arteri/o > Artery

Gastr/o > Stomach

Cardi/o > Heart

My/o > Muscle

NOTICE
The word root or its linking form cannot be used as a word in and of itself. **It needs the word root + linking vowel + a suffix** at the very least.

Kitchen lab

Think of all the commercials you have seen in the media. Knowing anatomical terms are medical terms, what terms can you identify?

1.5
Discuss your list with the instructor and classmates.

HISTORY OF NOMENCLATURE

Where exactly did these 'word roots' come from? Medicine is a language and it has had many influences over the millenn*ia* (plural). The oldest medical books are thought to be a set of papyri (plural) of Egyptian origin, dating back to 1950 BCE (Before Common Era). Several contain prescriptions and recommendations dealing with contraception, birthing methods, and tending to the care of infants. While hieroglyphics would not become part of the Western language of medicine, Arabic and others would contribute to the Greek and Latin.

The Greeks of Hippocrates's time (fourth–fifth century BCE) were anatomists and they began to name most of the many pieces and parts of the human body. Indeed, many word parts used every day are from the Greek. Roman physicians continued to define the body and its functions in Latin. Claudius Galen (129–200 CE) was an influential Greek physician doing his research in Rome and translating the Greek terms into Latin. He is credited with the development of several scientific disciplines: anatomy, physiology, pathology, pharmacology, and neurology.

LINKING VOWEL

The linking vowel is usually the 'o'. It is like the conjunction 'and' in a sentence; it links the word root to the suffix or the next word root. It is like the mortar between bricks, binding the terms and meanings together (Figure 1.4). **The 'o' joins the word root to any suffix which begins** with **a consonant.**

1.6
The suffix makes these word roots into complete words: nouns or descriptive adjectives:

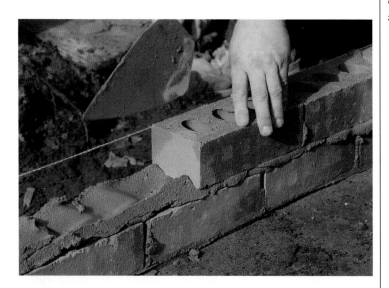

Figure 1.4

- **Cardi/o**: Cardiomyopathy (**Kar**-dee-oh-my-**op**-ath-ee) > disease of the heart muscle.

- **Cerebr/o**: Cerebrovascular (**ser**-eh-bro-**vas**-Q-lar) > pertaining to the brain's blood vessels. Cerebr/o > brain cortex, Vascul/o > blood vessels.

- **Enter/o**: Enterology (**en**-ter-**ol**-oh-gee) > studying the small intestines. Enter/o > small intestines (as a whole).

- **Ophthalm/o**: Ophthalmoscope (of-**thal**-moe-scope) > an instrument to look at the eyes. Ophthalm/o > eyes, one of the most frequently misspelled words because of the two 'h's. Alternate pronunciation is op-**thal**-moe-scope.

- **Arteri/o**: Arteriogram (ahr-**tier**-ee-oh-gram) > radiographic record of the arteries checking for blockage or injury.

- **Termin/o**: Terminology (**tur**-min-ol-**oh**-gee) > the study of words.

- Esophag/**o**/gastr/**o**/duoden/**o**/scopy (eh-**sof**-ah-go-**gas**-tro-**due**-oh-deh-**nos**-ko-pee) > procedure of looking at the esophagus, stomach and duodenum (**EGD**). This word is a **compound word** because it has two or more word roots > esophag/, gastr/, and duoden/.

-pathy > disease	
-ar > pertaining to	
-logy > study of	
-itis > inflammation	
-gram > record, the actual product	
-graph > the machine making the record or the record	
-graphy > the process of making a record	
-cyte > cell (as a suffix)	

✓ Mary needs to have an inspection of her eyes with a scope; construct this medical term. _____/_ /_____

1.7
Ophthalm/o/scope

✓ Hector has a disease of the muscle; construct this medical term. _____/_ /_____

1.8
My/o/pathy

Word building

*Using the word roots **with the linking vowel to build as many valid terms with the suffixes given. Please define each term.***

Rhin/o Cardi/o Cerebr/o

-logy -scope -graphy -itis -megaly -plasty -pathy

1.9
The instructor has the list!

When linking a word root with a suffix beginning with a vowel (a, e, i, o, u, or y) do NOT use 'o' as the linked vowel; omit it. Use the vowel of the suffix.

- **Arthr/itis** (are-**thri**-tis) > inflammation of the joints > (it is NOT, arthr/o/itis).

- **Lymph/oma** (lim-**foe**-ma) > tumor of the lymph tissue > (it is NOT, lymph/o/oma).

- **Chondr/o/my/algia** (kon-dro-**my**-al-gee-ya) > Pain of the cartilage and muscles > (it is NOT, chondr/o/my/o/algia).

- **Gastr/ectomy** (gas-**trek**-toe-me) > Surgical removal of the stomach > (it is NOT, gastr/o/itis).

- **Oste/itis** (**os**-tea-**eye**-tis) > Inflammation of the bone > (it is NOT, oste/o/itis).

- **Hepat/ic** (hep-**at**-ik) > pertaining to the liver > (it is NOT, hepat/o/ic).

✓ Heather has an inflammation of her nose. The proper term for this is?

✓ Aaron is 'studying words'. How is the term constructed? _____/ __/ _____

✓ The 'o' as a linking vowel is used with a suffix which begins with a _____ .

1.10
It seems this guideline should be true for word root + word root as well BUT it is not, most of the time.

Oste/**o**/arthr/itis

Gastr/**o**/enter/itis

Ot/**o**/encephal/itis

Suffixes
–oma > tumor

–algia > pain of

–ic > pertaining to

1.11
Rhinitis (no 'o')

1.12
Termin/o/logy

1.13
Consonant

MEDICAL RECORDS

Medical terminology is the process of studying the words of medicine. While the original word roots are primarily from the Greek and Latin, language is not static. French, German, Middle English, and other languages have affected the language. As science and technology has progressed, words have been added and others redefined. Medical terminology provides a standard language for all medical care worldwide; an appendicitis in Atlanta, Georgia, is the same appendicitis in Seoul, South Korea. This permits all medical providers to exchange information and research using a common language. It is vital to each of us, as the medical record is the story of health, illness, and injury. Today, the paper record of the personal medical story or history has become the **Electronic Health Record** (**EHR**). The story contains four main categories:

- **History (Hx)** or the **Subjective** section > the story of illness or injury or prevention efforts. It tells the story of how, where, and when a set of symptoms began, waxed, or waned, and what was done to alleviate the symptoms. It is based on what the patient tells the provider including a record of vaccinations, past medical history, previous surgeries, current medications, allergies, and more.

- **Physical exam (PE)** and other **Objective** findings > what a provider finds when a physical examination is conducted. It paints the picture of what is visualized or discovered. It tells the reader how the lungs and heart sound or what the rash looked like. It includes results from the laboratory, radiology, and any number of procedures giving a measured result. It is the facts as seen in a particular moment in time (Figure 1.5).

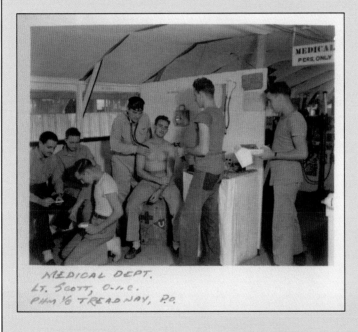

Figure 1.5

- **Diagnosis (Dx)** > also called the **Assessment** or problem list; it is what the provider believes is going on as indicated by the **Hx** and **PE** findings. It is the name of the problem: e.g., a viral upper respiratory infection or a broken fibula or hypertension. There may be one diagnosis or several. Sometimes, the provider is not exactly sure what is going on yet so the diagnosis area may contain the **R/O** (rule out) list: e.g., Abdominal pain R/O appendicitis.

- **Treatment (Tx) plan** > the plan is developed between the provider and patient to take a medication, or elevate the foot with an ice compress, or order an X-ray, or schedule a surgery. The treatment plan addresses all or some of the assessments. It should include prevention strategies which may include updating a tetanus vaccination, ordering a screening exam, or reminding the patient to use their seatbelt.

BEGINNING AT THE END: THE SUFFIX

Beginning at the end, the **SUFFIX** is the ending of a word which will change the meaning or function of the word. Attaching a suffix to the word root/linking vowel (linking form) makes a huge difference in a diagnosis. Let's look at the nose > Rhin/o:

- **Rhinoplasty** (**rye**-no-plas-tee) > surgical repair of the nose.

- **Rhinitis** (rye-**nigh**-tis) > inflammation of the nose.

- **Rhinorrhea** (**rye**-no-**ree**-ya) > discharge or flow from the nose (runny nose). Note the suffix -rhea when attached has two 'r's —rrhea.

- **Rhinoscopy** (rye-**nos**-kop-ee) > process of using an instrument to look in/at the nose.

1.14
'Suffix' > Latin for 'fastened under'

Suffix > singular

Suffixes > plural

There are about 120 suffixes for medical terminology added to the about 7,000 word roots. It seems like an insurmountable task to learn them all. The good news is many are known to you already! Think back to first grade, remember nouns and adjectives.

Nouns

A person, place, or thing. Most of the word roots are things (heart or nose), place (on the arm or in the lungs), or procedure (a surgery or an injection). The word root with linking vowel does not stand alone as a noun – it needs a suffix.

- -er -or Carpenter, doctor, photographer, porter, radiographer, engineer, builder, teacher, chiropractor, and many more. The —er, or -or suffix denotes a person who does something: builds, applies medicine, carries things, etc. A noun will always sound correct when used in a sentence as 'doing' something.
  - 'The photographer takes wedding photos'.
  - 'The doctor removed the skin lesion with cautery'.

- -ism Criticism, hypothyroidism, pessimism, Darwinism, symbolism. The suffix -ism is a process, a disease or condition caused by a specific set of signs and symptoms. It can be thought of as the *collective* noun for all the pieces making up a condition or concept versus an individual finding.
  - 'The criticism was valid because the doctor did not prove that Mrs. Stiller had Parkinsonism'.

- -ist Violinist, Orthopedist, Internist, Ophthalmologist. The suffix -ist is the person who specializes in a specific activity or study.

1.15
More noun suffixes
-ia > Condition, state or thing >

Anemia

Pneumonia

Bacteria

-itis > inflammation >

Tonsillitis

Gastritis

Pharyngitis

Cellulitis

-ics > Knowledge or practice of >

Pediatrics

Dietetics

Orthopedics

Gymnastics

– 'The Violinist specializes in playing the violin'.

– 'The Internist specializes in the internal organs of the body'.

• -logy Physiology, Rheumatology, Gynecology, Astrology, Ecology. The suffix -logy means the process of studying or the study of the specific area of interest.

– 'Astrology studies the stars in relationship to human events'.

– 'Rheumatology studies the specifics of joint disease'.

 Omar is studying to be a heart specialist. What is the term for the 'study of the heart'?

 Tony is an ultrasound technician; which part of this word makes him the person who does this work: Sonographer

Construct a word meaning 'to cut into muscle'.

Word building

 Using the word roots with linking vowel build as many valid terms with the suffixes given. Please define them too.

Oste/o My/o Gastr/o

-logy -rrhea -itis -ectomy -genesis -ics
-scopy -tomy

Adjectives

Adjectives describe things, telling the reader or listener what something is like. 'The pattern I am looking for is circular not linear'. The pattern, in other words, is like a circle, not like a line. Adding the suffix -ar, changes the noun into an adjective meaning 'like a circle' or 'like a line', respectively. These endings are used every day; they should be familiar.

• -ac or -ic > cardiac, amnesiac, colonic, cyanotic, maniac, lymphatic

• -al > intestinal, medical, critical, arterial, duodenal, renal, surgical

• -ary or -ory > urinary, pulmonary, literary, sedentary, circulatory, reactionary

Note: Depending on the book, it may be presented as:

-logy,-ology or o/logy. This is including the linking vowel (It is easier to say). The 'o' should not be used twice. It is not Rheumat**oo**logy

1.16
Cardiology

1.17
-er

1.18
myotomy

1.19
The instructor has the list!

1.20
There are words ending in –ic which may be used as NOUNS, including:

Critic

Medic

Fanatic

Fabric

- -ine or -ive > creative, uterine, digestive, excessive, corrosive

- -ous > jealous, venous (blood), mucous, famous, adventurous, conspicuous

- -oid > like or pertaining to: mucoid, rheumatoid, alkaloid, factoid, diploid

- -ile > virile, sterile, penile, antimissile, ductile, hostile

The **Urinary** system includes the bladder, ureters, and urethra. It stores and eventually evacuates the urine formed in the Renal system (Figure 1.6). *Notice, the word, 'urinary' is describing the noun, 'system'. Put it in a sentence. Does it describe? It is functioning as an adjective.*

Comic

Music

Panic

Arsenic

Cosmetic

Most still have the sense of 'pertaining to'. The medic is the person who is delivering medicine. It is a person, place, or thing versus a description.

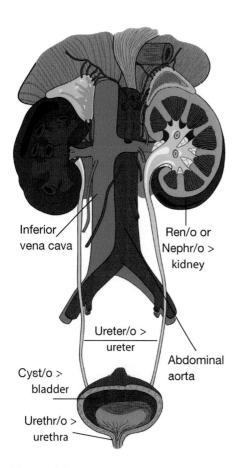

Inferior vena cava

Ren/o or Nephr/o > kidney

Ureter/o > ureter

Abdominal aorta

Cyst/o > bladder

Urethr/o > urethra

Figure 1.6

TOME

A little history on 'tome', both a word root and suffix; 'tome' is Greek meaning 'a section' or a roll of papyrus. In Latin, it meant 'to shear'. In Middle Irish it became 'to lop'. As a noun, a 'tome' is often defined as a large or scholarly book with many sections. In medicine, it is 'a cut', to make a 'section'.

- Tomogram (**toe**-moe-gram) > record of X-ray 'cuts', an X-ray set looking at sections of the body.

- Osteotome (**os**-tea-oh-tohm) > instrument which 'cuts' sections of bone.

As a **suffix**, 'tome' is seen in three endings: **-tomy** > to cut into.

- Craniotomy (**krany**-knee-**ot**-oh-me) > to cut into the skull. Crani/o > skull.

- Laparotomy (**lap**-ar-**ot**-toe-me) > to cut into the abdomen or loin area. Lapar/o > abdomen.

- Anatomy (a-**nah**-toe-me) > to cut into the body (dissection, cut apart).

-ec/tomy > -ec is out, -tomy is to cut > to surgically remove, to cut out.

- Embolectomy (**em**-bow-**lek**-toe-me) > surgical removal of a 'plug' (embolism). Embol/o > plug.

- Gastrectomy (gas-**trek**-toe-me) > surgical removal of the stomach.

-os/tomy > -os is opening, -tomy is to cut into > surgical creation of a new opening > usually brought out to the skin.

- Colostomy (ko-**los**-toe-me) > surgical creation of a new opening into the colon.

- Craniostomy (**krany**-knee-**os**-toe-me) > surgical creation of a new opening into the skull.

- Gastroduodenostomy (**gas**-tro-**due**-oh-de-**nos**-toe-me) > surgical creation of new opening between the stomach and duodenum (not brought to the skin). Duoden/o > C-loop of the small intestine, duodenum. This is also called an anastomosis (an-as-toe-moe-sis).

MORE SUFFIXES AND PREFIXES

There are two common suffixes meaning a condition (noun): –ia (as seen above) and –osis. By convention, attaching –osis to most word roots indicates *an abnormal condition*. Remember, because –ia and –osis begin with a vowel, they usually attach directly with the word root.

- **Endocytosis** (**en**-doe-**sigh**-toe-sis) > condition inside the cell (not necessarily abnormal). It is also used to describe the action of moving intracellular materials. Cyt/o is the word root for cell.

- **Diagnosis** (die-ag-**no**-sis) > discernment through knowledge, determination of the nature of the disease, injury, or medical need.

- **Acidosis** (as-i-**doe**-sis) > abnormal condition of blood acid levels, increased hydrogen ions.

- **Prognosis** (prog-**no**-sis) > condition of predicting knowledge, a forecast of outcome.

- **Sclerosis** (**sklar**-oh-sis) > abnormal condition of hardening. Scler/o is the word root for hardened.

✓ Construct a word meaning 'to cut into the artery'.
_____/__/_____

✓ Construct a word meaning 'abnormal condition of the joint'.
_____/_____

✓ What are three surgical suffixes involved in 'cutting'?

Word building

Using the word roots with linking vowel build as many valid terms with the suffixes given. Please define them too.

Cyt/o Arthr/o Chondr/o

–logist –itis –ectomy –malacia –scope –osis –al –centesis

1.21
These **–osis** words can mean a 'normal' condition or function as well:

Diagnosis

Prognosis

Pinocytosis

Anastomosis

Apoptosis

Phagocytosis

Zoonosis

Gnosis

Immunodiagnosis

Osmosis

1.22
Arteri/o/tomy

1.23
Arthr/osis

1.24
–tomy, –ostomy, –ectomy

1.25
The instructor has the list!

Back to the beginning, the **PREFIX**; it is attached before the word root. The prefix will also change the meaning of the word or its function. Again, prefixes are used every day.

- **Predict** > I predict the Green Bay Packers will make the playoffs this year. (Pre > before)

- **Promote** > Mia was promoted based on her hard work and innate intelligence. (Pro > before or forward)

- **Hyperactive** > Pepper, the dog, is so hyperactive it is like he is bouncing off the walls. (Hyper > too many, too much, increased)

- **Abnormal** > It is abnormal to have snow in Galveston Bay. (ab > away from center)

- **Microscopic** > Bacteria are microscopic. (micro > small, tiny, too small to see with the naked eye)

- **Epitome** > He is the epitome of charm. (Literally, a cut above) (epi > above, upon)

Placing an 'A-' in front of any word root beginning with a consonant will make it a negative. For word roots beginning with a vowel, the prefix is 'An-'. (Same grammar rule learned in 1st grade.) A- and An- > no, not, without, lack of, an absence of:

- **Amenorrhea** (a-**men**-or-**ree**-ah) > absence of the discharge of menses (monthly period).

- **Aplasia** (a-**play**-ze-ah) > absence of development (of an organ).

- **Anaerobic** (an-a-**roe**-bik) > no air (oxygen) available.

Anti- > against, opposing. Synonym: contra-

- **Antibiotic** (**an**-tea-buy-**ot**-ik) > literally, 'against life', this is the general term for the medication group which fights against bacterial infections.

- **Antidote** (**an**-tea-dote) > a substance (medication) neutralizing or counteracting poisons.

- **Antipyretic** (**an**-tea-pie-**ret**-ik) > a medication lowering or reducing fever.

1.26

ALERT
Spelling of prefixes is especially important as ONE letter can change the diagnosis

Ante- means before or forward *versus* **Anti-** means against.

A **Micro**-organism is much different than a **Macro**-organism.

To **Ab**duct is the opposite of **Ad**duct.

1.27
Notice there is no linking vowel for prefixes. They attach directly to the front of the word root.

Kitchen lab

Look around your home for these types of medications. What are their names? Share your findings with the instructor.

Ecto-, ec-, ex-, and **exo-** > outer, outside, external, or away

- **Ectopic** (**ek**-top-ik) > out of place (organ or pregnancy).

- **Eccentric** (ek-**sen**-trik) > away from the center, abnormal or different behavior.

- **Exogenous** (eks-**oh**-je-nus) > produced or originating from outside the organism.

- **Exposure** (eks-**poe**-zur) > contact with an element from the outside.

In-, En-, Endo- > inner, inside, part of, within, into

Intra- > within, in, inside

- **Incision** (in-**si**-zhun) > to cut into.

- **Intraorbital** (**in**-tra-or-bit-al) > within the orbit of the eye.

- **Injection** (in-**jek**-shun) > to push inside.

- **Endocrine** (**en**-doe-krin) > hormones traveling inside the blood stream.

- **Encephalitis** (en-**sef**-ah-lie-tis) > inflammation of the brain. Encephal/o is the linking form for brain, though literally it is 'inside the head'.

ALERT

In- has a different meaning as a prefix to many words. In fact, in-, im-, ir-, il- are used in medical terminology to indicate 'not within' or 'a lack of'.

- **In-** means no, not, less than, lack of (similar to an-): inactive, inadequate, injury, incompatible.

It is In- before most letters except:

- **Im-** also means no, not, less than; it used before 'b, m, or p': imbalance, impalpable, immaterial.

- **Ir-** also means no, not, lack of; it is used before an 'r': irregular, irrational, irreducible.

1.28
Discuss your findings with the instructor and class.

1.29
Exit > the way out during a fire

Excite > to take one out of norm

1.30
In-, Intra- are generally used for pushing something inside

En- and Endo- for inner layer or inner

1.31
LIKE ALERT!
There are several word parts which have exactly the same look but different meanings. Take care to understand the context when reading or using these 'like' word parts or words.

- **Il-** also means no or false; it is used before an 'l': illegal, illegitimate.

Prefix opposites

Hyper- > more than, elevated, increased, more of: hyperactive, hyperglycemia

Hypo- > less than, lower, decreased, under: hypodermic, hypothalamus

Brady- > slow: bradycardia, bradyphasia

Tachy- > fast: tachypnea, tachyarrhythmia

Epi- or **Supra-** > above, upon, on top of: epidermal, epidural, supracostal, suprapubic

Sub- > under, below, less than, underneath: sublingual, subliminal

Ante- or **Pre-** > before, forward, ahead of: antepartum, premature

Post- or **Retro-** > after, behind: postpartum, retroversion

Ab- > away from center or normal: ablation, aberrant

Ad- > toward the center, to add: adrenal, adduction

Eu- > good, normal, okay: euthyroid, euglycemic

Dys- > bad, difficult, painful, abnormal: dysmenorrhea, dyspnea

1.32
All of these terms are used on a regular basis in documentation and are the basis for coding as well. Look each one up!

 Construct two words meaning 'pertaining to the inside of the heart'.

_____/ _____/ __ac__ and _____/ _____/ __al__

1.33
Intra/cardi/ac
Endo/cardi/al

 Note all the prefixes meaning 'no, not, without, or absent'.

1.34
a-, an-, in-, and im-

Little Helen's heart is 'out of place'; the proper medical term is a/an _____ heart.

1.35
ectopic

Word building

 Using the word roots with linking vowel build as many valid terms with the suffixes given. Please define them too.

Col/o Dermat/o or Derm/o

-logy -itis -ectomy -genesis -scopy -al

1.36
The instructor has the list!

WHERE THE STORY IS TOLD

Basically, where a patient goes, the story follows. There are many facilities, agencies, and businesses seeing the patient over the course of a lifetime. They are all tasked to create the story. Here are a few of those places:

- **Inpatient facilities** > a patient is admitted for care for longer than 24 hours which may be medical, diagnostic, and/or procedural. They are staffed 7 days a week, 24 hours a day, 365 days a year.
  - Hospital: General, Pediatric, Burn Units, Transplant Units, and Research
  - Mental Health hospitals and Rehabilitation (Step-Down Units)
  - Skilled nursing care facilities (Nursing homes)
- **Same-day facilities** > admit patients for care which will be accomplished in less than 24 hours. This care may include procedures or diagnostic activities.
  - Surgical clinics: Orthopedics, Dermatology, Plastic surgery, Endoscopic, and more (Figure 1.7).
- **Ambulatory care** > from the family doctor or a consult for all kinds of issues.
  - Private offices and/or clinics including the dentist and many specialties
    - o Urgent care center (**UCC**) or Acute care clinics (**ACC**)
    - o Physical and/or Occupational therapy centers (**PT, OT**)

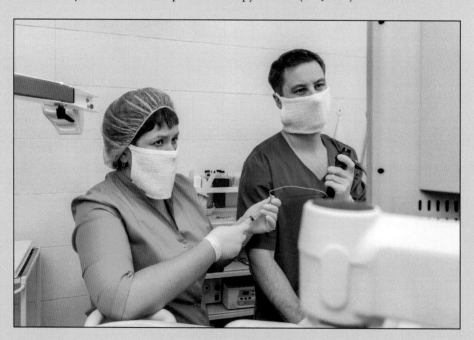

Figure 1.7

> o Independent Radiology and Laboratory centers
>
> o Child, Special needs, and Elder Day-Care facilities or programs; these provide therapy and activities for patients who may have Alzheimer's, autism, or special need disabilities.
>
> • Emergency care, Paramedics, Emergency Medical Technicians (EMTs), Life-flight organizations deliver emergency care.
>
> – Emergent care is defined as care required to prevent loss of life, limb, or eyesight. It is associated with an emergency department (**ED**) or area staffed and equipped for the reception and treatment of persons with conditions requiring immediate medical care such as a severe laceration or appendicitis.
>
> • **Home healthcare >** facilities or programs bring care to us at home.
>
> – Hospice is a facility or program designed to provide a caring environment with symptom management meeting the physical and emotional needs of the terminally ill person. Most patients are cared for at home with occasional facility admittance for symptom control.
>
> – Home health aides who help with activities of daily living (**ADLs**) and other tasks in the home.
>
> – Nursing and therapies of all types may help a patient recover from a surgery or medical condition at home.

ABBREVIATIONS, ACRONYMS, AND INITIAL SETS

Abbreviations: An abbreviation is the short form of a word or phrase. Differential is abbreviated 'diff' in the laboratory. While there are several 'shortened' words in use within medical terminology, the customary way to shorten the language is the use of the acronym or initials (see below).

ALERT

When learning and using this medical language students are tempted to make their 'own' abbreviations. There are standards used extensively such as those below. There are others on the **ISMP List of Error-Prone Abbreviations, Symbols, and Dose Designations** (USA) because their use often confuses and have caused injury and/or death.

In general there are no abbreviations with a single letter: e.g., Many students want to use 'D' to mean diarrhea or diabetes or dyspnea or double etc. . . . To the next reader a 'D' can be anything. Most

1.37
Abbreviations, acronyms, and initial sets like the language itself do change depending on the language of the country. There will be differences between the USA, the UK, Europe, Africa, and the Far East for instance.

Cesarean is also an eponym: delivery of a fetus via a hysterotomy.

facilities publish an acceptable abbreviations and acronyms list consistent with their primary focus of care.

- **Echo** > this might be an echocardiogram or any diagnostic ultrasound procedure

- **C-section** > short for cesarean section, a surgical procedure to deliver a child

- **Tx** > treatment

- **Fx** > fracture of a bone

- **Cardio** > cardiopulmonary

- **diff** > differential count, counts the cells on a slide, a laboratory procedure

- **crit** > hematocrit, a measure of the red blood cells; this is laboratory slang

Acronyms

These are quite common; they are made up of the first letter of each word in a phrase allowing the writer to shorten the language used. By definition an acronym can be said as a word: NASA, *National Aeronautics and Space Administration. With rare exception acronyms are usually written with upper case letters.*

- **MRSA (mer**-sa) > *Methicillin-r*esistant *S*taphylococcus *a*ureus

- **SOAP** note > Subjective, Objective, Assessment, Plan > standard format for documentation of a clinical visit

- **OSHA (oh**-sha) > Occupational Safety and Health Administration in the United States of America (USA)

- **HIPAA (hip**-ah) > Health Insurance Portability and Accountability Act, 1996. USA law on insurance portability and patient privacy

Initial sets are the shorthand for medical terms or procedures. Initial sets are the first letter of each word (similar to acronyms) but they are not spoken as words and they are also called **abbreviations**. They can have several meanings because of the different disciplines of medicine.

Understand the context of the use: e.g., **DM** is often used for 'diabetes mellitus' but it can also mean 'diastolic murmur'. Another is **PND**: 'post nasal drip' or 'paroxysmal nocturnal dyspnea'.

- **CBC** > Complete blood count

- **ISMP** > Institute for Safe Medication Practices

1.38

Look up these acronyms and share with the class:

AIDS

ARDS

CABG

IPAP

JAMA

MOM

1.39

Initial sets are typically capitalized. Combinations occur, such as:

pH > laboratory value concerning hydrogen ions.

- **RUQ** > Right upper quadrant (a location)

- **CVA** > Cerebrovascular accident (a condition)

- **RBC** > Red blood cell (erythrocyte)

- **PCN** > Penicillin (medication, antibiotic)

ALERT

Like abbreviations; there are initial sets which should not be used because they can confuse care. An example is **D/C** – for some this is **dis**charge from a body orifice but it can also mean **dis**charge as in to send the patient home or **dis**continue a therapy. This could prematurely stop a medication or send a patient home before care is complete. Medications are often written as initial sets; use with care!

✓ Kelly went to the UCC for care of her laceration. UCC is a/an _____, spelled out as _____ .

✓ The abbreviation for the treatment plan would be _____ .

✓ True or false: Medications written as acronyms or initial sets may be on the Error-prone list.

1.40 initial set Urgent Care Center or abbreviation

1.41 Tx

1.42 True

Eponyms

A 'proper name' given to a particular anatomical structure or disease is considered an 'eponym' (**ep**-oh-nims). This name is derived from the name of the person who discovered the particular structure or described the set of symptoms of the disease. Some eponyms note specific locations of anatomy, such as McBurney's point was used to find the appendix. While these GPS locators of the past can be useful, today many providers have forgotten or never learned 'McBurney's point'; for this reason eponyms denoting an anatomical location are no longer used.

The eponyms used today are the names by which a set of symptoms and objective findings are quickly identified. Parkinsonism, for instance, is a medical syndrome distinguished by progressive involuntary tremor, slowed movements (bradykinesia), muscle rigidity, and balance instability. The set of findings was noted even in ancient medical writing (papyri and Hippocrates for instance); but it was James Parkinson, an English physician, who first issued a thorough description in *An Essay on the Shaking Palsy* in 1817.

1.43 Common eponyms

Crohn's

Rickettsiosis

Addison's

Asperger's

Bell's palsy

Pott's Fx

Boxer's Fx

Adam's apple

Fallopian tube

Adson's forceps

Heimlich

Apgar scores

GOLGI APPARATUS
An eponym, named for the scientist

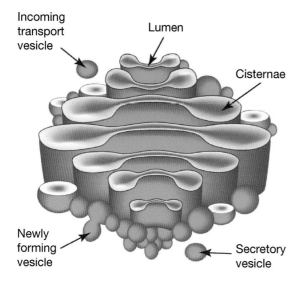

Figure 1.8

- **Golgi** (**goal**-gee) > Golgi apparatus in the cell and Golgi body, a muscle receptor. The Golgi apparatus is the packaging plant of every cell (Figure 1.8).

- **Alzheimer's** (**awlts**-hi-mers) > Degenerative disease of the neurons

- **Cushing** (**kus**-hing) > Hypersecretion of the adrenal cortex

- **Purkinje** (purr-**kin**-gee) > Refers to a specific set of cardiac electrical pathways

- **Swan–Ganz** (shawn-ganz) > Named for the two developers of the catheter used to monitor the heart and lung functions

Other types of abbreviations, acronyms, or initials

- The periodic table for elements is a specific list: Na^{++} > sodium; K^+ > Potassium . . .

- Latin abbreviations are used in charting: n.p.o. > nothing by mouth, usually in lower case.

- Measurements tend to be lower case initial sets: mm > millimeter (distance); ml > milliliters (fluid)

- Symbols: _ > increased, more; _ > decreased, less; † > death; # > pounds (No, it is not hash mark in medicine!)

- Initial sets or acronyms of professions, associations, and laws: AAFP > American Academy of Family Physicians

1.44

A '**cc**' is cubic centimeters and it is equal to '**ml**', milliliter. The use of 'cc' is not allowed in the USA as it can be confused with other 'CC' (Chief complaint) – always use 'ml'.

THE STORY OF ELDON

'Eldon died of consumption today, 31st day of July, in the year of the Lord, 1832'. How beneficial can this one statement be as a medical record? Why do we care and take the time to utilize medical terminology to express his or anyone's story?

- Eldon, a person, is dead. His story is complete.

- Eldon died of consumption. Consumption in those days was any disease which caused progressive **dyspnea** (shortness of breath). The commonplace disease was tuberculosis, but it could have been caused by any number of conditions, such as pneumonia, miner's lung, a cancer, or emphysema.

- These data could be used to track 'consumption' deaths in the region (Public Health, epidemiologist).

- These data could be useful in preventing or treating people close to Eldon (Infectious disease control).

- If Eldon was the first person to die with the consumption, he might be the original case which could explain the spread of the disease. The date might be important in tracking the illness (Forensic pathologist).

- This piece of information is part of Eldon's book. Every single sheet of data is essential to the story. To lose this part would deny the reader the last chapter of the novel. Every element and everyone has a story to tell.

CODING: ICD-10-CM

International Classification of Disease, 10th revision, Clinical Modification

Medical coding is the process of translating the story, the EHR results, including diagnoses, procedures, and materials used in the care of a patient, into a structured alphanumeric system to aid in a variety of areas. In the United Kingdom and Europe it is known as the *International Statistical Classification of Diseases and Related Health Problems* (ISD). In the United States of America it is the ICD-10-CM. For convenience, ICD will be used throughout the text.

The ICD is copyrighted by the World Health Organization (**WHO**), which owns and publishes the classification for worldwide use. It is an international process. This revision (10th) became effective for use in October 2015 in the USA. The specific codes for the United States are under the auspices of the CDC. The ICD provides:

- Standardization of diseases, injuries, procedures, and materials.

- The basis of statistical study (Health informatics) for
  - Morbidity and mortality

    Morb/o > sickness, illness

    Mort/o > death
  - Disease tracking
  - Procedure tracking
  - Injury cause and types
  - Poisoning and overdoses
  - Acts of terrorism.

- Logistics: All this medical care requires supplies, from needles and syringes to hospital beds and aspirins.

- Healthcare Policy and laws: HIPAA, fraud, Medicare, Medicaid etc. . . .

- Reimbursement data for insurance and other organization.

UNIT SUMMARY

1 Medical terminology is a standardized language permitting medical providers of all types and disciplines to communicate a patient's history, examination, diagnoses, treatments, and progress over the lifetime of the patient via the health record.

2 Much of the language used today is from the original Greek and Latin anatomists and scientists which accounts for some like words and definitions. Other influences include Arabic, French, German, Middle English and Irish.

3 The word parts of medical terminology allow for the creation of many terms which are easily linked to define anatomy and functions. They include the word root, linking vowel, suffix, and/or prefix.

4 The word root is the core of the word, it provides the basis or topic of the word; it seldom stands alone.

5 The linking vowel is the glue between the word root and suffix and is commonly the 'o'.

6 A compound word is formed with the use of two or more word roots. They are combined with the 'o' with either consonant or vowel. There is the occasional exception.

7 The suffix will change the meaning of the word root and is required to complete a linking form which cannot stand alone. The suffix will denote a word root as a noun or adjective or a procedure, plurals, therapy, and others. A suffix beginning with a vowel will not have an 'o' as the linking vowel, use the vowel of the suffix. e.g., arthr-itis.

8 The prefix will change the meaning of the word root as well and is attached directly in front of the word root.

9 Medical terminology is used to create the medical record tracking the wellness, illness, or injury of an individual. Collectively, these medical records also provide a number of agencies and industries statistics enabling research, immediate reaction to catastrophes, community health initiatives, and more.

10 Medical records are coded to allow for research and reimbursement. The coding method is via the ICD, International Classification of Disease produced by the World Health Organization and monitored by the US Centers of Disease Control.

11 Medical terminology has a shorthand with the use of acronyms, abbreviations, initial sets, symbols, and eponyms. It is important that all providers utilize the standard list to avoid confusion in the care of patients.

UNIT WORD PARTS

Word roots with linking vowel		
Anat/o > dissection	Arteri/o > artery	Arthr/o > joint
Bacteri/o > bacteria	Cardi/o > heart	Cellul/o or Cyt/o > cell
Cerebr/o > brain, cerebrum	Chondr/o > cartilage	Circul/o > circulation
Col/o or Colon/o > colon, large intestine	Crani/o > skull	Cyan/o > blue
Dermat/o, derm/o > skin	Duoden/o > duodenum	Enter/o > small intestines
Gastr/o > stomach	Hepat/o > liver	Lapar/o > abdomen, loin
Lymph/o > lymph, fluid	Medic/o > medicine, physician	My/o > muscle
Nas/o, Rhin/o > nose	Ophthalm/o > eyes	Orth/o > straight
Oste/o > bone	Pharyng/o > throat	Pulmon/o > lungs
Ren/o or Nephr/o > kidney	Splen/o > spleen	Steth/o > chest

Prefixes: attached to the front of the word root to change meaning		
A- or An- > no, not, absent, without	Ab- > away from the center or normal	Ad- > toward the center or normal
Ante- > before, forward, ahead of	Anti- > against, opposing	Brady- > slow
Dys- > bad, difficult, painful, abnormal	Ecto-, Ec- > outer, outside, external, away from	Endo-, En- > inner, inside, part of, within, into
Epi- > above, upon, on top of	Eu- > good, normal	Ex- or Exo- > outside, outer, external, away from
Hyper- > more than, elevated, increased, more of	Hypo- > less than, lower, decreased, under	In- > inner, inside, part of, within, into
In- and Im- > as a negative, not, less than	Intra- > within, inner, inside	Macro- > large
Micro- > small, tiny	Post- > after, behind	Pre- or Pro- > before, forward, ahead of
Retro- > after, back of, behind	Sub- > under, below, less than, underneath	Supra- > above, upon, on top of, superior
Tachy- > fast	Uni > one, single	

Suffixes change the meaning of the word, linking vowel is usually 'o' with consonants		
-ac, -ic > pertaining to	-al > pertaining to	-algia > pain
-ary, -ory > pertaining to	-centesis > removal of fluid	-cyte > cell
-ectomy > surgical removal	-gram > the record	-graph > a record, or machine making a record
-graphy > the process of recording	-ia > condition of	-ile, -ine, -ive > pertaining to
-ism > a process	-iatrist, -ist > specialist	-itis > inflammation
-logy > study of	-megaly > enlargement	-oma > tumor
-osis > condition of, often an abnormal condition	-ostomy > surgical creation of a new opening	-ous > pertaining to
-pathy > disease	-rrhea > discharge from	-scope > instrument to look
-scopy > process of looking	-spasm > involuntary contractions	-tomy > to cut into

Acronyms, abbreviations, and initial sets		
AAFP > American Academy of Family Physicians	ACC > acute care center	ADLs > activities of daily living
CBC > complete blood count	CDC > Centers for Disease Control and Prevention	Crit > hematocrit
C-section > short for cesarean section	CVA > cerebrovascular disease or costovertebral angle	Diff > differential count
DM > diabetes mellitus or diastolic murmur	Dx > diagnosis	ED > emergency department
EHR > electronic health record	EMT > emergency medical technician	FDA > US Food and Drug Administration
Fx > fracture	HIPAA > Health Insurance Portability and Accountability Act, 1996	Hx > history
ICD-10-CM > International Classification of Disease 10th revision, Clinical Modification	ISMP > Institute for Safe Medication Practices	Lab > short for laboratory
MRSA > Methicillin-Resistant *Staphylococcus aureus*	PCN > penicillin	PE > physical examination
PMH > past medical history	RBC > red blood cells	SOAP > Subjective, Objective, Assessment, Plan
Tx > treatment	UCC > urgent care center	WHO > World Health Organization

UNIT WORKSHEETS

Building terms: Use the proper prefix/word root/linking vowel/suffix as appropriate.

Example: To cut into the muscle > my/o/tomy

a) Pertaining to a small cell > _____

b) The study of skin > _____

c) Inflammation of the bone and cartilage > _____

d) Enlargement of the heart > _____

e) Surgical removal of the colon > _____

f) Pertaining to 'over the stomach' area > _____

g) Surgical repair of the joint > _____

h) Surgical removal of the spleen > _____

Which is it? Identify the word as either NOUN or ADJECTIVE based on the suffix AND define the word root.

Word	Noun or adjective	Definition of word root
Colonic		
Hyperthyroidism		
Mucous		
Cardiomyopathy		
Penile		
Sonographer		
Neuroma		
Pediatrics		
Circulatory		
Duodenal		

Best choice: Pick the most appropriate answer.

1 Which anatomist is credited with beginning several science disciplines?

   a) Hippocrates   c) Golgi

   b) Galen   d) Swan-Ganz

2 Ned's lab report revealed an elevated RBC count with many irregular cells. His WBC count was also abnormal. His TSH was normal. Which part of a medical record would include this information?

   a) Treatment Plan   c) Physical Exam or Objective

   b) Diagnosis or Assessment   d) History or Subjective

3 What is the meaning of the suffix -ostomy?

   a) Tumor of   c) Create a new opening

   b) Flow from   d) To cut into

4 What is the meaning of the prefix anti-?

   a) Before   c) Within

   b) Against   d) After

5 Which of the following is a true abbreviation of a word?

   a) Cardio   c) ICD-10-CM

   b) EHR   d) MRSA

6 What is the meaning of the prefix tachy-?

   a) Slow   c) Sticky

   b) After   d) Fast

Multiple correct: Select ALL the correct answers to the question given.

1 Which of the following are considered ambulatory care options?

   a) Private office   e) Physical therapy agency

   b) Day-care for Alzheimer patients   f) Dental office

   c) Skilled nursing care facility   g) Research hospital

   d) Burn unit

2 Which of these suffixes mean 'pertaining to'?

   a) –er   d) –ist

   b) –ile   e) –megaly

   c) –al   f) –ous

3 Which of the prefixes mean 'inner, inside, part of . . .'?

   a) Sub-   d) Post-

   b) Intra-   e) Endo-

   c) Exo-

4 Use of the ICD helps provide statistics for which of the following?

a) Morbidity and Mortality   d) Acts of Terrorism

b) Procedure tracking   e) EMGR data

c) Hiring recommendations   f) Injury types and cause

Spelling challenge: Circle the correct spelling based on the definition given.

1 'Enlargement of the liver'

        Hepotomegally   Hapatomegaly   Hepatomegaly   Hepatomagely

2 'Abnormal condition of the skin'

          Dermetosis   Dermatosis   Dirmatosis   Durmatossis

3 'Repair of the nose'

        Rinoplastie   Rhinoplasty   Rhiniplasy   Rhinaplasty

Define the term: Spelling *does* count in your definition too!

1 Microbacterial >   _____

2 Laparotomy >   _____

3 Renopathy >   _____

4 Myoma >   _____

5 Antibiotic >   _____

6 Gastroenteritis >   _____

7 Arteriogram >   _____

8 Lymphoid >   _____

Find it and build it: Using the word elements in the table, build the term that matches the definition given or answers the statement. Some may be used several times and some may not be used at all. SPELLING COUNTS.

-al	Pharyng/o	Encephal/o	-tome	-osis	Neur/o
Arthr/o	-scope	Col/o	Cyt/o	-dynia	-logy
Cyan	Oste/o	Endo	Dermat/o	-pathy	-itis
Exo-	-megaly	Micro-	Cardi/o	-ostomy	-ectomy

1 _____   Pertaining to the inside of the heart

2 _____   Condition of blueness

3 _____   Study of nerves

4 _____   Inflammation of the throat

5 _____   Enlargement of the brain

6 _____   Painful joint(s)

7 _____   Surgical removal of the colon

8. _____   Abnormal condition outside the cell

Deconstruction: Using the format given here, deconstruct the terms by their word parts.

1 Rheumatology   _____/_____/_____

2 Venous   _____/_____

3 Craniotomy   _____/__/_____

4 Splenectomy   _____/_____

5 Endocytosis   _____/__/_____

6 Anaerobic   __/____/__/___

7 Encephalitis   _____/_____

8 Epidermal   ____/_____/____

Matching: Medical abbreviations, acronyms, and initial sets. Some will not be used.

FDA	a. slang for hematocrit
Lab	b. methicillin-resistant *staphylococcus aureus*
Crit	c. location, right upper quadrant
CBC	d. U.S. Food and Drug Administration
UCC	e. short for laboratory
MRSA	f. past medical history
Hx	g. counter-ballistic corners
PMH	h. urgent care center
	i. complete blood count
	j. history

An essay: Explain the two different definitions for the prefix, in- and give at least 3 examples of each.

Translation challenge: Translate the short note below: Note the meaning of the terms (*underlined*) and expand the abbreviations/acronyms/initial sets (They are *underlined* too). Use your dictionary or appendix to look up words as needed.

A reminder, these case studies are developed to provide context for your learning. They are incomplete and should not be considered standard of care!

UCC SOAP NOTE

Briar is a 23-year old woman with severe pharyngeal pain for four days. She is having dysphagia now and complaining of enlarged lymph nodes in the neck. She has had a fever of 101°F for most of today with no response to over-the-counter acetaminophen. She works at a day-care center. The patient is allergic to PCN.

PE: Vital signs reveal respirations of 24, labored with a slight wheeze noted; heart rate is 123; blood pressure 110/64; and a temperature of 101.8°F. Her anterior neck is positive for lymphadenomegaly and tenderness. Inspection of the pharynx reveals tonsillar enlargement and redness with exudates. The epiglottis appears swollen as well. A CBC reveals ↑ lymphocytes.

Diagnosis: 1. Tonsillitis 2. Epiglottitis 3. Tachycardia 4. Febrile

Tx: Admit to the hospital for respiratory observation

Keep patient n.p.o.

No use of instruments on oral exams

Blood cultures prior to antibiotics

Start an IV and give 2 gm of Ancef

Consult Pulmonologist and Infection Control

Unit 2

Systems, directions, and numbers

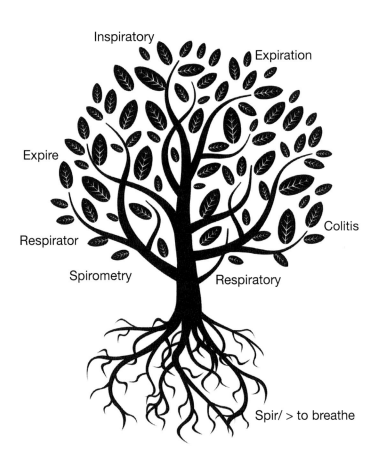

Inspiratory

Expiration

Expire

Colitis

Respirator

Spirometry

Respiratory

Spir/ > to breathe

TARGETED LEARNING

1   Identify the systems, directions, and numbers terms as they apply to the human body.

2   Correctly construct, define, pronounce, and spell medical terms.

3   Correlate X-ray and UCC records with the key learning concepts.

4   Distinguish components of the SOAP note.

5   Relate numbers and abbreviations to medication prescriptions.

6   Link the Index of Disease and Injury of ICD with directions and injury.

KEY WORD PARTS

Word roots with linking vowel	Prefixes	Directions
Arteri/o > artery	Ab-	Anterior
Cardi/o > heart	Ad-	Posterior
Cephal/o > head	Bi-, Di-	Lateral
Coron/o > crown	Centi-	Medial
Gastr/o > stomach	Deca-, Deci-	Ventral
Home/o > same, unchanging	Hemi-	Dorsum
Immun/o > protector, immune	Milli-	Superior
Intestin/o > intestines	Mono-	Inferior
Lymph/o > watery, fluid	Multi-	Pronate
Muscul/o > muscle	Non-	Supinate
Neur/o > nerve	Nulli-	Sagittal
Path/o > disease	Poly-	Proximal
Physi/o > nature/physical	Quadri-	Distal
Radi/o > X-rays	Quint-	Cephalad
Spir/o > breathe	Semi-	Caudal
Thorac/o > chest	Trans-	Ipsilateral
Ur/o > urine	Tri-	Contralateral
Vertebr/o > spinal bone	Uni-	Recumbent

RADIOLOGY REPORTS

Radi/o is the linking form for the energy generated by radiation or rays. X-rays or Roentgen waves were detected for the first time in 1895 by Wilhelm Röntgen, a German physicist. The radiology department uses the same imaging technology to diagnose and treat diseases 'seen' within the body. Plain X-rays are still taken to evaluate a fractured arm or pneumonia. Other imaging techniques are contrast images, ultrasound (**US**), computed tomography (**CT**), nuclear medicine, positron emission tomography (**PET**), and magnetic resonance imaging (**MRI**).

Radiology reports include the procedure ordered; the reasons for the exam, including a short history of the complaint; the technique used; the comparison study or film if available; the definition and exact location of the findings; and finally the impression. The planes, anatomical directions, and numbers of medical terminology are essential to communicating results and ensuring the continuity of care.

SYSTEMS OF THE HUMAN BODY

The human body has 12 distinct yet collaborative systems to maintain homeostasis (Figure 2.2). Home/o > same, alike > homeostasis (**hoe**-me-oh-**stay**-sis). To be exact, homeostasis means 'to stop or stay the same'. In the human body this is a dynamic balance between opposing systems sustaining living. The goal of the body systems is to synchronize the many facets of maintaining life.

2.1
A system is a set of linked elements creating a complex whole:

Respiratory

Digestive

Urinary

Lymphatics

Skeletal

Muscular

Integumentary

Nervous

Endocrine

Immune

Circulatory

Reproductive

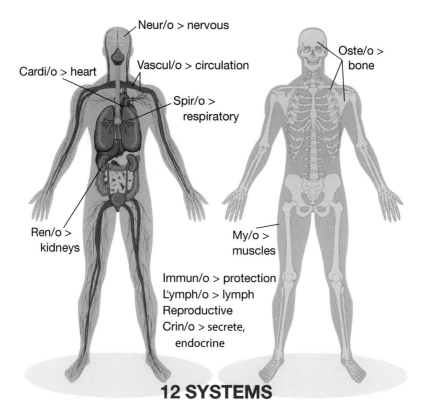

Figure 2.2

The Coming and Going Systems move something into the body such as oxygen or food AND move wastes out of the body such as urine and carbon dioxide (CO_2). These systems include: *Respiratory system, Urinary or Renal system, Digestive system, and the Lymphatic system.*

- **Spir/o** > to breathe, to move gases > to respire (**res**-pyre) is to move oxygen in and push CO_2 out with each breath. Other terms: respirations, inspiration, expiration, and respiratory system.

- **Gest/o** > to carry; add di- > two, double > digest (**die**-jest) > to separate or dissolve as it is carried. Other terms: digestant, digestive tract, and digestive system.

- **Ur/o** > urine (**your**-in) > waste product of the kidneys (ren/o) which filters blood to remove excess water and waste products such as urea and creatinine. Another linking form for urine is urin/o.

- **Lymph/o** > life fluid > the lymphatic (lim-**fat**-ik) system helps defend the body against pathogens and other foreign material.

2.2

LIKE TERMS!

Gest/o means to carry or bear, and it forms the root of the word digestion, which means to break up and carry nutrients. Di- means two, in this case two ways to digest food: chemical and mechanical.

We also get 'gestation' to carry or bear a pregnancy.

It is essentially our vacuum cleaner pulling in debris and leftovers, cleaning them, and returning the clean fluid to the heart via the veins. Other terms: Lymphedema, lymphadenopathy, lymph nodes, and lymphatic system.

The moving and grooving systems allow stretching, reaching, and lifting; they also protect: Skeletal system, Muscular system, and Integumentary system.

- **Skelet/o** > dried up (bones) > skeletal (**skel**-et-al) system forms the basic framework for the body, protects, and supports our internal organs such as our brain, heart, and lungs.

- **Muscul/o** > muscle > muscular (**mus**-Q-lar) system is the highly specialized elastic tissue which binds our skeleton, allows movement, generates heat, and helps maintain body posture cushioning falls. There are three types: Skeletal, smooth, and cardiac. Other terms: Musculature, muscularity, and the musculoskeletal system. Other linking form: my/o or myos/o > muscle.

- **Dermat/o** > skin > also called the integumentary (in-**teg**-U-**men**-tar-ee) (covering or skin) system, which forms a relatively waterproof cover for our body regulating body temperature, keeping bugs out, and it contains part of our sensory net. Other linking forms are derm/o, cutane/o, and cut/i. Other terms: dermatitis, dermatology, dermatome, dermoplasty, and subcutaneous.

 Who is the scientist who discovered and first used X-rays?

 Which of the following terms is using two word roots, making a compound word?

    Lymphedema Urology Lymphadenopathy Muscular Inspiration

Word building

 Using the word roots with the linking vowel to build as many valid terms with the suffixes given. Please define each term too.

    Dermat/o Urin/o or Ur/o Cardi/o

    -logy –scope –graphy –itis –megaly –plasty –pathy

Spir/o > also means coil, or coil like: spirochete

2.3
Linking forms for skin include:

Dermat/o (Greek)

Derm/o

Cutane/o (Latin)

Cut/i

Integumentary is used almost exclusively to denote the system.

2.4
Wilhelm Röntgen

2.5
Lymphadenopathy

2.6
The instructor has the list!

The linkers and roadways are the systems carrying information back and forth within the body: Nervous system, Endocrine system, and Circulatory system.

- **Neur/o** > nerve or neuron (**nur**-on) > system brings the world to us up the afferent (**af**-air-ent) nerves to the brain allowing us to respond with motion via the efferent (**ef**-air-ent) nerves. Neurons are the actual brain cells whereas nerves are a collection of nerve fibers (axons). Other terms: neurocytoma, neuroblast, neuroanatomy, neuroglia, and nervous system.

- **Endocrin/o** > secreting or separating internally > actually endo- (inside) + crine (Greek for separating) > endocrine (**en**-doe-krin) system are hormone compounds circulating via the blood stream acting on target organs. Other terms: Endocrinologist, endocrine glands, and endocrinoma.

- **Circul/o**: to circle, as in a closed loop > the circulation (**sir**-Q-**lay**-shun). The heart (cardi/o) is the pump and the arteries and veins are the pipes (arteri/o; ven/o). Synonym: cardiovascular.

The specialists: These systems use tissue and functions of the other systems to maintain homeostasis; they are the Immune system and Reproductive system.

- **Immun/o** > protector or exempt > immunity (i-**mew**-nee-tea). The immune system has many facets from the keratin secretions helping waterproof the skin and fight bacteria to the very smart T-lymphocytes which locate bacteria and cancer cells to destroy them.

- **Reproductive** (**ree**-pro-**duk**-tiv) > act of forming again > reproductive system is not actually required to survive or protect or communicate BUT as a species it is imperative. The gonads produce specific hormones to allow reproduction. The gonads are Oophor/o > ovary > to bear eggs in women and Test/i > testis > the male gonad produces sperm.

2.7

Afferent means 'to travel to the center'. The afferent nerves carry sensations to the brain. The afferent vessels carry blood or lymph into an organ.

Efferent means 'to carry away from the center'. The efferent nerves carry the actions required back to the body.

2.8
Multiple linking forms

O/o > egg, ovum

Ov/o > egg cell

Ovul/o > egg cell

Ovari/o > ovary

Oophor/o > ovary

Test/i > testicle

Testicul/o > testicle

Orchid/o > testicle

Orchi/o > testicle

PROFESSIONALS

Healthcare providers specialize in various body systems. They sometimes sub-specialize. These are a few:

- Urinary system: Urologist, Nephrologist (kidneys), Dialysis technician

- Respiratory system: Pulmonologist (pulmon/o > lungs), Respiratory therapist (**RT**), Speech–Language therapist (**SLT**)

- Digestive system: Gastroenterologist, Internal medicine, Proctologist (rectum/anus), Bariatric surgeon, Colorectal surgeon, Dietician

- Circulatory system: Cardiologist, Vascular surgeon, Cardiac electrophysiologist, Hematologist

- Endocrine system: Endocrinologist, Diabetologist

- Immune system: Immunologist, Pathologist, Infectious disease, Rheumatologist

- Reproductive system: Gynecologist (**gyn**), Obstetrics (**OB**), Urologist (men)

- Skeletal system: Orthopedist, Podiatrist, Hand surgeon, Chiropractor rheumatologist, Physical therapist (**PT**)

- Integumentary system: Dermatologist, Cosmetic surgeon, Plastic surgeon

- Nervous system: Psychiatrist, Neurologist, Neurosurgery, Psychologist, Psychotherapist

DIRECTIONS

Someone standing in anatomical (an-a-**tom**-mi-kal) position is in the standard position to relate locations of structures and injuries. It is a person standing as noted in Figure 2.2 above. Of course, most people do not land in this position following an injury. No matter the configuration of the patient, the injury is noted from this position.

- The directions of anatomy are used extensively in medicine. Instead of 'on the arm', a more specific phrase is 'distal humerus'. It is especially important to communicate the exact location of an injury or lesion whether seen on the person or on an image (Figure 2.3).

- Most directions are in relationship to the reference point. The head is superior to the neck, but if we are speaking of only the neck, C1 is most superior (Figure 2.4).

2.9
Anterior > front, in front, ventral > what is seen in a mirror

Posterior > back, in back, dorsum

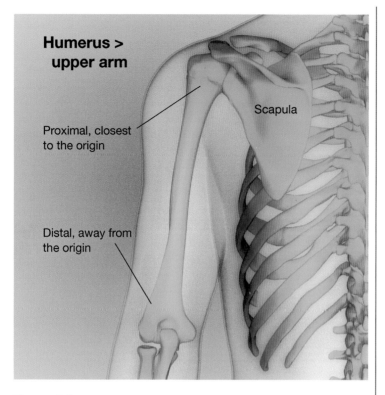

Figure 2.3

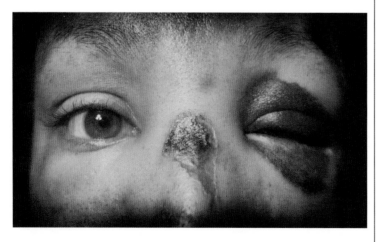

Figure 2.4
The Physical Exam would read 'Ecchymosis and swelling of L eye orbit. Abrasion superior aspect of nasal bridge'.

Directional terms are used in the anatomical position. These are the common opposites (Figure 2.5).

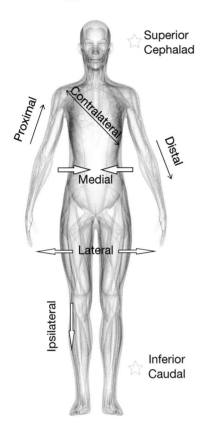

Figure 2.5

2.10
Mes/o also means middle, mean, or intermediate. It is used in embryology and to describe internal anatomy such as mesentery.

Sometimes anter-, later-, super-, and proxim- are designated as prefixes and other times as word roots. This is because they can be used as both depending on the context: e.g., anterolateral. Radiology uses anteroposterior (**AP**) to shoot a film front to back; or posteroanterior (**PA**), back to front for chest X-rays and other areas.

Oblique > taken at an angle (usually 45 degrees)

- **Super**ior (sue-**peer**-ee-or) > at the top, uppermost, directed upward, excess, or above. The shoulder is superior to the hip. It is opposite of inferior. Synonyms: **Proximal or Cephalad**

- **Infer**ior (in-**fear**-ee-or) > below, under, less than, or directed downward. The ankle is inferior to the knee. Opposite of superior. Synonym: **Distal**

- **Medial** (**me**-dee-al) > relating to the middle or center of the body or part. The belly button is on the median (middle) of the body. A movement to the center is called ad**duction** (ad-**duk**-shun), adding to the center.

- **Lateral** (**lat**-er-al) > 'on the side'. A lateral view will look at the body or object from the side. It is the furthest away from the center of the body or area. The movement of a limb away from the center is ab**duction** (ab-**duk**-shun).

- **Proximal** (**prok**-si-mal) > nearest to the trunk or center or point of origin. The elbow is proximal to the wrist. Opposite of distal. Synonym: **Superior**

- **Distal** (**dis**-tal) > away from the center. It is a directional term pertaining to a part of the body furthest from the point of origin. The fingertip is the most distal portion of the finger. Opposite of proximal. Synonyms: **Inferior or Caudal**

- **Deep** (deep) > interior, toward the back. The pancreas is located behind the stomach, making it deeper. It is in the retroperitoneal space. It is opposite of superficial.

- **Superficial** (**sue**-pur-**fish**-al) > toward the surface, on top. The scratches were superficial. Opposite of deep.

- **Anterior** (an-**tier**-ee-or) > front of the structure, or more to the front (**ventral**). Opposite of posterior, back, or dorsal.

- **Posterior** (pos-**tier**-ee-or) > back of the structure, or more to the back (**dorsal**). The back of the hand is called the dorsum. It is the opposite of anterior, front, or ventral.

- **Ipsilateral** (**ip**-see-**lat**-er-al) > structures or effects are on the same side. Opposite of **contralateral**.

- **Contralateral** (**kon**-tra-**lat**-er-al) > structures or effects are on the opposite side. A stroke in the right brain area may cause loss of function of the left body. It is contralateral. Opposite of **ipsilateral**.

 What is the proper direction term for the back side of the hand?

2.11
Dorsum or dorsal

 The nipple line is more _____ than the navel. (Direction)

2.12
superior or proximal

True or false: The ankle is both inferior and distal to the knee.

2.13
True, both are away from the top

Word building

 Using the word roots with the linking vowel to build as many valid terms with the suffixes given. Please define each term too.

Muscul/o Immun/o Neur/o

–logy –ar –al –itis –pathy –oma –tomy –logist

2.14
The instructor has the list!

Kitchen lab

Look around your home. Which things are presented in the different views? Where is the anterior side of your TV? What view do the bookends present? What is the most distal thing in your kitchen from where you are standing? What is the most proximal? Looking at the table and chairs, what is most lateral? What is in the midline of the table? Are the window curtains more superior or inferior to the other objects in a room? Do you have a chair sitting at an oblique angle?

2.15
Discuss your findings with the instructor and class.

The SOAP note

This acronym stands for **S**ubjective-**O**bjective-**A**ssessment-**P**lan. The **SOAP** note is like illustrating a short story. It is the snapshot of the patient at specific moment in time. It is used extensively in emergency departments, private offices, mass casualty events, and in the back of ambulances to name a few arenas. The SOAP note communicates the story to all who read it in the future and it will provide a continuity of care which would otherwise not exist; if it is not documented it never happened.

The SOAP note delivers information essential to patient care, practice workflow, coding, billing, insurance, and reimbursement. It can be used as evidence in legal proceedings and should follow the patient for a lifetime to provide continuity of care.

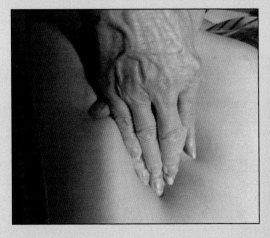

Figure 2.6

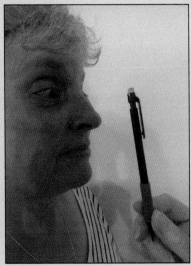

Figure 2.7

Subjective: This is the story of an illness or injury *as told by the patient*. It is what the patient explains happened or is happening. The **how**, **what**, **when**, **where**, **how long**, **why**, and **who** of the story is central to treating the right illness or injury AND it will be used to properly record and code the illness or injury for insurance, statistics, and reimbursement.

Objective: This is the area where the **tangible discoveries of the examination** are documented. The objective section provides the facts, **only the facts**. The physical: seen, heard, felt, smelled or tasted, labs, X-rays, and procedure results of any kind (Figures 2.6 and 2.7).

Assessment: A decision will be made here as to what the patient has – **a diagnosis (Dx)**. Some providers call it the problem list.

Plan: The plan concludes the SOAP note. This is where the course of therapy is written out, a collaborative effort between the provider and the patient.

MORE DIRECTIONS AND PLANES

- **Prone or pronate** (pron or **pro**-nate) > the turn of the lower arm or entire body to face the floor, turn down. When lying on the stomach we are prone. We pronate our forearm to pour the seeds into the garden.

- **Supine or supinate** (**sue**-pine or **sue**-pi-nate) > the turn of the forearm or entire body to face the sky, turn up. Lying on the back makes us supine. Supinating the hand allows the hand to hold 'soup'.

2.16

Two memory tricks to remember these opposites.

1) Supine is looking up, **sUPine**, from the anterior position.

2) You can hold a bowl of soup in your hand when it is **SOUPine**.

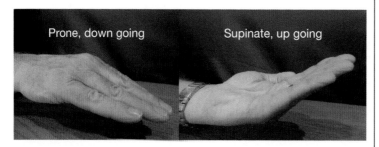

Prone, down going   Supinate, up going

Figure 2.8

- **DIP, PIP, MCP or MTP >** these initial sets are a method to name the *joints* of the fingers or toes (Figure 2.9). The **DIP** is the *d*istal *i*nter*p*halangeal (**in**-tur-fa-**lan**-gee-al) joint, the most distant knuckle of the finger (phalanx) or thumb (pollex > **pol**-lex) or great toe (hallux > **hal**-lux). The **PIP** is the *p*roximal *i*nter*p*halangeal joint, the middle knuckle of the four fingers or toes. The **MCP** is the *m*eta*c*arpal (**met**-ah-**car**-pal) inter*p*halangeal joint, the top knuckle of the hand. The thumb and great toe only have two bones thus 2 joints. At the great toe, it is the **MTP**, *m*eta*t*arsal (**met**-ah-**tar**-sal) inter*p*halangeal joint.

2.17
phalang/o > digits, finger or toe bones

digit/o > finger or toe bones

carp/o > wrist

tars/o > ankle

meta- > beyond

inter- > between

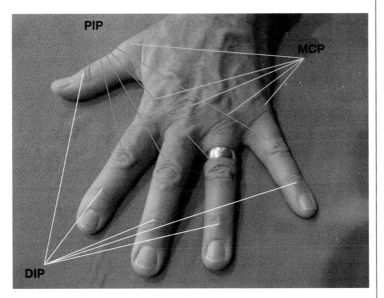

Figure 2.9

- **Dorsal** (**door**-sal) > as a *direction*, pertains to the feet and toes. The top of the foot looking down is the dorsum of the foot even though looking from the anterior (front) position. Dorsiflexion is

2.18
As above, dorsum means back, behind or posterior. This is ONE of those exceptions to the rule. Called the 'back of' but really appears on the front.

The palm of the hand may be designated 'palmar'.

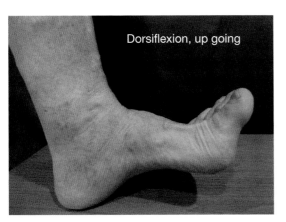

Dorsiflexion, up going

Figure 2.10

pulling the foot or toes up toward the head. When hyperextending the wrist, it is also called dorsiflexing.

- **Plantar** (**plant**-ar) > as a *direction*, pertains to the feet and toes. It is the sole of the foot; planting it on the ground. When stepping on the gas pedal or brake, plantar flexion is employed.

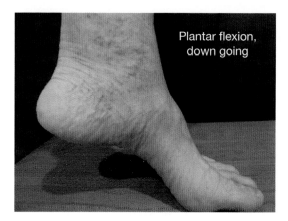

Plantar flexion, down going

Figure 2.11

- **Recumbent** (re-**come**-bent) > lying down to rest is recumbent. In medicine, laying a patient down in the left or right lateral recumbent position (Figure 2.12) is to put them on their side. For example, a pregnant woman should lie in the left lateral recumbent position to keep the weight of the baby off of her inferior vena cava during the last trimester.

2.19
Fowler's position is the patient lying in semi-upright and supine position.

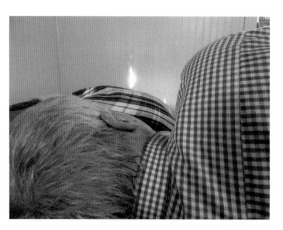

Figure 2.12

Body planes

These planes are basically 3-D directions describing how we slice and dice the human body. These are cuts, slices, or sectional directions. Locating a lesion in the small intestines requires three angles to locate it in space, like outer-space coordinates (Figure 2.13).

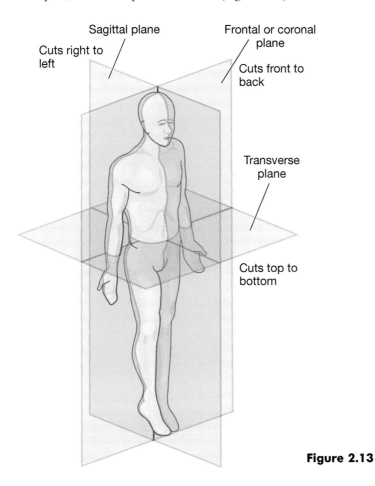

Sagittal plane

Cuts right to
left

Frontal or coronal
plane

Cuts front to
back

Transverse
plane

Cuts top to
bottom

Figure 2.13

Sagittal plane (**saj**–it–tal) > divides the body lengthwise into right and left portions. It is a vertical plane cutting the body from head to toe. A common marker is the MCL, mid-clavicular line (Figure 2.14).

Frontal plane > divides the body into front or anterior and back or posterior portions. It is a vertical plane, often depicted as cutting the body head to toe through the ears (Figure 2.15). It is also known as the coronal (**kore**-row-nal) plane because the head was dissected (die-**sek**-ted) in this manner by the early anatomists.

2.21
The frontal plane gives us two regions: anterior and posterior OR ventral and dorsal.

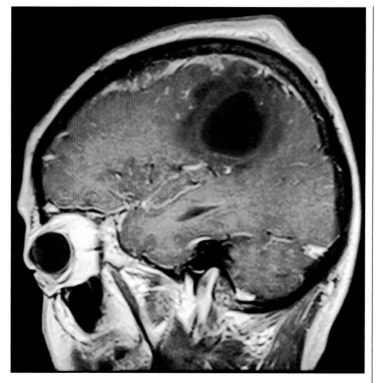

Figure 2.14

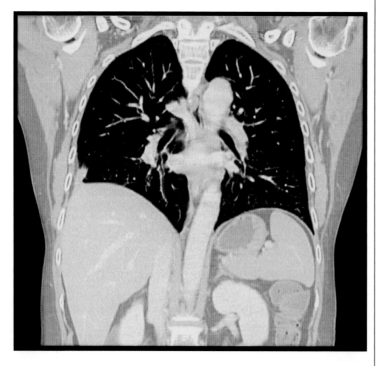

Figure 2.15

Transverse plane > divides the body horizontally into upper and lower portions. Trans- is the prefix for 'across', and 'verse' means to slice across like slices of bread; this is the origin of the term 'cross-sections'. Diagnostic procedures can cut (tom/o) the body in the transverse plane (Figure 2.16).

2.22
Other trans-words:

Transcellular
Transcription
Transdermal
Transection
Transfixion
Transformation
Transient

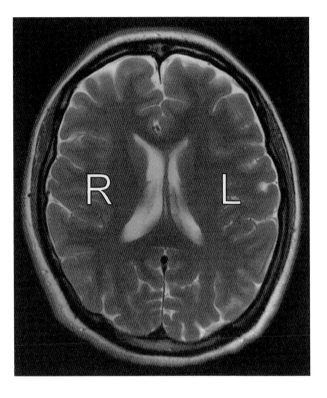

Figure 2.16

✓ Looking at the rib cage at a 45-degree angle would be which of the following views? Lateral, Oblique, Anterior, Posterior

2.23
Oblique

✓ During the preoperative set up the patient is placed on the operating table face down to allow access to the latissimus dorsi muscle. The position is best described as _____ .

2.24
prone

✓ A surgeon is preparing to make an incision to deliver a child by C-section. The cutting line will be from right to left across the pubic area. This is a/an _____ incision.

2.25
transverse

Word building

*Using the word roots **with the linking vowel to build as many valid terms with the suffixes given. Please define each term too.***

Carp/o Tars/o Mening/o

-al -ectomy -itis -tomy -pathy -us -oma

2.26
The instructor has the list!

Numbers

It is in the numbers! Numbers give perspective; a human hair is approximately 0.00065 inches wide while the longest nerve axon can be between 1 to 2 feet long in humans. Some of our nerves conduct signals at 80 meters a second. In this short discussion of numbers, decimals are demonstrated (0.00065) and the Household measure system and the Metric system of enumeration are seen. Numbers are used everywhere: to measure length and speed, weigh trace metals and medications, and count children and fingers. Numbers are used as labels, in serial numbers, social security numbers, catalogs such as the ISBN numbers on books, and the alphanumeric of the ICD. This list of prefixes is related to a specific number. Note the Latin symbols are still used by pharmacies.

- **Bi-** or Di- > Two > 2 or **ii**. Bicipital (**buy**-sip-**it**-al), having two heads. Bi- is a suffix and number designator. The trachea will bifurcate (**buy**-fur-kate), splitting into two main bronchi.

- **Tri-** > Three > 3 or **iii**. Triad (**try**-ad), a group of three elements having things in common or associated with a syndrome.

- **Quadr-** or Tetra- > Four > 4 or **iv**; Quadrant (**kwad**-rant) > 25% of an area like the four quadrants of the abdomen. Quadruplets (kwad-**rup**-lets) > four infants born at one birth. Tetra- (Greek) seen with tetradactyl (**tet**-rah-**dak**-teal), having four toes on one foot or hand.

- **Quinta-** or Penta- > Five > 5 or **v**. Quintuplets (kwin-**tup**-lets) > single birth of five infants. Pentad (**pen**-tad) > Greek, a group of 5 elements relating to or perhaps signifying a syndrome.

- **Sexta-** or Hexa- > Six > 6 or **vi**. Sextuplets (sex-**tup**-lets) > single birth with six infants.

2.27

Conversion of weights:

2.2 pounds (2.2#) = 1 kilogram (kg)

Kilogram (**kill**-oh-gram) is used exclusively for weighing infants and children to ensure the correct dose of medication by weight.

An infant who weighs 24.25 pounds is 24.25 / 2.2 = 11.02 kg

Other bi-, tri-, and quad- words:

Bilateral > 2 sides

Bicuspid > 2 cusps

Bifid > 2 tips

Bilobate > 2 lobes

Bimanual > 2 hands

Triplet > 3 items

Trifocal > 3 foci

- **Septi-** or Hepta- > Seven > 7 or **vii**. Septi- > seldom seen as a number designator because septa is the plural of septum, the thin wall or walls dividing a cavity like the sinuses of the face.

    – Heptachromic (**hep**-ta-**crow**-mik) > seeing in seven colors.

LIKE ALERT!

Septic is pertaining to sepsis, an infection spreading via the bloodstream.

This next set of prefixes are seen less often within medical documents but are frequently used in chemistry and pharmacotherapeutics.

- **Oct-** or Octa- > Eight > 8 or **viii**. The Latin and the Greek almost agreed here; while not seen often in medical documents there have been octuplets (ock-**tup**-lets) born in one birth. An octan (**ock**-tan) > fever reoccuring every eight days.

- **Nona-** or Noni- > Nine > 9 or **ix**. Nonigravida (**no**-knee-**grav**-ee-da) > history of nine pregnancies.

- **Deca-** > Ten > 10 or **x**. It is for whole numbers of 10, such as living for five decades is being alive for 50 years or more.

- **Deci-** signifies 1/10th or 0.1 like deciliter is 1/10th of a liter. A liter is 10 deciliters. Both deca- and deci- are **SI (Standard International)** and **metric** designation for 10.

The metric system is the international standard for medicine and science!

- **Cent(i)** > 1/100th (10^{-2}) > 0.01. Centi- > SI and Metric designation of 1/100th. There are centimeters (**sen**-teh-**me**-ters) > 1/100th of a meter. Centigrade (**sen**-teh-grade) > temperature range of 100 units used initially to differentiate melting and boiling points of water.

- **Mill(i)** > 1/1000 (10^{-3}) > 0.001. Millimeter (**mil**-ee-**me**-ter) > measure of a length, 1/1000th of a meter. A milligram (**mg**) > weight measure, 1/1000th of a gram. A milliliter (**ml or cc**) > volume measure, 1/1000 of a liter.

- **Kilo-** > SI and metric designation for 1000, a measure of mass, length, or weight. Kilograms are used extensively in many areas of science and specifically as weight in medicine. One (1) kg = 2.2 pounds. A kilometer is a measure of distance.

Tricyclic > 3 cycles

Trigone > 3 sides

Quadriceps > 4 muscles

Quadrate > 4 sides

2.28

LIKE ALERT!

Hepta- can be confused with the word root for liver, hepat/o.

The prefix for '9' nona or noni, may be confused with the prefix non- which indicates none, opposite, no, or negative.

Other metric measures:

Millimicron

Millisecond

Millivolt

Milliampere

Kilocalorie (**kcal**)

Kilovolt peak (**kVp**)

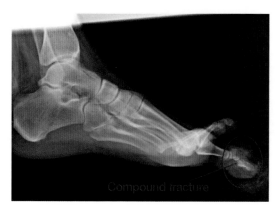

Compound fracture

Figure 2.17

✓ Radiology report

#000000000000 03/12/2013 12:27 P FOOT 3 VIEW LEFT

TECHNIQUE: AP, Lateral, Oblique. 54 kVp, 2 MAS, 4 cm

FINDINGS:

PROCEDURE: FOOT 3 VIEW LT

COMPARISON: None.

INDICATIONS: BIG TOE LAC/PAIN, Hyperflexion of the left great toe, joint exposed with dislocation.

FINDINGS:

There is a displaced <u>fracture</u> of the <u>proximal</u> diaphysis of the first <u>distal phalanx</u> with <u>inferior</u> displacement of the <u>distal</u> fracture fragment.

CONCLUSION: Displaced fracture of the distal phalanx of the left great toe.

2.29
Use the X-ray and radiology report to answer the following questions.

Discuss your answers with the instructor.

a) Look at the Technique line: There are three 'directions' listed. What views does each represent?

b) What measurement does *4 cm* represent on the distance used to shoot the foot X-ray?

c) What is the abbreviation for fracture?

d) What are the definitions for *proximal*, *distal*, and *inferior* as related to this X-ray?

e) What is the *phalanx*? What is the term's plural spelling?

f) What does the initial set **kVp** stand for? What measurement system is **kVp** found in?

g) The radiology result would be included in which section of the SOAP note?

PHARMACY CORNER

The precision of names and numbers is as important to quality care of a patient as is the delivery of medications. An error in spelling or in the placement of the decimal point can mean life or death. Even with the advent of computer entry for medications, errors can still occur. Consider this example:

> A busy provider is inputting medications for a diabetic patient. The 'T' medications pop up, then the 'To', and finally 'Tol', at which point the provider selects and orders Tolectin®. The only problem is Tolectin® is an anti-inflammatory medication. The provider needed Tolinase®, an oral diabetic medication. The pharmacy team filled the medication and the patient used it for 5 days and was admitted to the hospital with hyperglycemia. The pain medication did not lower the blood glucose level. In fact, there are currently 15 medications beginning with the letters 'Tol'. **Short cuts can be deadly.**

A decimal point should not appear naked or alone (.5 mg). The decimal point may be mistaken as a period, making the dose 5 mg, 10 times too much. When noting fractions on the computer or in writing, be sure to use a 'zero' before the decimal point, e.g., 0.5 mg.

Measurements in pharmacy are a challenge as there are four systems. The SI and Metric system are slowly taking over most measures. These are the milligram (mg), kilogram (kg), and microgram (mcg) for weight.

• The Apothecary System is increasingly historical. It is the source of dram (dr), ounce (oz), and pound (lb or #). Today, there are only a few medications measured via the Apothecary System.

• The Household measure system is what is found at home for making dinner or mixing cake batter. But as measures of volume, 'cup', 'pint', 'teaspoon', 'tablespoon', and 'drop' fail to indicate by their names alone precisely how much each contains. Yet many liquid prescriptions continue to be written in the following way: 'Give 1 tablespoon by mouth every 12 hours'. A tablespoon converts to 5 ml but most patients are unaware of this fact.

• Units and Milliequivalents (**mEq**) are used to illustrate the strength of the medication or element. Natural salts, such as potassium and sodium, are measured in **mEq**. Insulin, heparin, and some vitamins are calculated in units which is a calculation of strength with a base of 1 ml of normal solution. Units and milliequivalents cannot be converted to the other systems, making how a number is written or medication name crucial to quality patient care.

MORE NUMBERS

Kitchen lab

Look around your home and workplace and find all the measuring tools in your environment. What are the measurements listed for your over-the-counter liquid medications? What measuring system is being used for all the items you find? How do you keep it all straight?

2.30
Share your findings with the instructor and class.

NONE, ONE, and MANY

There are several prefixes indicating none, one, or many. Some are interchangeable and others are used by convention.

- **Non-** > none, no, not, opposite, or negative. Not to be confused with noni- > 9.
    - Noncompliance (**non**-come-**ply**-ants) > person who fails to follow directions.
    - Nonproductive (**non**-pro-**duk**-tiv) > pertaining to a cough which is not getting the thick sputum up and out.
- **Null or Nulli-** > nothing, empty, absence of > a null cell has no significant landmarks; it looks empty.
    - Nulligravida (**nul**-ee-**grav**-ee-da) > woman who has never been pregnant.
    - Nulliparous (nul-**ip**-ah-rus) > woman who may have been pregnant but did not deliver a child.

2.31
Other NONE words:

Nonverbal

Nonavailability

Nonpenetrating

Nonpitting edema

'Convention' is the accepted usage of a term or process.

- **Mono-** > single, one element > Monocyte (**mon**-oh-sight) > white blood cell with one, large nucleus.
    - Mononeuralgia (**mon**-oh-**nur**-al-gee-ah) > pain of one nerve.
    - Monoplegia (**mon**-oh-**play**-gee-ah) > paralysis of one or a single limb.
- **Uni-** > one, single, alone > Unicellular (**u**-knee-**sell**-u-lar) life has just one cell, e.g., the protozoa.
    - Unilateral (**u**-knee-**lat**-er-al) > occurring on one side of the body.

2.32
Mononucleosis

Monoxide

Unifocal

Unilocular

Unipolar

- **Multi-** > many, several, increased number > Multiform (**mul**-tea-form) > having many forms or shapes. It is used interchangeably with polymorphic (many shapes).

  – Multinodular (**mul**-tea-**nod**-u-lar) > pertains to having many nodules; a kidney or ovary may be multinodular.

  – Multisynaptic (**mul**-tea-si-**nap**-tik) > pertains to having many nerve connections.

- **Pan-** > all, entire, whole > a panacea (**pan**-ah-**see**-a) > something curing everything.

  – Pancolectomy (**pan**-co-**lek**-toe-me) > surgical removal of the entire colon.

  – Pancytopenia (**pan**-sigh-toe-**pee**-knee-ah) > a distinct decline in the number of all the blood cells: RBCs, WBCs, and platelets being produced by the bone marrow.

- **Poly-** > many, multiple, too many to count, increased > Polyarticular (**pol**-ee-are-**tik**-u-lar) pertains to multiple joints.

  – Polycythemia (**pol**-ee-sigh-**thee**-me-ah) > abnormal and marked increase in the number of red blood cells.

  – Polycystic (**pol**-ee-**sis**-tik) > presence of many cysts.

Semi- and **Hemi-** are prefixes which are often interchanged to mean 'one half', a measurement. Use hemi- to mean a precise 'half'. Use semi- when the quantity or measure is less precise.

- **Hemi-** > Greek for one-half as in hemisphere, half the sphere (Earth). Hemiplegia (**hem**-ee-**play**-gee-ah) > paralysis of half the body.

- **Semi-** > Latin for one-half or partial > semicomatose (**sem**-ee-**ko**-mah-tose) > a vague term concerning the loss of consciousness or drowsiness. A semipermeable (**sem**-ee-**pur**-me-able) membrane lets only certain elements through by size.

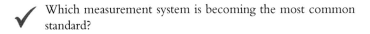 Hector has an inflammation involving many arteries. Construct the correct medical term: _____/_____/ _____ .

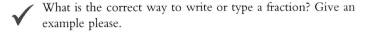 Which measurement system is becoming the most common standard?

What is the correct way to write or type a fraction? Give an example please.

2.33
Of the three prefixes meaning many, more often, increased, poly- is used most often:

Polyuria

Polydipsia

Polyhidrosis

Polyadenitis

Polypharmacy

Polyplastic

Polymorphic

Polypeptide

Polyphagia

Polysaccharide

Polyspermia

2.34
Semi- depending on region may be pronounced

sem-eye-**ko**-mah-tose *or* **sem**-ee-**pur**-me-able

Both are seen.

2.35
Poly/arter/itis
Multi/arter/itis

2.36
Metric

2.37
With a 0 before the decimal point, 0.05

Word building

Use number prefixes with word roots and suffixes to build as many valid terms as possible. Please define these too.

Bi- Tri- Poly-

uria pedal focal furcated geminal dipsia lobar phagia

2.38
The instructor has the list!

CODING: INDEX FOR DISEASE AND INJURY*

The current ICD took four decades to create. It replaced the ICD-9 which had approximately 17,000 primary terms. ICD has approximately 176,000 diagnoses and procedures. The huge increase is a measure of not only the number of diagnoses but procedures wrought by the ever-changing landscape of technology. The hundreds of contributors to the update worldwide have even left room for more. Navigating all these codes takes a fair amount of training and patience. It is important for all readers to have an understanding of the link between the documenting and coding of SOAP note, operative record, radiology report, laboratory finding, and more while learning medical terminology.

The Index for Diseases and Injury is the first and largest index of the book. It is arranged alphabetically with related subheadings to help the coder find the initial diagnosis with a key word such as 'fracture', 'infection', or 'aberrant'. Example:

'Displaced fracture of the distal phalanx of the great toe'. This is the diagnosis for the fractured toe seen above (Figure 2.17). The search could start with 'toe', 'fracture', 'displaced', or 'phalanx'.

• 'Displaced' does not have a category for bone or toe: it does have 'orthopedic NEC' and advises the finder to look in orthopedics.

• 'Toe' yields the advice to see 'condition'.

• 'Phalanx' is not listed at all and 'bone' instructs the reader to see 'condition'.

• 'Fracture' yields the most useful results. It has 'fracture, burst'; 'fracture, chronic'; 'fracture insufficiency'; 'fracture, pathological'; and finally, most relevant to our purpose, 'fracture, traumatic'.

  – Fracture, traumatic

    o Toes S92.91

      o Great (displaced) YEAH! We found it! No, not yet.

        o Distal phalanx (displaced) S92.53-

S92.53- is the alphanumeric code for the fracture noted above right? Not quite yet! The dash at the end is waiting for the number designator for right or left great toe. The Index to Disease and Injury is essentially like the white pages of a phone book (even on a smart phone); it gives the coder a beginning point. There are lots of 'Joneses' and 'Smiths' in the white pages; the first name, second initial, and even the address give the clues to find one specific Jones or Smith. The compilers have gone to great lengths to ensure cross-referencing will get the reader to the right diagnosis. What does this have to do with learning the medical language, directions, and numbers? Let's look at the UCC note on this toe injury:

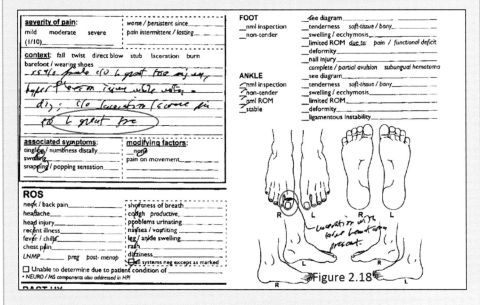

Figure 2.18

The hand-written SOAP note of the UCC provider states the injury involves the left great toe in the HPI (**H**istory of **P**resent **I**llness), but the illustration places the injury on the right great toe. In the surgery suite, prior to repair, the surgeon needs to know which toe to fix! As this injury will be tracked by several agencies they need to know it was the left great toe. It matters. **Precision in terminology, spelling, and numbers matter.**

★ IMPORTANT NOTE: The reader is notified that these examples are from an online search made in 2016. Do **not** use these codes for patient care episodes; look up the new ones!

REGIONS AND CAVITIES

REGION is defined as an area, usually continuous. Like directions, an area is what it is defined by. The anterior view of the body may be considered the front or ventral region, and medicine has had millennia to redefine an area into many smaller regions with several names in most cases, as noted by Figure 2.19. Here are some of the regions defined by multiple terms.

2.39
Common terms:

Trunk or **core** refers to the chest and abdomen

Shoulder is the upper arm/shoulder blade area

Hip is the upper leg/pelvic area

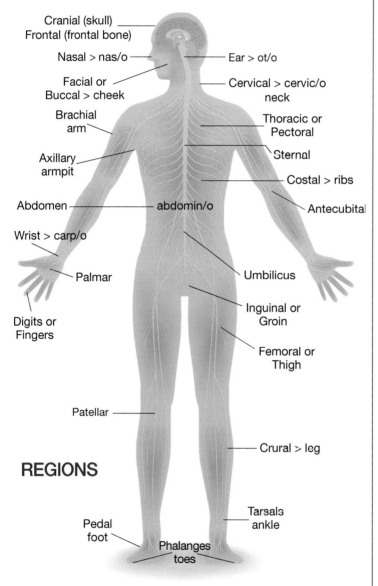

Cranial (skull)
Frontal (frontal bone)
Nasal > nas/o
Facial or
Buccal > cheek
Brachial arm
Axillary armpit
Abdomen
Wrist > carp/o
Palmar
Digits or Fingers
Patellar
REGIONS
Pedal foot

Ear > ot/o
Cervical > cervic/o neck
Thoracic or Pectoral
Sternal
Costal > ribs
abdomin/o
Antecubital
Umbilicus
Inguinal or Groin
Femoral or Thigh
Crural > leg
Tarsals ankle
Phalanges toes

Figure 2.19

- Cranial (**kray**-knee-al) > pertaining to the **skull** and we also call it the cranial cavity and the head. Cephal/o is another word root for head, as a direction and pertaining to what is in the head.

- The chest is properly called the **thorax** (**tho**-raks) or thoracic (thor-**as**-ik) region or cavity. The term pectoral (**pek**-tor-al) region is also used because of the underlying muscles, the Pectoralis major and minor. Overlying the muscle in the same region is the breast, which is termed mammary (**mam**-ah-ree). It all depends on the focus of the examination and findings.

- The **sternum** is the breast bone and it comprises three parts: manubrium (ma-**new**-bree-um), the sternum (**stir**-num) or sternal body, and xiphoid (**zeye**-foyd).

- The larger, less protected area of the trunk is the **abdomen** (ab-doe-men) or abdominal cavity, and it lies between the chest and pelvis or the thoracic and pelvic regions.

A **CAVITY** is a hole, an enclosed space, or a hollow place. Just as the body comprises several regions, it also has several cavities, large and small, and some of the cavities have cavities within them.

- **Thoracic cavity** > encased by the spinal column posteriorly and the rib cage, which is mobile by virtue of costal margin and the sternum. Some of the structures within the cavity are the lungs, heart, great vessels, esophagus, trachea, lymphatics, and the thymus. Within the cavity are cavities or niches which are unique:
  - The **mediastinum** (**me**-dee-ah-**sty**-num) > area of the chest midline, protected by the sternum anteriorly and spine posteriorly with the heart, great vessels, and lymphatics.
  - The entire surface of the lungs are covered with a membrane, the **visceral pleura** (**vis**-ur-al **plur**-ah). At the hilum (where the main bronchi and main blood vessels enter the lungs) the visceral pleura turns back on itself and forms the **parietal** (pah-**rye**-eh-tal) **pleura** which adheres to the mediastinum, the inner surface of the rib cage, and the diaphragm. This makes a continuous sac and an enclosed space called the **pleural cavity**, see Figure 2.20.

**2.40
Other regions linking forms**

Ot/o > ear

Ocul/o > eye

Crani/o > skull

Cervic/o > neck

Brachi/o > arm

Umbilic/o > belly button, umbilicus

Carp/o > wrist

Tars/o > ankle

Ped/o > foot

Nas/o or Rhin/o > nose

Stern/o > breast bone

2.41

Viscer/o > internal organs. The visceral membrane will touch the actual organs it protects. The heart, lungs, and abdominal peritoneum have this double layer covering.

Pariet/o > wall of the body. It is the membrane outermost yet continuous with the visceral layer.

Pleurisy is an inflammation of the pleural membranes. Instead of moving easily, their movement is more like moving across Velcro®. It hurts.

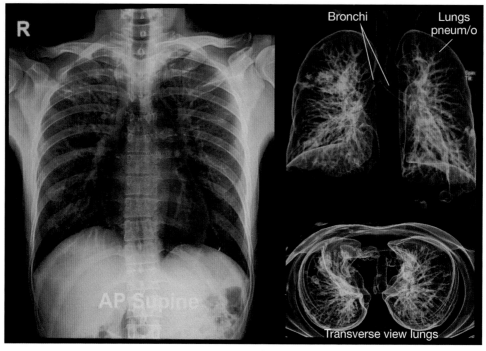

Figure 2.20

Kitchen lab

 Build a lung – if you check the internet or the book website you will find the instructions on how to build your own model of a lung. It will be a fun family activity and allows you to associate word roots and functions.

2.42
Share your creation with the class.

✓ Russell needs a tetanus vaccination. It will be given in his upper arm. This region is called the _____ region.

2.43
brachial or shoulder

✓ Nellie has found enlarged lymphatic nodes in her right arm pit area. This area is properly called the _____ area.

2.44
axillary

✓ Maria has been diagnosed with costochondritis. What index is used in the ICD to begin coding this visit?

2.45
Index to Disease and Injury

Word building

Using the word roots with the linking vowel to build as many valid terms with the suffixes given. Please define each term too.

Thorac/o Abdomin/o Cervic/o

-ic -tomy -centesis -al -scope -dynia
-plasty -stomy

Can you build one compound word?

2.46
The instructor has the list!

• The **abdominal cavity** begins at the diaphragm, which acts like a roof, and really ends at the strong muscles of the pelvic floor, which keep our abdominal and pelvic contents inside!

2.47
Peritone/o is the linking form for the peritoneal cavity. Peri- is around, about, or near.

A peritoneocentesis is a procedure to remove fluid from the sac for evaluation or as a therapy.

A peritoneoclysis is a procedure that uses sterile fluids to flush the peritoneal sac to remove debris.

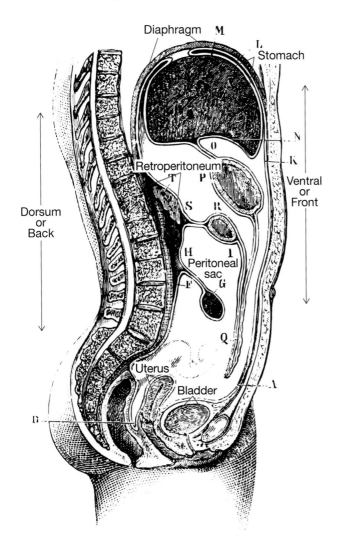

Figure 2.21

Within this cavity there are distinct areas which are more ventral (anterior) and dorsal (posterior). Some are found within the peritoneal sac of the abdomen and others are more retroperitoneal.

- The **peritoneum** (**pear**-i-toe-**knee**-um) > double-layered membrane surrounding and supporting the various structures of the abdominal cavity: the stomach, liver, gallbladder, spleen, the jejunum and ileum, and the transverse and sigmoid colon. These organs are more ventral in the abdominal cavity.

• The **retroperitoneum** (**ret**-row-**pear**-i-toe-**knee**-um) > 'behind' the peritoneum providing cushioned protection and stability for these structures: kidneys, adrenal glands, duodenum, pancreas, the ascending colon with its hepatic flexure, descending colon with its splenic flexure, and the great vessels (abdominal aorta and inferior vena cava).

The **four quadrants of the abdomen** are typically used to localize organs.

• Right Upper Quadrant (**RUQ**) > liver, a portion of the ascending colon with hepatic flexure, upper pole of the right kidney, a section of duodenum.

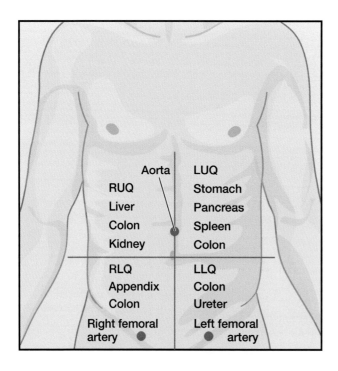

2.48
Like the thoracic cavity, examination includes inspection; auscultation for bowel and vessel sounds; percussion for organ size and air/fluid levels; and palpation.

Figure 2.22

- Left upper quadrant (**LUQ**) > Stomach, spleen, pancreas tail, portion of descending colon with splenic flexure, upper pole of left kidney.

- Right lower quadrant (**RLQ**) > Ascending colon, appendix, lower pole of the kidney, ovary and uterine tube in women.

- Left lower quadrant (**LLQ**) > Descending colon, sigmoid colon, lower pole of kidney, ovary and uterine tube in women.

The regions seen in Figure 2.23 are often used to localize pain or findings which pertain to the nine sections of the abdomen.

- The epigastric (**ep**-ee-**gas**-trik) > above the stomach. In fact the pyloric region of the stomach is transitioning to the C-loop of the duodenum. Under these structures are the head of the pancreas, common bile duct, and the abdominal aorta with no fewer than 4 major branches, which deliver blood to the liver, stomach, pancreas, and spleen.

- The **umbilical** (um-**bill**-ee-kal) region > middle square with lots of small intestines, specifically the 2nd section called the jejunum cushioning the abdominal aorta. The aorta branches to the kidneys and intestines and the inferior vena cava.

- The **pubic** (**pew**-bik) area > above the pelvic cavity with the ureters, urinary bladder, urethra, sigmoid colon, rectum, and anus. In men, this will include the prostate and in women, the uterus. Region synonym is suprapubic (**sue**-pra-**pew**-bik).

2.49
The middle row of the tick-tack-toe board is utilized most often. The middle square is the umbilicus area and the right and left lateral areas are often called the right and left flank, respectively.

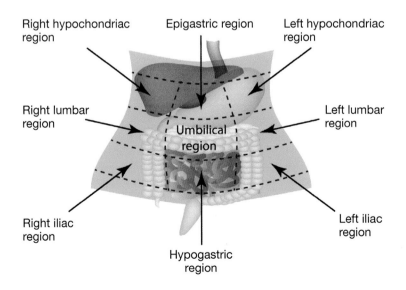

Right hypochondriac region

Epigastric region

Left hypochondriac region

Right lumbar region

Umbilical region

Left lumbar region

Right iliac region

Left iliac region

Hypogastric region

Figure 2.23

The **cranial cavity** contains the brain and the brain stem, which does fill the majority of the skull. Within the skull there are several smaller cavities unique in their purpose:

- There are two **otic** (oh-tik) **cavities**. The **middle ear** is a chamber containing the smallest bones of the body, the incus, stapes, and malleus. The **inner ear** is a bony chamber giving us both hearing and balance (Figure 2.24).

- The **sinus cavities** of the facial area give us phonation and foreign body protection via the frontal, ethmoid, and maxillary sinuses. The conchae (**kong**-kay) of the nose are considered nasal cavities.

- The **oral cavity** is the mouth with its many structures and functions performed by the teeth, tongue, mucosa, palate, and uvula.

Linking forms

Gastr/o > stomach

Hepat/o > liver

Duoden/o > duodenum

Jejun/o > jejunum

Ile/o > ileum

Pub/o > pubic

**2.50
Linking forms**

Ot/o > ear

Gloss/o > tongue

Dent/o > teeth

Palat/o > palate

Uvul/o > uvula

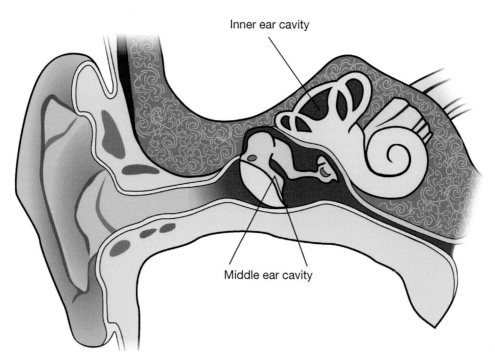

Inner ear cavity

Middle ear cavity

Figure 2.24

UNIT SUMMARY

1   The human body is a complex organism functioning via the interactions of 12 body systems. These systems work together to maintain homeostasis, an intricate set of negative and positive feedback loops keeping things the 'same'.

2   The systems which have things coming and going are the Respiratory, Digestive, Urinary, and Lymphatic systems. The systems permitting us to move and groove are the Skeleton, Muscular, and Integumentary systems.

3   The linking systems include the Circulation, Endocrine, and Nervous systems. And the specialists are the Immune and Reproductive systems.

4   The human body can be sliced for imaging purposes in 4 directions at almost any point on the body. This enables a lesion or illness to be pinpointed more precisely: sagittal, frontal, transverse, and oblique.

5   The body can also be divided into regions, some small such as the ear and others larger such as the chest, the thorax. The region designations give the provider the opportunity to think about which structure lives in a particular area such as skin, muscles, tendons, ligaments, blood vessels, and nerves in the antecubital region.

6   Numbers give us amounts, weight, lengths, and volume. The precision used to document these is imperative to patient care and medication delivery. Numbers are also used to label and sort like the alphanumeric of the coding system. Typically, in the United States, we use the Metric and Household Measurement Systems.

7   SOAP notes are used extensively to relate a patient encounter of one or two issues. The subjective is the history or the story as told by the patient as to what is happening to bring them to care. The objective section is for the facts! The assessment is one or more diagnosis and other pertinent findings. The plan is the action the provider and patient agree to accomplish from taking a medication to starting a diet.

8   If it is not documented, it never happened! Medical terminology, its correct spelling, correct locations, and correct numbers form the structure of the medical encounter facilitating quality care for each patient. The documents allow continuity of care and coding to be done via the ICD which determine reimbursement, illness and injury tracking, and even environmental and building projection, training needs, and so much more.

UNIT WORD PARTS

Word roots with linking vowel		
Arteri/o > artery	Brachi/o > arm	Cardi/o > heart
Carp/o > wrist	Cephal/o > head, brain	Circul/o > circulation
Coron/o > crown	Crin/o > secreting, separate	Cutane/o or Cut/i > skin
Derm/o or Dermat/o > skin	Gest/o > to bear, to carry	Hem/o or Hemat/o > blood
Home/o > same, unchanging	Immun/o > protector	Lymph/o > lymph fluid
Mamm/o > breast	Ment/o > chin or mind	Mes/o > middle, median
Muscul/o or My/o > muscle	Neur/o > nerves	O/o > egg
Ocul/o > eye	Orchid/o or Orchi/o > testicles	Ot/o > ear
Ovari/o or Oophor/o > ovary	Pariet/o > inner wall	Path/o > disease
Ped/o > foot or child	Phalang/o > fingers or toes	Physi/o > function
Pulmon/o > lungs	Radi/o > X-ray	Skelet/o > dried up (bones)
Spir/o > breath	Stern/o > sternal, breast bone	Tars/o > ankle
Test/i or Testicul/o > testicles	Thorac/o > chest	Tom/o > cut, section
Umbilic/o > belly button	Ur/o or Urin/o > urine	Ven/o > vein
Vertebr/o > spinal bone	Viscer/o > internal organs	Xiph/o > sword tip, distal bone of sternum

Prefixes: attached to the front of the word root to change meaning		
Ab- > away from the center	Ad- > toward the center, add	Anter- > front, ventral
Bi- or Di- > two, double	Centi- > 0.01, 1/100th, 10−2	Deca- > ten Deci- > 1/10th, 0.1
Dist- > away from, furthest from point of origin	Hemi- > precisely half	Hepta-, Septi- > seven
Hexa-, Sexta- > six	Infer- > below, under, directed downward	Inter- > between

Prefixes: *continued*		
Kilo- > 1000	Later- > to the side, furthest from the center	Medi- > middle, center, closest to center
Meta- > beyond	Milli- > 0.001, 1/1000th, 10^{-3}	Mono- > one, single
Multi- > many, more, excess	Non- > none, no, not, opposite, or negative	Noni- or Nona- > nine
Nulli- > no, none, never	Oct-, Octa- > eight	Pan- > all, entire, whole
Poly- > many, more than, too often	Poster- > back, dorsum	Proxim- > nearest to the trunk or point of origin
Quadri- > four	Quinta-, Penta- > five	Semi- > half, less than
Super- > at the top, uppermost, directed upward	Trans- > across	Tri- > three
Uni- > one, single		

Acronyms, abbreviations, and initial sets		
AP > anteroposterior	cm > centimeter, 1/100th, a measure or length	CT, CAT > computed tomography scan
DIP > distal inter-phalangeal joints	HPI > history of present illness	kcal > kilocalorie (energy)
kg> kilogram, a weight	kVp > kilovolt peak (energy)	mcg > microgram, 10^{-6}
MCL > mid-clavicular line	MCP > metacarpo-phalangeal joints	mEq > milliequivalent
mg > milligram, 1/1000th, 10^{-3}; a weight	ml > milliliter, 1/1000th, 10^{-3}; a volume	mm > millimeters, 1/1000th, 10^{-3}; a length
MRI > magnetic resonance imaging	MTP > metatarso-phalangeal joints	OB/Gyn > obstetrics and gynecology
PA > posteroanterior	PET > positron emission tomography	PIP > proximal interphalangeal joint
PT > physical therapy or therapists	RT > respiratory or radiology therapist	SpT > speech therapist

UNIT WORKSHEETS

Building terms: Use the proper prefix/word root/linking vowel/suffix as appropriate. Example: To cut into the muscle > my/o/tomy

a) Pertaining to the side or a view from the side > _____

b) Like a 'sword tip' > _____

c) Condition of complete absence of all blood cells _____

d) Pertaining to many joints involved > _____

e) The study of X-rays _____

f) Pertaining to an 'inside' organ or the membrane touching it > _____

g) A specialist in the system which secretes internally > _____

h) A pain in one nerve > _____

Number reference: For the word given, what number is involved? Spell the number please, e.g., eleven.

1 Bilobate _____

2 Unilateral _____

3 Tetralogy _____

4 Trigeminal _____

5 Diplopia _____

6 Decade _____

7 Nonigravida _____

8 Sextuplets _____

Best choice: Pick the most appropriate answer.

1 The eponym, Fowler's position, places the patient in which of following positions?

   a) Right lateral recumbent   c) Pronation

   b) Dorsiflexion   d) Semi-upright

2 This system includes the microglia of the brain, the spleen and lymph nodes, and a bevy of white blood cells.

   a) Nervous   c) Endocrine

   b) Immune   d) Circulation

3 A prefix which is a synonym of 'multi' is?

   a) Dys–   c) Poly–

   b) Mono–   d) Pan–

4 During the preoperative set up, the patient is placed on her right side. This is the _____ position?

   a) Fowler's   c) Lateral recumbent

   b) Dorsal   d) Prone

5 The movement of the leg away from the body is best described as?

   a) Proximal   c) Flexion

   b) Supination   d) Abduction

6 'Ned states he has a bad cold. He has had a fever, cough, and chills for 3 days'. Which section of a SOAP note does this sentence belong in?

   a) Subjective   c) Assessment

   b) Objective   d) Plan

Where in or on body? Based on the word or linking form given what region or area of the body is noted?

1 Femoral   _____

2 Pectoral   _____

3 Cervic/o   _____

4 Antecubital   _____

5 Ot/o   _____

6 Phalanges   _____

7 Armpit   _____

8 Ribs   _____

Multiple correct: Select ALL the correct answers to the question given.

1 Which of these are part of the work of the digestive system?

a) Mechanical chewing

b) Consolidation of waste

c) Filtering the blood

d) Chemical churning in the stomach

e) Production of blood cells

f) Maintenance of our body position

2 Which of these indicate the front of the body?

a) Ventral

b) Lateral

c) Dorsal

d) Anterior

e) Superficial

3 Which of these systems are considered 'linkers or roadways'?

a) Immune

b) Circulatory

c) Integumentary

d) Endocrine

e) Reproductive

f) Nervous

Spelling challenge: Circle the correct spelling based on the definition given.

1 'Plane divides the body right to left'

Sachital   Sajittal   Saggittal   Sagittal

2 'Specialist in blood conditions'

Hemotolojist   Hemmatology   Hematologist   Heematologist

3. 'Pertaining to the digits'

Phalangeal   Falangeal   Phalanxgeal   Phelangeal

Define the term: Spelling *does* count in your definition too!

1 Milliequivalent > _____

2 Nulligravida > _____

3 Supination > _____

4 Electrocardiogram > _____

5 Colorectal > _____

6 Adduction > _____

7 Polycythemia> _____

8 Thoracic > _____

Find it! Using the words in the table – match the definition given or answer the statement. Some may not be used. It is recommended you know all the choices.

retroperitoneum	dorsiflexion	skeletal	decimal	compound
transdermal	bifurcation	frontal	tongue	superior
prone	supinated	adduction	visceral	distal
polyneuropathy	parietal	sagittal	respiration	immunity

1 _____ This term can mean the forehead or the plane to slice the body anterior to posterior.

2 _____ The pancreas, ascending and descending colon, and kidneys are found here.

3 _____ To breathe over and over again.

4 _____ This 'point' should never stand alone or naked to avoid medication errors.

5 _____ Turning the hand down from anatomical position.

6 _____ The farthest structure from the origin.

7 _____ Membrane lining the walls of a cavity, such as the thorax.

8 _____ Pertaining to crossing the skin.

9 _____ The linking form is gloss/o.

10 _____ When a medical term has two or more word roots.

Matching: Medical abbreviations, acronyms, and initial sets, some will not be used.

	Letter	Defined as
SOAP		a) 1/1000th of a meter
DIP		b) metacarpophalangeal joint
kcal		c) posteroanterior
mcg		d) Subjective, Objective, Assessment, Plan
CT		e) microgram
AP		f) proximal interphalangeal joint
mm		g) distal interphalangeal joint
MCP		h) kilocalorie
		i) anteroposterior
		j) computerized tomogram

An essay: Explain the function of each of the sections making up a SOAP note in your own words.

Note challenge: Define the underlined terms. You may need to look up a few. Answer the questions which follow. Student is reminded this is an incomplete SOAP note used for the learning experience. Do not use this for patient encounters.

> Matteo is a 23-year old man who was playing basketball when another player came down on his left ankle. He is complaining of 5/10 pain at rest and more with any motion of the ankle. He has no previous history of ankle injury. He is allergic to penicillin. No current medications. He smokes 1 pack of cigarettes a day.
>
> 23-year-old man with edema over the lateral aspect of the left ankle with bruising and point-tenderness. Good dorsalis pedis pulse and nail perfusion. No deformity noted. X-ray of left ankle reveals:
>
> 1 Distal tibial fracture of the medial malleolus slightly displaced posteriorly.
>
> 2 Distal diaphysis spiral fracture of the fibula slightly displaced anteriorly.

Questions:

1 Which portion of this note is the objective section? What does it include?

2 What key words could you use to look this injury up in the ICD?

3 What section of the ICD do you start with?

4 What is the linking form for *dorsalis pedis*?

Unit 3

Cells, tissues, and pathology

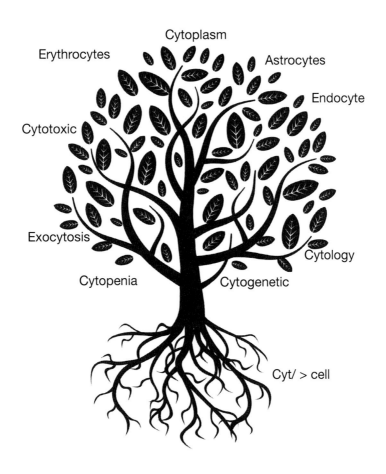

TARGETED LEARNING

1 Correlate elements of cells and tissues as they pertain to the human body and medical terminology.

2 Correctly construct, define, pronounce, and spell medical terms.

3 Distinguish symbols, acronyms and terms to pathology, genetics, and electrolytes.

4 Link pathology findings, oncology, and pharmacotherapeutics within medical records.

5 Demonstrate how to find pathology elements associated with patient care via the ICD.

KEY WORD PARTS

Word roots with linking vowel	Prefixes	Suffixes
Adip/o; Lip/o > fat	Ana-	-ase
Chem/o > chemical	Cata-	-blast
Cyt/o; Cellul/o > cell	Dys-	-cidal
Electr/o > electricity, charge	Endo-	-clast
Gluc/o; Glyc/o > glucose, sugar	Epi-	-dystonia
Hist/o > tissue	Exo-	-gen, -genesis, -genic
My/o > muscle	Hyper-	-glia
Myel/o > spinal cord or bone marrow	Meta-	-lysis
Nucle/o; Kary/o > nucleus, center	Micro-	-oma
Onc/o > cancer	Mono-	-osis
Path/o > disease	Neo-	-pathy
Plasm/o > tissue, living substance, gel-like fluid	Oligo-	-plasm
Prote/o > protein	Poikil-	-plasty
Sarc/o > flesh	Poly-	-poiesis
Thel/o; Theli/o > cellular layer or nipple	Sym-	-tomy

PATHOLOGY REPORTS

Pathology is the study of disease. The suffix -pathy indicates 'disease of': e.g., adenopathy, disease of the glands. A pathology (pah-**thol**-oh-gee) report details the inspection of cells and tissues via gross examination and under the microscope. A pathologist (pah-**thol**-oh-jist) is the specialist who studies disease by describing the cells and tissue in terms of size, shape, or its morphology (more-**fol**-oh-gee) using samples (Figure 3.2).

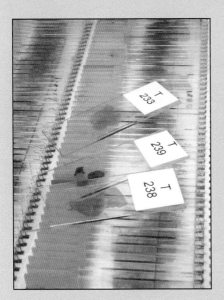

Pathology reports can convey both normal and abnormal findings. Thus, a pathology report does not necessarily mean a 'disease' is present. A pathology report is considered the gold-standard in defining normal or disease processes such as cancer, Alzheimer's, multiple sclerosis, myositis, and so many more. Defining the changes in cells and tissues permits staging of a disease such as cancer, which helps establish care alternatives.

Figure 3.2

ELEMENTS AND CELLS

ELEMENTS are the small stuff of life. 'Atomos', Greek for indivisible or uncut. Today, it is called the 'atom', the functional unit of all **elements**. All living organisms are a collection of chemicals and all the chemicals are made of trillions of atoms, which build **compounds**. We breathe oxygen and our cells use sodium (Na^{++}) and potassium (K^+) to create an electrical charge running our cells. The elements controlling the chemistry of the human body have several names, the first is electrolytes.

Electr/o > linking form for electricity or charge; the spark of energy moving our body and much of the world around us. Many of the elements in our body are **electrolytes** (ee-**lek**-tro-lites) because they carry an electrical charge. Most are found in our environment: e.g., sodium salt, potassium salt, and magnesium.

The ability to carry an electrical charge requires an atom or group of atoms to lose or gain one or more electrons, which makes them **ions** in the body, having the ability to exchange and dissolve. These form the ionic basis of resting membrane potential of all cell interactions (Figure 3.3). In medical terms, they are called **anions** and **cations**.

3.1

A/tom > not cut, unable to be cut

electr/o terms

Electricity

Electrode

Electrolysis

Electrocautery

Electrocardiogram

Electroshock

Electrophoresis

Ionic Basis of the Resting Membrane Potential

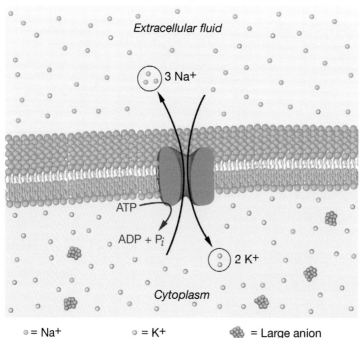

Extracellular fluid

3 Na+

ATP

ADP + P$_i$

2 K+

Cytoplasm

○ = Na+   ○ = K+   🟤 = Large anion

Figure 3.3

- **Anion** (**an**-eye-on) > ion with a negative charge (*no ion*, literally) gives it more electrons. It will attract positive ions to form compounds. Chloride (Cl⁻) is negative, an anion; it is attracted to cations, such as sodium (Na⁺⁺). Sodium chloride (so-**dee**-um **klor**-ide) is table salt.

- **Cation** (**cat**-eye-on) > ion with a positive charge; more positive protons will attract the negative anions.

- Using many ions or elements to build larger compounds is called **anabolism** (a-**nah**-bowl-ism) such as taking the amino acids from food to build proteins which function throughout the body.

- Breaking down the many elements so they may be used is called **catabolism** (ka-**tab**-oh-lizm), such as chewing food to get the nutrients into the body.

- **Metabolism** (meh-**tab**-oh-lizm) > the sum of the give and take of the chemical and physical changes of the body. Meta- > change, beyond.

Anions and cations are investigated on a daily basis via the other limb of the pathology department–laboratory science. Electrolytes are found on the 'basic metabolic panel' (**BMP**), also referred to as a 'Chem 6' or the larger **CMP**, complete metabolic panel. Abnormal findings may denote pathology, the presence of disease. Take note of the symbol for each element, these are seen on laboratory reports and medical documentation (Chart 3.1).

3.2

Did You Know?

Ionization is the process of breaking apart or disassociating the ions from each other in a solution. The solution is usually water, such as in the blood. Radioactive ions are used as tracers in nuclear medicine to find or track disease.

3.3

Other chemical symbols found in medical reports:

H > Hydrogen

Cr > Chromium

Fe⁺⁺⁺ > Iron

Zn > Zinc

C > Carbon

P > Phosphorus

I > Iodine

Pb > Lead

Hg > Mercury

O > Oxygen

Mg⁺⁺ > Magnesium

Electrolyte	Symbol	Ion type	Chemical weight	Function in the body
Sodium	Na^{++}	Cation	11	Extracellular ion > all cells
Potassium	K^+	Cation	19	Intracellular ion > all cells
Chloride	Cl^-	Anion	17	Travels equally to maintain electrical neutral
Calcium	Ca^{++}	Cation	20	Essential to muscle, nerve, and heart function
Magnesium	Mg^{++}	Cation	12	Vital to energy production for muscles, nerves, and bone health
Carbon dioxide	CO_2	A covalent bond reflects HCO3 (bicarbonate)	Compound with Carbon 6 Oxygen 8	Helps maintain a stable pH (acid-base level)
As a comparison, the smallest normal protein of the body, albumin, has a chemical weight of 63,000.				

Chart 3.1 Assembled by author

✓ Najib's Chem 6 report reveals an elevated Na^{++}. This symbol indicates which element?

3.4
Sodium

✓ The term 'cardiopathy' means _____ .

3.5
disease of the heart

✓ A cation such as potassium, will have a/an _____ electrical charge.

3.6
positive

Kitchen lab

Look around your environment. Which processes in your daily life represent anabolism, the process of building? Explain how. Which processes represent catabolism? Explain how. Are there any processes resembling metabolism? Explain how.

3.7
Share your findings with your instructor.

Cells

Cyt/o > cell > cytology (sigh-**tol**-oh-gee) > study of cells. Cyt/o, Greek for 'a hollow'. The human body has an estimated 35 trillion cells at any given moment. The cell is the smallest structural and functional living unit. Each cell is an operational neighborhood of working components as noted in Figure 3.4. The suffix –cyte(s) allows cells to be described as individual types.

3.8 Prefixes

Poly > many, frequent

Micro > small

Macro > large

Poikil > various

Mono > single

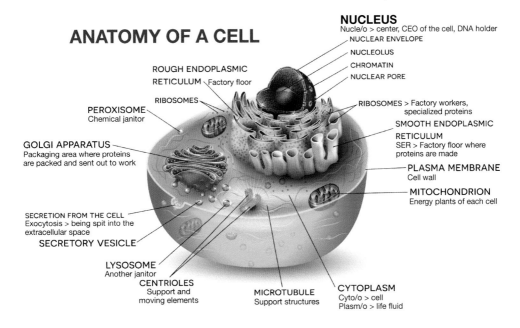

Figure 3.4

- Cyt/o/plasm > sigh-**tol**-plazm > fluid or gel-like filling of the cell. Intracellular environment floating the organelles > small organs.

- Cyt/o/lysis (sigh-**tol**-ee-sis) > breakdown or dissolution of the cell.

- Cyt/o/toxin (**sigh**-toe-**tok**-sin) > identifiable substance which inhibits or destroys the cell.

- Erythr/o/cytes (eh-**rith**-row-sites) > red blood cells (**RBC**), carry oxygen to cells.

- Phag/o/cytes (**fag**-oh-sites) > white blood cells (**WBCs**) literally eat (phag/o) debris and foreign bodies.

Suffixes

–logy > study of

–meter > measure

–penia > less than or fewer

–chrome > color

–logist > specialist

–lysis > break up

–scope > instrument to look

–osis > abnormal condition

–plasm > fluid/gel

–genic > production of, development

–cidal > causing death

Pathology reviews are done on cells or tissues. These cells and tissues are retrieved by a variety of methods. Biopsy (buy-**op**-see) is the removal of cells or tissue for inspection via scraping the surface, excisional, incisional, punch or syringe aspiration. The word root is Bi/o > life and the suffix -opsy > vision; therefore, a biopsy literally means to 'view life'.

Look at the report (Figure 3.5) and answer the following questions:

1 What kind of medical record or report is this?

2 Please note all the terms appearing as medical terms, acronyms, and abbreviations. Look them up, define or explain them as appropriate.

3 If this record was lost in the system would it be a concern? Why?

Discuss your findings with the instructor and class.

Specimen source	Vaginal cytologic material
LMP:	1991
IUD:	
BC pills:	
Weeks pregnant:	
Weeks post-partum:	
Post-menopausal:	
Hysterectomy:	Yes
Hormone therapy:	
Cytotoxic therapy:	
Radiation therapy:	
Comments/HCP:	no lesions of cuff
Previous Dx/HCP:	no abn
Diagnosis:	NEGATIVE
Estrogen invalid:	
SNOMED codes:	T-8X210/M-00120: Vaginal
Pathologist:	xxxxxxxx

Figure 3.5

✓ Construct a word meaning 'a large cell'. (n)
_____/_____

3.9
Macro/cyte

✓ Construct a word meaning 'condition of too few small cells'. (n) _____/_____/_____/_____

3.10
Micro/cyt/o/penia

✓ Navin works in the local hospital in the laboratory where she looks at slides having cellular changes from infection or cancers. Navin is a _____ (n).

3.11
cytotechnician

Word building

Using the word roots with the linking vowel to build as many valid terms with the suffixes given. Please define each term too.

Electric/o Cyt/o Erythr/o

–phoresis –megaly –toxin –genesis –lysis
–al –logy

3.12
The instructor has the list!

HUMAN CELLS

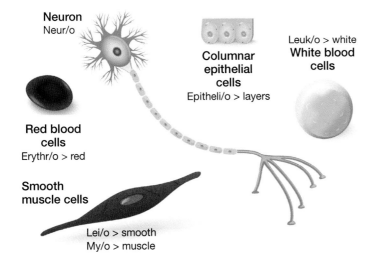

HUMAN CELLS

Neuron
Neur/o

Columnar epithelial cells
Epitheli/o > layers

Leuk/o > white
White blood cells

Red blood cells
Erythr/o > red

Smooth muscle cells

Lei/o > smooth
My/o > muscle

Figure 3.6

There are about 200 cell types divided into four large tissue categories. Figure 3.6 demonstrates a few of the shapes and functions. Human cells have three principal components:

- **Plasma membrane** (**plaz**-ma **mem**-brain) or the cell wall > flexible, outer boundary.

- **Cytoplasm** > intracellular fluid containing organelles and nucleus.

- **Nucleus** (**new**-klee-us) > control center of all cells with the exception of erythrocytes. Mature red blood cells carry only the hemoglobin (**he**-moe-**glow**-bin) protein which binds oxygen for use in all cells (Figure 3.7).

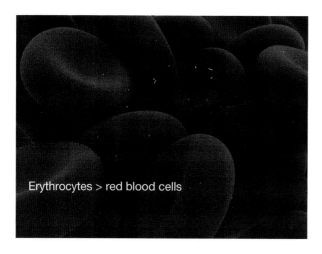

Erythrocytes > red blood cells

3.13
Linking forms of cell organelles

Plasm/o > gel-like internal milieu of the cell

Cyt/o > cell

Cellul/o > cell

Organ/o > organ

Nucle/o > center

Kary/o > center, nucleus

Gene- > functional unit of heredity

Reticul/o > network

Figure 3.7

The cell neighborhood is filled with several structures. Some are designated by a dissectible medical term and others are not. In some cases, by eponyms: e.g., Camillo Golgi, an Italian physician, gave us the Golgi apparatus and Golgi bodies.

The nucleus is considered the chief construction engineer of the cell as it contains the DNA, deoxyribonucleic acid, which carries the genetics (je-**net**-iks) making each individual different.

- Nucle/o > center or core > nucleus is singular. Nuclei (**new**-klee-eye) is plural.

- Nuclear (**new**-klee-ar) > pertaining to the nucleus.

- Nucleoplasm (**new**-klee-oh-plazm) > protoplasm (fluid) environment of the nucleus itself.

3.14
Multinucleate > many nuclei

Mononuclear > one nucleus

Nucleated > possessing a nucleus

The factory of the neighborhood is the **endoplasmic reticulum** (**en**-doe-**plaz**-mik re-**tik**-you-lum) (**ER**) > attaches to the nucleus in a semi-circle taking the 'construction blueprint' into a series of inter-connected canals or networks to assemble the proteins for use by the cell itself and the rest of the body – just like an assembly line (Figure 3.8). The workers on the line are **ribosomes** (**rye**-bow-soms).

ENDOPLASMIC RETICULUM

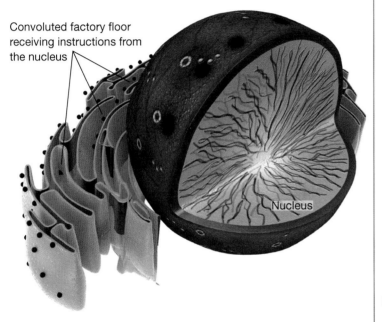

Convoluted factory floor receiving instructions from the nucleus

Nucleus

3.15

Endo- > inside, within

Prote/o > protein

Figure 3.8

Proteins are wrapped and shipped by the cell's packaging center, the **Golgi apparatus** (**goal**-gee **app**-are-**rat**-us). When the proteins stay in the cell the process is called **endocytosis**. The term endocytosis is also used when something outside the cell is brought *into* the cell. If the proteins are destined for other places, the package make its way through the cytoplasm to the cell wall and the packaged proteins are pushed in the bloodstream. This is called **exocytosis** (**eks**-oh-sigh-**toe**-sis), see Figure 3.9.

3.16

Golgi is an eponym

Exo- > outside, outermost

Endo- > inner, inner most, interior

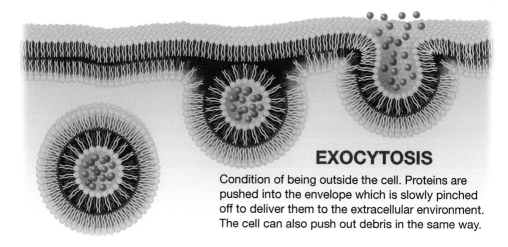

EXOCYTOSIS

Condition of being outside the cell. Proteins are pushed into the envelope which is slowly pinched off to deliver them to the extracellular environment. The cell can also push out debris in the same way.

Figure 3.9

The **mitochondria** (**migh**-toe-**kon**-dree-ah) > among the many organelles of the cell neighborhood (Figure 3.10). The role of the mitochondrion (singular) is the production of cell energy; these are the energy power plants for the cell. The fuel for the mitochondria is glucose (glyc/o or gluc/o) and oxygen (O) for running the factories and the transportation systems of the cells.

3.17
Glucose (**glue**-kose) and oxygen work together in the mitochondria to maximize the production of **ATP**, adenosine triphosphate, the energy compound used for all cell activity.

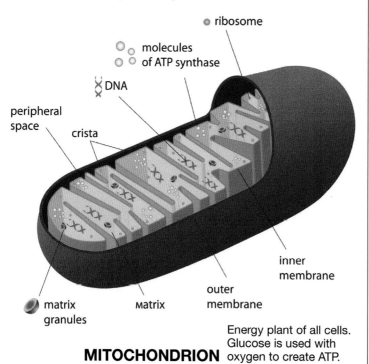

- ribosome
- molecules of ATP synthase
- DNA
- peripheral space
- crista
- matrix granules
- matrix
- outer membrane
- inner membrane

Energy plant of all cells. Glucose is used with oxygen to create ATP.

MITOCHONDRION

Figure 3.10

✓ The fluid inside the cell is called _____ .

3.18
cytoplasm

✓ Sodium is a positively charged ion, this makes it a _____ .

3.19
cation

✓ Construct a term meaning 'pertaining to two nuclei'.
_____/_____/_____

3.20
Bi/nucle/ar

Word building

Using the *word roots* with the linking vowel to build as many valid terms with the *suffixes given.* Please define each term too.

Nucle/o

–ic –lysis –ar –ase –oid –plasm –us

3.21
The instructor has the list!

Some of the other players of the intracellular neighborhood get the labor done. They are essentially the workers at the factories, energy plants, and around the neighborhood.

- **Ribosomes** > most abundant; each cell will have up to 2,000 ribosomes. The ribosomes are a combination of proteins and RNA; they receive the instructions from the nuclear DNA to build the proteins specific to the cell type.

- **Lysosomes** (**lie**-so-soms) > cleanup workers of the cell neighborhood. They contain lysozymes (**lie**-so-zimes); enzymes digest cellular debris, foreign bodies, and invaders inside the cell.

- **Peroxisomes** (pear-**ock**-see-soms) > town janitors too; they contain oxidative enzymes to destroy debris in the intracellular environment.

- **Microvilli** (**my**-krow-**vil**-lie) > tiny finger-like or hair-like structures on the surface of the cells (Figure 3.11). They move fluids and absorb nutrients depending on their location. Synonym: **Cilia** (sea-**lee**-ah).

3.22
RNA comes in three types

mRNA > messenger RNA carries the DNA instructions to the ribosomes.

tRNA > transfer RNA carries the specific amino acids to the ribosomes to build the protein.

rRNA > ribosomal RNA is actually part of the ribosome allowing communication.

✓ Which of the three types of RNA will carry the DNA message to the ribosomes hanging out in the endoplasmic reticulum?

3.23
mRNA > messenger

✓ Construct the word meaning 'condition of being outside the cell'. _____/_____/_____

3.24
Exo/cyt/o/osis

✓ The meaning of 'phagocytes' is _____ . What is the linking form?

3.25
eating cells; Phag/o

CILIA

Cilia or microvilli come in many sizes. From those that help move the cells or the villi of the GI tract which absorb nutrients. Cilia > finger-like, thread

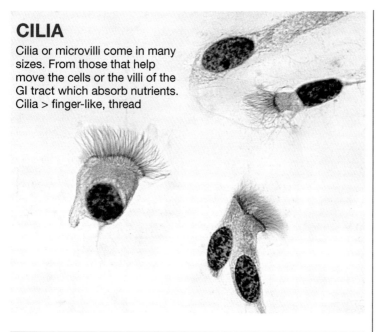

Figure 3.11

Word building

Using the prefixes to build as many valid terms with the terms given. Please define each term too.

Micro- Macro-

-cyte -villi -graph -fibril -ic -some -scope

3.26
The instructor has the list!

A SHORT HISTORY OF GENETICS

Charles Darwin was one of the first scientists to propose that natural selection allowed a population to survive and pass on characteristic traits, the task of genes (Figure 3.12). Shortly after, in 1866, Charles Mendel published his inheritance results on the traits of the pea plant. These were the beginnings of genetic research. As far back as 1908, scientists believed there were 'inborn' errors of metabolism with the absence or insufficient amounts of specific enzymes. It was not until 1973 that recombinant DNA could be replicated and maintained. From this point, oncogenes (cancer genes) and disease genes have been slowly discovered and investigated. Gene-therapy was hit and miss in the 1990s, and in 2000 the differentiation of the **human genome** was completed. Since then the number of genetic testing opportunities has risen from BRCA1 for breast cancer in 1990 to over 1,200 possible gene analyses currently listed in the *current procedural terminology (cpt®)* standards with many more likely to come. What does this have to do with medical terminology?

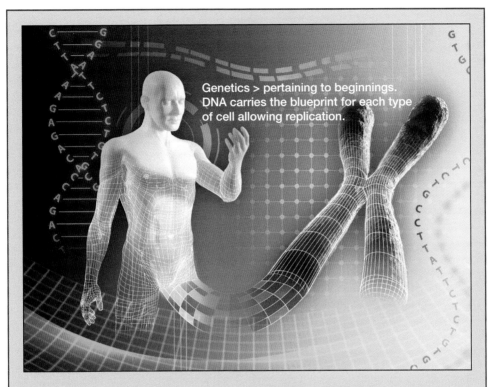

Genetics > pertaining to beginnings. DNA carries the blueprint for each type of cell allowing replication.

Figure 3.12

Medical history and breakthroughs are occurring almost daily as these genetic analyses allow for gene-therapy. Genesplicing is allowing providers to build person-specific fixes for both metabolic and immunologic diseases. New words are being constructed, this is just a sample:

- Proteomics (**pro**-tea-oh-miks) > related to how proteins are expressed by human genes; in other words, proteomics is the study of how and why proteins are built and function in the body based on the DNA in the nucleus.

- Metabolomics (**met**-ah-**bol**-oh-miks) > methodical study of the individual chemical fingerprints which cellular processes leave behind, the **metabolites**.

- Immunostaining (i-**mew**-no-stain-ing) > biochemistry term used for any antibody-based approach to detect specific proteins in a specimen. This is part of many pathology reports looking for the presence of carcinomas.

Diseases which are caused by mutations of the tRNA may have a cure in our lifetime. The readers of this text will see these genetic terms, findings, and solutions within the SOAP notes now and into the future.

TISSUES

The study of tissues is histology (his-**tol**-oh-gee). Tissue types are divided by their general function and/or location. The epithelial tissue types outnumber the rest because they are most likely to replicate (mitotic), repair, and replenish their numbers day-in and day-out.

Epithelial (**ep**-ee-**the**-lee-al) > Greek for above or on top of the cell layer. These are the surface cells of the skin, the inside of the bladder, the inside of the bronchial tubes, stomach and intestines (Figure 3.13), and more. In general, the functions are protection, absorption, filtration, excretion, and part of the sensory net.

Kitchen lab

Collagen is the protein making up egg whites. Look around your kitchen for other proteins or products which are really tough to eat or clean up. This is a function of their connective tissues. Discuss your results with your instructor.

Connective tissues support and connect other tissues and systems and are grouped into six categories. Some connective tissues are hard, such as the bone and cartilage of our limbs. Yet, blood and lymph are fluids.

• Fibr/o > fiber, thread > fibroblasts (**fie**-bro-blasts) > produces the **collagen** and elastic fibers giving connective tissue strength and flexibility (Figure 3.14).

• Chondr/o > cartilage > chondroblasts (**kon**-dro-blasts) produces cartilage cells which will make the knee meniscus or the tip of the nose.

• Oste/o or osse/o > bone > osteoblasts (**os**-tea-oh-blasts) > immature cells for the bone; they are the builders.

• Areol/a > small place, delicate > areolar (a-**re**-oh-lar) tissue is loose tissue like a cotton ball, providing padding and protection to many areas.

• Reticul/o > network, delicate > the spleen has reticular (re-**tik**-U-lar) tissue; it is delicate, almost spider-web like allowing support and free-motion of the leukocytes and lymphatics.

• Adip/o or lip/o > fat, fatty > adipocytes (**ah**-dee-poe-sites) have room for a nucleus and fat; they are the packing peanuts of the body providing energy and cushioning.

GASTROINTESTINAL EPITHELIAL TISSUE

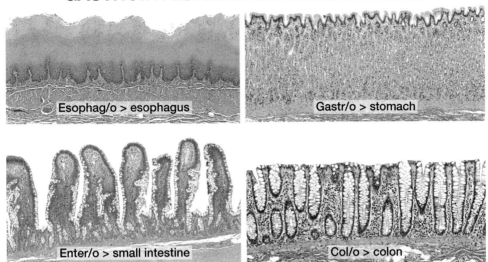

Esophag/o > esophagus

Gastr/o > stomach

Enter/o > small intestine

Col/o > colon

Figure 3.13

CONNECTIVE TISSUES

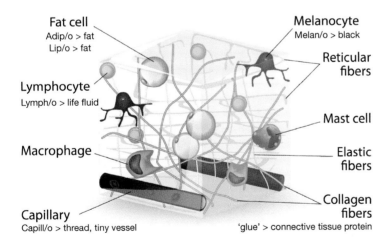

Fat cell
Adip/o > fat
Lip/o > fat

Melanocyte
Melan/o > black

Reticular
fibers

Lymphocyte
Lymph/o > life fluid

Mast cell

Macrophage

Elastic
fibers

Collagen
fibers

Capillary
Capill/o > thread, tiny vessel

'glue' > connective tissue protein

Figure 3.14

- Derm/o or dermat/o > skin > dermis (**dur**-mis), the active layer of skin providing blood and lymphatic support of the epidermis. It is here some nerve endings, blood vessels, and glands reside.

- Hem/o or hemat/o > blood > actually a mix of water, solid cells such as erythrocytes, leukocytes, platelets, and many electrolytes, nutrients, and hormones.
  - Hemophobia (hee-moh-**foe**-bee-ah) > fear of blood.

- Lymph/o > lymph > lymphatic (lim-**fat**-ik) vessels are like vacuum cleaners picking up the trash and debris of the interstitial (between cells) environment.

 What is the appropriate medical term for a 'reticular cell'?

3.29
Reticulocyte

 The term 'adipose' pertains to which connective tissue type?

3.30
Fat

Word building

 *Using the word roots **with the linking vowel to build as many valid terms with the suffixes given.** Please define each term too.*

Hemat/o Oste/o Chondr/o

–blasts –osis –logist –genesis –lysis –al
–logy –algia –plasty

3.31
The instructor has the list!

Muscle

Muscle comes in three varieties; the most abundant is **skeletal muscle** > the moving and grooving type – strong, resilient, and trainable because it is involved in voluntary motions. The fibers are long, cylindrical, and striated as noted in Figure 3.15.

- Sarcomere (**sar**-ko-meer) > functional unit of the skeletal muscle cells.

- Myofibrils (**my**-oh-**fie**-brils) > tiny muscle fibers, it takes 100s to 1000s of tiny threads to build a muscle fiber – a single muscle cell.

Smooth muscle is not linear like skeletal muscle; it is spindle-like and configured to allow it to work in relative unison, contracting to push things along. Smooth muscle is found in GI tract, lungs,

3.32
Skelet/o > dry (bones)

Lei/o > smooth

Cardi/o > heart

My/o > muscle

Muscul/o > muscle

Fibr/o > fiber, thread

–oma > tumor

–dysplasia > bad or poor formation

bladder, and blood vessels – it is involuntary, smooth, and flat (sheet-like).

- Leiomyoma (**lie**-oh-my-**oh**-ma) > neoplasm of the smooth muscle. These occur in the uterus, small intestines, and esophagus; they are usually benign.

Cardiac muscle is specialized for the heart only; the heart muscle is a blend of the striated skeletal – tough and resilient and the smooth muscle of the internal organs, which tend to work as a unit, in unison.

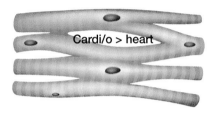

Cardi/o > heart

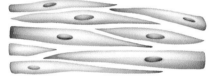

Leiomy/o > smooth muscle

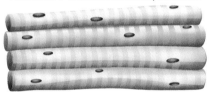

Rhabd/o > skeletal muscle, striated

-clonus > jerking, tumult

-dystonia > slow relaxation

-oid > resembling, similar to

Remember many of these terms were defined by how they appear to the naked eye. Sarc/o > is flesh, because several layers of tissue are torn or cut through.

Figure 3.15

Neurons

The 4th group of tissues are the **neuron** and **neuroglia** (**nur**-oh-glee-al) cells of the nervous system. Neurons are the densely packed cells of the brain and spinal cord carrying sensory input to the brain and motor output to the rest of the body. The neuroglia cells are the supporting cast for the neurons. Neuroglial cells perform the functions of the connective tissue and immune cells in the brain and spinal cord.

- **Neurons** (nur-ons) > functional cells of the entire nervous system (Figure 3.16). They have extreme longevity (optimally 100+ years) and there are about 8 billion in the brain alone.

3.33

Neur/o > nerve

Ax/o > axon or axis

Astr/o > star shape

-glia > glue

Myel/o > spinal cord and brain stem

Dendr/o > relating to a tree, branching

Oligo- > too few, scant

BASIC NEURON TYPES
Neur/o > nerve, neurons

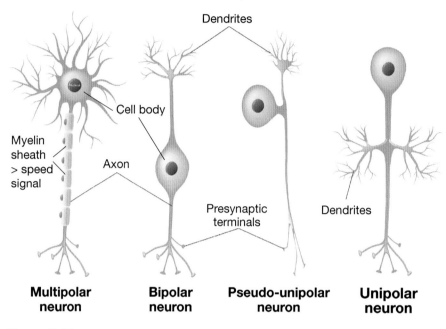

Dendrites

Cell body

Myelin
sheath
> speed
signal

Axon

Presynaptic
terminals

Dendrites

**Multipolar
neuron**

**Bipolar
neuron**

**Pseudo-unipolar
neuron**

**Unipolar
neuron**

Figure 3.16

GLIAL CELLS
'Glue' neural cell types

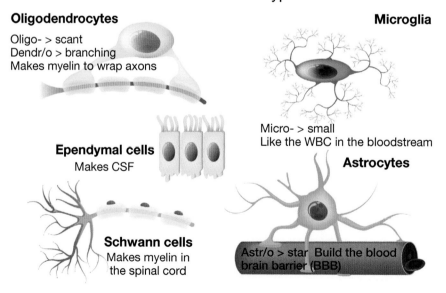

Oligodendrocytes

Oligo- > scant
Dendr/o > branching
Makes myelin to wrap axons

Microglia

Micro- > small
Like the WBC in the bloodstream

Ependymal cells
Makes CSF

Astrocytes

Schwann cells
Makes myelin in
the spinal cord

Astr/o > star Build the blood
brain barrier (BBB)

Figure 3.17

They are amitotic (**a**-my-**tot**-ik); they cannot replicate or duplicate; therefore, repair is quite limited.

- **Astrocytes** (**as**-tro-sites) > Greek for 'star'. These are the most abundant and have many functions in the brain. They form the blood–brain barrier (**BBB**) keeping toxins and many medications out of the brain.

- **Oligodendrocytes** (**ol**-ee-go-**den**-dro-sites) > build and apply their fibers around brain axons producing the insulating cover called the myelin sheath. This speeds up the transmission of the nerve's messages to the body.

- **Ependymal** (eh-**pen**-dee-mal) **>** cells line the central canals of the spine and brain ventricles; they serve to produce the cerebral spinal fluid (**CSF**).

- **Microglia** (my-**krow**-glee-ah) > act as the leukocytes of the brain; they fight bacteria, viruses, fungi, and other foreign bodies. They are very tiny, as seen in Figure 3.17. They are the janitors of the brain and spine.

LIKE ALERT!

Myel/o is the linking form for three different structures. At the time of naming, the tissues looked similar: spinal cord, bone marrow, and brain stem. Today, the linking form typically references the spinal cord or bone marrow.

TABLE OF NEOPLASMS (ICD)*

Mrs. Symone found a lump in her left breast 2 months ago. Because of the size of the lesion, a wide excision biopsy was performed. The microscopic description follows:

> Slides B6–B7 are comprised of a section of breast tissue in which is found an infiltrating ductal carcinoma of the breast. The malignancy is differentiated by infiltrating grouping of malignant cells. The cells reveal a fair degree of nuclear pleomorphism (shapes), with some of the cells having central nucleoli. The mitotic rate is less than 0.5 mitosis per 10 high power fields. The carcinoma is grade II. Bordering to the carcinoma are areas of ductal carcinoma in situ. Histologically, the tumor is 3 mm from excision margins, clear margins. Part two demonstrates 5+ lymph nodes positive for carcinoma from the 12 sampled from the left axilla.

Diagnosis:

- Infiltrating ductal carcinoma of the breast, Grade II
- Foci of ductal carcinoma in situ
- Tumor is 3 mm from the excised margins, margins are clear, no repeat excision required
- Fibrocystic disease of the breast
- Metastatic cancer in 5.5 lymph nodes

In ICD there is the Table of Neoplasms (**knee**-oh-plazm) > new growth. It is based on the histology of the cells, immunostaining, and the morphology. Genetic markers may be part of the examination as well. The table is set up on the anatomical location of the neoplasm. In our scenario, the lesion is from the left, upper outer quadrant of the breast. The codes will begin here:

- Infiltrating ductal carcinoma of the breast: C50.4- The dash is for laterality and will found in the tabular table.

- Foci of ductal carcinoma in situ: D05.- This is a cancer which has not spread yet, beginning at the site.

- Metastatic disease in lymph nodes: C77.3. This is the spread of the breast cancer to a secondary anatomical location, the left axilla, a secondary malignancy.

There will be other codes for the patient associated with this visit; these are specific to the pathology report. The pathology report supplies the diagnosis and the Table of Neoplasms provides codes for approximately 1,000 anatomical locations noting six possible conclusions:

1 Primary malignancy > where the neoplasm began; it is the origin of the cancer or tumor.

2 Secondary malignancy > spread of the malignancy away from the origin; called metastasis (**meh**-tah-**stay**-sis) > 'beyond stopping' (Figure 3.18).

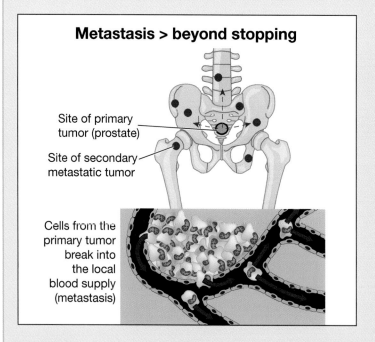

Metastasis > beyond stopping

Site of primary tumor (prostate)

Site of secondary metastatic tumor

Cells from the primary tumor break into the local blood supply (metastasis)

Figure 3.18

3   Carcinoma in situ > cancerous changes are seen in these cells but they have not spread to other cells yet; they are not metastatic (**meh**-tah-**sta**-tik).

4   Benign > while the growth of the cells takes up space, they are not malignant or likely to metastasize.

5   Uncertain behavior > pathologist is not sure of the behavior based on the cellular morphology – the shape.

6   Unspecified behavior > similar to uncertain behavior, it is more like a working diagnosis. A repeat biopsy might be needed on a time line to determine behavior.

Individuals with any carcinoma will be tracked for the remainder of their life by the pathology department of the facility where the biopsy was done. This provides many agencies and pharmacotherapeutic companies with statistics on the value of the treatment options and reoccurrence of disease. Breast cancer is one of those cancers where the genetics of cells are being manipulated and tailored to each patient with some success.

*The reader is notified these examples are from an online search carried out in 2016. Do not use these codes for patient care episodes; look up new ones!

ONCOLOGY

Greek for 'bulk' or 'mass', oncology is the study of tumors. Figure 3.19 depicts the different way chromosomes can change the function and wellness of cells, creating abnormal tissues.

- Oncogene (**on**-ko-jean) > family of genes coding proteins for cell growth. In carcinoma, this rapid cell growth adds to the size of the carcinoma.

- Oncogenesis (**on**-ko-**jen**-ee-sis) > production or development of a neoplasm. Triggers include carcinogens such as tobacco, radiation, or viruses effecting cell DNA.

- Oncolysis (ong-**ko**-lie-sis) > process of destroying or reducing the size of a tumor or mass.

3.34
Did You Know?

Prevention and Screening are not the same thing!

Prevention is using common sense to avoid injury or illness such as using sunscreen and wearing seat belts.

Screening is checking for the presence of early disease in an effort to stop it early. This includes mammograms or blood glucose levels.

CHROMOSOMAL TRANSLOCATION

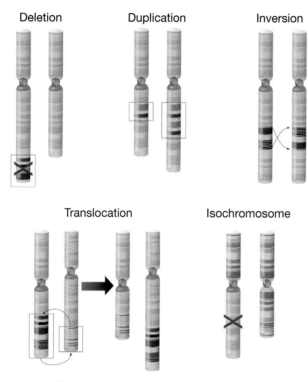

Deletion   Duplication   Inversion

Translocation   Isochromosome

Figure 3.19

Symptoms

Carcinomas of all types come with a variety of symptoms. These symptoms are not exclusive to cancers, and this is a good place to review the terms likely to appear in the Subjective section of a SOAP note or history of an admission report (Figure 3.20).

- **Sym-** > together > **symptoms** (**simp**-toms) > a collection of feelings or a departure from normal as *perceived by the patient*.

- **Nausea** (**naw**-zee-ah) > sensation of a queazy stomach, the sensation of needing to vomit. One can be nauseated without vomiting.

- **Vomiting** (**vom**-it-ing) > spewing of stomach contents via the mouth (yuck!) There are two medical terms for this symptom and action: emesis (**em**-e-sis) tends to be forceful; and regurgitation (ree-**gur**-jeh-**tay**-shun) is more of a reflux, bubbling up. Vomiting is a defense mechanism to empty the stomach of irritants.

3.35
Symptoms are what the patient describes. There are many conditions presenting with this set of symptoms. During acute illnesses these will resolve within a short period of time. Patients with carcinoma tend to have symptoms which are chronic or wax and wane for weeks at a time.

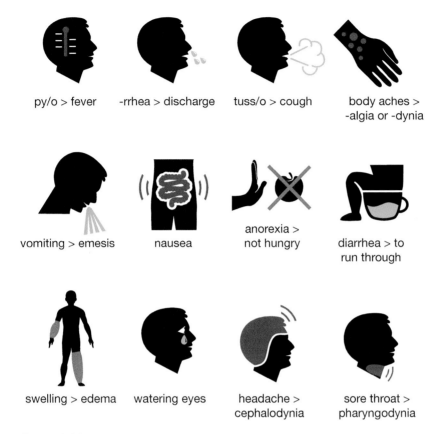

py/o > fever   -rrhea > discharge   tuss/o > cough   body aches >
-algia or -dynia

vomiting > emesis   nausea   anorexia >
not hungry   diarrhea > to
run through

swelling > edema   watering eyes   headache >
cephalodynia   sore throat >
pharyngodynia

Figure 3.20

- **Cough** (kawf) > sudden, forceful expulsion of air from the trachea past the glottis and out the mouth. Like vomiting, coughing is a defense mechanism to clear the airway of irritants.

- **Anorexia** (**an**-oh-**rek**-see-ah) > steep decline in appetite. When the body is not feeling well, the appetite decreases so energy can be used to fight infection or injury; this is another defense mechanism. In carcinoma, the appetite drops drastically and what food the patient does eat is not well digested and/or absorbed.

- **Fatigue** (fa-**teeg**) > tired, less capacity to do normal activities, weariness, or a lack of energy. Fatigue can also be a defense mechanism by slowing the body down to rest and recover.

- **Weight loss** > steady or sudden loss of weight without an effort to lose the weight. Anorexia contributes to this weight loss and the carcinoma literally steals the nutrition for its growth. Of the symptoms on this list, weight loss is most worrisome for the presence of cancer.

The search for a possible carcinoma includes all the regular blood work and imaging used for other conditions.

- **Complete blood count > CBC >** checks the status of the erythrocytes (red blood cells, **RBC**), the leukocytes (white blood cells, **WBC**), and thrombocytes (platelets). A CBC can demonstrate an anemia or a change in WBC activity. It is not specific to cause – just an indication of change.

- **Complete metabolic panel > CMP >** 14 to 20 tests for the electrolytes: minerals, such as calcium and magnesium; glucose; and liver and kidney function. Again, change does not diagnose
  a cancer but may give an indication of abnormal functions.

- **UA >** urinalysis (**yur**-in-**al**-i-sis) > set of tests done on the urine, collected by clean catch. It should be clear of all cells with a **pH** of around 6.0. Hematuria, proteinuria, or glycosuria may help define a carcinoma or effects of it.

- There are some carcinomas found (presumed) and tracked by laboratory studies; these are also described as tumor markers: e.g.,
  - **PSA >** Prostate-Specific Antigen > Prostate cancer.
  - **CA-125 >** Cancer Antigen > Ovarian cancer, some Lymphomas.
  - **CA-19–9 >** Cancer Antigen > Colon, pancreatic, and breast cancers.
  - **CD30 >** tumor necrosis (**nek**-row-sis) factor receptor, thought to be involved the regulation of apoptosis of cells > Lymphomas.

Imaging studies include plain X-ray (bone tumors), CT scans, MRI, PET scans, nuclear medicine scans, and ultrasound studies. Like the laboratory studies, these imaging studies can confirm the presence of a mass, but the mass or lesion is not defined until it is biopsied.

 A process which 'break down a tumor' is properly termed
_____ .

 True or False – John is going to cut an acre of thick grasses and he is putting on his sunscreen and mosquito repellent. This is an example of screening.

Kaylin has a code of C18.2, indicating a primary malignancy of the ascending colon. This comes from which area of the ICD?

3.36
Erythr/o > red

Leuk/o > white

Thromb/o > blood clot

Prostat/o > prostate

Ovari/o > ovary

Lymph/o > lymph

Col/o > colon

Pancreat/o > pancreas

Mamm/o > breast

Bi/o > life

Necr/o > death

Carcin/o > cancer

-emia > condition of blood, pertaining to blood.

-uria > condition of urine, pertaining to urine.

Apoptosis
(ah-pop-toe-sis) > programmed death of cells like the natural shelf-life for a product.

3.37
oncolysis

3.38
False: it prevents the bites and sunburn.

3.39
Neoplasm table

Word building

Using the word roots with the linking vowel to build as many valid terms with the suffixes given. Please define each term too.

Col/o Pancreat/o Leuk/o

-tomy –osis –itis –penia –lysis –algia –plasty – ectomy –cytes

3.40
The instructor has the list!

Therapy for carcinoma includes four basic types or combinations of therapy.

- **Surgical** (**sur**-gee-cal) > physical removal or destruction of the tumor. Two surgical procedures include (there are more):
  - Ablation (ab-**lay**-shun) > ab- > to take away from, the destruction of tissue by heat, radiation, or chemicals applied directly to the tissue. Ablation is used as a therapy for hepatic, prostate, uterine, bladder, and cervical cancers.
  - Excision (ek-**sizh**-un) > removal of the tumor with some normal tissue (clean margins). Therapy for colon, lung, breast, prostate, and melanoma frequently includes excision.
- **Radiation therapy** > use of X-rays or photodynamic rays to destroy the tissue. This destroys the cancer and may damage surrounding tissues. Radiation is used for breast and prostate cancers, and some brain cancers.
- **Chemotherapy** > uses chemical combinations via the bloodstream to kill cancer cells anywhere in the body. Used for metastasis of almost all carcinomata (plural). It can and does damage healthy tissues as well. These may include the hormonal (e.g., anti-estrogen) therapies or **molecular** therapies targeting the carcinoma more directly.
- **Biological therapy** are the highly specific gene-therapies and immunotherapies designed to destroy the cancer but leave the healthy tissue undamaged. To date, there is some success with controlling cancer.

3.41

Did You Know?

Surgery and surgeon are from the Latin *chirurgia* meaning 'hand work'. In the time of Hippocrates a surgeon operated or manipulated the body with his hands to heal. The Greek is chir/o > the source of today's 'chiropractor'.

Radi/o > X-rays

Chem/o > chemicals or medications

Therapy is Greek for medical treatment.

PHARMACY CORNER

There are several conditions and medications which put a person at risk for a change in electrolyte status. The homeostasis of these body ions or salts is imperative to life and there is a small window of normal. Disease processes disrupt this homeostasis:

- Alcoholism and/or cirrhosis of the liver > the liver detoxifies everything. Over time, alcohol and other toxins damage the liver's ability to clear the body of toxins.

- Congestive heart failure (**CHF**) > the heart is the body's pump; anything making it work harder sets the body up for failure.

- Kidney diseases > the kidneys process approximately 180 liters of blood a day, removing toxins and balancing the electrolytes; disease and infections disrupt this vital function.

- Trauma, such as burns or severe bleeding > injuries deplete the volume of active blood and loss of electrolytes strains the function of major organs.

- Thyroid and parathyroid disorders > these two hormone tissue types are vital to calcium (Ca^{++}), phosphorus (P^-), and magnesium (Mg^{++}) function, which in turn, run the nerves, muscle, and bone activities. Medications can disrupt this homeostasis.

Any medication can disrupt the electrolytes unless used carefully. These medications are often part of the therapy for the disease processes noted above.

- Furosemide (fur-**oh**-see-mide) > Lasix blocks the reabsorption of Na^{++} and Cl- in the kidneys. This causes a **diuresis** > 'running through'. Furosemide causes the body to release more water, decreasing the volume in the bloodstream. It can also cause hypokalemia (hi-**poe**-kay-**lee**-me-ah), too little potassium in the bloodstream.

- Hydrochlorothiazide (**hi**-dro-**klo**-row-**thigh**-ah-side) > blocks the reabsorption of Na^{++} and Cl^- in the kidneys. This causes a mild diuresis. It is used for **hypertension**, mild **heart failure**, and hepatic fluid retention. It can cause a **hyperuricemia** (hi-**purr**-ur-ee-**see**-me-ah) > elevated uric acid is associated with gout, pancreatitis, and can disrupt diabetes control.

- Spironolactone (**spear**-oh-no-**lak**-tone) > Aldactone blocks the reabsorption of Na^{++} and spares K^+ in the kidneys. It causes a mild diuresis, and it is not used often because it promotes **hyperkalemia** (hi-**purr**-ka-**lee**-me-ah). A change in intracellular K^+ levels up or down (hyper/hypo) can become lethal all too quickly.

These medications have **drug–drug** interactions, meaning they can enhance or negate other medications in negative ways. An example, using over-the-counter pain medications such as ibuprofen, may increase the hyperkalemia risks. They also have **drug–food** and **drug–herb** interactions; citrus fruits in particular can increase the risk of hyperkalemia. Licorice, an herb, can cause an unexpected potassium loss, hypokalemia. Dandelion and ginseng may prevent these medications from performing as intended to decrease edema, decrease blood pressure, and lessen stress on the heart.

* IMPORTANT NOTE: This list is incomplete and is gleaned from the current standard of care. Medicine is always in evolution. Do <u>not</u> use this information for patient care.

UNIT SUMMARY

1   The human body (indeed all structures) is made up of atoms. Atoms of the same type are called elements. Elements combine to make compounds which build cells. Cells build tissues and tissues will build organs. Organs will work with other tissues and organs to build systems allowing us, the organism, to function.

2   There are approximately 200 cellular types with unique forms and functions permitting the body to function. Similar cells build tissues, which are broken into four general form and function categories: Epithelial, Connective, Muscle, and Nervous tissues.

3   Electrolytes are the elements gaining or losing one or more electrons, thus producing an electrical charge. This charge powers the movement of the body via the nervous system tissue interacting with all the other tissues, especially the muscles.

4   Cells and tissues are inspected by pathologists for changes indicating health or illness. A pathology report, like a laboratory report, give the findings, good or bad, as to what the cells look like and how they may have changed in shape (morphology). A biopsy of tissue with its pathology report is considered the most definitive for diagnosis and prognosis for health and illness.

5   The examination of the nucleus of cells has yielded a broad range of information on the genetics of the human organism. New testing and therapies effecting positive changes are evolving by the day.

6   Histology, the study of tissue is vital to oncology, the study of tumors. Oncology involves the study, testing, and treatment of carcinomas and sarcomas. The new genetic and immunotherapies offer hope of new and individual therapy which may control the tumor without damaging the surrounding normal tissues. The classification of neoplasm is found and coded by anatomy location in the ICD, Table of Neoplasms.

7   Disease and injury are evaluated and noted on documents via the results of laboratory findings and pathology reports. Laboratory tests include the CBC, CMP, mineral assays, liver and renal functions, and genetic analyses. Imaging studies are used to identify the mass effect of abnormal cell growth, e.g., CT scan, MRI, US, or PET scan.

8   Some of the symptoms associated with carcinoma are nausea, vomiting, weight loss, anorexia, fatigue, and cough. These can be symptoms of any number of illnesses or even injuries.

9   There are several conditions which affect and are affected by electrolyte imbalances. Medications used to control some of these conditions can impact electrolytes in a negative manner. All medications and therapies should be used with their side-effect profiles in mind.

UNIT WORD PARTS

Word roots with linking vowel		
Aden/o > gland	Adip/o or Lip/o > fat	Areol/a > small place, delicate
Astr/o > star	Bi/o > life	Carcin/o or Onc/o > cancer
Cardi/o > heart	Chem/o > chemical	Chondr/o > cartilage
Cyt/o > cell	Dermat/o, Derm/o > skin	Electr/o > electrical
Erythr/o > red	Fibr/o > fiber, thread	Gene- > functional unit of heredity
Gen/o > beginning	Gluc/o, Glyc/o > sugar	Hem/o, Hemat/o > blood
Hist/o > tissue	Ion/o > ion, atom	Lei/o > smooth
Lymph/o > lymph, watery	Metabol/o > change	My/o > muscle
Myel/o > spinal cord or bone marrow	Neur/o > neuron, nerve	Nucle/o, Kary/o > nucleus, center
Oste/o or Osse/o > bone	Path/o > disease	Phag/o > devour, eat
Plasm/o > tissue, living substance	Prote/o > protein	Radi/o > X-ray, radiating
Reticul/o > network	Sarc/o > flesh	Skelet/o > dried up (bone)
Thel/o, Theli/o > cellular layer, nipple		

Prefixes: attached to the front of the word root to change meaning		
Ana- > up, building up	Cata- > down, breaking down	Dys- > bad, abnormal, painful, difficult
Endo- > within, inside, innermost	Epi- > on top, upon	Exo-, Ex- > outside, outer, outermost
Hyper- > increased, more of, elevated, excessive	Hypo- > decreased, less than, depressed, insufficient	Meta- > change, beyond
Micro- > small, tiny	Mono- > one, single	Neo- > new
Oligo- > scant, few	Poikil- > irregular, varied	Poly- > many, abundant, often
Sym-, Syn- > together, joined		

Suffixes change the meaning of the word, linking vowel is usually 'o' with consonants		
-ase > break down, enzyme that destroys	-blast > immature, building cell	-cidal > an agent that kills
-clast > to break into pieces	-dystonia > abnormal muscle tone	-esis > condition, process or action
-gen, -genesis, -genic > beginning, origin, or development	-glia > glue, glue-like	-lysis > to break up
-oma > tumor	-osis > condition of, abnormal usually	-pathy > disease
-phobic, -phobia, -phobe > to fear, not attracted to	-phoresis > carrying, assisting with transportation	-plasia > development or formation of
-plasm > living tissue, fluid	-poiesis, -poietic > production	-villi > finger-like projections or tiny hair-like

Acronyms, abbreviations, and initial sets		
ATP > adenosine triphosphate	BUN > blood urea nitrogen	CA-19–9 > cancer antigen
CA-125 > cancer antigen	CBC > complete blood count	CD 30 > tumor necrosis factor receptor
Chem 6 or Basic metabolic panel (BMP)	CMP > complete metabolic panel	DNA > deoxyribonucleic acid
PSA > prostate-specific antigen	RBC > red blood cells	RNA > ribonucleic acid
WBC > white blood cells	H > hydrogen	Fe > iron
C > carbon	Cr > chromium	Hg > mercury
O > oxygen	Ca > calcium	Mg > magnesium
I > iodine	P > phosphorus	

UNIT WORKSHEETS

Building terms: Use the proper prefix/word root/linking vowel/suffix as appropriate.

Example: To cut into the muscle > my/o/tomy

a) A condition of having many cells > _____

b) White blood cells which 'eat' or 'devour' debris > _____

c) The condition 'inside the cell' > _____

d) Pertaining to the 'dry bones' > _____

e) The production or development of a neoplasm > _____

f) A cell clotting the blood > _____

g) A specialist in the 'study of life' > _____

h) Pertaining to the area 'above the cell layer' > _____

Element recognition: For the symbol given, write the correct element name. Spelling counts.

a) Fe _____

b) Na _____

c) Cl _____

d) K _____

e) Mg _____

f) O _____

g) H _____

h) Pb _____

Best choice: Pick the most appropriate answer.

1 The specialist who looks at the morphology and behavior of cells is called a

    a) Cardiologist

    b) Pathologist

    c) Anatomist

    d) Endocrinologist

2   Which of the following is **NOT** considered a connective cell/tissue?

   a) Osteocyte   c) Reticulocyte

   b) Chondrocyte   d) Astrocyte

3   A tumor involving the linking form for 'flesh' is called

   a) Sarcolemma   c) Sarcoma

   b) Epithelioma   d) Leiomyoma

4   The give and take process of the body helping maintain homeostasis.

   a) Anabolism   c) Metabolism

   b) Catabolism   d) Embolism

5   The endoplasmic reticulum is the cell factory which builds

   a) Fats   c) Carbohydrates

   b) Proteins   d) Blood cells

6   To code a 'carcinoma in situ' of the left breast, which table should you refer to in the ICD?

   a) Table of External Causes   c) Table of Neoplasms

   b) Alphanumeric Index   d) Table of Laboratory Findings

Name the organelle! Based on the description and/or function name the cell organelle. Spelling counts.

a) The construction engineer of the cell. _____

b) Uses glucose and oxygen to produce energy (ATP). _____

c) The cell janitor, using enzymes to break down debris. _____

d) Tiny projection moving fluid or increase absorption. _____

Multiple correct: Select ALL the correct answers to the question given.

1   Which of the following are connective tissue linking forms?

   a) adip/o   d) fibr/o

   b) my/o   e) areol/a

   c) prote/o   f) neur/o

2   Which of the following suffixes pertain to 'breaking up or dissolving'?

   a) –osis   d) –clasts

   b) –ase   e) –lysis

   c) –ous   f) –blasts

3 Which of the following is a morphology choice in the Table of Neoplasms?

a) Secondary malignancy

b) Tertiary metastasis

c) Benign

d) Uncertain color

e) Primary malignancy

f) Unspecified behavior

Spelling challenge: Circle the correct spelling based on the definition given.

1 Diminishing the function of bone marrow

Myosuppression   Mylodepression   Myelosuppression   Meylodepression

2 Plural form of cancers

Carcinomata   Onchomata   Carcenogens   Carcenosis

3 Cells building myelin sheaths around neuronal axons

Polydendrosites   Oligodentricytes   Oligodendrocytes   Ependymal

Define the term: Spelling *does* count in your definition too!

1 Leiomyoma > _____

2 Mitochondria > _____

3 Microvilli > _____

4 Lysosomes > _____

5 Endocytosis > _____

6 Leukocytes > _____

7 Morphology > _____

8 Microglia > _____

Find it! Using the words in the table – match the definition given or answer the statement. Some may not be used. It is recommended you know all the choices.

proteolysis	metabolic	exocytosis	erythrocytes	K
nucleus	reticulosis	microglia	organelles	Golgi
macrocytes	Pb	neuritis	chondroblasts	skeletal

1 _____   Inflammation of the nerves

2 _____   Red blood cells

3 _____   Pertaining to the center of the cell

4 _____ Pertaining to the 'dried up' bones

5 _____ Symbol for the intracellular cation

6 _____ Large cells

7 _____ Small organs

8 _____ Breaking down protein

Matching: Match the terms, some will not be used.

	Letter	Defined as
Pathology		a) a type of WBC eating debris
Phagocytes		b) having several nuclei
Biopsy		c) steep decline in appetite
Multinucleated		d) study of how proteins are built and function
Epithelial		e) procedure to capture cells or tissue for review
Ependymal		f) these tissue protect and absorb and secrete
Metastasis		g) the study of disease
Anorexia		h) support the cytoskeleton of a specific cell type
		i) the spread of a carcinoma, beyond stopping
		j) line interior of the ventricles of the brain and central canal of the spinal cord

An essay: Explain the common symptoms associated with carcinoma:

• State the symptom (example: cough)

• Define the symptom (example: Coughing is the sudden expulsion of air from the lungs.)

• Relate to symptoms you may have had – was your symptom set acute or chronic? Why?

Please write in complete sentences with correct spelling.

Pathology note challenge: Define the underlined terms. You may need to look up a few. Answer the questions which follow. *The student is reminded this is an incomplete Pathology note used for the learning experience. Do not use this for patient encounters.*

Clinical information:
Reason for procedure: Lump on right ankle

Gross description:
A soft tissue mass right ankle
The specimen consists of an un-oriented, fairly well-outlined <u>lobular</u> portion of soft tissue measuring 3.4 × 2.9 × 1.8 cm. The <u>surgical</u> margin is marked in black ink. The specimen is subsequently serially sectioned revealing mostly uniform tan cut surface throughout. Representative sections are submitted as A1–7.

Microscopic examination:
It is composed of bland spindle cells, mixed with <u>inflammatory</u> cells. It has characteristic <u>virocyte</u>-like cells with large <u>nuclei</u> and some with <u>nucleoli</u> and with abundant <u>eosinophilic cytoplasm</u> which has some vacuolated spaces. The latter resembles <u>lipoblasts</u>. <u>Mitoses</u> are scarce. These are negative with <u>immunostains</u> for viruses. Tumor is noted at the inked margins.

Assessment: In both appearance and <u>immunophenotype</u>, this is a

1 <u>Dermatofibrosarcoma</u> protuberans, malignant
2 <u>Lymph</u> nodes: negative
3 Tumor is present in the inked margins, indicating the need for re-<u>excision</u>.

Questions:

1 Note all the linking forms associated with the pathology report with definitions.

2 In the Table of Neoplasms, which category would be chosen from the assessment given?

Unit 4

Skin and soft tissues

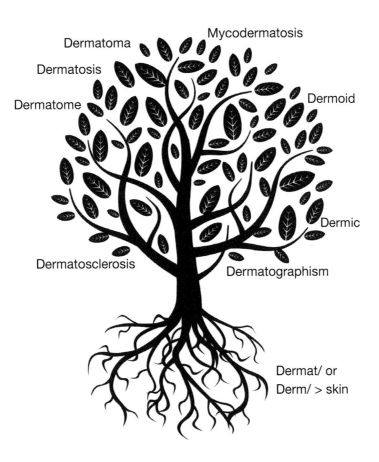

Mycodermatosis

Dermatoma

Dermatosis

Dermatome

Dermoid

Dermic

Dermatosclerosis

Dermatographism

Dermat/ or
Derm/ > skin

TARGETED LEARNING

1 Recognize word parts and the assembly of medical terms as related to skin and soft tissues.

2 Correctly construct, define, pronounce, and spell medical terms.

3 Link skin and soft-tissue diseases and injury with appropriate diagnostic evaluation, pharmacotherapeutics, surgical, and non-surgical treatments.

4 Relate skin and tissue injuries to documentation using medical terminology.

5 Explore the use of the ICD Index of External Causes with skin injuries.

KEY WORD PARTS

Word roots with linking vowel	Prefixes	Suffixes
Adip/o or Lip/o > fat	A-, An-	-clysis
Corne/o; Kerat/o > fibrous protein, horny layers	Anti-	-ectomy
Cutane/o; Cut/i > skin	Dys-	-iasis
Elast/o > flexibility	Epi-	-lysis
Fasci/o > a band, connective tissue	Ex-, Exo-	-malacia
Pil/o; Trich/o > hair	Hyper-	-oid
Sarc/o > flesh, combined tissues	Hypo-	-oma
Seb/o; Sebace/o > oil	Mal-	-plakia
Thel/o; Theli/o > cell layers or nipple	Para-	-plasty
Ungu/o; Onych/o > nails	Sub-	-rrhaphy

TATTOOS

Archeology and anthropology (**an**-throw-**pol**-oh-gee) have confirmed humans have been 'inking' their skin for a variety of reasons since about 5000 BCE. In some cultures, women tattoo tiny dots in a semi-circle across their abdomen; it is thought these were prayers for a safe pregnancy. Tattoos have been used to solicit the spirits for a happy and healthy life and/or used as a measure of beauty or status (Figure 4.2).

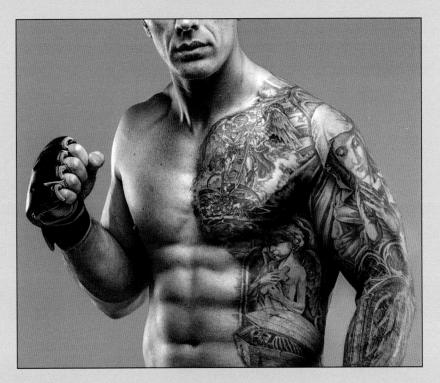

Figure 4.2

Today, tattooing the skin is no less prevalent. Cultures still use tattoos for adornment, religious statements, and even as a form of acupuncture. The ink is placed into the dermis, the second layer of the skin where it will permanently color the tissue. Yes, it hurts, more or less depending on the location. Yes, there are risks and consequences. The ink is permanent, short of laser ablation, at a cost to the skin and the pocketbook. Infections occur because there are currently no standards of care from shop to shop. Poor sterilization or technique can set up hepatitis B or C, staphylococcal or streptococcus infections and worse, a chronic inflammation. Inks with metal particles can interfere with **MRI**s. As with all invasive procedures, serious consideration of all the risks and benefits is imperative before receiving a tattoo.

SKIN ANATOMY AND CELLS

Skin is our protective barrier from the world. It is waterproof, helps regulate our temperature, and is somewhat bug resistant. It has a full sensory net. The skin is one of the largest organs of the body and vital to homeostasis. Loss of too much skin can make a person vulnerable to infection and death.

Epidermis > Derm/o > skin > top layer of the skin. Epi- > means 'on top of', thus epidermis (**ep**-ee-**dur**-miss) is 'on top of the skin'. As noted in Figure 4.3 the epidermis has several thin layers. The basal layer is where millions of new skin cells begin their journey each day.

Notice the layers of the epidermis, like other types of epithelial cells, have **NO** blood supply as the capillary beds are absent. The nutrients and oxygen for the epidermis diffuse up from the dermis.

- Derm/o or Dermat/o > skin
  - Dermatitis > inflammation of the skin.
- Dermoid > like the skin.
- Dermabrasion > procedure to remove scars or pits.

4.1 Linking forms

Derm/o > skin

Dermat/o > skin

Cutane/o > skin

Cut/i > skin

Trich/o > hair

Fasci/o > fascia, band-like connective tissue

Hidr/o > sweat

Neur/o > nerve

Theli/o > cell layer

Suffixes

–itis > inflammation

–tome > cut, slice

–oma > tumor

–lysis > destruction

–ous > condition of fullness, having much

–oid > like, resembling

–phyte > fungal elements

–plasty > repair

The dermis

The dermis is a very busy place; its tissue is soft and a little spongy with collagen and elastic fibers. The matrix provides strength and flexibility to the skin and holds water well (Figure 4.4).

The tiny capillary beds formed by the arterioles (arteri/o) bring oxygen and other nutrients to the dermis and by diffusion to the epidermis. The waste is taken away by the venous (ven/o) side of the capillary beds. Sebaceous glands live here supplying oily lubrication to the hair shaft and skin. Where there is hair (trich/o), there are sebaceous glands. When these sebaceous glands get plugged up, the result is acne, otherwise known as pimples or zits.

4.2 The matrix

The substance of the dermis is called the matrix. It is a combination of fibers giving the dermis its 'soft tissue' feel. It is collagen fibers, elastic fibers (elastin), and

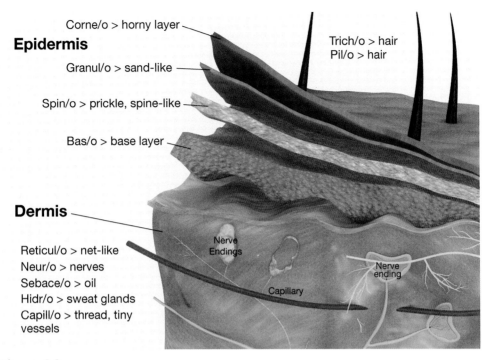

Epidermis

Corne/o > horny layer

Granul/o > sand-like

Spin/o > prickle, spine-like

Bas/o > base layer

Trich/o > hair
Pil/o > hair

Dermis

Reticul/o > net-like
Neur/o > nerves
Sebace/o > oil
Hidr/o > sweat glands
Capill/o > thread, tiny vessels

Nerve Endings

Nerve ending

Capillary

Figure 4.3

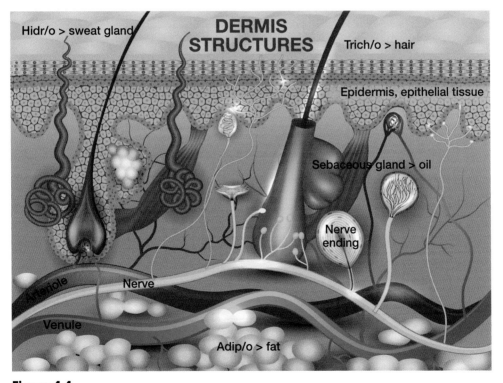

Hidr/o > sweat gland

DERMIS STRUCTURES

Trich/o > hair

Epidermis, epithelial tissue

Sebaceous gland > oil

Nerve ending

Arteriole

Nerve

Venule

Adip/o > fat

Figure 4.4

There are millions of sweat (hidr/o) glands as well regulating body temperature. While the hair and sebaceous glands are invaginated into the dermis, they are actually part of the stratum basale of the epidermis.

There are tiny nerve (neur/o) endings picking up the smallest breeze. Other types of nerve endings will pick up pressure, sharp, heat and cold. The tiny **arrector pili** (ah-**rek**-tor **pee**-lie) muscles are attached to the hair roots to lift the hairs with the perception of cold or stress. Arrector pili literally mean 'erect hairs'.

Subcutaneous tissue > supporting soft tissues below the dermis, also called the hypodermis (**hi**-poe-**dur**-mis). It is not skin tissue but it does provide support and cushioning for the skin and the underlying structures too. Built of fat > adip/o and connective tissue structures such as fascia, tendons, ligaments, and retinacula (**reh**-tea-**nak**-u-lah). It provides the anchor for the skin; without it, the skin would just slide off.

When a laceration goes through to the subcutaneous (**sub**-Q-**tay**-knee-us) tissue it is termed a full-skin-thickness laceration (**FST**). The fascia is thick connective tissue binding muscle tissues as groups. It also binds the dermal layers allowing everything to work in unison for movement > **fash**-ee-ah. Fascia, while tough, can also be delicate, like a spider-web, wrapping individual muscle fibers and other structures.

✓ Construct the medical term for 'skin repair'. ____/__/___

✓ Construct the medical term for 'inflammation of the skin'. _____/_____

✓ The matrix of the dermis is produced by _____ and _____ .

Word building

*Using the word roots **with the linking vowel** to build as many valid terms with the **suffixes given**. Please define each term.*

Dermat/o Trich/o Fasci/o

-itis -logy -ist -plasty -lysis -oma -tomy -ectomy

---

delicate reticular fibers with water.

The matrix is produced by the fibroblasts and chondroblasts. The matrix resembles a soft eraser in texture and bounce.

4.3

Did You Know?

Many of the meats we eat include the skin (epidermis and dermis) and the subcutaneous layer, fascia, and muscle, such as fried chicken.

4.4
Derm/o/plasty or Dermat/o/plasty
4.5
Dermat/itis
4.6
fibroblasts; chondroblasts

4.7
The instructor has the list!

Skin cells

While the majority of the epidermis is epithelial cells tightly packed and stacked, there are several specialized cells in the epithelial tissue providing protective elements.

- **Keratinocytes** (ca-**rat**-in-oh-sites) > supply the hardening protein for the epithelial cells which essentially waterproof the compacted cells like the wax on a car. These will form the hair and nails too.

- **Dendritic cells** (den-**drit**-ik) > part of the first line of immune defenses against microorganisms. Eponym: Langerhans cells

- **Melanocytes** (**mel**-ah-no-sites) > interspersed within the basal layer providing each person with skin tones, ranging from red-yellow to brown-black (Figure 4.5).

Melanocytes > 'black cells'

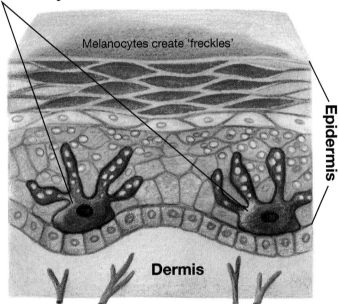

Melanocytes create 'freckles'

Epidermis

Dermis

Figure 4.5

- **Tactile cell** (**tak**-till or **tak**-tile) > tiny nerve receptors have a stellate shape. These mechanoreceptors (Figure 4.4) give us soft touch sensation. They are abundant in our fingertips. Eponyms: Merkel cells.

4.8 Linking forms

Kerat/o > horny, scaly

Melan/o > black

Squam/o > scale

Dendr/o > branching

Tanning occurs with exposure to UV light. The light stimulates the keratinocytes to ask for shielding from the melanocytes. The darkening protects the regenerating basal cell layer from radiation and heat damage.

Sunscreen adds to this protection and is recommended no matter how many melanocytes you have.

Cutane/o or **Cut/i** > Latin for skin. By convention, cutaneous is frequently used to describe location of the tissue versus the tissue itself.

- **Cutane**ous **horn** (Q-**tay**-knee-us horn) > hard, scaly, protruding growth of skin.

- **Cuticle** (**Q**-tea-cal) > outer, thin layer of the horny composition securing and protecting the proximal nail.

- **Subcutane**ous > under the skin layer, a frequent placement of a needle as noted in Figure 4.6. In the past, this had several abbreviations but because of persistent medical errors, the word must be spelled out for safety.

4.9
Derm/o and Dermat/o are used for disease or injury, e.g., dermatomycosis > abnormal condition of fungus on the skin.

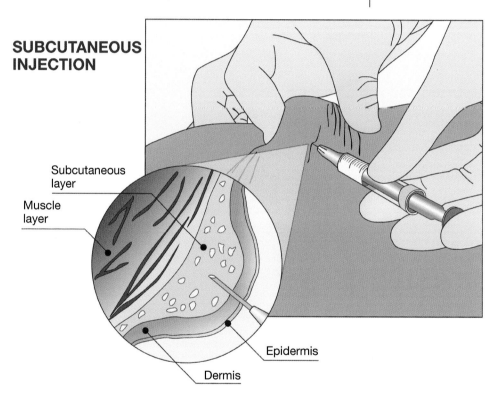

SUBCUTANEOUS INJECTION

Subcutaneous layer

Muscle layer

Epidermis

Dermis

Figure 4.6

Kitchen lab

Look around the house for familiar items with layers like the skin and may even have similar functions as skin. Also, find things having the same consistency of skin and soft tissues.

4.10
Discuss your findings with the instructor.

Dermatitis (**dur**-mah-**tie**-tis) > inflammation of the skin > comes in a huge variety of types often heard of or seen in the media.

- **Atopic dermatitis (**ay-**top**-ik **dur**-mah-**tie**-tis**)** > genetically regulated condition of hypersensitivity to the environment. It is associated with asthma, eczema, and food allergies, as seen in Figure 4.7.

- **Atopy** (a-**top**-ee) > Greek for 'strangeness (of a) place'. It is known for its lichenification (**lie**-ken-ee-**fi**-kay-shun) > thickening of the skin with prominent skin lines. 'Eczema' (**ek**-zeh-ma) > used interchangeably for this type of dermatitis.

- **Contact dermatitis >** inflammatory reaction of the skin to an exogenous source such as poison ivy, nickel, or latex. This is called the wet or edematous type (Figure 4.7). Contact dermatitis can also be chronic and present with dry, thickened, and scaly skin changes.

- **Stasis dermatitis (stay**-sis) > acutely inflamed area found over the distal leg or foot area. It is crusty, reddened skin with ulceration due to slow blood flow as seen in Figure 4.7.

4.11

Did You Know?

The description of 'lichen' (**like**-en) is Greek for the stippled composition of lichen growing on rocks, an eruption of growth.

Exo- > outside

Anti- > against

Gen- > production of, development

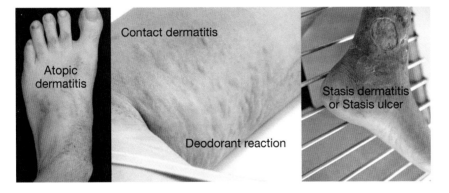

Contact dermatitis

Atopic dermatitis

Deodorant reaction

Stasis dermatitis or Stasis ulcer

Figure 4.7

- **Seborrheic dermatitis (seb**-or-**rhee**-ik) > chronic disorder similar to another skin condition known as psoriasis. Seborrhea (flowing sebum) presents as oily scaling or plaques.

The treatment for these conditions includes a number of topical applications or oral medications. Corticosteroids may be used as well.

DOCUMENTING SKIN

To the average person on the street, skin is to be washed, pinched, poked, pierced, and/or decorated with applied make-up. Skin gets insect repellent, sunscreen, and lotions smeared on daily. Medical documentation is full of descriptives of how skin appears. For example, the color of skin can be described as red, blanched, pink, purple, blue, yellow, and even green. How the skin feels to the touch of a provider is described as hot, cold, scaly, smooth, leathery, waxy, greasy, dry, wet, hard, horny, pitted, and bumpy. Lesions or 'funny-looking rashes' are described as eruptive, edematous, herpetic, serpentine, atrophied, macerated, raised, elevated, depressed, ulcerated, or compared to lichen. And this is a *short* list ☺.

With so many possible descriptors it is important to continuity of care to qualify lesions as accurately as possible, thus all the terminology.

An example

Figure 4.8 depicts multi-layered skin infection, cellulitis (**sell**-U-**lie**-tis), and gangrene (**gan**-green) secondary to a mosquito bite. It is the progression of the erythema and/or blackened (necrotic) skin which will help the providers decide when and how much skin will be excised.

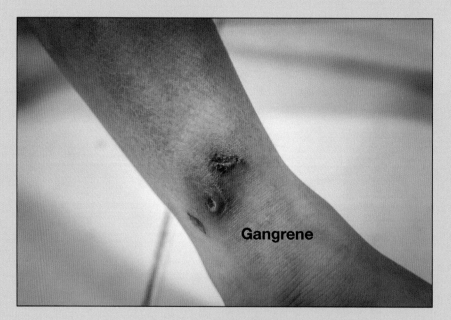

Figure 4.8

COLOR DESCRIPTIVES

The skin is the window on illness and injury for the body. Inflammation has four hallmarks: redness, edema (swelling), heat, and pain. Redness leads off our discussion on color terms.

- **Eryth/o** > red > erythema (**eh-ree-thee-**ma) > redness of the skin, Greek for 'flushed'. An infection's spread or retreat can be measured in millimeters (**mm**) via the location of the erythematous edge on the skin.

- **Cyan/o** > blue > cyanosis (**sigh-an-oh-**sis) > bluish color of the skin and nail beds in the absence of oxygen filling the RBCs. It is seen in infants with respiratory distress.

- **Xanth/o** > yellow > xanthoma (zan-**though-**ma) > yellow appearing nodule full of fat or lipid cells. This yellow is different from yellow skin and the membrane coloration of jaundice.

- **Jaundice** (**jahn-**dis) > yellow staining > collection of bile pigments in the dermis, oral mucosa, and eye sclera indicating liver malfunction and/or excessive destruction of red blood cells (Figure 4.9). A synonym is **icterus** (**ick-**tur-us), Greek for yellow.

4.12

LIKE TERMS!

Erythr/o > red, is the other word root used to describe red blood cells.

Cyan/o > blue AND is the prefix for compounds containing cyanide.

4.13

Lip/o > Fat

Or/o > oral

Muc/o > sticky liquid

Scler/o > hardened, also the whites of the eye

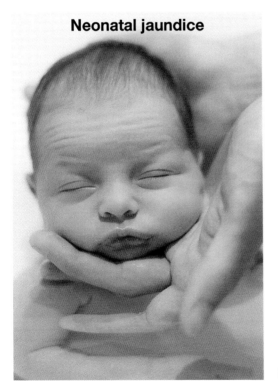

Neonatal jaundice

Figure 4.9

- **Leuk/o** > white > leukocytes > set of blood cells vital to immunity.
- Leukemia (**lew**-key-**me**-ah) > progressive proliferation of abnormal white blood cells; it is a type of malignancy.
- Leukoplakia (**lew**-ko-**play**-key-ah) > condition typified by a white patches on the oral mucosa which cannot be scraped off. -plakia > thick, plaque-like.
- **Albino** (al-**buy**-no) > without color, dim white > albinism is the marked decline or absence of pigment formation. Individuals will present with white/pinkish skin over the entire body and gray irises.

4.14
Suffixes used with Leukocyt-
-penia > low numbers
-osis > abnormal condition

- **Melan/o** > black or brown black > melanin (**mel**-a-nin) > dark hue pigments coloring the skin, iris of the eyes, and hair. As we age, the melanocytes (Figure 4.5) decrease or become less functional, softening skin and eye colors, and graying the hair.
- **Eosin/o** > dawn or rosy coloration > eosinophil (**ee**-oh-**sin**-oh-fil) > one of the WBC types. The color designation is due to the staining characteristics.
- **Bas/o** > base, basis of, lower layer > a basophil (**bay**-sew-fil), another WBC type, will stain deep blue or purple in basic stain.

4.15
Melanoma is a malignant carcinoma which develops on the skin and eye areas, a function of sun damage. It is known to metastasize quickly via the regional lymph nodes.

- **Chlor/o** > green > chlorine or chloride gas has a greenish hue and of course, chlorophyll is what makes plants green.
- **Carotene** (**kare**-oh-tin) > yellow-orange > like chlorophyll, these lipochromes (fat colors) are derived from food. Eating a lot of carrots can give the skin an orange hue.

4.16
Chlorophyll is the light energy absorber in green plants. It converts light energy into food nutrients.

✓ Construct the word for 'too few white blood cells'.
_____/__/_____/__/_____

✓ The proper term for a yellow skin discoloration due to liver malfunction is _____ .

✓ An 'erythrocyte' will be what color?

4.17
Leuk/o/cyt/o/penia
4.18
jaundice
4.19 Red

Word building

*Using the word roots **with the linking vowel to build as many valid terms with the suffixes given. Please define them too.***

Erythr/o Leuk/o Melan/o
-cyte -penia -lysis -plakia -osis -phils

4.20
The instructor has the list!

CODING INJURIES

The ICD has produced a precision tool for defining and classifying injuries from simple contusions to burns and fractures. A coder begins as usual in the Index of Disease and Injury with the injury types. When dealing with a burn, for example, the coder would look up 'burn', and then, note the anatomy burned – the fingers. The alphanumeric is T23. It is possible to code to more specificity in this index but it is best to go to Chapter 19 in the ICD, the **Injury, Poisoning and Certain Other Consequences of External Causes** for the complete coding list. T23 is the category area for Burn (from heat source) and Corrosion of the wrist and hand. This is where the exact description of the injury is so important – it defines the anatomy and depth of the burn to be coded.

There is a different code for just one finger or for multiple fingers. The code also includes the level of burn: 1st, 2nd, or 3rd degree. A second degree burn to multiple fingers without the thumb on the right hand (Figure 4.10) would be coded T23.241. A final 7th digit is added to indicate if the visit is the initial visit (A), a subsequent visit (D), or a visit for consequence of the injury (S). The final code would be T23.241A for the photo. All of this is based on the objective section of the note, which describes the injury and its severity.

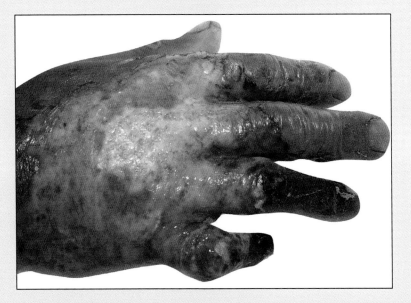

Figure 4.10

Additional injury codes are included based on the subjective section of the note – how did the injury occur and where. This specificity is used to track types of injuries, causes, and location so a better car or bike or stove can be built to avoid injury.

Chapter 20 of the ICD contains a wide assortment of **External Causes of Morbidity (V00–Y99)**. X10–X19 is the section for contact with heat and hot substances, in our example, hot oil while cooking – the code will be X10.2A. Finally, a third code can be applied, location and activity existing at the time of the injury occurred. This note was not specific to actual location, thus we use Y93.G3 – Activity, cooking and baking.

Precision of coding is dependent on documentation using proper terms, providing clear and correct directions, and gauging the severity of injuries accurately. All injuries are tracked by a variety of agencies including the Department of Health and Human Services (DHHS); Centers of Disease Control and Prevention (CDC); and Occupational Safety and Health Administration (OSHA). Tracking the consequences of burns or falls via coding allows for better ways to 'fall proof' or 'burn proof' the environments for all of us.

★ **IMPORTANT NOTE: The reader is notified that these examples are from an online search done in 2016. Do <u>not</u> use these codes for patient care episodes; look up the new ones!**

PRIMARY SKIN LESIONS

The need to consistently describe skin findings led to a set of standard terms. The majority do not come with word roots. This is the primary skin lesion list as published in any number of medical textbooks.

- **Macule** (**mak**-yule) > discoloration of the skin is flat and small – less than 2 cm. With eyes closed, touch cannot tell where the 'spot' is. This is a freckle – it might be brown, red, or bluish.

- **Patch** (pach) > small (larger than 2 cm) flat discoloration of the skin. It is a larger freckle or the old term is 'liver spots'.

Kitchen lab

Time to take an inspection tour of your skin! Find all your freckles (macules) and patches, and papules as defined by size on your face/neck and both arms.

4.21

- **Papul**/o > solid elevation of the skin > papule (**pap**-yule) can be felt readily with eyes closed. It is firm, like the end of an eraser and smaller than 0.5 cm. Papules are seen with acne or milia (keratin-filled papules) as seen in Figure 4.11.

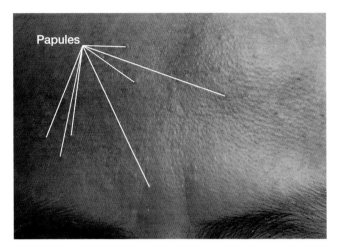

Figure 4.11

- **Nodule** (**nod**-yule) > Latin for 'knot' > firm, elevated lesion like a papule larger (0.5 to 5 cm). These have a variety of names and locations: enlarged axillary glands are called lymph nodes; keloid scars tend to be nodular; and there are skin, thyroid, lung, and pancreatic nodules.

- **Tumor** (**too**-mur) > another term for swelling; by convention, it is an abnormal growth, solid, and larger than 5 cm.

- **Plaque** (**plak**) > larger (greater than 1 cm), raised lesion with a flatter top and well demarcated edges. A 1 cm plantar wart is a plaque, as are eczema lesions, psoriasis (Figure 4.12), and pityriasis rosea.

The rest of the primary skin lesions switch from the solid lesions above to those which are fluid-filled or vascular in nature.

- **Vesicles** (**ves**-ee-kels) > small (less than 0.5 cm), raised, with fluid which is usually clear or translucent.

- A **bulla** (**bull**-ah > singular) > larger vesicle (greater than 0.5 cm) is fluid-filled and generally translucent too. Figure 4.13 depicts a contact or abrasion burn, **a blister**. (**bul**-lee > plural)

4.22

Did You Know?

Acne vulgaris is seen in teens because of the increase in hormone levels activating the sebum glands in the face, neck, and chest. The overproduction of oily sebum, keratin plugs, and bacteria set up teens for **comedones**.

4.23

Plaques also occur in the arteries, cholesterol causing atherosclerosis.

Multiple sclerosis is caused by plaques on the myelin sheaths.

4.24

Sunburns are classified by the presence of vesicles or bullae.

1st degree is the redness only.

2nd degree is the redness with clear vesicles or bullae.

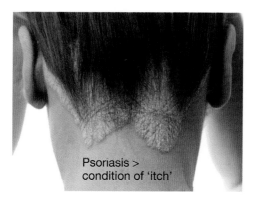

Psoriasis >
condition of 'itch'

Figure 4.12

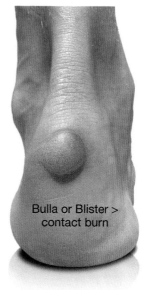

Bulla or Blister >
contact burn

Figure 4.13

- **Pustules** (**pust**-yule) > vesicles are full of the debris of inflammation including leukocytes (WBCs) – otherwise known as **pus**. There is no size limit on the use of the term 'pustules' although **boil** is used for the larger lesions.
    - There are several terms for the contained or walled-off fluid and pus-filled lesions: **boil**, **abscess**, **furuncle**, and **carbuncle**. These are treated with an incision and drainage (**I&D**), cleaned > dermatoclysis and packed to encourage healing.

- **Wheals** (wheels) > raised papules or plaques representing capillary swelling or permeability (weeping). They tend to be the shape of the area irritated by contact, and are well-defined and short-lived. Itchy wheals is called an **urticarial** (**ur**-tea-**kare**-ee-al) reaction. Urticaria occurs ordinarily with systemic allergic reactions. Synonym: **Hives**

- **Telangiectasia** (tel-**an**-gee-ek-**taz**-ee-ah) > dilation of a tiny vessel previously not seen on the surface of the skin. Tel- is the prefix for 'end', as in 'end point' or terminal vessel in this case. Angi/o > vessel and the suffix -ectasia is Greek for 'stretching out'. Thus this term is the very description of the tiny vessels visible on the skin.

4.25
The causes of **urticaria** are many:

Sudden exposure to cold; allergic reactions both contact and systemic; hepatitis B or C; and vasculitis associated with autoimmune diseases.

4.26
Telangiectasias are tiny varicose veins.

✓ Pustules are full of debris and white blood cells. The WBCs are properly called _____ .

4.27
leukocytes

✓ The difference between a papule and nodule is the _____ .

4.28
size. Papule is
0.5 cm or less.

✓ The best medical term to describe a freckle is _____ .

4.29
macule

BURN UNIT DOCUMENTATION

Burn units are specialized intensive care units caring for patients with burns or similar skin disruptions. Burns occur via fire or another heat source, but they can also result from chemicals or corrosives, radiation, electrical sources, and abrasion. A burn unit will employ many professional caregivers from doctors to respiratory therapists and counselors. The mainstay for the unit is the Registered nurse (**RN**). This documentation box will review the nurse's duties in documenting the progress of a recovering burn patient.

- Specific to the injury, the burns being cared for are described daily in regards to swelling, weeping of fluids, size, and progress of debridement and healing, and evidence of deep, thick, coagulated scabbing called an **eschar** (**es**-kar). When appropriate these descriptions are actually measured in millimeters (mm).

- Debridement is a process of removing the damaged and dead skin tissue to promote healing. It is a day-to-day procedure that can entail pain for the patient, which is also precisely documented.

- Bandage type and quantity is documented as a measure of improvement. Sterile procedures are followed to minimize the chance of infection of the exposed skin and soft tissues of the burn.

- Respirations are evaluated every day because as the skin heals a contraction of the scars may stop or restrict breathing if the burns occurred around the chest.

- Because healthy skin provides a barrier against loss of bodily fluids and helps regulate temperature, one of the most dangerous effects of a burn is the loss of fluids and temperature control. Its absence requires a precise measurement and evaluation of fluid replacements literally hour-to-hour.

- Pain control is an important part of quality care and documentation. Healing, sleep, and the psychological well-being of the patient depend on adequate and regular pain control.

As always, documentation allows for continuity of care for the patient by providers as they interact to achieve improvement. Loss of or lack of documentation sets the patient up for gaps in care, which can slow recovery or worse. Every step, every person, every record, affects the recovery.

SECONDARY SKIN LESIONS AND TERMS

These terms describe lesions as well – illustrating their texture and sometimes their shape.

- **Scale** > scaly like a snake or reptile > actually an increase in the thickness and dryness of the top layer. It appears flaky.

- **Annular** (**an**-yule-ar) > ring shaped lesions > annular is usually 'ring worm', which is not a worm at all but a fungal infection.

- **Nummular** (**num**-yule-ar) > coin like > lesion will look like a stack of coins and is usually seen with eczema.

- **Burrows** (**bur**-rows) > tunnel-shaped > lesion looks like a subway pathway in the skin and linked with scabies.

- **Crust** > dried serous fluids or exudates from opening vesicles or pustules. Conditions making a crust are **impetigo** or **shingles**.

- **Cyst** (sist) > soft, raised, and encapsulated lesion > typically deep in the dermis or even in the subcutaneous layer. It is generally filled with a semisolid fluid. A **ganglion cyst** is a classic example.

- **Ulcer** (**ul**-sir) > loss of the epidermis and portion of the dermis > associated with poor circulation. A 'bed sore' is a decubitus ulceration. Squamous cell carcinoma often presents with an ulcer.

- **Atrophy** (**at**-row-fee) > loss of thickness or matrix > skin looks flatter, more depressed, paler. A scar can take years to remodel. It ends up being thinner, flatter, and less mobile skin (Figure 4.14).

- **Scar** > fibrous tissue replacing healthy tissue > the injury is sufficiently severe that instead of the dermis and epidermis resuming full recovery, a scar develops. It will may be raised, have a nodular feel (Figure 4.14), and be discolored or hypopigmented initially. Synonym: **Cicatrix** (**sik**-ah-tricks)

4.30

Did You Know?

There are many systemic conditions which present with a rash or skin lesions including:

Chickenpox > varicella virus

Herpes zoster > shingles

Lyme disease > from deer ticks

Ringworm > fungal infections

MRSA > *Staphylococcus aureus* resistant to antibiotics

Impetigo > *Staph* or *Streptococcus* infections

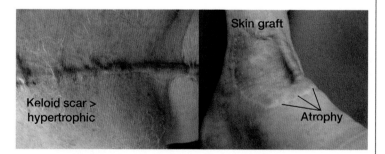

Skin graft

Keloid scar > hypertrophic

Atrophy

Figure 4.14

The skin is a crowded place with several structures interacting and supporting the function of the skin on many levels.

HAIR ANATOMY

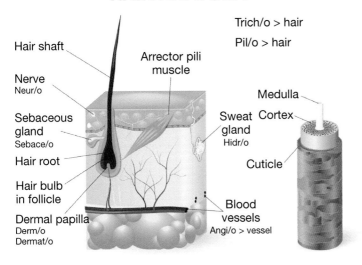

Figure 4.15

4.31

LIKE ALERT!

Trich/o > hair is also used to describe microorganisms such as Trichomonas, a parasitic protozoan flagellate because its tail looks like a hair.

There are several fungal infections carrying the designation as well.

- **Trich**/o or trich/i Greek and **Pil/o** > Latin. Hair protects the skin, adds to sensation recognition, and warms.
  - Trichomycosis (**trik**-oh-**my**-ko-sis) > abnormal condition of the hair caused by fungi, *Nocardia* or *Corynebacterium*.
  - Trichorrhexis (**trik**-oh-**rek**-sis) > disorder in which the hairs tend to break or split.
  - Pilonidal (**pie**-low-**nigh**-dal) > presence of hair in a dermoid (skin-like) cyst.
  - Pilomotor reflex (**pie**-low-**mow**-tur re-**flex**) > goose bumps or goose flesh.

- **Alopecia** (al-oh-**pee**-see-ah) > loss or absence of hair. The word is from the old French for 'fox mange'; another example of nature providing a term description.
  - Alopecia areata (ah-ree-**ah**-tah) > well-defined and non-scarring loss of hair on the scalp, eyebrows, or facial areas.

Exocrine (**ek**-so-krine) > gland secreting to the outside via a duct. The exocrine glands of the skin are broken up into two categories.

LIKE ALERT!

Hidr/o > sweat

Hydr/o > water

Other word parts

Ec– > outer

Apo– > strange, unusual

Crin/o > secrete

SKIN GLANDS

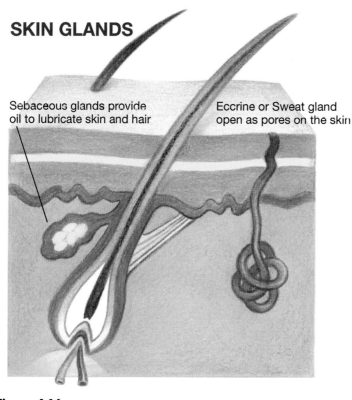

Sebaceous glands provide oil to lubricate skin and hair

Eccrine or Sweat gland open as pores on the skin

Figure 4.16

- **Sebaceous** > seb/o or sebace/o > each hair shaft has one or two sebaceous (sey-**bay**-shus) glands. These collect sebum (**see**-bum) until it bursts like a tiny balloon to release the oils, lubricating skin and hair.

- **Sweat** > hidr/o > sweat glands come in two types.
  - **Eccrine** (**ek**-krin) > sweat glands depositing the secretions on surface of the skin.
  - **Sudoriferous** (**su**-door-**if**-ur-us) or **apocrine** (**ap**-oh-krin) > specialized sweat glands known from their odor. These glands tend to be deeper in the dermis and are related to the hair bulb and produce molecules called pheromones (**fair**-oh-monz).

- **Ceruminous** (se-**rue**-min-us) **glands** > specialized apocrine glands found in the ear. Along with some sebaceous secretions, cerumen is produced to moisturize and protect the ear canal.

Did You Know?

Aging skin loses moisture because the exocrine glands decrease their activities and the subcutaneous adipose tissue is slowly lost.

This change causes wrinkles, and deepening of skin lines > Rhytid/o

✓ If exocrine is secreting outside, build a term meaning to secrete inside.

4.33
Endocrine

✓ Of the following suffixes which means to split or break?
-osis –iasis –rrhexis –monas

4.34
-rrhexis

✓ What is the medical term for 'an abnormal condition of sweat glands'?

4.35
Hidrosis

Word building

Using the word roots with the linking vowel to build as many valid terms with the suffixes given and define them. Be sure to check in your dictionary.

Pil/o Hidr/o Sarc/o

–osis –oid –itis –oma

Try some *prefixes* ***too!*** *Hyper- Hypo-*

4.36
The instructor has the list!

Our fingernails and toenails, like our hair, are keratinized skin cells. Keratinization is the key to the strength of the nails which protect our fingertips and contribute to our ability to pick up pins.☺

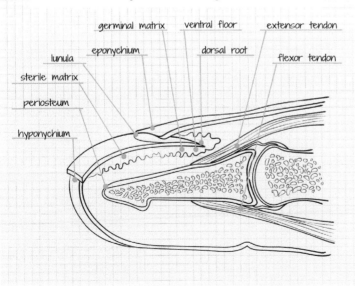

ANATOMY OF THE NAIL
Onych/o or Ungu/o

germinal matrix   ventral floor   extensor tendon

eponychium   dorsal root   flexor tendon

lunula

sterile matrix

periosteum

hyponychium

Figure 4.17

130 SKIN AND SOFT TISSUES

The linking form used most often for the nails is onych/o.

- Onychomalacia (**on**-ee-ko-mah-**lay**-she-a) > nail softening.

- Onychomycosis (**on**-ee-ko-**my**-ko-sis) > abnormal condition of the nails due to fungal infection (Figure 4.18).

- Onychia (oh-**nik**-ee-ah) > inflammation of the nail. Synonym: onychitis (**on**-ee-**keye**-tis)

- Paronychia (**pair**-oh-**knee**-key-ah) > inflammation or infection of the nail fold surrounding the nail bed (Figure 4.18).

Ungual (**ung**-wal) > Latin for nail. It is seen with these terms and/or conditions.

- Subungual (sub-**ung**-wal) > under the nail.

- Subungual hematoma > blood under the nail (Figure 4.18).

- Subungual melanoma > melanoma malignancy under the nail.

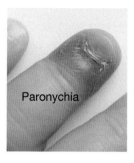 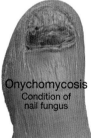 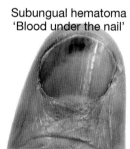

Subungual hematoma 'Blood under the nail'

Paronychia

Onychomycosis
Condition of nail fungus

Figure 4.18

4.37

LIKE ALERT!

Onch/o > tumor

Onych/o > nail

These can be confused via spelling errors. Be careful.

Suffixes

-malacia > softening

-lysis > destruction

-rrhexis > split or rupture

-itis > inflammation

-dystrophy > poor growth

-oid > like, resembling

-oma > tumor

-pathy > disease

-schizia or -schisis > splitting in layers

-tomy > to cut

-ectomy > to remove

PHARMACY CORNER

Needling the skin

Syringes and needles pair up to remove blood to determine a serum level or to inject a medication. In research labs, the tiniest of needles gather nuclear materials or combine sperm with ovum in a culture medium (in vitro fertilization). The skin is a natural barrier easily penetrated by a sharp needle.

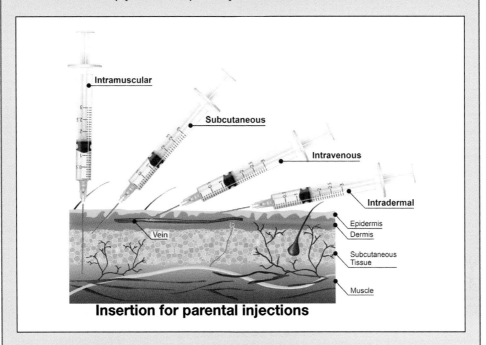

Insertion for parental injections

Figure 4.19

Intradermal (in-tra-dur-mal) > within the dermis > a mosquito bite, a tuberculosis (TB) test, allergen testing, and Botox® injection are all intradermal injection types. When done correctly, an intradermal injection will form a wheal.

Subcutaneous (sub-Q-tay-knee-us) > under the skin > an insulin or heparin injection, most vaccinations, and other medications are introduced to the fatty soft tissue just below the dermis.

Intramuscular (IM) (in-tra-mus-Q-lar) > within the muscle > antibiotics, pain medications, Vitamin B$_{12}$, some vaccinations, and steroids are medications delivered via IM injection. IM injections go deep to the muscle.

Intravenous (IV) (in-tra-vee-nus) > within the veins > adding volume to the bloodstream, blood, specific antibiotics, and steroids are medications delivered via IV. The IV approach is also used to draw blood for evaluation.

COMMON SKIN INJURIES AND CONDITIONS

By virtue of its large surface area and location, the skin is a normal place for injury. Let's start with the simplest.

- **Abrasion** (ah-**bray**-shun) > removal of the superficial layers of skin > Ouch! The everyday words to describe these injuries are **scratch**, **scrape**, **strawberry**, and **rug burn**. Another medical term is **excoriation** > eks-**kor**-ee-**a**-shun. These injuries bleed a little (capillaries are broken) and they weep the first 24 hours.

- **Penetrating wounds** > puncture wounds are caused by ice picks, thorns, nails, splinters – any number of possibilities. Punctures can be deceptive because it is hard to know how deep they go. And the deeper the puncture goes into the dermis or subcutaneous soft tissue, the better the chance for pathogens to get started in the warm, dark recesses of the wound.

- **Lacerations** (**las**-ur-**a**-shuns) **>** 'to tear apart', it is also used for cuts caused by paper to kitchen knives to broken glass, to sheet metal – again any number of possibilities. Lacerations are classified by thickness:
  - **Partial-skin-thickness (PST)** > hurts like an abrasion because only the epidermis/part of the dermis is involved. **Avulsion** lacerations involve both layers as it cuts the skin at a shallow angle. Elders are prone to this type of laceration due to thinning skin and slight strike injury occurs more often.
  - **Full-skin-thickness (FST)** laceration goes all the way through the dermis, into the soft tissues. PST's may bleed or not; FST's always bleed. They will heal as the other injuries do from the bottom up (Figure 4.20).

4.38 CODING
ICD Index of Disease and Injury alphanumeric exist for all these skin issues:

Abrasions

Burns

Blisters (non-thermal)

Excoriations

4.39
Foreign bodies

Bites

Punctures

Contusions

Lacerations

Purpura

4.40
Injury

Skin ulcers

Skin infection

Coding starts with the description: laceration, puncture or even injury.

The index then gives the coder numerous types and locations.

Remember, injury cause is found in Chapter 20 of the ICD.

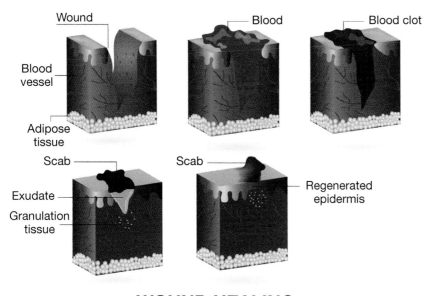

Wound

Blood

Blood clot

Blood vessel

Adipose tissue

Scab

Scab

Exudate

Regenerated epidermis

Granulation tissue

WOUND HEALING

Figure 4.20

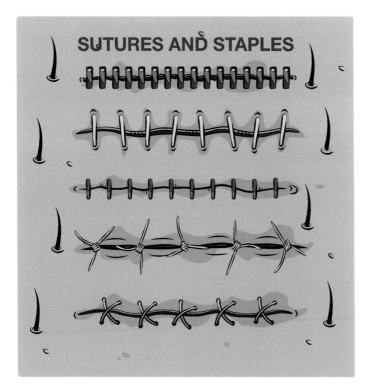

SUTURES AND STAPLES

Figure 4.21

- Lacerations may be repaired at home or in an operating room depending on their severity. Stopping the bleeding is the goal of the repair.
  - **PST** lacerations are usually easily closed with an adhesive bandage, butterfly stitches, or skin glue.
  - **FST** lacerations may be closed by intermittent sutures, continuously running suture, or staples. The method of closure is dependent on location (Figure 4.21).

4.41
Hemostasis > to stop bleeding may be done by the use of a hemostat, heat, cold, chemicals, and direct pressure.

- **Burns** > loss of tissue from heat > fire is an obvious heat source but any heat source – friction, corrosive agent, and electricity – can cause burns. Burns are categorized by the level of damage to the skin and soft tissue layers. Figure 4.22 gives examples of the three levels. A 3rd degree burn will have areas of both 1st and 2nd degree burns.

4.42
Terms of repair
-plasty > surgical repair
-pexy > surgical fixation
-rrhaphy > suture
Allograft
Autograft
Xenograft
Dermatome
Debridement
Sutures
Staples
Surgical drains
Sterile packing materials

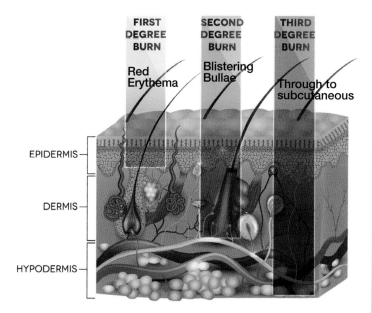

Figure 4.22

- Treatment of burns depends on their depth, location, and total surface area involved. Debridement (dee-**breed**-ment) > to remove devitalized tissue is the first treatment.
  - **FST** grafts continue to be an option for the facial areas burn repair because the **FST** will have the sweat glands, sebaceous glands and blood supply intact. The graft is taken with the 'skin cutting instrument', the dermatome.

- **FST and PST** grafts may be taken from the patient (autograf) or donors (allograft). Human skin cells with collagen in gel-type products can be very useful as well.
- Research continues on using collagen, silicone, and a combination product called lipidocolloid.

✓ Which of the following lesions is most likely to get infected because of the type of injury? One or more may be correct.

Contusion   Puncture   Excoriation
2nd degree burns   PST laceration

✓ Construct a word meaning 'the surgical repair of the skin'.

_____/___/_____

_____/___/_____

✓ The tissue below the dermis with fat and fascia is called the _____ .

4.43
Puncture and
2nd degree burns

4.44
Derm/o/plasty
Dermat/o/plasty

4.45
Subcutaneous or
Hypodermis

Word building

Using the word roots with the linking vowel to build as many valid terms with the suffixes given. Please define them too.

Orchid/o Col/o

-plasty -rrhaphy -pexy -tomy -ectomy

4.46
The instructor has the list! Note this set tests your recall and a word root you have not seen yet.

Skin infections

Skin infections can indicate a discrete skin condition or a systemic infection or infestation. Testing for skin lesions include biopsy or scraping for microscopic review. Lesions can also be cultured with sensitivities **(C&S)** checking for response to treatment options. Fung/o > Latin for mushroom, fungus is used as a general term.

Fungal infections are often identified on the skin > myc/o or mycet/o > fungus (singular). Synonym: **tinea** (**tin**-ee-ah) Latin for worm or moth. **Fungi** (plural) are the same plant species as mushrooms. Fungal infections are detectable with a simple microscope exam with **KOH** (potassium hydroxide) to visualize the branching **hyphae** (**hi**-fee) (Figure 4.23).

- **Tinea pedis** (**tin**-ee-ah **ped**-is) > athletes foot > distinguished by redness, peeling skin, itching, and blisters. Ped/o > foot.

4.47
Fungal infections of the skin, hair, and nails are from the genus families of:

Trichophyton

Microsporum, and

Epidermophyton

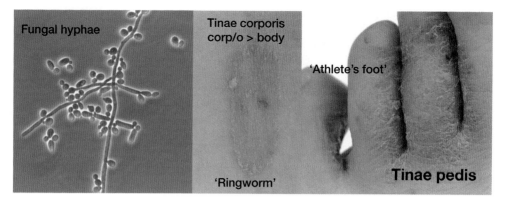

Figure 4.23

- **Tinea cruris** (**tin**-ee-ah **krew**-is) > jock itch > damp, warm area of the genitalia can be a home for the same fungus as the foot. Crur/o > thigh.

- **Tinea corporis** (**tin**-ee-ah **kor**-pore-sis) > ringworm > NOT a worm, this is typified by a raised, scaly, red, circular lesion. Corp/o > body.

Exanthem (eg-**zan**-them) > skin eruption secondary to viral or bacterial systemic infection. These are usually the soft red slightly papular rashes of measles (Figure 4.24); examples are 5th-disease

Pityriasis rosea (pity-rye-**ah**-sis **ro**-zee-ah) is quite similar to tinea corporis, but it has a softer pink lesion and has no known cause. It is self-limiting.

4.48
You may see this term as **exanthema**.

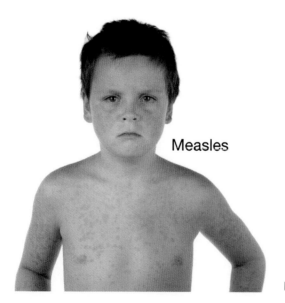

Measles

Figure 4.24

(Epstein–Barr virus (**EBV**)), early HIV changes, West Nile virus, and cytomegalovirus (**CMV**). Early bacterial infections include scarlet fever, meningococcemia, typhoid, syphilis, and some *Rickettsia* infections. Synonym: Morbilliform

* There are many medications exhibiting a soft red, generalized rash: Penicillins, sulfonamides, and phenytoin to name a few.

Human papilloma (pap-il-**low**-ma) **Virus (HPV)** > over 100 HPV varieties – all of them can cause trouble. Warts are the most common!

Warts are actually neoplasms and come in an assortment of lesions.

* **Verruca vulgaris** (**vair**-u-kah vul-**gah**-ris) > dome-shaped lesion on fingers and knees. It looks like wax thrown onto the skin. (Figure 4.25) Synonym: **Common warts**

* **Verruca plana** (**vair**-u-kah **play**-nah) > dome-shaped lesion which gets flattened and penetrates deeper into the skin on the feet > **plantar warts** (Figure 4.25) Synonym: **seed-warts** (trapped blood in the capillaries)

* **Filiform** (**fil**-lee-form) **warts** > tiny papules found on the face, neck, and creases of the body. These are seen in infants and are self-limiting. Synonym: **milia**

* **Genital warts** > tiny papules too but they tend to fungate and easily spread to the vagina and cervix in women and penis and testicles in men. Synonym: **Condylomata acuminata**

**4.49
Destruction
methods**

Ablation
Fulguration
Curette
Curettage
Cryosurgery
Cautery
Electrodessication
There is NO cure for **HPV**, in fact any virus. Avoiding contact with these viruses is the recommended prevention along with vaccination if available.

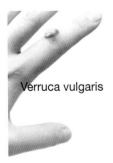

Verruca vulgaris

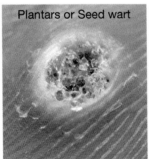

Plantars or Seed wart

Figure 4.25

Herpes viruses > involving the skin come in many forms. Like HPV, **HSV** has no cure, but medications can slow it down. HSV are easily spread.

- **Herpes simplex** (**her**-pees **sim**-plex) **virus-1** > canker sore or fever blister.

- **Herpes simplex virus-2** > genital herpes > painful, itchy, blisters on erythematous bases in the genital areas.

- **Varicella-Zoster** (**vair**-ee-**sell**-ah **zos**-tur) **Virus** (**VZV**) > Shingles are the result of remnants of the chickenpox virus (varicella) in a spinal root (Figure 4.26). The rash follows the natural nerve root dermatome (Figure 4.27). A vaccination is available to limit both chickenpox for children and **VZV** in adults.

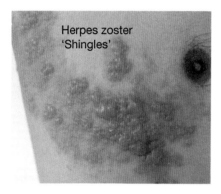

Herpes zoster
'Shingles'

Figure 4.26

Bacterial skin infections range from the very mild to the deadly. The skin, like our internal mucosal surfaces, has lots of bacteria present all the time. Most of them are good bacteria, useful to keeping all things balanced. Skin infections have a range of descriptives and causes; this is only a partial list!

- **Bullae** > *Staphylococcal* (**staff**-ee-low-**kock**-us) scalded-skin syndrome (**SSSS**) > abbreviated 'staph' or 'S. aureus'.

- **Crusted lesions** > honey colored crusts from staph species and streptococcus species > impetigo (**im**-peh-**tie**-go)

- **Folliculitis** (foe-**lick**-ule-**eye**-tis) > inflammation of the hair follicles > also from S. aureus. A **furuncle** (**fir**-un-kel) is a larger lesion and when several furuncles merge, the result is termed a **carbuncle** (kar-**bun**-kel).

4.50

Did You Know?

Some skin infections are considered sexually transmitted disease (**STD**) because of their location.

C-sections may be recommended with uncontrolled HSV-2, syphilis, GBS, HIV, and HPV to protect the infant from cross-contamination.

4.51
Linking forms
Necro- > death

Follicul/o > hair follicles

Fasci/o > band, fascia, soft tissue sheath binding muscles and other structures

Py/o- > pus, suppurative

Aer/o > air, as in breathing air

Strept/o > curved or twisted

Cocci/o > round

Staphyl/o > looks like a cluster of grapes

Vir/o > virus

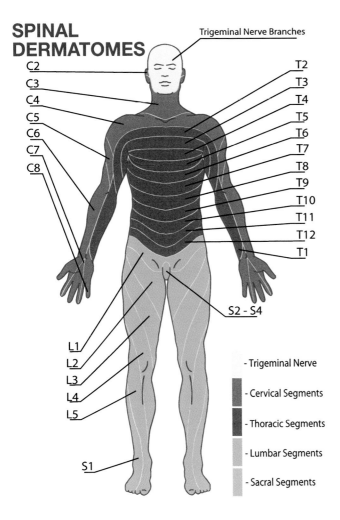

SPINAL DERMATOMES

Trigeminal Nerve Branches

C2
C3
C4
C5
C6
C7
C8

T2
T3
T4
T5
T6
T7
T8
T9
T10
T11
T12
T1

S2 - S4

L1
L2
L3
L4
L5

S1

- Trigeminal Nerve
- Cervical Segments
- Thoracic Segments
- Lumbar Segments
- Sacral Segments

Figure 4.27

STAPHYLOCOCCUS AUREUS

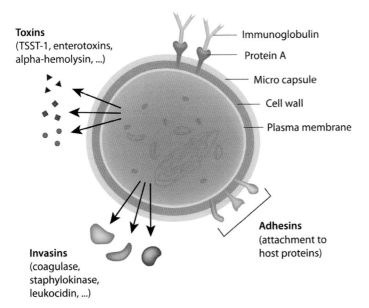

Toxins
(TSST-1, enterotoxins, alpha-hemolysin, ...)

Immunoglobulin
Protein A
Micro capsule
Cell wall
Plasma membrane

Adhesins
(attachment to host proteins)

Invasins
(coagulase, staphylokinase, leukocidin, ...)

Figure 4.28

- **Ulcers** > *Bacillus anthracis* (anthrax) and *Yersinia pestis* (yur-**sin**-knee-ah **pest**-is) > Bubonic plague.

- **Cellulitis** > inflammation of the deep dermis and soft tissues > *Staph* and *Streptococcus*, (**strep-toe-kock**-us) abbreviated *Strep* > **GBS** are the initials for Group B *Streptococcus*.

- **Necrotizing fasciitis** (**nek**-row-**tie**-zing **fash**-ee-**eye**-tis) > inflammation of the fascia, death of tissue > *Staph pyogenes* and **MRSA**, Methicillin-resistant *Staph aureus* and mixed anaerobic and aerobic pathogens.

 True or false: Viral infections are easily treated and cured.

4.52
False, we can slow them down but there are no cures.

 What is the proper medical term for 'athlete's foot'? What is this infection caused by?

4.53
Tinea pedis
Fungus or Fungi (plural)

Word building

 Using the word roots with the linking vowel to build as many valid terms with the suffixes given. Please define them too.

Follicul/o Arteri/o Py/o

-rrhea -itis -cele -cyst -derma -oid -genic

4.54
The instructor has the list!

PHARMACY CORNER

Pharmacy options for treatment of the skin are numerous. They range from simple over-the-counter (**OTC**) topical creams all the way up to complex IV antibiotics, antifungal, and antiviral medications. This is a short list of treatments for skin infections!!

Bacterial skin infections treatment may include the

- OTC antibacterial ointments or creams: Bacitracin or Neomycin.

- Simple *S. aureus* or *Strep* therapy may include oral antibiotics such as Amoxicillin, Erythromycin, Zithromax, or Ampicillin.

- Acne is often treated with oral Tetracycline or Doxycycline.

- Serious skin infections may be treated with IV Vancomycin, Nafcillin, Penicillin, Ciprofloxacin, and Clindamycin. These may not be enough to cure a resistant infection; often several medications are needed to treat a necrotizing fasciitis or similar. The use of stronger antibiotics or the use of several antibiotics increases the risk of adverse side effects.

Viral infections cannot be cured but they can be slowed down by decreasing the viral shedding.

- Topical creams for canker or cold sores (HSV-1) include Acyclovir and Penciclovir.

- Herpes virus: Oral Acyclovir, Famciclovir, and Valacyclovir.

- **HPV**: Wart may be destroyed by liquid nitrogen, ablation, or excision but none of these treatments is a cure. There is an HPV vaccination to avoid getting the HPV variety.

Fungal infections are treated with topical, oral, or IV therapy depending on their severity.

- Athlete's foot OTC medications abound: Tolnaftate, Haloprogin, Nystatin, and ketoconazole preparations.

- Nail fungal infections may respond to oral medications such as Mycostatin, Diflucan, Griseofulvin, Nizoral, and Amphotericin.

- IV antifungals are all similar but as a medication moves from topical to IV the adverse side-effect profile goes up. All medications have a potential for side effects; keep that in mind when you or a patient are using them.

A note about antibiotic resistance. In the 70+ years since antibiotics were first developed millions of lives and limbs have been saved. Antibiotics were considered the 'magic bullet'. The problem is we (collectively) have overused them from treating viral colds with penicillin to feeding them to our animals to make them fatter and infection-free before butchering them for food. This overuse has led to bacterial mutations protecting the bacteria from our antibiotics. This is the source of **MRSA** and **CRE** (carbapenem-resistant *Enterobacteriaceae*) infections. The result is that bacteria are not controlled and people are dying from lack of functional antibiotics.

⋆ IMPORTANT NOTE: Medicine is always in evolution. Do <u>not</u> use this information for patient care.

Kitchen lab

Time to investigate your medicine drawers and cabinet. Find all the topical creams, ointments, lotions, or drops you have for your skin issues. Find them and note which skin condition they match in this unit. Share your findings with the class.

SKIN TUMORS

Skin cancer is one of the most numerous types of cancer. With rare exception, the cause of skin cancer is too much exposure to the sun, specifically to UV-A and UV-B light over time (Figure 4.29). The damage to the skin from sun is cumulative. Occupations involving water add to the risk because of the intensity of the light off the water.Individuals with darker skin tones have less risk of skin cancers.

4.55
Skin cancer lesions are different from benign macules and papules. An annual skin exam is recommended yearly for adults.

UV PENETRATION INTO THE LAYERS OF THE SKIN

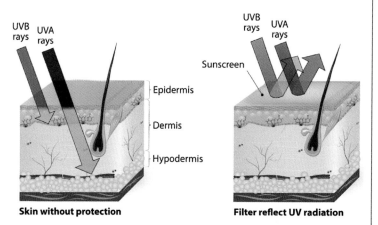

Skin without protection

Filter reflect UV radiation

Figure 4.29

BASAL-CELL CARCINOMA

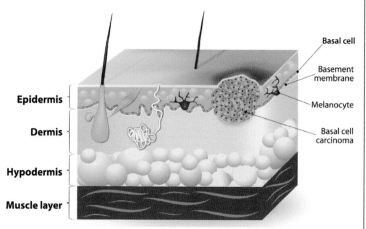

Figure 4.30

Basal cell carcinoma (**BCC**) > abnormal growth of the basal layer of the epidermis > most common skin cancer (Figure 4.30).

- Treatment includes destruction via electrodesiccation and curettage (**ED&C**), excision, cryotherapy, laser therapy, and occasionally radiation; Mohs micrographic surgery (**MMS**) and topical chemotherapy.

Squamous cell carcinoma (**SCC**) > malignant neoplasm of the keratinized epidermal cells > known for its rapid growth and metastatic behavior. It typically presents as an ulceration on an erythematous base with poorly demarcated edges (Figure 4.31).

SQUAMOUS-CELL CARCINOMA

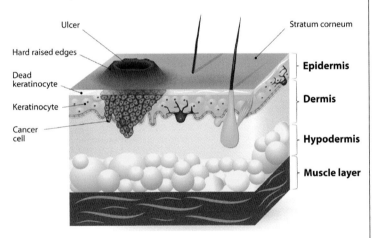

Ulcer

Hard raised edges

Dead keratinocyte

Keratinocyte

Cancer cell

Stratum corneum

Epidermis

Dermis

Hypodermis

Muscle layer

- Treatment includes surgical excision, Mohs micrographic surgery, and radiation therapy. Since SCC is likely to become metastatic, evaluation of the local lymph nodes is required.

Melanoma (**mel**-ah-**no**-ma) > pigmented lesion with an aggressive malignant behavior can arise from any melanic cell be it in the skin or eye or under the nails. Sun-exposed areas with normally benign lesions can turn malignant 5 to 20+ years later (Figure 4.32).

- Early detection is a must and biopsy of any changing lesion is recommended.

- Treatment depends on the pathology report and stage of the melanoma based on tumor location, size, and lymph node metastases. Gene-therapy with targeted therapy holds new hope for a cure.

4.56
Actinic keratoses and cheilitis (inflammation of the lips) are pre-cancerous lesions almost everyone will have over the hands, face, or arms.

Figure 4.31

4.57
The best way to avoid skin cancers is to protect your skin > Prevention.

Wear a hat with neck covering.

Wear light, long sleeves and pants for hikes, biking, etc.

MELANOMA

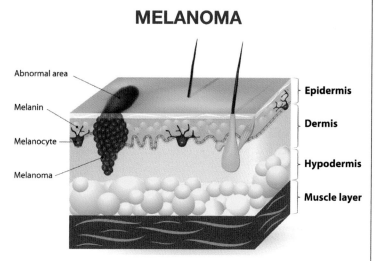

Abnormal area

Melanin

Melanocyte

Melanoma

Epidermis

Dermis

Hypodermis

Muscle layer

Sunscreens do help, specific to UV-A and –B. Apply liberally and often.

Figure 4.32

UNIT SUMMARY

1   The integumentary system is built of the epidermis and dermis. Each performs functions protecting the human body from the external environment. The epidermis is uppermost, taking the effects of everyday living from scratches to burns and lacerations. This is a protective mechanism including the melanocytes, which protects from UV light and provides skin tones.

2   The dermis is the deeper and thicker of the skin layers containing the nerve endings giving us fine touch, pressure, heat, and vibration sensation. The capillary beds supply the matrix of the dermis with oxygen and nutrients which diffuse to the epidermis. The sweat and sebaceous glands also take up space along with the hair follicles with their tiny arrector pili muscles.

3   The subcutaneous layer has the packing peanuts – adipose tissue cushions the skin, and it also provides the fascial sheets and connections anchoring the skin to the underlying structures.

4   The skin receives its color from a variety of sources. The key component to skin tones and protection is the melanin. Erythema is the redness associated with inflammation.

5   Skin 'lesions' come in a variety of shapes and sizes: flat, elevated, solid, fluid-filled, pus-filled, and wounds. Size determines the name such as a

papule versus a nodule or a vesicle versus a bulla. Scaling is a finding on lesions which may be dry or oily.

6   The skin protects from any number of infections or infestations: scabies, bacterial, viral, and fungal infections to name a few. Systemic disease often presents with a wide variety of skin manifestations ranging from soft red rashes (exanthems) to melanoma lesions.

7   All three common skin cancers occur due to over-exposure of the skin to UV-A and UV-B light. The effects are cumulative over a lifetime.

8   Skin conditions are treated with topical, oral, and IV medications. IV medications are delivered via a puncture in the skin to the underlying vein. Testing and medications are delivered intradermally and subcutaneously. Some skin conditions are treated with light therapy and chemotherapy.

UNIT WORD PARTS

Word roots with linking vowel		
Adip/o or Lip/o > fat	Arteri/o > artery	Bas/o > base, neutral
Capill/o > capillary	Chlor/o > green	Cocci/o > round
Coll/a > collagen, connective	Corne/o or Kerat/o > hard, horny scale	Cutane/o or Cut/i > skin
Cyan/o > blue	Dendr/o > branching	Derm/o or Dermat/o > skin
Elast/o > elastic, connective	Eosin/o > rosy color	Eryth/ or Erythr/o > red
Fasci/o > band, connective	Fibr/o > fiber, thread	Follicul/o > follicle
Hidr/o > sweat	Leuk/o > white	Melan/o > black
Myc/o or Mycet/o > fungus	Onych/o or Ungu/o > nails	Ped/o > foot or child
Py/o > pus, suppuration	Rhytid/o > wrinkle	Seb/o or Sebace/o > oil
Squam/o > scaly	Staphyl/o > grape cluster	Strept/o > curves, twisted
Theli/o > cell layers, nipple	Trich/o or Pil/o > hair	Xanth/o > yellow

Prefixes: attached to the front of the word root to change meaning		
A- or An- > no, not, absent, without	Anti- > against, opposing	Dys- > poor, difficult
Epi- > on top of, upon	Ex- or Exo- > outside, outer, external, away from	Hyper- > greater than, increased, more than, higher
Hypo- > less than, lower, decreased, under	Inter- > between	Intra- > within, inside
Mal- > poor, bad	Para- > abnormal	Sub- > under, below, less than

Suffixes change the meaning of the word, linking vowel is usually 'o' with consonants		
-clysis > infusion of fluid, washing	-ectomy > to cut out	-iasis > condition of infestation, usually abnormal
-lysis > destruction	-malacia > softening	-oid > resembling, like
-oma > tumor	-phil > to like	-phyte > fungal element
-plakia > plaque, unmoving	-plasty > repair of	-rrhaphy > suture
-rrhexis > split or rupture	-tomy > to cut into	

Acronyms, abbreviations, and initial sets		
BCC > basal cell carcinoma	C&S > culture and sensitivity	CDC > Centers for Disease Control and Prevention
CHF > congestive heart failure	DHHS > Department of Human and Health Services	ED&C > Electrodessication and curettage
FST > full skin thickness	GBS > Group B strep	I&D > incision and drainage
HIV > Human immunodeficiency virus	HPV > Human papilloma virus	HSV 1 & 2 > Herpes Simplex
IM > intramuscular	IV > intravenous	NCI > National Cancer Institute
OSHA > Occupational Safety and Health Agency	OTC > over-the-counter	PST > partial skin thickness
SCC > squamous cell carcinoma	VZV > Varicella-Zoster virus	

UNIT WORKSHEETS

Building terms: Use the proper prefix/word root/linking vowel/suffix as appropriate.

Example: to cut into the stomach > gastr/o/tomy

a) An instrument slicing skin layers >   _____

b) Pertaining to a large, solid elevation of the skin > _____

c) Condition of thick white plaque on the tongue > _____

d) An abnormal condition involving fungus   _____

e) Split ends on hair >   _____

f) Pertaining to the oil glands of the skin >   _____

Know your initials or acronyms! For the initial set given, spell each out correctly.

a) IV   _____

b) FST   _____

c) PST   _____

d) I&D   _____

e) C&S   _____

f) OSHA   _____

g) IM   _____

h) VZV   _____

Best choice: Pick the most appropriate answer.

1   This skin gland type secretes our sweat:

   a) Eccrine

   b) Apocrine

   c) Ceruminous

   d) Tactile

2   The suffix for splitting in layers is:

   a) –rrhexis

   b) –schism

   c) –clysis

   d) –rrhaphy

3 Staphylococcus aureus is a:

   a) fungus

   b) virus

   c) bacterium

   d) parasite

4 Which of the following is spelled correctly?

   a) Zenigraft

   b) Xanthelasma

   c) Ikterus

   d) Eccymosis

5 A burn involving the subcutaneous layer is considered a:

   a) Minor burn

   b) 3rd degree

   c) 2nd degree

   d) 1st degree

6 A simple laboratory test for fungal infections is a:

   a) KOH slide

   b) CBC

   c) C&S

   d) Electrophoresis

Name the skin lesion! Based on the description and/or function, name the skin lesion.

a) Tiny, round, solid elevation _____

b) Walled off, greater than 5 cm mass full of debris and pus _____

c) Like a subway pathway in the skin usually associated with scabies _____

d) Firm, solid, elevated lesion like a papule but larger (0.5 to 5 cm) _____

e) An inflammatory reaction of the skin to an exogenous source such as poison ivy or latex _____

f) Small (less than 0.5 cm), raised, with fluid which is usually clear or translucent _____

g) Dried serous fluids or exudates from opening vesicles or pustules _____

Multiple correct: Select ALL the correct answers to the question or statement given.

1 Which of the following can produce viral infections of the skin?

   a) HPV

   b) HSV

   c) GBS

   d) EBV

   e) MRSA

2 Which of the following are considered secondary descriptions of skin lesions?

   a) Alopecia

   b) Cyst

   c) Nodule

   d) Bullae

   e) Nummular

   f) Scale

Spelling challenge! Circle the correct spelling based on the definition given.

1 'Softening of the nail'

   Onycomycosis   Oncorrhexis   Onychomalacia   Onycoclysis

2 'Disease of the hair caused by fungi'

   Trichomycosis   Pilomyosis   Tricomycitis   Pilomycotic

3 'Removal of the superficial layers of skin'

   Avrasion   Ecchymosis   Excoriation   Petichia

Define the term: Spelling *does* count in your definition too!

1 Leukocytopenia > _____

2 Cyanosis > _____

3 Dermatofibrosarcoma > _____

4 Hyperhidrosis > _____

5 Eschar > _____

6 Rhytidectomy > _____

7 Atrophy > _____

8 Keloid > _____

Find it! Using the words in the table – match the definition given or answer the statement. Some may not be used. It is recommended you know all the choices.

arrector	subungual	dermatoplasty	nummular	endocrine
exocrine	dermoid	trichosis	dysplasia	lichenification
onychitis	dyspnea	intramuscular	dermabrasion	subcutaneous

1 _____ under the nail

2 _____ pertaining to 'into the muscle'

3 _____ difficult breathing

4 _____ secreted from outside

5 _____ poor or bad development

6 _____ repair of the skin

7 _____ inflammation surrounding the nail

8 _____ skin-like

Matching: Skin lesions or conditions, some will not be used.

	Letter	**Defined as**
Jaundice		a) denting of the skin secondary to excess fluids
2nd degree		b) frequent sun-induced skin cancer
Urticaria		c) larger than 2 cm flat discoloration of the skin
Condyloma acuminata		d) small (less than 0.5 cm), raised, with fluid
Basal cell carcinoma		e) this burn type will have vesicles or bullae
Exanthem		f) inflammation and/or infection of a hair follicle which is large and growing
Patch		g) an eruption of itchy wheals
Furuncle		h) yellow discoloration of skin and mucous membranes
		i) generalized soft red, papular rash
		j) HPV infection involving the genitalia

An essay: Explain why an injury can have two or more codes from the ICD? Please write in complete sentences with correct spelling.

Note challenge: Define the underlined terms. You may need to look up a few terms. Answer the questions which follow. Student is reminded this is an incomplete SOAP note used for the learning experience. Do not use this for patient encounters.

S. Shalonda was washing dishes in her kitchen when a glass she had in her hand broke, cutting her right hand. She has no allergies, no current medications, and no previous history of this type of injury.

O. 42 yo woman in no acute distress. VS are 128/68, P – 88, R – 16, Temp – 97.2, and Pulse ox of 97%. The right hand has a FST laceration of the thenar area of the palm. Total length is approximately 6 cm. There is no evidence of foreign bodies and the wound appears clean. Pulses in the right wrist are intact and there is good nail perfusion. Fingers have FROM and touch and vibratory sensation is intact.

Procedure note: Patient signed the consent form. The patient was seated with her right hand on the procedure table. The hand was draped in a sterile manner. 2% Xylocaine, 5 ml, was instilled subcutaneous into the wound for local anesthesia. Once the area was numb, the wound was re-examined (no FB) and cleansed well. The hand was then redraped and six (6) interrupted sutures of 3-O Prolene were placed to approximate the edges. The wound was cleaned, dried, and bacitracin applied before being dressed. Instructions for care were given to the patient. There were no complications and the patient tolerated the procedure well. Her tetanus status is up to date.

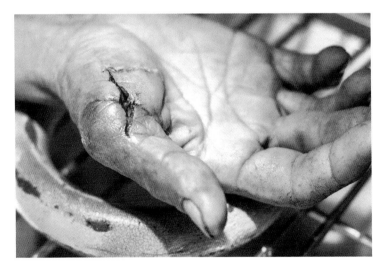

Figure 4.33

A: Laceration, FST, right hand

Questions:

1 Translate all the initials or acronyms and give meaning to the words which are underlined in the SOAP note.

2 What information do you need to code this injury properly?

3 Which layers of the skin are involved in a FST laceration?

4 Use the coding sets below to pick out the correct codes for this injury.*

Chapter 19 examples	Chapter 20 examples	Location at time of injury: examples
S61.401 Unspecified open wound right hand S61.402 Unspecified open wound left hand S61.402 Unspecified open wound of unspecified hand	W23.XXX Caught, crushed, jammed between objects W24.XXX Contact with lifting devices W25.XXX Contact with sharp glass	Mobile home Y92.029 Bathroom Y92.022 Kitchen Y92.020 Yard Y92.090
S61.411 Laceration without foreign body of right hand S61.412 Laceration without foreign body of left hand	W26.XXX Contact with knife W27.2XX Contact with garden tool	Residence Y92.009 Bathroom Y92.091 Kitchen Y92.090 Yard Y92.096
S61.421 Laceration with foreign body of right hand S61.422 Laceration with foreign body of left hand		

* **IMPORTANT NOTE: The reader is notified that these examples are from an online search carried out in 2016. Do not use these codes for patient care episodes; look up the new ones!**

Unit 5

The skeleton

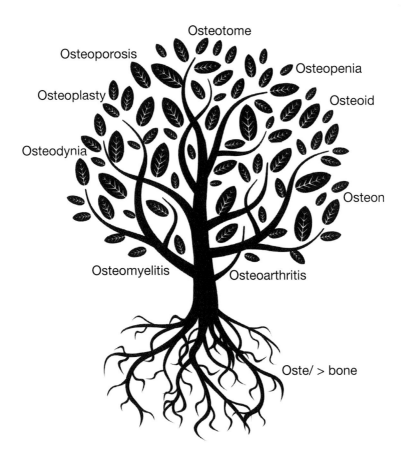

Osteotome

Osteoporosis

Osteopenia

Osteoplasty

Osteoid

Osteodynia

Osteon

Osteomyelitis

Osteoarthritis

Oste/ > bone

TARGETED LEARNING

1 Recognize word parts and the assembly of medical terms as related to the skeleton and joints.

2 Correctly construct, define, pronounce, and spell medical terms.

3 Link bone and joint diseases and injury with appropriate diagnostic evaluation, pharmacotherapeutics including pain medications, surgical, and non-surgical treatments.

4 Utilize the medical terms to describe movement directions and pain medications.

5 Explore the use of the Healthcare Common Procedure Coding System (HCPCS) using bone and joint injuries.

KEY WORD PARTS

Linking forms	Prefixes	Suffixes
Articul/o; Arthr/o > joint	A-, An-	-algia
Carp/o > wrist	Ambi-	-blasts
Cervic/o > neck	Bi-	-clasts
Chondr/o > cartilage	Dia-	-dynia
Cost/o > ribs	Dys-	-dystrophy
Crani/o > cranium, skull	Endo-	-genic
Fasci/o > band, fibrous connective	Hyper-	-malacia
Orth/o > straight	Hypo-	-oma
Oste/o; Osse/o > bone	Mal-	-penia
Rachi/o; Spondyl/o > spine	Meta-	-plasty
Sarc/o > flesh	Non-	-poiesis
Tars/o > ankle	Para-	-poikilo
Ten/o, Tend/o, and Tendin/o > tendon	Peri-	-porosis
Vertebr/o > back bone (spine), spinal bone	Poly-	-sclerosis

LEGACY OF THE CIVIL WAR BETWEEN THE STATES

Unfortunately, war is an event mankind as a whole has not been able to avoid. Yet, despite the devastation and destruction war brings, occasionally it is the source for the phrase, 'Necessity is the mother of invention'. While the United States worked out many political issues across the Mason–Dixon Line, orthopedic surgery was learning how to deal with severe injuries to the skeleton. In fact, they were drinking from a fire hose; they had far too many injuries and they quickly had to come up with ways to save life and limb.

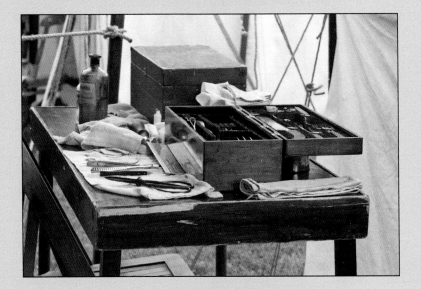

Figure 5.2

The importance of having a field hospital where injuries could be evaluated and treated immediately was a definite lesson learned from the conflagration. Orthopedic surgeons learned to triage injury, set bones, and perform amputations in a cauldron of need. The instruments and techniques developed in those killing fields would translate to civilian care for decades to come. Finally, sanitation and hygiene rose to a 'respected' level during this war – before this time hand washing was thought to be a waste of time. Today, the sterile field for orthopedic surgery remains a mandate to avoid infection in the bones, osteomyelitis.

THE BONES

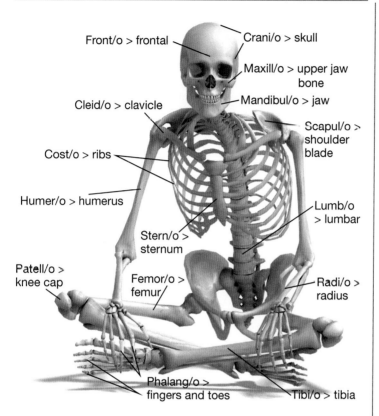

Front/o > frontal
Crani/o > skull
Maxill/o > upper jaw bone
Cleid/o > clavicle
Mandibul/o > jaw
Scapul/o > shoulder blade
Cost/o > ribs
Humer/o > humerus
Lumb/o > lumbar
Stern/o > sternum
Patell/o > knee cap
Femor/o > femur
Radi/o > radius
Phalang/o > fingers and toes
Tibi/o > tibia

Figure 5.3

5.1
In Figure 5.3 most word roots are used exclusively for the bone itself, thus they are not technically a word root. They are used as locators of bone to bone.

Just a pile of bones – place them in the right order and you have a strong, resilient support system for the human body. The skeletal system is composed of the bones, joints, cartilage, ligaments, and bursae. The bones utilize the muscles and tendons to bind, support, and move the skeleton. **Skelet/o** > dried up (bone) > framework of bones.

- Support, protection, and movement not unlike all the pieces of a car or the frame of a home.

- Mineral and growth factor storage area for calcium (Ca^{++}) and phosphorus (**P**). Both are used for bone, muscle, nerve, and cell metabolism.

- Blood cell formation via the bone marrow (myel/o) in the long and flat bones.

- Triglyceride > fat storage in the yellow marrow.

LIKE ALERT!
Myel/o is used for the bone marrow and spinal cord.

Oste/o or Osse/o > bone > matrix of collagen fibers, hydroxyapatite (Ca^{++} + P), water, and trace magnesium (**Mg^{++}**), sodium (**Na^{++}**), and bicarbonate (**HCO$_3$**). The building block or functional unit of bone is the osteon (**oz**-tea-on) (Figure 5.5).

- **Compact** (com-**pakt**) bone > tough outer shell of the bones surrounded by tough connective tissues, which allows blood, nerve, and lymph flow. Synonym: cortical or cortex (outer zone of an organ)

- **Trabecular** (tra-**bek**-U-lar) bone > architectural webs and arches of the bone interior; it is also termed 'spongy'. The tensile strength comes from the arches while decreasing the weight of the bone.

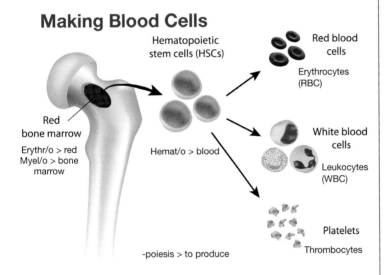

Making Blood Cells

Hematopoietic stem cells (HSCs)

Red bone marrow

Erythr/o > red
Myel/o > bone marrow

Hemat/o > blood

-poiesis > to produce

Red blood cells

Erythrocytes (RBC)

White blood cells

Leukocytes (WBC)

Platelets

Thrombocytes

Figure 5.4

Kitchen lab

The osteon is built of successive rings of calcium resembling tree rings. A single tube or column is not strong, but bind them together and the strength is evident. Check it out – take a single straw, stand it on end and see how easily it bends. Now take a handful of straws, bind them with a rubber band. You will find it much harder to bend.

5.2

INTERNAL STRUCTURE OF A BONE

Oste/o > bone -cyte > cell

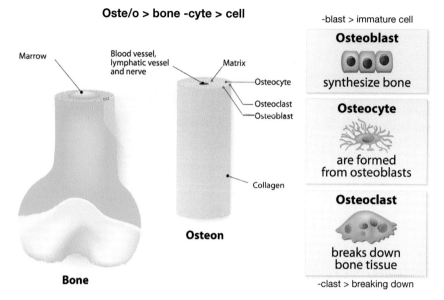

Figure 5.5

Osteogenic (os-tea-oh-**jeh**-nik) **>** origin of bone, producing bone. These cells come from stem cells surrounding the periosteum like a sock.

Osteoblasts (os-tea-oh-blasts) > produce the bone matrix spreading in all directions in the trabecular bone and more linearly in the compact bone (Figure 5.5).

Osteocytes (os-tea-oh-sites) > bone cells contain the nucleus and organelles of the osteon. When the osteocyte is finished with its individual duties (5–10 years) it will be reabsorbed by the osteoclasts.

Osteoclasts (os-tea-oh-klasts) > similar to the phagocytes of WBCs. They break up calcium and recycle it into the bloodstream. Synonym: osteolysis (**os**-tea-**ol**-eye-sis) > destruction of bone.

5.3

Suffixes

–blast > producing

–clast > breaking

–lysis > breaking

–oma > tumor

–dystrophy > abnormal or bad development

–malacia > softening

–penia > too few

–porosis > condition of pores

–poiesis > production of

–sclerosis > hardening

–scope > instrument to look at

✓ What are the two linking forms for 'bone'?

✓ Construct a medical term for 'too few bone cells'.

✓ Construct a medical term for 'bone pain'.

5.4
Oste/o and osse/o

5.5
Osteocytopenia

5.6
Osteodynia
Ostealgia

Word building

Using the word roots with the linking vowel to build as many valid terms with the suffixes given. Please define them too.

Oste/o Myel/o (bone marrow)

–itis –logy –ist –plasty –lysis –oma –ectomy –blast –cyte

5.7
The instructor has the list!

Toddlers' and children's bones slowly harden, lengthen, and eventually widen to support adult body weight. Figure 5.6 demonstrates the bone structures referred to in X-ray and orthopedic SOAP notes on a regular basis.

BONE STRUCTURE

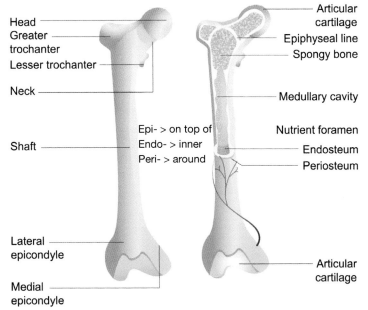

Figure 5.6

- **Epiphysis** (eh-**pif**-ee-sis) > upon growth > the distal and proximal ends of the bone provide attachments for tendons and ligaments and are covered with hyaline cartilage.

- **Diaphysis** (die-**af**-ee-sis) > between or through growth > shaft of the bone carrying red marrow from fetal development until the end of life. The nutrient blood flow is an important element with the long bones because an injury can cause substantial blood loss.

- **Periosteum** (**pear**-eh-**os**-tea-um) > around the bone > combination of the connective tissues – wrapping the bone like a sock, the fascia and bone tissue will protect the bone and bind muscle to bone as well.

- **Medullary** (**med**-U-**lar**-ee) canal > central core of the bone > inner core or 'medulla' is the inner layer of an organ.

- **Endosteum** (en-**dos**-tea-um) > inner layer of bone > inner membrane of cells, lining the inner core of the bone.

About every 10 years we have a fresh skeleton.
Like the skin, the old cells are pushed out by the new. The calcium and phosphorous are recycled.

✓ Epiphysis means _____ .

✓ Construct the medical term for cells meaning 'build bones'.
_____ / __ / _____

✓ The meaning of the prefix 'dia-' is _____ .

5.8

Did You Know?

By weight the cortical bone is about 80% of our total skeletal weight but the trabecular bone has about 10× the surface area.

Hardest: Mandible

Longest: Femur

Tiniest: Stapes, an ear bone

5.9
upon growth

5.10
Oste/o/blasts

5.11
through or between

BONE 'STRAIGHTENERS'

Orth/o > straight > used to discuss the many providers who 'straighten' bones. A practitioner is called an orthopedist (**or**-tho-**pee**-dist) – orthopaedist is also correct. An orthopedist will care for the joints and bones with surgical and non-surgical methods. An osteopath (**os**-tea-oh-path) (**DO**) originally designated a provider who cared for muscle and bone, but today, most practice the full-scope of medicine. Dentists and orthodontists deal with the bone of the jaw and face, indeed, orthodontist (**or**-tho-**don**-tist) means 'straightener of teeth'. Other practitioners who help treat bone and muscle include:

- Physical therapist (**PT**) and their assistants (**PTA**) treat patients before and after surgery; they focus on rehabilitation and decreasing pain.

- Podiatrists (poe-**die**-ah-trists) diagnose, treat, and perform surgery on the feet exclusively.

- Orthopedic assistants, technicians, and orthotists are skilled in casting, splinting, and fitting orthopedic appliances such as knee braces, back supports, and more.

- Chiropractors (**DC**) > Chir/o > hand > these practitioners work with their hands to manipulate bone and muscles.

- Prosthetists (**pros**-the-tist) are specialists who develop and fit a **prosthesis** (pros-**thee**-sis), an artificial device or appliance replacing a missing body part. Working with patients who have lost a limb takes an interdisciplinary team of healthcare professionals including surgeons, physical therapists, occupational therapists and their assistants (**OT and OTA**), and psychologists.

THE AXIAL SKELETON

An **axis** is the center on which an object turns. The **axial** (**ak**-see-al) skeleton pertains to the central bones of the human body, the core. They house and protect the delicate internal organs: the brain by the cranium; the heart and lungs by the thoracic cage; and the spinal cord by the spinal column.

The **cranium** > crani/o > composed of 22 bones, 8 making up the 'skull' cap protecting the brain and 14 facial bones shielding and interacting with the environment. The cranium is also considered a cavity.

- **Craniectomy** (kray-knee-**ek**-toe-me) > excision of part of the skull, usually to access the brain for surgery.

The **spinal column** is a stack of bones called vertebrae (**vur**-teh-breh) (plural). There are 33 with 5 distinct areas and shapes. They

5.12
Skull bones
Frontal and
Occipital
Parietal (2)
Temporal (2)
Sphenoid and
Ethmoid

Facial bones
Zygomatic (2)
Maxilla (2)
Nasal (2)

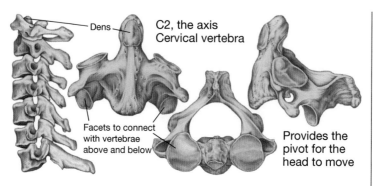

Dens — Facets to connect with vertebrae above and below

C2, the axis
Cervical vertebra

Provides the pivot for the head to move

Figure 5.7

Lacrimal (2)
Vomer (1)
Palatine (2)
Inferior concha (2)
Mandible (1)
Middle ear bones (3)

protect the neural tissues of the spinal cord to about L2 as it transitions to the cauda equina. Rachi/o > spine and Spondyl/o > spine or vertebra are other linking forms. A single back bone is a vertebra (**vur**-teh-brah).

- **Rachiocentesis** (**rah**-key-oh-sen-**tea**-sis) > lumbar puncture.

- **Spondylolisthesis** (**spon**-di-low-lis-**thee**-sis) > slipping, falling of the vertebra.

- **Spondylolysis** (**spon**-dee-**low**-lie-sis) > degeneration of the vertebra.

- **Ankylosing** (**ang**-key-los-ing) **spondylitis** > term used for arthritis of the spine. Ankyl/o > bent or crooked (Greek).

- From C2 to L5 each vertebra has a cartilage disc, the intervertebral disc cushions the body of the vertebra, allowing for motion, and protecting the peripheral nerves as they leave via the spinal cord.

Figure 5.8 demonstrates an exaggerated kyphosis (kyph/o > hump) of the thoracic spine occurring due to osteoporosis or infection. The effected vertebrae are crushed or compressed. Space is lost and the spinal nerves become trapped causing some level of symptoms.

5.13
Lordosis: the normal anterior curvature of the lumbar spine. It is aggravated during pregnancy, called hyperlordosis > **hi**-purr-lor-**doh**-sis

Scoliosis (sko-lee-oh-sis): an abnormal lateral curvature of the spine, S-shaped.

The thoracic (thor-**as**-ik) rib cage consists of 12 (sometimes 13) ribs articulating with the thoracic vertebrae and track around to the anterior chest. They do not go bone to bone with the sternal bone (breast bone). They transition to cartilage, then attach to the sternum, at least the first seven, true ribs.

5.14
Cartilage: is found throughout the body – rib cage, tip of the nose, and

KYPHOSIS

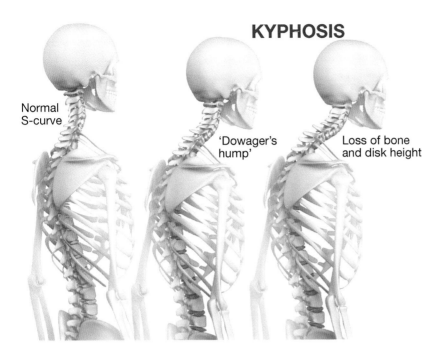

Normal
S-curve

'Dowager's
hump'

Loss of bone
and disk height

Figure 5.8

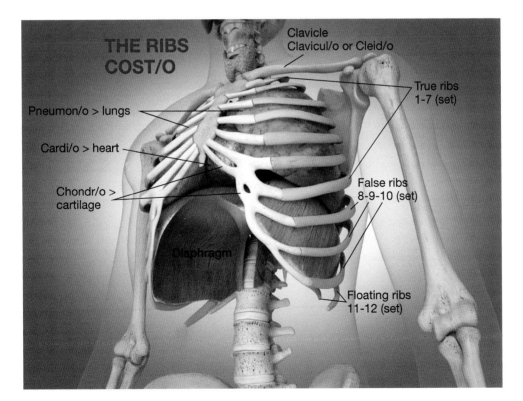

THE RIBS
COST/O

Clavicle
Clavicul/o or Cleid/o

True ribs
1-7 (set)

Pneumon/o > lungs

Cardi/o > heart

Chondr/o >
cartilage

False ribs
8-9-10 (set)

Diaphragm

Floating ribs
11-12 (set)

Figure 5.9

- Cost/o > ribs > 7 true ribs connect to the sternum (manubrium + body of sternum). The 3 false ribs will connect via cartilage to the 7th rib cartilage. The 2 floating ribs end in the deep muscles of the abdominal muscle sets (Figure 5.9).

- Chondr/o > cartilage > heavy collagen matrix permitting for the flexibility of the thoracic wall, letting the chest move in and out with respiration.

  - **Costochondritis** (**kos**-toe-kon-**dry**-tis) > inflammation of the rib cartilage, anterior chest wall pain.

  - **Sub**costal (**sub**-kos-tal) > under the ribs.

  - **Chondromalacia** (**kon**-dro-ma-**lay**-shah) > cartilage softening.

cushioning the ends of the long bones. It is avascular tissue like epithelial tissue. It gets its nourishment via diffusion.

Other terms are:

Chondrodysplasia

Chondroma

Chondroplasty

Chondrofibroma

 The suffix '-malacia' means _____ .

5.15
softening

 The spinal column has _____ vertebrae.

5.16
33

 Construct the medical term meaning 'surgically remove part of the skull bone'. _____/_____

5.17
Crani/ec/tomy or Crani/ectomy

Word building

 Using the word roots with the linking vowel to build as many valid terms with the suffixes given. Please define each term.

Chondr/o Crani/o Thorac/o

-itis -plasty -lysis -oma -tomy -ectomy
-centesis -malacia

5.18
The instructor has the list!

PHARMACY CORNER

Bone pain*

Injured bones (fractures or bruising) hurt because of the bone's tremendous blood and nerve supply. Bone pain is often described as dull, achy, and hard to localize. The surrounding periosteum is very sensitive to pain, whether it be from a break or expansion of a tumor or carcinoma in the closed system of the bone.

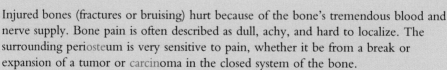

A bone fracture creates intense pain but it will recede with rest and bone healing. Chronic bone pain from osteoarthritis is a dull, gnawing pain which is worse with weight bearing. Metastatic cancer to the bone tends to be unremitting and fractures are more likely due to loss of cohesiveness of the bone. Paget's disease, osteoporosis, and sarcoma may cause neurological type pain as well. What can be done for bone pain?

- **NSAIDs** > **N**on-**S**teroidal **A**nti-**In**flammatory **D**rugs > all inflammation, be it in the bone or skin or blood vessels, is moderated by prostaglandin, a localized cell hormone. The healing process brings with it the generation of pain. This is a protective mechanism to keep an individual at rest. NSAIDs are anti-prostaglandins; they decrease inflammation. Medications include aspirin, ibuprofen, naproxen, celecoxib, diclofenac, ketoprofen, sulindac, and piroxicam. These do help with most bone pain, however, their side-effect profile may cause more trouble when used regularly. Chronic use is not recommended.

- **Corticosteroid therapies** > work to decrease inflammation and the reaction of the immune system to pain. Steroids are helpful for rheumatoid arthritis, psoriatic arthritis, SLE, and gout. Whether given orally or injected, steroids can cause susceptibility to infection, bleeding, rupture of tendons or ligaments, and joint necrosis. Steroids include triamcinolone, cortisone, prednisone, and methylprednisolone.

- **Radiation therapy (RT)** > a pain-control option for metastatic bone cancer or bone tumors. Shrinking the bulk of the tumor decreases the pain. It is usually delivered by external-beam radiation (**EBRT**). It can set up the healthy bone tissue for osteoporosis and spontaneous fractures.

- In the presence of severe osteoporosis or Paget's disease, bisphosphonates (bis-**fos**-fo-nats) decrease the bone tissue breakdown (osteolysis) thus pain is diminished.

- **Opioids >** such as morphine, oxycodone, tramadol, and hydromorphone work well because they interact at the cell receptors well and they relieve some of the anxiety associated with pain. For acute injuries they should be used carefully because addiction can occur. For chronic, terminal bone pain, they can help. Dosing should be titrated to relief of pain.

- Medications used for neuropathy may help with bone pain because of the sensitivity of the periosteum. Tricyclic antidepressants such as amitriptyline have been used successfully for years.

- Proper nutrition, biofeedback, ice- and -heat therapy (thermotherapy), water-therapy, electrostimulation, and massage are all part of the regimen to control bone pain. Find the source and treat it.

★ IMPORTANT NOTE: Medicine is always in evolution. Do <u>not</u> use this information for patient care.

THE APPENDICULAR SKELETON

Appendicular or appendix is Latin for 'to hang something on'. The arms and legs are literally hung on the core, the axial skeleton. In fact, the arms are connected at only one spot, the sternoclavicular joint (collar bone and sternum). The pelvis attaches at the sacroiliac joint and the legs attach to the pelvis at the acetabulum.

5.19
Linking forms
Humer/o > arm bone
Carp/o > wrist
Radi/o > radius
Uln/o > ulna
Brachi/o > arm

Wrist bones
Hamate
Triquetrum
Capitate
Pisiform
Lunate
Scaphoid
Trapezoid
Trapezium

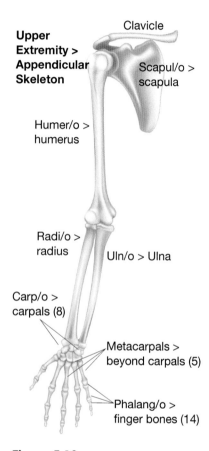

Clavicle

Upper Extremity > Appendicular Skeleton

Scapul/o > scapula

Humer/o > humerus

Radi/o > radius

Uln/o > Ulna

Carp/o > carpals (8)

Metacarpals > beyond carpals (5)

Phalang/o > finger bones (14)

Figure 5.10

- The **clavicle** (**klav**-ee-kel) > collarbone.

- The **scapula** (**skap**-U-la) > shoulder blade. They provide attachment surfaces for many neck and chest muscles.

- The **humerus** (hue-mur-us) > upper arm bone and it sits in the **glenoid fossa** (**glen**-oyd **foz**-ah), a ball and socket joint. This joint allows the greatest range of motion of any other joint in the body.

- The forearm has the **ulna** (**ul**-nah) (medial) and **radius** (**ray**-dee-us) (lateral). The **olecranon** (oh-**lek**-rah-non) process (proximal ulna) and fossa (distal humerus) is the funny bone. It forms our elbow and allows us to rotate our forearm in **supination** and **pronation**.

- The eight **carpals** (**car**-pahls) > wrist bones. The short, squarish bones slide slightly over each other and give the hand motions for waving, writing, typing, etc. Following the carpals are the five metacarpals (**met**-ah-**car**-pohls), literally, 'beyond the wrist'. These are the bones of the hand (palm). Finally, the 14 finger bones are the **phalanges** (fay-**lan**-geez) (plural) > fingers; phalanx (**fay**-langks) (singular).

The **pelvis** is a fusion of three fairly flat bones: ilium (**il**-ee-um), ischium (**is**-key-um or **is**-he-um), and pubis (**pew**-bis) (Figure 5.11). The pelvis protects the abdominal and pelvic organs. The iliosacral joint is where the axial skeleton joins with the lower extremities. The coxal (**koks**-al) or pelvic girdle is a huge muscle attachment area for the strong abdominal and back muscles.

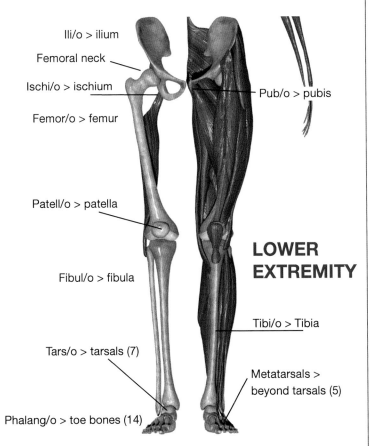

Ili/o > ilium

Femoral neck

Ischi/o > ischium

Pub/o > pubis

Femor/o > femur

Patell/o > patella

LOWER EXTREMITY

Fibul/o > fibula

Tibi/o > Tibia

Tars/o > tarsals (7)

Metatarsals > beyond tarsals (5)

Phalang/o > toe bones (14)

LIKE ALERT!

Ileum > last section of the small intestines; *Ilium* > largest, proximal section of the pelvis. They are pronounced the same.

- The **femur** (**fee**-mur, **fem**-oh-ra (plural) > thigh bone and has a well-defined femoral neck and femoral head. It is rounded to fit in the **acetabulum** (as-eh-**tab**-U-lum).

- The **tibia** (**tib**-ee-ah) (medial), the shin bone, and the **fibula** (**fib**-U-la) (lateral) make up the lower leg. The tibia is the second longest bone of the body and bears all the weight of the femur via the two **menisci**, the cartilage pads. The fibula bears no weight although it is essential to muscle and ligament attachments at the tibiofibular joint (proximal) and fibulotalar joint (distal).

- The seven bones of the ankle are called the **tarsal** (**tar**-sol) bones. There are two discussed often, the **talus** (**tay**-lus), which articulates with the tibia and fibula and receives most of the weight of standing. The **calcaneus** (cal-**kay**-knee-us) is our heel bone, posterior to the forefoot and takes the rest of the weight of walking. The other five tarsals are the navicular, cuboid, and three cuneiform (wedges).

- Following the **tarsals** are the five **metatarsals** (**met**-ah-tar-sols) > literally, 'beyond the ankle'. These are the bones of the foot. Finally, the 14 toe bones are the phalanges.

- The **patella** (pah-**tel**-lah) > also called the knee cap and is tucked inside the patellar tendon which originates with the thigh's large quadriceps (4 muscles) and attaches to the tibial tuberosity. It is considered a **sesamoid** bone and protects the femorotibial joint during kneeling and flexing activities.

Word building

Construct the bone connection words.

- Pertaining to the leg bone + lower leg bone joint (the big one)
- Pertaining to the arm bone + smaller lower arm bone
- Pertaining the 'beyond the wrist' + fingers
- Pertaining to the cartilage + ribs

5.21
The instructor has the answers!

ANATOMY OF THE KNEE

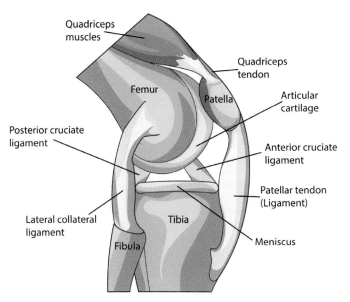

Figure 5.12

The skeletal system includes the connectors and joints made of strong connective tissues formed by fibroblasts and chondroblasts: **tendons**, **ligaments**, and **cartilage**. Figure 5.12 represents the most complex joint of the body, the knee. It gives us a look at the connective tissues at work.

- **Ligaments** (**lig**-ah-ments) > tough fibrous tissue connecting bone to bone. Most ligaments are thick, short, wide bands holding the joints together. A sprained ankle is stretching these to their maximum and may involve tears.

- **Tendons** > tough, fibrous cords joining muscle to bone. They are made of the same fascial sheets wrapping the muscle. They terminate as the connective cord to the bone. There are three linking forms: ten/o, tend/o, and tendin/o.
  - **Tendinitis** (**ten**-din-**nigh**-tis) > inflammation of the tendon.
  - **Tendolysis** (ten-**doh**-lie-sis) > release of a tendon.
  - **Tenosynovitis** (**ten**-oh-sin-oh-**vie**-tis) > inflammation of the tendon and enveloping sheath (synovium).

5.22
Linking forms
Arthr/o > joint

Burs/o > bursa

Chondr/o > cartilage

Synov/i > synovia

Ten/o > tendon

Tend/o > tendon

Tendin/o > tendon

Singular/plural
Meniscus

Menisci

Bursa

Bursae

Tendon

Tendinea or tendons

- **Hyaline** (**hi**-ah-lin) **cartilage** > coats the end of the long bones to protect the ends. It is tough, avascular tissue which look like frosted glass – firm, smooth, and with some give. Loss of this cartilage is the beginning of osteoarthritis.

- **Meniscus** (me-**nis**-kus) > crescent-shaped cartilage cupping the distal femoral epiphysis. Menisci (me-**nis**-keye) is plural.

- **Bursa** (**burr**-sah) > joints have one more structure designed to protect surfaces from the constant motion of life. Like jelly-filled donuts with gel on the inside it is a tough connective tissue sac. It is designed to provide for smooth motion and to cushion movement. Bursae (**burr**-say) is plural.

✓ What is the plural term for the cartilage pad between the femur and tibia?

✓ What is the medical term for 'inflammation of the fascia of the plantar surface of the foot'?

Word building

Using the word roots with the linking vowel to build as many valid terms with the suffixes given. Please define each term.

Ten/o Synovi/o Burs/o

-itis -plasty -rrhaphy -oma -tomy -ectomy

Can you make any compound words or add a prefix?

Joint motion terminology is about the movement occurring at the joint in anatomical position. Most of the directions have to do with the appendicular skeleton as they are the most mobile. In anatomical position the back, legs, and arms are all at 180 degrees. Increasing the degree is **extension** and decreasing the degree is **flexion** (Figure 5.13).

- **Abduction** (ab-**duk**-shun) > moving away from the center, away from the body in a lateral direction. The arm, leg, hand, foot, fingers, and toes can abduct from the center.

- **Adduction** (ad-**duk**-shun) > moving to the center, to the body, in a medial direction. The arm, leg, hand, foot, fingers, and toes can all adduct to the center but to a lesser degree than abduction.

- In the ankle, **eversion** (ee-**vur**-zhun) > the great toe is outgoing, moving away from the center.

5.23

Did You Know?

Prior to birth, most bones are really cartilaginous prototypes to the bone, permitting the fetus to be pliable in its snug living conditions.

5.24
Menisci

5.25
Plantar fasciitis

5.26
The instructor has the list!

5.27
Our lumbar spine has several motions including: flexion, hyperextension, lateral motion, and twist motion (rotation).

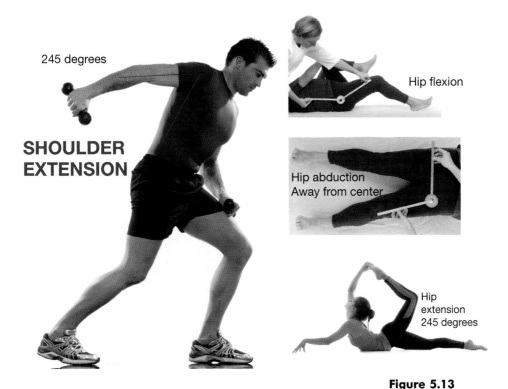

245 degrees

SHOULDER
EXTENSION

Hip flexion

Hip abduction
Away from center

Hip
extension
245 degrees

Figure 5.13

- In the ankle, **inversion** (in-**vur**-zhun) > 'turning' the ankle, as the great toe is ingoing, moving more inward to the center. This is a frequent injury to the ankle, an inversion or turned ankle.

Kitchen lab

Did you realize when you use your hand to trace a 'turkey' for Thanksgiving you are abducting your fingers? Get some tracing paper, abduct your fingers as wide as you can, trace your hand. Now, do your toes. Compare the angles.

- **Extension** (eks-**ten**-shun) > straightens the joint to anatomical position, the distal end moves away from the proximal. The elbow extends to 180 degree, no further (safely). The knee can hyperextend just a bit with effort, otherwise it is 180 degrees in extension.

- **Flexion** (**flex**-shun) > bends the distal end to the proximal end; decreases the angle. Figure 5.13 demonstrates the **goniometer** (**go**-knee-**om**-ee-tur); it is used to measure joint motion exactly and vital to documenting improvement post injury or surgery.

5.28
The thoracic spine has only elevation and depression motion as related to breathing.

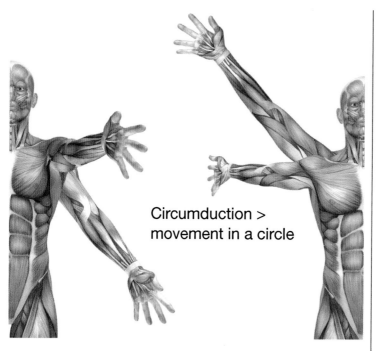

Circumduction >
movement in a circle

Figure 5.14

- **Circumduction** (**sir**-kom-**duk**-shun) > ability to turn the joint in a circle. The shoulder has the best ROM (Figure 5.14). The hip can circumduct as well but to a lesser degree. The thumb motion is not a pure circumduction.

- The neck can move our cranium in many directions. **Lateral** is ear to shoulder; **rotation** is chin to shoulder; **extension**, chin up; and **flexion**, chin down.

- The mandible can **protract** (pro-**trakt**) > to push forward, anteriorly. It can also **retract** (ree-**trakt**) > to pull inward, posteriorly. This is used more than most of us realize with facial expressions, laughing, and chewing.

- The shoulders via the trapezius muscles can **elevate** > the shrug and **depress** > breathing out hard. We use both of these often, as well without much thought.

- **Ambidextrous** (**am**-bi-**deks**-trus) > ability to use either hand equally.

5.29
Initial sets
FROM > full range of motion
DIP > distal IP
PIP > proximal IP
MCP > metacarpal phalangeal
MTP > metatarsal phalangeal
C1–7 > cervical vertebrae
T1–12 > thoracic vertebrae
L1–5 > lumbar vertebrae

✓ The motion of the shoulder in a lateral motion away from the body is called _____ .

5.30
abduction

✓ What is the medical term for 'removal of the bursa'?

5.31
Bursectomy

✓ The femorotibial synovial joint is found where on the body?

5.32
Knee or femur and tibia

Word building

Note the correct direction or motion.
- Pulling the jaw backward _____
- Putting your arm behind your back is

  _____

- Turning your chin to your shoulder

  _____

- Closing your hand into a fist is _____
  of your fingers

  Getting up from a squat is _____ the
  knees

5.33
The instructor has the answers!

PHYSICAL THERAPY NOTES

S Rolin is a 27 yo man who had a lumbar fusion between L4–L5 after a basketball injury. He is here for his 4th PT appointment. He reports better sleep, waking only twice with mild pain. His current low back pain is 5/10 with walking or shifting and 2/5 at relative rest. He did try to pick up his daughter this morning but it hurt a little too much. He reports using Tylenol #3 (1) at bedtime only now.

O Gait is even and steady. He was able to climb on the exam table easily. I demonstrated a good sleeping position (again) and how to move from that position to upright without stressing the back. 1) Patient repeated the process with limited increase in pain. 2) Lumbar flexion is up to 55%, better from 45% 2 days ago. 3) Tolerated US 1.5 w/cm2 for 10 minutes and he moved easily when getting up from the prone position.

A S/P Lumbar fusion L4–L5, steady improvement. Patient appears compliant with home activities:

P 1 Interferential electrical stimulation 80–150Hz X-set up through pain × 20 min. prone.

2   Educated patient on good body mechanics with 15lb. box lift for 10 reps. twice a day.

3   Prone lumbar extensions x 20 reps. Twice a day.

Again discussed safe activities at home. Slow, steady progress will ensure continued healing to full recovery. Avoid lifting 50# daughter for now. May drive for 5–10 minutes twice a day. Reinforced importance of proper posture and movement decisions. Next appointment in 2 days.

This is a good physical therapy SOAP note. It has full statements on how the patient is feeling, sleeping, his limitations and successes in the subjective section. It includes the measurable progress in the objective section. The assessment and plan clearly states current goals, therapy, and patient instructions.

BONE INJURY

INJURIES – When it comes to injuries, bones and joints are easy targets. The good news is, like the skin, bones heal readily with the constant process of bone building and remodeling. Joints can be more problematic because the protective ligaments, tendons, and cartilage structures are avascular. They do not repair easily or at all.

Fractures to any bone in the body are usually mechanical; something hits the bone or creates torsion to the bone. Because the appendicular skeleton is linear, it generally takes a significant transverse blow. These are **traumatic fractures**. **Pathological fractures** occur spontaneously secondary to disease such as osteoporosis, bone cancers, or infection.

- **Stress** fracture, non-displaced, microfractures due to overuse. This injury is seen in the metatarsals.

- **Transverse** fracture, non-displaced, most likely a lateral hit.

- **Oblique** is at an angle and is usually a torsion injury.

- **Spiral** is like opening a can of biscuits – it requires a twist.

- **Greenstick** is seen in children because their bones are like a new branch on a tree. You can break the edge but it does not go all the way through.

- **Comminuted or compacted** fracture includes several pieces. Impacted or compressed fractures are comminuted and they occur by landing on them – jumping out of a burning building or falling while rock climbing, etc. Impact fractures are also seen in pathological conditions such as seen in the spine with collapsed vertebrae.

5.34

There are four ways to describe a fracture for the next reader:

1 Open or Closed

2 Simple (two pieces) or comminuted (several pieces)

3 Trauma or pathological

4 Location and type of fracture.

In children, the involvement of the epiphyseal growth plate is vital to note as it can slow or stop growth of the bone if not repaired properly.

These descriptives help with evaluation and treatment options for the patient.

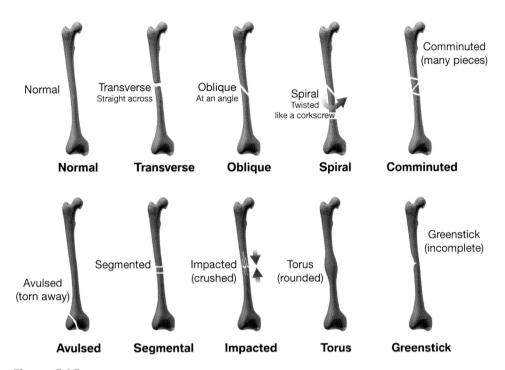

Figure 5.15

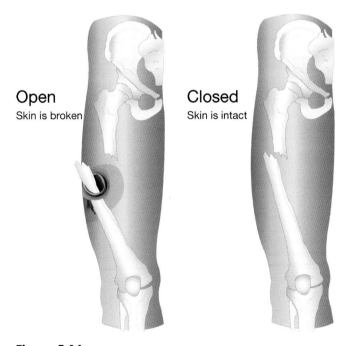

Figure 5.16

There are two other classifications of the fracture: **Open or compound**, the injury has damaged the skin (Figure 5.16) and all the soft tissue and bone are exposed to external contaminates. If a fracture does NOT involve open skin it is considered **closed**.

A **fractured bone** can be set in a closed mode by casting the joint above and below to help decrease motion while providing traction. The closed fracture may need an open reduction with internal fixation (**ORIF**) to pin or plate the fracture (Figure 5.18). When the bone is set with external pin(s), it is an open reduction with external fixation (**OREF**) such as a halo-fixator. The open fracture is cleaned, pinned or plated, and drains are placed to avoid a warm, dark, wet place for opportunistic bacteria to grow.

On average, over the next 6 to 8 weeks the bone heals to its original strength. In children and young adults the bone will remodel to absolute normal in 6 months. The older we are the longer it will take, thus the 60-year-old who breaks his leg falling off his bike will take 8–10 weeks to heal (Figure 5.17).

5.35

Terms of bone healing
Hematoma
Granulation tissue
Neovascularization
Callus
Remodeling
ORIF
OREF

REPAIR OF FRACTURES

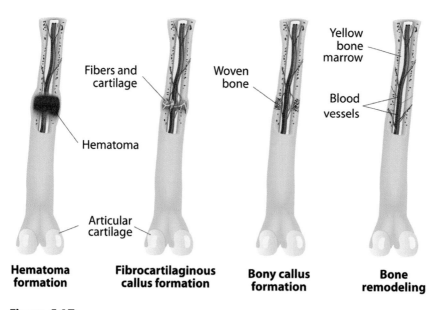

Fibers and cartilage

Hematoma

Articular cartilage

Woven bone

Yellow bone marrow

Blood vessels

Hematoma formation

Fibrocartilaginous callus formation

Bony callus formation

Bone remodeling

Figure 5.17

✓ The tough connective tissue linking muscle to bone is called a
_____ .

5.36
tendon

✓ A fracture which does not break through the skin is
considered a _____ fracture.

5.37
closed

✓ Arthritis is inflammation of a _____ .

5.38
joint

CODING ALL THE PIECES AND PARTS*

If you wanted to pick a system or specialty using a large number of durable items in the care of patients, it would be orthopedics. Fixing the strains, sprains, bursitis, torn rotator cuffs, fractures, and torn ACLs, the types of orthotics equipment are numerous. There are two coding books used to look up hardware used in orthopedic injury or disease: the ICD-10-PCS and the HCPCS. Some of the items are included in the cost of the surgery or reduction. This is called a bundle. A short story:

> Jorge was riding his bicycle when a dog startled him and he fell and fractured his left arm. A BLS (Basic Life Support) ambulance transported him to a local hospital where he was seen in the ER. They took an X-ray, started an IV, drew some blood for lab tests, and called the orthopedic surgeon to set his Colles fracture.

The ICD-10-PCS (Procedure Coding System) is used for surgical repair and includes codes for the hardware. If Jorge needed ORIF, his operative codes would include some of the following:

- Joint fixation plate, joint liner, or joint spacer

- Fusion screws (compression, lag, locking)

- Kirschner wire (K-wire) to wire a joint or bone together

Jorge is not going to need ORIF. A closed reduction and casting will be performed in the ER. Many of the supplies will be coded from the HCPCS (**hik**-piks). It covers every imaginable function and device for patient care from crutches to needles to catheter bags and prosthetics. Jorge will need codes for the following:

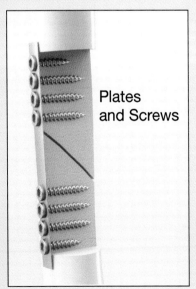

Plates and Screws

Figure 5.18

- Ambulance ride, BLS with routine disposable supplies > A0382H
- Syringe with needle, sterile 5 cc > A4209
- Morphine sulfate up to 10 mg > J2270
- Fluids, normal saline, 500 cc > A4217
- Casting supplies > A4580

Proper documentation and descriptions make an enormous difference on how the record is coded and reimbursed.

Non-durables are items used only once and thrown away properly after use. They all cost money. They include needles, syringes, tissues, 4 by 4 gauge pads, surgical masks, suture kits, and medications such as morphine sulphate as given above.

Durables are items which can be used again such as wheelchairs, crutches, halo-devices, semirigid braces, and even artificial limbs.

- Crutches are coded E0112 for wood and E0114 for other than wood.
- A prosthetic for a below the knee (**BK**) amputation is L5100 for a molded socket, shin, and SACH (solid ankle cushion heel) foot.

Coding is a complex activity which depends on the medical terms, directions, and documentation of materials used in a specific setting being properly documented. It is a system, which despite much regulation, continues to have providers who creatively 'unbundle' a procedure so they can charge more for their care. This is called **fraud** and is quite illegal. Accurate documentation is necessary, not only for the care of the patient but for the dollars they will pay for their care. Do it well!

⋆ **IMPORTANT NOTE: The reader is notified that these examples are from an online search done in 2016. Do <u>not</u> use these codes for patient care episodes; look up new ones!**

BONE AND JOINT DISEASE

Osteoporosis (**os**-tea-oh-pore-**oh**-sis) > loss of bone mineral density (Figure 5.19). This can occur to some degree with aging, making elders more susceptible to bone breaks from relatively benign trauma. It can also occur due to the lack of use. Exercise stimulates the osteoblasts; being lazy or bedridden encourages the osteoclasts. Osteoporosis is associated with women due to hormone changes.

5.39

Prevention of osteoporosis

Stop smoking.

Avoid long-term steroid use.

Get regular exercise and some sunshine daily.

Eat a healthy diet.

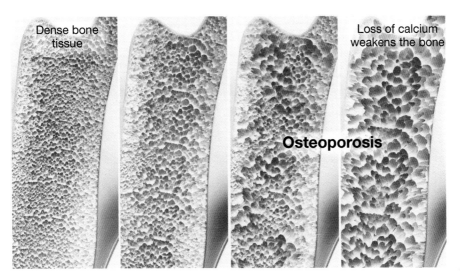

Figure 5.19

- It is evaluated with a **DEXA** (dual-energy X-ray absorptiometry) scan. It is an easy, inexpensive, and non-invasive procedure.

Oste**odystrophy** (**os**-tea-oh-**dis**-trow-fee) > defective bone formation. This is the result of renal disease or failure.

Paget's disease > pathologic process where both the osteoclasts and osteoblasts are working too hard creating patches of osteomalacia and osteosclerosis (**os**-tea-oh-sklar-**oh**-sis). Treatment for Paget's (**pah**-jets) includes low-dose IV bisphosphonates for symptomatic pain.

- Osteopoikilosis (**os**-tea-oh-poy-keye-**low**-sis) > description of mottled bone effect associated with Paget's.

Sarc**oma** > tumor of the flesh > rare (less than 1%) and classified as soft tissue and bone sarcoma. Bone sarcomas are more dangerous especially if they occur in children because they metastasize easily.

- **Ewing's** (**U**-wings) > occurs in the diaphysis of the long bone or in flat bones. Targeted therapy with an anti-IGF1 receptor has been useful to date; otherwise chemotherapy will usually put this metastatic cancer into remission.

- **Osteosarcoma** (**os**-tea-oh-sar-**ko**-ma) > spindle cell neoplasm producing osteoid (bone-like) bone. These occur with children and elderly in the long bones. It presents similarly to Paget's disease.

Suffixes

–malacia > softening

–sclerosis > condition of hardening

–poikilo > many changes, mottled

5.40

Most bone diseases can be inferred from their characteristic plain X-ray appearance. **MRI** and **CT** scans may be done for more precision.

A **bone scan** is a nuclear medicine examination used to define metastatic disease.

- **Chondrosarcoma** (**kon**-dro-sar-**ko**-ma) > arise from the periosteum among the chondroblasts. It presents with slow, unremitting, dull bone pain usually in the flat bones.

✓ Hugo had the misfortune to walk into a swinging bat; it hit his L humerus. The X-ray revealed a comminuted fracture of the diaphysis. What do comminuted and diaphysis mean?

✓ Mr. Patrick is heading home from the rehab unit following hip replacement surgery. Which book is used to code the walker he will use at home?

✓ The proper spelling for the 'weakening or loss of bone mass'. Osteoclysis Osteopoikosis Osteoporosis Osteomalasia

---

ARTHRITIS > inflammation of the joint, like dermatitis, is used for several conditions. While orthopedists take care of injury to joints, disease of the joints is the purview of the rheumatologist (**roo**-mah-**tol**-oh-jist).

Rheumatology is a specialty under the internal medicine areas of study. Rheumatologists concentrate on clinical problems involving joints, autoimmune diseases, genetics, soft tissue and vasculitis issues.

Rheumatoid arthritis (RA) > systemic disease thought to be similar to autoimmune disease (Figure 5.20). It causes marked inflammation of the synovial joints, bone, and connective tissues throughout the body. Rheum/o is Greek for 'flux', fluid changes. Testing includes a combination of old tests and new ones:

- **Rheumatoid factor** (**RF**) > by itself it is not conclusive.

- **Erythrocyte sedimentation rate** (**Sed rate**) > helps assess disease activity.

- **C-reactive protein** (**CRP**) > helps assess disease activity.

- **Antinuclear antibody** (**ANA**) > present in many autoimmune diseases.

- **Anti-cyclic citrullinated peptide antibody** (**ACPA** or **anti-CCP**) > helps confirm the diagnosis and may project risk of severe disease.

The severe deformities and disability of the past are yielding to the new therapies today.

Laboratory studies are used, and then a biopsy.

5.41
Comminuted = many pieces
Diaphysis = shaft of the long bone

5.42
HCPCS

5.43
Osteoporosis

5.44
New science on protein behavior has yielded a new test for **RA**.
The **ACPA**s are antibodies working against a patient's own proteins. They appear in the majority of RA patients.

Linking forms
Arthr/o > joint
Rheum/o > flux
Oste/o > bone
Myel/o > bone marrow or spinal cord

Suffixes
–ic > pertaining to
–oid > like, similar
–logy > study
–scope > instrument to look
–scopy > process of looking

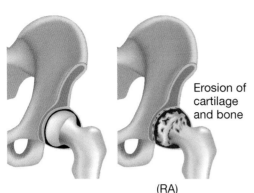

Erosion of
cartilage
and bone

Healthy hip joint   (RA)
                     Rheumatoid arthritis

Figure 5.20

- **D**isease-**M**odifying **A**nti-**R**heumatoid **D**rugs (**DMARD**s) have significantly decreased the inflammation and damage done to the bones, joints, and systems. These include methotrexate, leflunomide, hydroxychloroquine, and sulfasalazine.

- Biological **DMARD**s are protein therapies targeting the inflammatory trigger, cytokines. These include TNF-α-inhibitors, Rituximab, Anakinra, and Abatacept.

Gout arthritis (gowt) > disorder of purine (protein) metabolism. If the uric acid of muscle and protein activity is not adequately cleared via the kidney, the salts tend to gather at joints. The MTP joint of the great toe is the most common involved joint. (**MTP** > metatarsophalangeal joint)

Osteoarthritis (OA) > wear and tear arthritis; it is also called degenerative joint disease (**DJD**). It is the erosion of the articular cartilage (like sanding down a piece of wood) until there is little or no protection of the bone with loss of joint space (Figure 5.21). The vertebrae, knees, and hips are the usual areas of **OA**. They are weight-bearing joints.

5.45

- NSAIDs and corticosteroid injections can help decrease inflammation.

Obesity makes OA worse. Losing weight is a major change which can really help treat OA. For each 1 pound of weight the pressure loading across the knees is increased three to six fold. **What helps?** Regular exercise, healthy diet, drinking water, and no smoking.

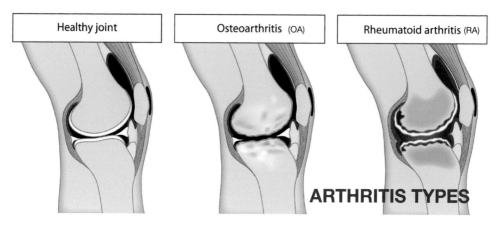

| Healthy joint | Osteoarthritis (OA) | Rheumatoid arthritis (RA) |

ARTHRITIS TYPES

Figure 5.21

Joint injury and illness

Muscles are flexible and trainable, tendons and ligaments, less so.

Ligament sprains are all too familiar. As seen in Figure 5.22, a ligament sprain is forcibly distended or stretched or even torn.

5.46
Ligament tears create a lax joint. In the ankle, there is

ANKLE SPRAINS

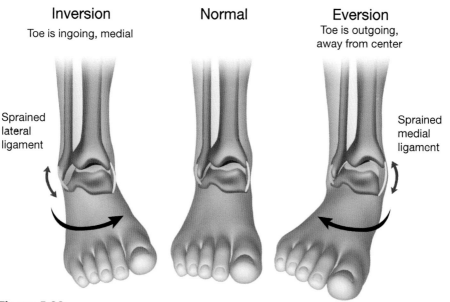

| Inversion | Normal | Eversion |
| Toe is ingoing, medial | | Toe is outgoing, away from center |

Sprained lateral ligament

Sprained medial ligament

Figure 5.22

Over-stretching is grade 1, micro-tearing is grade 2, and a partial or complete tear is a grade 3. A ligament tear may also pull off a piece of the bone. This is an avulsion fracture. The therapy for the initial injury is RICE: *r*est, *i*ce, *c*ompression, and *e*levation to decrease pain and inflammation.

- **Anterior cruciate** (**krew**-she-ate) **ligament (ACL)** > one of the two major ligaments in the middle of the knee. It links the femur to the tibia in the knee (Figure 5.23).

- **Posterior cruciate ligament (PCL)** > second major ligament in middle of the knee linking the femur to the tibia, making an X pattern at the center of the knee.

- **Lateral collateral ligament (LCL)** connects the femur to the fibula on the outer side of the knee. It gets more work from going up steps, a slight lateral motion.

- **Medial collateral ligament (MCL)** also connects the femur to the tibia on the medial or inside of the knee, working harder when we go down steps.

Evaluation of joints is done via plain X-ray, **MRI**, and a procedure, **arthroscopy**. Joint fluid can be sent to the lab for evaluation for blood, infections, and specific changes.

a redundancy of ligaments so losing one will most likely not cause dysfunction.

However, the loss of one of the knee's internal ligaments (ACL or PCL) can disrupt knee function. Therapy is to reattach the ligament with a screw. Recovery depends on the extent of the injury, good rehab, and what your job is. Obviously, playing football for a living or soccer puts you at risk for repeat injury.

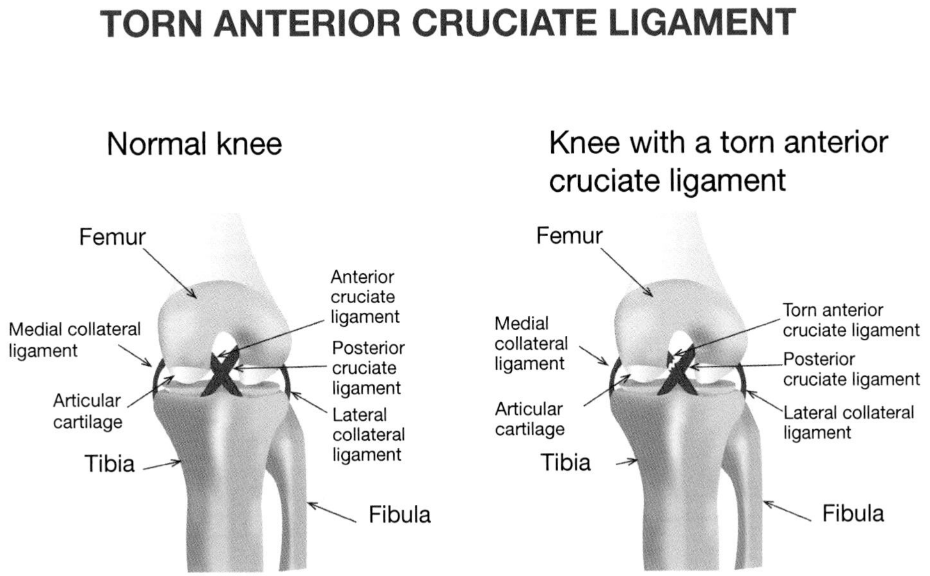

TORN ANTERIOR CRUCIATE LIGAMENT

Normal knee

Knee with a torn anterior cruciate ligament

Femur — Anterior cruciate ligament — Posterior cruciate ligament — Medial collateral ligament — Articular cartilage — Lateral collateral ligament — Tibia — Fibula

Femur — Torn anterior cruciate ligament — Posterior cruciate ligament — Medial collateral ligament — Articular cartilage — Lateral collateral ligament — Tibia — Fibula

Figure 5.23

✓ The term meaning a 'tumor of the cartilage and flesh'.

✓ In gouty arthritis, there is an elevated _____ .

✓ The term meaning 'repair of the skull'.

5.47
Chondrosarcoma

5.48
uric acid

5.49
Cranioplasty

More joint terms

These are linked with joint pain and/or findings that are not necessarily involve the ligaments or tendons.

*   **Crepitus** (**krep**-ee-tus) > palpation technique of placing a hand over the joint during motion and *feeling* the crackling of an inflamed joint. Tendinitis often presents with crepitus. Crepitus can also be auscultated (heard).

*   **Dislocation** (**dis**-low-kah-shun) > two articular surfaces are malaligned. Fingers are easily dislocated because there is little ligament support.

*   **Subluxation** (sub-**luks**-ay-shun) > similar to dislocation but it is slighter, the joint does not separate completely. This can occur between the rib head and vertebra.

*   **Contracture** (kon-**trak**-shur) > scar tissue or tight fascia locks tissue in place stopping complete motion. A tendon can contract enough making the patient use their other hand to extend the affected finger.

*   **Deformity** (dee-**form**-it-ee) > any abnormal joint or bone change such as an enlarged joint or deviated bone.

*   **Epicondylitis** (**ep**-ee-kon-dee-**lie**-tis) > inflammation of the condyles of the joint epiphysis such as the elbow or ankle.

Kitchen lab

Most of us have experienced a bursitis, sprain, dislocation, or fracture. Recount one of your injuries: what is the proper name for the injury? What therapies were used? How long did it take to get well? Did you use any equipment which could be coded in HCPCS?

5.50

Aerobic, anaerobic infections, and prosthetic issues are benefit or risk variables in the management of the skeletal and joints systems even as our technology improves. This statement may seem backward as technology is usually a friend; but the more artificial joints and hardware placed in the body to repair injury and disease, the more infections tend to occur. Any time the skin and soft tissues are interrupted to fix trauma or disease – the opportunistic bacteria, viruses, and even fungus can cause an infection.

- **Osteomyelitis** (**os**-tea-oh-my-eh-**lie**-tis) > infection of the bone (bone marrow) leading to tissue death. Osteomyelitis is a very hard infection to treat because of the incredible blood supply the bone represents. Even without skin interruption, an infection can get started due to the slowed circulation of the injury area.
  - A foot puncture in a diabetic patient increases the risk of osteomyelitis.
  - **MRSA** is an enemy to saving limbs because of the resistance to antibiotics.

- Viral arthritis or **polyarthritis** (**pohl**-ee-are-**thri**-tis) > inflammation of multiple joints secondary to viral illness. West Nile virus, Parvo-virus B-19, rubella, and hepatitis are among the many viruses causing a sudden and severe arthritis.

- **Disseminated fungal** or tubercular infections can infect the joint, its fungal growth taking up space and destroying tissue.

- *Rhizobium radiobacter* is a pathogen associated with **medical devices** such as prosthetic joints and the hardware of fracture repair. Figure 5.24 shows a colorized illustration of an infection

5.51
Pathogens associated with osteomyelitis

Staphylococcus aureus (from skin)

Streptococci can spread through soft tissues quickly

Pseudomonas aeruginosa > increasingly resistant to treatments.

CT scans may be used to evaluate for joint disease and injury but **MRI**s are considered better as they define the soft tissues of the joints well.

US may be used to determine the status of fluid in a joint.

SPECT > Single photon emission computed tomography is sensitive to bone abnormalities.

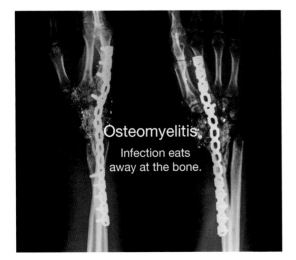

Osteomyelitis
Infection eats
away at the bone.

Figure 5.24

following fracture repair. This is one of the many reasons orthopedic surgery is done under the strictest of sterile procedures.

Spinal column disc disease/injury comes in many forms and terms. Figures 5.25 (close up) and 5.26 (as a column) illustrate disease or injury to the spine.

- **Disc/o** > denoting a disc, roundish and thick. It is also seen as 'disk'.

- **Disc**ogenic (**dis-ko-jen**-ik) > originating from the intervertebral discs.

- **Disc**ectomy (disc-**ek**-toe-me) > to remove the disc.

- **Disc**oplasty (dis-**kop**-as-tea) > repair of the disc.

5.52
Spinal injury or disease is evaluated most often now with **MRI** because it reveals the soft tissue down to the myelin sheaths surrounding the nerves.

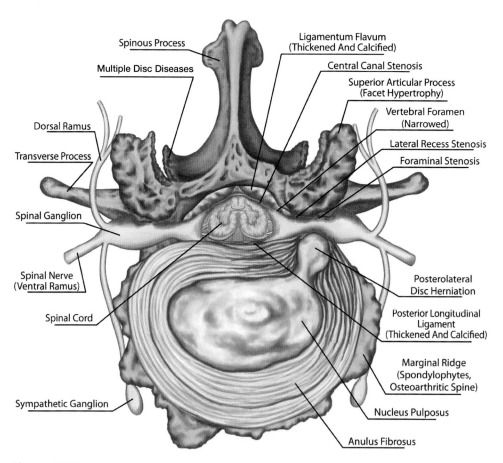

Spinous Process
Multiple Disc Diseases
Dorsal Ramus
Transverse Process
Spinal Ganglion
Spinal Nerve (Ventral Ramus)
Spinal Cord
Sympathetic Ganglion

Ligamentum Flavum (Thickened And Calcified)
Central Canal Stenosis
Superior Articular Process (Facet Hypertrophy)
Vertebral Foramen (Narrowed)
Lateral Recess Stenosis
Foraminal Stenosis
Posterolateral Disc Herniation
Posterior Longitudinal Ligament (Thickened And Calcified)
Marginal Ridge (Spondylophytes, Osteoarthritic Spine)
Nucleus Pulposus
Anulus Fibrosus

Figure 5.25

- **Spinal stenosis** (**sten**-oh-sis) > condition of narrowing. As the herniated disc protrudes, the space for the passage of the spinal cord diminishes.

- **Lumbar sprain** is not about the spinal column but the strong back muscles working to keep us upright. The paravertebral muscles will be tender and there may be spasm with motion.

Occasionally, a myelogram is done with a lumbar puncture for **CSF** review. The myelogram uses a series of plain X-rays to track injected dye.

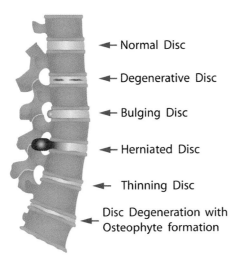

Normal Disc

Degenerative Disc

Bulging Disc

Herniated Disc

Thinning Disc

Disc Degeneration with Osteophyte formation

Figure 5.26

Genetics plays an important role in the proper development of our bones and joints. Stem cell research, gene therapy, and biological therapies are being developed as you read this to impact these conditions in positive ways.

- **Osteogenesis imperfecta** (**os**-tea-oh-**jen**-eh-sis **im**-purr-**fek**-tah) > group of inherited connective tissue disorders with abnormal collagen synthesis. Associated with brittle bone, blue sclera, bowed legs, lax joints, and fragile skin – all the places collagen is working are affected (Figure 5.27).

- **Osteopetrosis** (**os**-tea-oh-peh-**tro**-sis) > massive but fragile bone disorder due to the lack of osteoclasts. The bone just gets bigger and heavier, taking up spaces including the spinal cord and skull because there are no functional osteoclasts to carve the bone out.

- **Dwarfism** (**dworf**-izm) > individual who is unusually short, with short limbs. There are three major expressions of this growth hormone deficiency.

5.53
Imperfecta > lack of perfection

-petrosis > condition of stone

-plasia > development

Genetic identifications are written as:

Chromosome 5q sulfate transporter

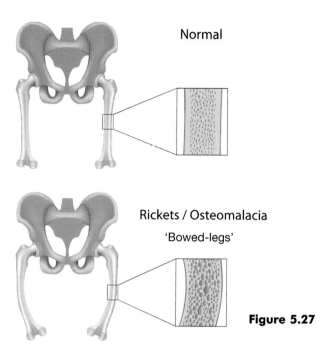

Normal

Rickets / Osteomalacia
'Bowed-legs'

Figure 5.27

- **A**chondr**o**plasia (ah-**kon**-drow-**play**-zee-ah) > abnormality in conversion of cartilage to bones particularly in the limbs. These individuals have a longer torso and large head (similar to taller persons) but shortened legs and arms.

- **S**pondyl**oepiphyseal** dysplasia (**spon**-di-low-**ep**-i-**fizz**-ee-al dis-**play**-zee-ah) > growth deficiency effecting the vertebral column as well as the arms and legs.

- **Diastrophic** dysplasia (**die**-ah-**stro**-fik dis-**play**-zee-ah) > widespread malformations of all the bones with calcification, chondritis, clubbed foot, and scoliosis.

DTDST is responsible for the changes in diastrophic dysplasia. For those who are using medical terminology and documentation these genetic markers will become part of the EHR with increasing regularity.

Limb amputation is often the duty of the orthopedic surgeon. Amputation is required for a variety of reasons including: frostbite, trauma, infection, bone tumors, and anything compromising blood supply such as diabetes or vascular disease. Limb amputation engages a team for recovery and rehabilitation. Prosthetist from Greek for 'one who adds'. This professional creates and helps patients with the artificial limb prosthetic.

- **AE** or **A-E** > above the elbow

- **BE** or **B-E** > below the elbow

- **AK** or **A-K** > above the knee

- **BK** or **B-K** > below the knee

5.54
Prosth/e > one who adds an appliance to replace a limb or other body part. An artificial eye is a prosthesis as well.

UNIT SUMMARY

1   The skeletal system includes 206+ bones stacked and configured to protect and support the rest of the body with the help of ligaments, bursae, tendons, and muscles. It is the framework for the human form. It has several other functions including producing all the blood cells over a lifetime.

2   Bone is a connective tissue built with calcium, phosphorus, water, and other trace elements forming a hard shell (compact or cortical bone) with a core at the center (medullary canal). Trabecular bone is light but strong, with arches at the proximal and distal areas of the long bones and flat bones.

3   Linking forms for bone are oste/o and osse/o. Osteoblasts are the osteon-building cells which deposit calcium to the bone. Osteoclasts carve out the calcium on demand to leach calcium into the bloodstream for use by the cells of the body.

4   The skeleton is divided by the axial and appendicular bones. The axial skeleton is the core of the body: cranium, spinal column (back bone), and rib cage. The appendicular bones make up the upper and lower extremities which are 'hung' on the axial skeletal. It takes ligaments, tendons, and muscles to keep it all together and mobile.

5   Bone has a strong blood and nerve supply allowing it to conduct its business. Bone pain may be triggered by inflammation, pressure (growing tumor), or neuropathy. Medications, radiation therapy, and biofeedback all have the potential to limit pain.

6   Bone fractures (Fx) are common. There are four injury characteristics to be considered: 1) Open or closed; 2) Simple or comminuted; 3) Trauma or pathological; and 4) Type and location of the fracture. Repair of fractures may be closed by casting and/or an operative procedure. Any 'hardware' used will be coded and tracked via the ICD-10-PCS and HCPCS.

7   Bones are susceptible to cancers, infections, and several genetic diseases. After injuries, the most commonplace condition of the bone is osteoporosis – the loss of the calcium matrix weakening bone.

8   Disease and injury of the joints may involve the bone but more often it is a function of the synovial joints with their joint space and ligaments giving way to a variety of concerns. Arthritis, inflammation of the joint, comes in many types from the very destructive rheumatoid arthritis to a reactive viral polyarthritis.

9   Orthopedists, rheumatologists, physical and occupational therapies are experts in prosthetics and orthotics. These are some of the professionals who help those with injury or illness of the bones and joints.

UNIT WORD PARTS

Word roots with linking vowel		
Adip/o or Lip/o > fat	Ankyl/o > bent, crooked	Articul/o or arthr/o > joint
Burs/o > bursa	Calcane/o > heel bone	Carp/o > wrist
Cervic/o > neck	Chondr/o > cartilage	Cost/o > ribs
Crani/o > skull, cranium	Dent/o or Odont/o > teeth	Disc/o > disc, round/thick
Fasci/o > fiber, fascia, band	Ili/o > Ilium	Ischi/o > ischium
Myel/o > bone marrow or spinal cord	Orth/o > straight	Oste/o; osse/o > bone
Phag/o > to eat	Prosth/e > to add on, appliance	Pub/o > pubic
Rachi/o or Spondyl/o > spine	Radi/o > radiating, arm	Sarc/o > flesh
Tal/o > talus	Tars/o > ankle	Ten/o, Tend/o, Tendin/o, and Tenon/o > tendon
Tibi/o > lower leg, tibia	Uln/o > ulnar	Vertebr/o > back bone

Prefixes: attached to the front of the word root to change meaning		
A-, An- > no, not, absent	Ambi- > two ways	Bi- > two
Dia- > through or between	Dys- > poor, bad, difficult	Endo- > inner, inside
Hyper- > more than, increased	Hypo- > less than, decreased	Mal- > poor, bad
Meta- > beyond, change	Non- > none, absent	Para- > near, beside, departure from normal
Peri- > around, about, near	Poly- > many	

Suffixes change the meaning of the word, linking vowel is usually 'o' with consonants		
-algia, -dynia > pain	-blast > building, immature cells	-clast > carving out, a breaking-down cell
-dystrophy > poor development	-lysis > to destroy, break down	-malacia > softening
-oma > tumor	-penia > less than, not enough	-petrosis > condition of stone

Suffixes *continued*		
-physis > growth	-plasty > repair	-poiesis > condition of making
-poikilo > mottled, varied	-porosis > condition of pores	-sclerosis > condition of hardening

Acronyms, abbreviations, and initial sets		
ACL > anterior cruciate ligament	AE > above the elbow	AK > above the knee
BE > below the elbow	BK > below the knee	Ca^{++} > calcium
CMS > Centers of Medicare and Medicaid Services	CSF > cerebral spinal fluid	DC > doctor of chiropractor
DIP > distal interphalangeal	DJD > degenerative joint disease	DMARDs > disease-modifying rheumatoid arthritis drugs
DO > doctor of osteopath	EBRT > external beam radiation therapy	FROM > full range of motion
Fx > fracture	GH > growth hormone	HCPCS > Healthcare Common Procedure Coding System
LCL > lateral collateral ligament	MCL > medial collateral ligament	MCP > metacarpophalangeal
MRSA > methicillin resistant staphylococcus aureus	MTP > metatarsophalangeal	NSAIDs > nonsteroidal anti-inflammatory drugs
OA > osteoarthritis	OREF > open reduction external fixation	ORIF > open reduction internal fixation
OT > occupational therapist	OTA > OT assistant	P > phosphorus
PCL > posterior cruciate ligament	PCS > Procedure coding system	PIP > proximal interphalangeal
PT > physical therapist	PTA > PT assistant	PTH > parathyroid hormone
RA > rheumatoid arthritis	RICE > rest, ice, compression, and elevation	RT > radiation therapy (in this context)
Spinal numbering: C1 to C7 cervical T1 to T12 thoracic L1 to L5 lumbar	Tib/Fib > tibia and fibula	TMJ > temporomandibular joint

UNIT WORKSHEETS

Building terms: Use the proper prefix/word root/linking vowel/suffix as appropriate.

Example: to cut into the stomach > gastr/o/tomy

a) To repair cartilage > _____

b) Disease of the joints > _____

c) Inflammation of the bone and bone marrow > _____

d) A cell building bone > _____

e) Inflammation of the ribs and cartilage > _____

f) A specialist in joint disease > _____

Know your acronyms and initial sets! For the acronym/initial sets given, spell it out correctly.

a) MRSA   _____

b) ORIF   _____

c) DMARD   _____

d) PTA   _____

e) ACL   _____

f) DIP   _____

g) OA   _____

h) RICE   _____

Best choice: Pick the most appropriate answer.

1 The femoral head fits into the
   a) Patella fossa   c) Glenoid fossa
   b) Iliac crest   d) Acetabulum

2 The shaft of the long bone is the
   a) Epiphysis   c) Biaphysis
   b) Diaphysis   d) Physis

3 Only mobile bone in the cranium
   a) Hyoid   c) Maxilla
   b) Ethmoid   d) Mandible

4 The functional unit of the bone is the
   a) Osteon   c) Glomerulus
   b) Alveoli   d) Chondrocytes

5 The best book to code non–durable medical materials is the
   a) ICD-10-CM   c) HCPCS
   b) ICD-10- PCS   d) HIPAA

Name the bone or joint condition! Based on the description and/or function, name the bone or joint condition.

a) Fracture at an angle across the bone _____

b) Inflammation of the connective tissue sac with gel-like middle _____

c) Abnormality in conversion of cartilage to bones particularly in the limbs _____

d) Narrowing of the spinal canal is _____

e) Fracture which is crushed, compressed, or in several pieces is _____

f) Place a hand over a joint and 'feel' the crackling _____

g) *Rhizobium radiobacter* is a pathogen associated with _____

Multiple correct: Select ALL the correct answers to the question or statement given.

1 Which of the following linking forms are specific for 'spine > backbone'
   a) ungu/o   c) myel/o   e) vertebr/o
   b) spondyl/o   d) rachi/o   f) xiph/o

2 Which of the following bones are part of the axial skeleton?
   a) Zygomatic   c) Xiphoid process e) Parietal
   b) Scapul   d) Coccyx   f) Maxilla

3 Which of the following are part of the appendicular skeleton?
   a) Patella   c) Talus   e) Inferior concha
   b) Vomer   d) Ulna   f) Femur

Spelling challenge! Circle the correct spelling based on the definition given.

1 'Growth deficiency of the vertebral column and limbs'

   Achrondroplasia   Vertebrodisplagia   Rachiosystis   Spondyloepiphyseal

2 'Slight dislocation of a joint'

   Asymmetric   Subluxation   Hypovursion   Retroluxation

Define the term: Spelling *does* count in your definition too!

1 Subluxation > _____

2 Periosteum > _____

3 Kyphosis > _____

4 Erythropoietin > _____

5 Menisci > _____

6 Inversion > _____

7 Osteosarcoma > _____

8 Hyoid > _____

Find the bone to build a skeleton! Using the words – match the definition given. Some may not be used. It is recommended you study all of the choices.

C1	maxilla	occiput	teeth	carpals
pollex	clavicle	mandible	coxal	humerus
metatarsals	calcaneus	vertebrae	stapes	femur
sternum	C2	temporal	phalanges	acetabulum
parietal	scapula	fibula	tibia	

1 _____ Heel bone

2 _____ Shoulder blade

3 _____ Foot bones

4 _____ Back of the skull

5 _____ Breast bone

6 _____ Collar bone

7 _____ Hold the upper teeth

8 _____ Smallest bone

9 _____ Saucer in Latin

10 _____ Bears all the weight of femur

Matching: Bone terms or conditions, some will not be used.

	Letter	Defined as
Greenstick		a) associated with TMJ pain
Osteoporosis		b) associated with high uric acid
Cartilage		c) incomplete fracture in children
Manubrium		d) flat bone suture
Osteomyelitis		e) DEXA scan can evaluate this bone condition
Mandible		f) this can decrease the pain of bone metastasis
Sarcoma		g) heavy collagen matrix on the end of bones
Gout		h) superior section of the breast bone
		i) inflammation of the bone marrow
		j) Ewing's is this type of tumor

An essay: What are the goals of the physical therapy team in helping a patient post-orthopedic surgery? Who makes up the team?

Note challenge: Define the underlined terms and spell out the acronyms/initial sets. You may need to look up a few terms. Answer the questions which follow. Student is reminded this is an incomplete SOAP note used for the learning experience. Do not use this for patient encounters.

S. Mia is a 67 yo woman with a history of <u>HTN</u>; breast cancer, disease free × 5 yrs; and <u>OA</u>. She is seen for a preop physical prior to knee joint replacement. Left knee is worse than right knee per the patient. Patient has lost 50# prior to surgery. Currently 180# at home. No previous joint surgeries. Has successfully added exercise to daily activities.

O. Mia is a well appearing 67 yo in NAD. VS: 132/76, 16, 72, 98.6, pulse ox 97%.

Left knee with marked <u>crepitus</u> and palpable <u>osteophytes</u>. Knee is tender without <u>erythema, edema</u>, or heat. Pain with full <u>extension</u>. <u>Flexion</u> to 95 degrees. Pulses at the <u>dorsal pedis, posterior tibial</u>, and <u>popiteal</u> pulses are full and regular. <u>No evidence of vascular or infectious diseases.</u> X-ray: Left Knee <u>lateral</u> view with total loss of joint space, multiple osteophytes and some early calcifications of the patellar tendon (Figure 5.28).

OA KNEE LEFT

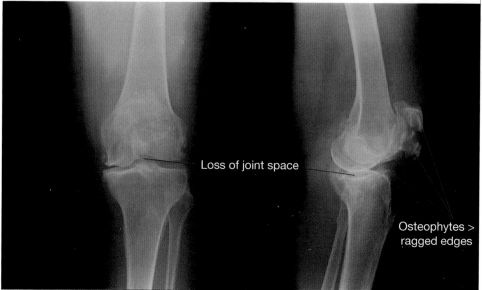

Loss of joint space

Osteophytes > ragged edges

Figure 5.28

A. Osteoarthritis, ready for total joint replacement, Left Knee

P. Schedule surgery

- Anticipate need for ambulatory scooter and then walker post-surgery.

- Arrange for pneumatic leg compression for home use in 1st week of recovery.

- Arrange post op PT visit 24 hours after surgery.

- Consent discussed and signed.

Questions

1 As above, define the underlined terms and spell out the acronyms or initial sets.

2 'No evidence of vascular or infectious diseases', based on the focus on this sentence, why is this important prior to a joint surgery?

3 What is the importance of noting the weight loss of this patient in this setting?

4 What HCPCS materials will this patient need based on the note? Are there other things the patient may need? (Think dressings)

Unit 6

The muscles

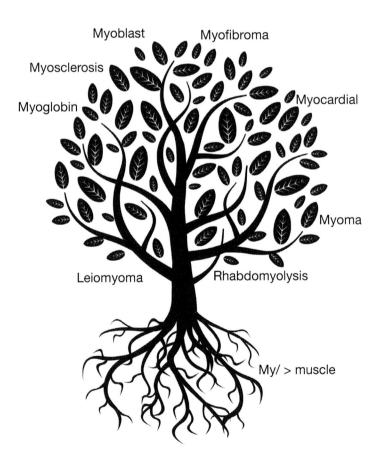

Myoblast

Myofibroma

Myosclerosis

Myocardial

Myoglobin

Myoma

Leiomyoma

Rhabdomyolysis

My/ > muscle

TARGETED LEARNING

1 Recognize word parts and assemble medical terms as related to the anatomy of the muscles and motion.

2 Correctly construct, define, pronounce, and spell medical terms.

3 Relate muscle and motion conditions with appropriate diagnostic evaluation and pharmacotherapeutics.

4 Link muscle illness and injury with documentation for rehabilitation and long-term care facilities.

5 Associate the *current procedural terminology* (**cpt**®) use for outpatient settings in the care of patients with muscle illness or injury.

KEY WORD PARTS

Word roots with linking vowel	Prefixes	Suffixes
Condyl/o > condyle	A- or An-	-algia
Erg/o > work	Apo-	-cele
Fasci/o > fascia, connective band	Auto-	-gram or -graphy
Kines/o, Kinesi/o > movement	Bi- or Di-	-ity
Lei/o > smooth	Brady-	-lysis
Muscul/o; My/o or Myos/o > muscle	Dys-	-plegia
Neur/o > nerve or sinew	Epi-	-rrhaphy
Rhabd/o > striated, skeletal	Iso-	-spasm
Tendin/o, Ten/o, or Tend/o > tendon	Peri-	-sthenia
Ton/o > tone, stretch	Polio-	-trophy

MUSCLEMEN AND -WOMEN

Muscle building eons ago was more about survival than a feat of strength or achieving the perfect body form. The beginnings of weight lifting as a sport return to the same Greeks who were writing the first anatomy books. The ancient Olympic Games were all about strength and perhaps some aesthetics too. Most cultures have a history of those who enjoy the sport and the look of a hard six-pack. In India, using particular equipment to focus on specific muscles goes back to the eleventh century. It would be transformed into many of today's equipment types.

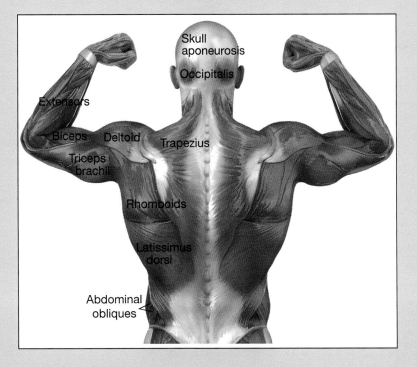

Figure 6.2

In North America, musclemen started in the circus (circa 1790s) but over time the sport and the aesthetics of Greece prevailed. The value weight lifting could provide to wellness became increasingly evident. Regular exercise including weight lifting is good for our bone, muscle, cardiac, and pulmonary health. Elders are encouraged to continue weight lifting to improve strength and balance. As with all activities, finding the equilibrium of health, body form, and strength is the goal. Slow, steady, progressive weight resistance is the way to go to avoid injury.

THE MUSCLES

The muscles move us, generate heat, allow flexibility, move our blood around and wastes out, and cushion the body. Moving is more than walking or throwing a ball. The smooth muscles of the body move air into the bronchial tubes and push food through the gastrointestinal tract. The unique cardiac muscle moves blood through a closed system of vessels.

Skeletal muscles provide the leverage to move the bones via contraction. Skeletal muscles perform all of our *voluntary* action (Figure 6.3).

- **Rhabd/o** > resembling a rod, striated > formal word root for skeletal muscle. It is used for specific skeletal muscle conditions such as rhabdomyolysis (**rab**-doe-my-**oh**-lie-sis). Rhabdomyolysis is the destruction of skeletal muscle tissues, which may lead to renal failure.
  - Rhabdomyosarcoma (**rab**-doe-**my**-oh-sar-**ko**-ma) > an aggressive malignant muscle tumor.

- Ton/o > stretching, tension > constant skeletal muscle function supports posture and potential movement even during sleep. **Tonicity** (toe-**nis**-i-tea) is the quality of having tone.
  - **Atony** (**at**-oh-knee) > no tone or tension, it also seen as atonia or atonic.

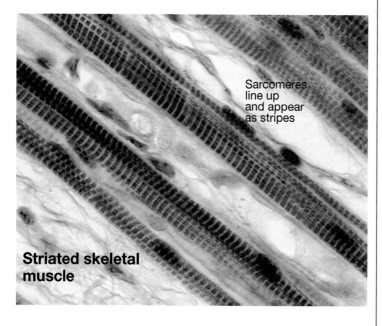

Sarcomeres line up and appear as stripes

Striated skeletal muscle

6.1
Skeletal muscle >
Striated muscles are attached to the skeleton

Skelet/o > dried-up (bones)

Rhabd/o > striated

My/o > muscle

Myos/o > muscle

Muscul/o > muscle

Electr/o > spark

Contract > Latin for 'draw together'

Functions

Motion

Posture

Body heat

Respiration

Communication

Bind and cushion

Stores myoglobin

Muscle tone is measured by a

Myogram > the record, product of a muscle recording

Myography > the process of recording muscle

Myograph > the instrument used

Figure 6.3

- **Dystonia** (dis-**toe**-knee-a) > poor tone or tension, is also seen as dystonic.
- **Isotonic** (**eye**-sew-**tohn**-ik) > same tension > contraction where the tone stays the same as the length of the muscle changes. This is dynamic tension; there is motion at the joint.
- **Isometric** (**eye**-sew-**met**-rik) > same measure > contraction where the tone increases without changing the length of the muscle. Isometric is static tension, creating tension with no motion.

• Pyr/o > heat, temperature > skeletal muscles generate most of our heat via catabolism.

LIKE ALERT!

Pyr/o is heat or temperature; Py/o is pus.

• The skeletal muscles store the muscle protein, **myoglobin**, helping with sudden energy needs. It supplies extra oxygen and fuel. Myoglobin also gives our skeletal muscles their deep red coloration.

Smooth muscles are involuntary muscles, lei/o > smooth. These muscles are often called the visceral muscles. They move the contents of the bladder, digestive, respiratory, circulation, and reproductive tracts.

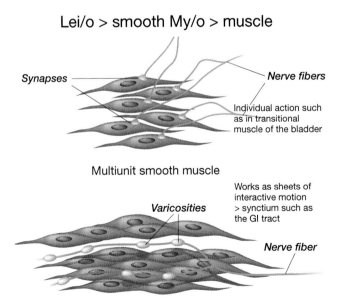

Lei/o > smooth My/o > muscle

Synapses

Nerve fibers

Individual action such as in transitional muscle of the bladder

Multiunit smooth muscle

Varicosities

Works as sheets of interactive motion > synctium such as the GI tract

Nerve fiber

Single-unit smooth muscle

6.2
Smooth muscle >

Lei/o > smooth

Viscer/o > body organs

The word root, lei/o is seen with

Leiomyoma > smooth muscle tumor

Leiomyofibroma > smooth muscle and fibrous tumor

Functions
Move the walls of hollow organs such as mixing in the stomach.

Contributes some body heat especially during sleep.

Figure 6.4

The visceral smooth muscles are single-units joined in large sheets to rhythmically move in sequence.

- Cells working together in near simultaneous action is called a **syncytium** (sin-**sish**-ee-um).

- As the muscles contract they push contents along the path, this is called **peristalsis** in the GI tract.

- These muscles have a degree of auto-rhythmicity (aw-toe rith-mis-i-tea), making them 'self-starters'. Examples: the GI tract and urogenital tract.

The **cardiac muscle** is exclusive to the heart – it has qualities of the other types. The tissue looks a little striated but the pieces are short and irregular – interlocking like puzzle pieces. This enables the muscle to contract as one, thousands of times a day.

- **Cardi/o** > heart > weighs about 3/4 pound and is the size of a fist.

- **Cardiac** (**kar**-dee-ak) > pertaining to the heart.

- **Cardiomyopathy** (**kar**-dee-oh-my-**op**-ath-ee) > disease of the heart muscle.

6.3
Cardiac muscle >
Cardi/o > heart

Function
Moves the walls of the heart to circulate blood.

The left is stronger than the right as it pumps blood to the entire body.

Word parts
-ac > pertaining to
-al > pertaining to
-dynia > pain
-ectasia > dilatation
-cele > herniation
-centesis > remove fluid

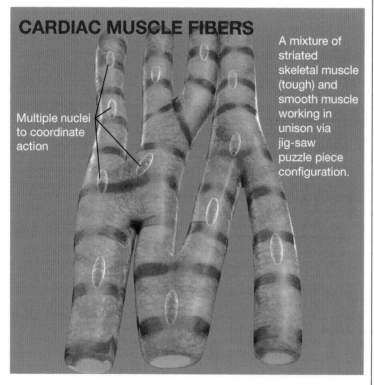

CARDIAC MUSCLE FIBERS

Multiple nuclei to coordinate action

A mixture of striated skeletal muscle (tough) and smooth muscle working in unison via jig-saw puzzle piece configuration.

Figure 6.5

– **Cardiodynia** (**kar**-dee-oh-**dine**-ee-ah) > pain in the heart.

– **Cardiogram** (**kar**-dee-oh-gram) > tracing record of the heart's electrical impulses.

✓ Construct a medical term for 'destruction of skeletal muscle' ____/__/__/__/_____

✓ The linking form for 'smooth' and 'muscle' are _____ and _____ .

✓ The primary function of the cardiac muscle is _____ .

6.4
Rhabd/o/my/o/lysis

6.5
lei/o and my/o

6.6
to circulate blood

Word building

Using the word roots with the linking vowel to build as many valid terms with the suffixes given. Please define each term.

My/o Cardi/o Rhabd/o

–itis –ist –dynia –lysis –oma –tomy –ectomy –blast –pathy

Can you make any compound words?

6.7
The instructor has the list!

With **640 muscles** it can be a challenge to learn them all, the key is understanding the nomenclature which follows. Most muscles are paired (bilateral), taking the challenge down to about 320. The single muscles tend to occur around the head and neck such as the frontalis, occipital, and platysma.

Few muscles work independently of all the others. They work as **synergists** (**sin**-er-jist) to get the work of the day done. They also work opposite of each other as **antagonists** (an-**tag**-oh-nist) such as the quadriceps of the anterior leg and hamstrings of the posterior leg. They take turns contracting allowing us to walk or jump without interruption.

• There are many sets at angles to each other such as the internal and external intracostals; the exterior and interior obliques of the abdominal muscles; and the anterior serratus superior set and the posterior inferior set.

• There are layers of muscles we never think about – both large and small. These are some of the deep muscles:

– The tiny interosseus muscles abduct/adduct our fingers and toes.

6.8
Synergist > Aids in the action of another muscle.

Agonist > a muscle that produces a specific motion, a primary mover.

Antagonist > a muscle that provides resistance to the primary mover.

Linea alba > the confluence aponeurosis of four abdominal muscle sets in the mid-sagittal line:

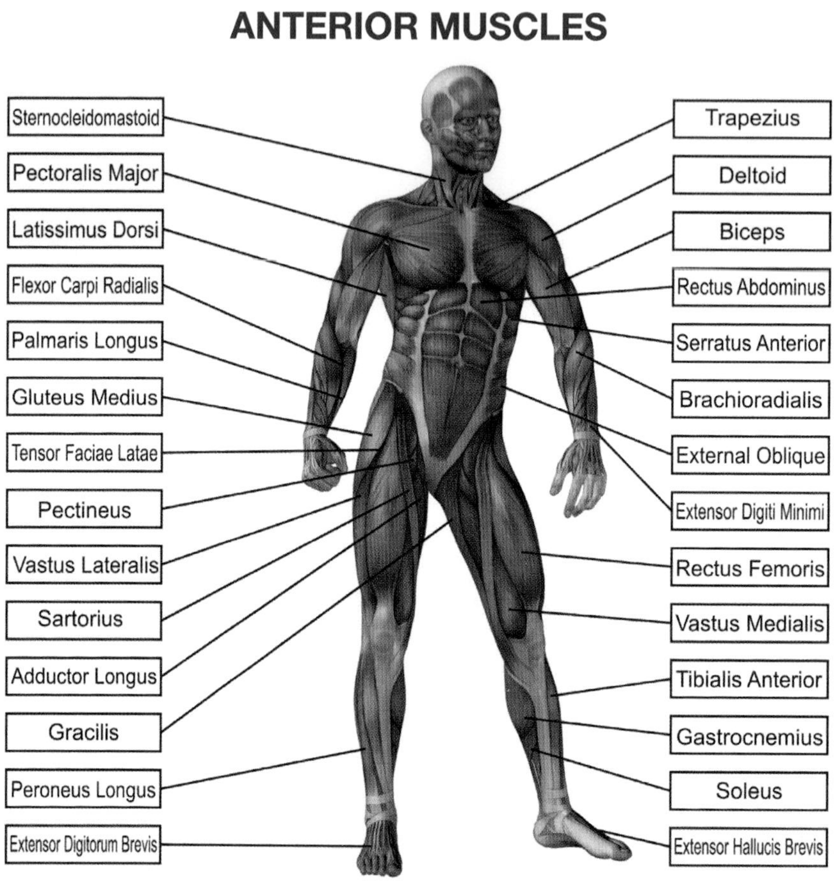

ANTERIOR MUSCLES

Sternocleidomastoid	Trapezius
Pectoralis Major	Deltoid
Latissimus Dorsi	Biceps
Flexor Carpi Radialis	Rectus Abdominus
Palmaris Longus	Serratus Anterior
Gluteus Medius	Brachioradialis
Tensor Faciae Latae	External Oblique
Pectineus	Extensor Digiti Minimi
Vastus Lateralis	Rectus Femoris
Sartorius	Vastus Medialis
Adductor Longus	Tibialis Anterior
Gracilis	Gastrocnemius
Peroneus Longus	Soleus
Extensor Digitorum Brevis	Extensor Hallucis Brevis

Figure 6.6

For a medical terminology course knowing the location and function of all the muscles is not necessary. Knowing their names *is* important.

- Long, slender muscles meshing in and around the length of the spine.
  - o Iliocostalis thoracis > **il**-ee-oh-kos-**tah**-lis.
  - o Semispinalis thoracis > **sem**-ee-spy-**nah**-lis.
  - o Spinalis thoracis > **spy**-nal-is tho-**ray**-sis.
  - o Interspinales > **in**-tur-spy-**nah**-les.
  - o Multifidus > mul-**tif**-i-dus.
- Many muscle groups are linked with others via the wide, strong **aponeurosis** (ap-oh-**nur**-oh-sis). In the abdomen, these interconnect the four sets of muscles like a girdle, keeping the body parts stable yet mobile.

External oblique, Abdominal rectus, Internal obliques, and Transverse abdominis.

This is a favorite surgical incision site as it avoids significant muscle damage.

APONEUROSIS

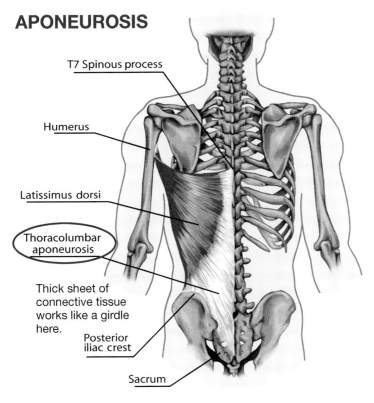

T7 Spinous process

Humerus

Latissimus dorsi

Thoracolumbar aponeurosis

Thick sheet of connective tissue works like a girdle here.

Posterior iliac crest

Sacrum

Figure 6.7

As with the skin and skeleton, many of the terms related to muscles are descriptive concerning their form and function. In the case of skeletal muscles, the configuration (Figure 6.8) of the muscle fibers will have much to do with the action performed by the muscle.

- **Convergent** (kon-**vur**-jent) > tending to a common point > this muscle will have a broad origin point inserting into a common point such as the pectoralis major.

- **Parallel** (**par**-ah-lel) > fibers running side by side, equidistant. These muscles are also called **strap** muscles such as the rectus abdominis; many of the neck muscles and the sartorius muscle of the leg. Rect/o > straight, upright > 'to stand erect' is to stand straight up.

- **Circular** (sir-**Q**-lar) > forms a circle > these muscles help form our orifices such as the mouth, anus, and eye orbits.

- **Fusiform** (**fue**-see-form) > spindle shaped > these muscles are bulky and have a muscle belly. A fusiform muscle belly generates the 'muscle bump' when we are showing off the biceps brachii. Check out your fusiform muscle now ☺.

6.9
Origin > Latin for 'source'. It is the least mobile and the most stable attachment of the muscle.

Insertion > Latin for 'planting in'. This is the most mobile muscle attachment; it is where the action of moving the skeleton occurs.

MUSCLE TYPES

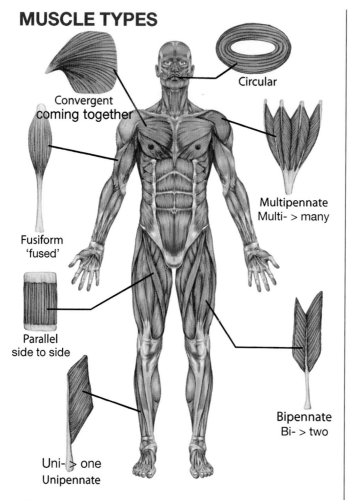

Figure 6.8

- **Pennate** (**pen**-nate) > resembling a feather > as there are different feathers so there are three pennate muscle types.

  – Unipennate (**U**-knee-**pen**-nate) > one or a single feather > these muscle fibers will attach to only one side such as the soleus of the leg.

  – Bipennate (buy-**pen**-nate) > two feathers > these muscles will have fibers on both sides in a chevron pattern such as the rectus femoris (part of the quadriceps).

  – Multipennate (**mul**-tea-**pen**-nate) > many feathers > these are quite similar to the convergent muscle type but the fascicles or fibers are in a more distinct feather pattern as seen at the deltoid. This configuration allows the muscle to drape the 'corner'.

Fascicles > from the word root fasci/o > band or bundle of muscle fibers (or nerve). The directions of the fascicles help determine function.

- **Spiral** (**spy**-ral) > twist or curving > these muscles are similar to the convergent as well and include a slight twist on the way to the insertion. The latissimus dorsi of the posterior chest is an example.

Kitchen lab

Put your muscles to work for you. For each action below note which muscle type is at work?

1 Make a fist and flex your elbow strongly like Popeye.

2 Rotate your head hard to the right. What kind of muscle is your sternocleidomastoid muscle?

3 Squint your eyes.

Muscle naming has had many inputs over the centuries and it continues even today as anatomists redefine individual muscles which were not noted in the past. In fact, in the anatomy books of the 1960s humans are reported to have about 600 muscles and today it is up to 640 muscles. Science and medicine are always evolving.

- **Number of heads** or origins – these have two, three, or four points of origins usually grouped together.
    - Biceps > two heads > anterior arm muscle > **buy**-seps **break**-ee-i. There is also a biceps femoris in the leg.
    - Triceps > three heads > posterior arm muscle > **tri**-seps **break**-ee-i.
    - Quadriceps > four heads > anterior set of leg muscles > **qwa**-dree-seps **fem**-or-is.
    - Digastric (die-**gas**-trik) > having two bellies > muscle of swallowing attached to the hyoid bone in the neck.

- **Direction** of fascicles, as seen with the body planes and directions.
    - Internal **oblique** > at an angle.
    - **Rectus** abdominis > straight.
    - **Trans**verse > across.

- **Location** is another naming process
    - **Ster**nocleido**m**astoid (**SCM**) > sternum, clavicle, and mastoid process > **stir**-no-**klie**-eh-doe-**mas**-toyd (Figure 6.9).
    - **Pectoralis** major (**pek**-tor-al-is) > chest.
    - **Ex**ternal oblique > outside > abdominal muscle.

6.10

Did You **Know?**

Some muscles were named by how people use them.

Sartorius > is based on how a tailor sits cross-legged when sewing or the Lotus position in yoga. Sartor > Latin for tailor

6.11

Did You **Know?**

A crooked trumpet > Latin is 'buccina', the source of the name of the cheek muscle, the **buccinator** (**buk**-see-**nay**-tor).

STERNOCLEIDMOMASTOID MUSCLES (SCM)

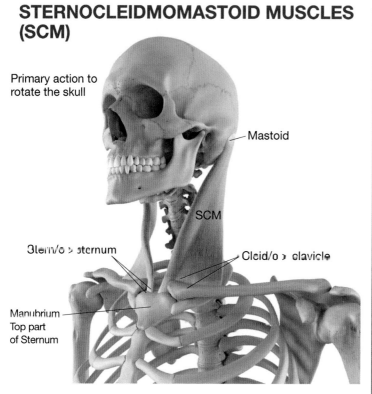

Primary action to rotate the skull

Mastoid

SCM

Stern/o > sternum

Cleid/o > clavicle

Manubrium
Top part
of Sternum

Figure 6.9

- **Brachial**is (**bray**-key-al-is) > pertaining to the arm.
- **Glute**us minimus (glue-**tea**-us min-ee-mus) > buttocks.
- **Tibial**is anterior (tib-ee-a-lis) > tibia.

- **Function** is another nomenclature method – how it moves the skeleton by extension, flexion, abduction, or adduction.
  - **Extensor** digitorum (eks-**ten**-sor dij-i-**tor**-um) > extends the digits.
  - **Flexor** carpi radialis (**fleks**-or **kar**-pee ray-dee-a-lis) > flexes the index finger.
  - **Ad**ductor magnus (ad-**duk**-tor **mag**-nus) > moving the thigh toward the center.
  - **Ab**ductor hallucis (ab-**duk**-tor **hal**-u-sis) > moving the great toe away from the center.
- The **size** of a muscle is a naming method.
  - Pectoralis **major** > large.
  - Gluteus **maximus** > maximum, largest, larger.

When an animal was cut for meat and it was hung by the tendons, the posterior leg muscles were called the **hamstrings**.

6.12

Did You Know?

The largest, strongest, and widest tendon of the body is the **Achilles** tendon, which attaches the gastrocnemius and soleus muscles of the calf to the calcaneus (heel bone). It is named for the place

- **Vastus** lateralis > vast, huge.
- Adductor **magnus** > vast, huge.
- Teres **minor** > small, smaller.
- Gluteus **minimus** > tiny, smallest.
- Gluteus **medius** > middle.
- Extensor pollicis **brevis** > short.
- Adductor **longus** > long.
- **Latissimus** dorsi > very wide.
- **Longissimus** capitis> very long.

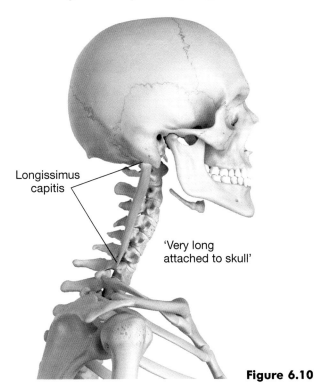

Longissimus
capitis

'Very long
attached to skull'

Figure 6.10

- The final nomenclature scheme is by **shape** as defined from the Latin and some geometry.
  - Deltoid (**del**-toyd) > triangular.
  - Trapezius (tra-**pee**-zee-us) > trapezoid.
  - Serratus (seh-**rate**-us) > notched.
  - Teres (**tear**-ez) > rounded, smooth.
  - Pectinate (**pek**-tea-nate) > comb-like.
  - Quadratus (qwah-**dra**-tus) > square-like.

of 'vulnerability' in Achilles of Greek mythology. Today, it is properly called the **calcaneal tendon**.

A modern slang phrase concerning muscles is '**six pack abs**'. These are the rectus abdominis muscles which have five tendinous anchors to keep the muscle from buckling up with motion.

6.13

Muscle abbreviations:

Quads > quadriceps of the anterior leg

Pecs > pectoralis major and minor of the chest

- Platys (platz) > flat, wide.
- Rhomboid (**rohm**-boyd) > geometric rhomboid.
- Gracilis (**gras**-i-lis) > slender.
- Orbicularis (or-**bik**-U-**la**-ris) > round, circular.
- Piriformis (**peer**-ee-**form**-is) > wedge-shaped.

Abs > abdominal muscles

Hamstrings > posterior leg muscles

Gluts > gluteus set

✓ What is the term for movement toward the center?

6.14 Adduction

✓ 'Pectoralis' pertains to this region?

6.15 Chest

✓ A muscle set with four elements is the _____ .

6.16 quadriceps

REHABILITATION

Re-habilitas > Latin for 'bring back to normal, to make fit again'. Whether a patient is recovering from a hip replacement, a stroke, a heart attack, or an abdominal surgery all the muscle types need to mend, to be made fit again. When the human body sustains injury or illness with or without a surgery, the muscles need to recover.

- Skeletal muscles lose some level of strength, tone, and endurance within 3 days of illness or injury.

- The heart must accommodate an increase in adrenaline, inflammation changes, and excess fluids associated with illness or injury.

- The smooth muscles of the gut slow. The intestine may even stop (an ileus) secondary to illness or trauma leading to constipation and even bowel blockage.

- The lack of activity slows the movement of bronchial secretions and the ability to cough is lessened. This puts the patient at risk of pneumonia.

Rehabilitation facilities and programs address all these muscle issues with a team approach. They will work simultaneously to decrease the strain of the injury or illness while improving the activity level of the patient.

- Respiratory therapy (**RT**) will assist the patient in 'exercising' the diaphragm to open up sticky alveoli and move air regularly. From the simple spirometer (breath meter) to **CPAP** (continuous positive airway pressure) for sleep apnea, the goal is to improve gas exchange.

- Physical therapy (**PT**) focuses on restoring mobility skills, flexibility, and strength of tired or injured joints and muscles.

- Occupational therapy (**OT**) aid the patient's return to the activities of daily living (**ADL**s) such as dressing, grooming, and moving around the house safely.

- Speech and language pathology (**SLP**) is committed to helping an injured or ill patient get back to clear speech and safe swallowing.

- Therapeutic recreation (**TR**) is designed to put all the work of recuperation into a fun and useful recognition, strengthening, and coordination activity.

- Pharmacy has a role in rehabilitation too. Many medications create a sluggish gut or cause sedation, and this can retard the activity of the patient. The pharmacist will work with providers to eliminate medications which may slow improvement while providing pain and other symptom control.

As always, the documentation of all this therapy is vital to the continuity of care for the patient. The daily SOAP notes must reflect the actual status of the patient and objective measurements of their improvement.

MOTION

Motion depends on the functional units of the muscle, the sarcomere (**sar**-ko-meer). Its many proteins build an elastic, linear muscle fiber called the myofibril (**my**-oh-**fie**-brils) > tiny muscles. Each muscle has millions of fibrils wrapped in fascia (**fash**-ee-ah); the tough connective tissue makes up tendons and ligaments too.

When the muscle is weak or not moving at all, discovering the source of the blockage includes several possibilities – the brain, spinal cord, muscles, circulation, hormones, or any combination of the systems. The linking form for motion or movement is kine/o or kinesi/o.

- **Kinesis** (ki-**knee**-sis) > movement induced by a stimuli.

- **Kinesiology** (ki-**knee**-see-**ol**-oh-gee) > the science or study of motion.

- **Kinesalgia** (**ki**-neh-**sal**-gee-ah) > painful movement.

- **Dyskinesia** (**dis**-key-**knee**-see-ah) > difficult or poor movement.

- **Bradykinesia** (**braid**-ee-ki-knee-**see**-ah) > slow to motion, halting movement. Parkinsonism is a brain deficiency of the neurotransmitter, dopamine, and characterized by bradykinesia, the rigidity of motion, cogwheeling, muscular tremors, and droopy posture (Figure 6.12). The brain signals are not connecting consistently with the muscle junctions.

6.17
The major muscle proteins include:
Actin
Myosin
Troponin
Tropomyosin
Titin

Cogwheeling >
while actively resisting movement the muscle 'stutters'. The provider pulls the arm down and it gives like it is stuck in a cogwheel, giving intermittently.

STRUCTURE OF SKELETAL MUSCLE

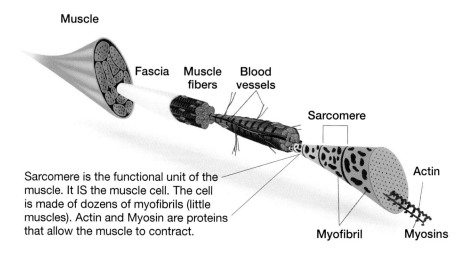

Muscle

Fascia   Muscle   Blood
         fibers   vessels

Sarcomere

Actin

Sarcomere is the functional unit of the
muscle. It IS the muscle cell. The cell
is made of dozens of myofibrils (little
muscles). Actin and Myosin are proteins
that allow the muscle to contract.

Myofibril   Myosins

Figure 6.11

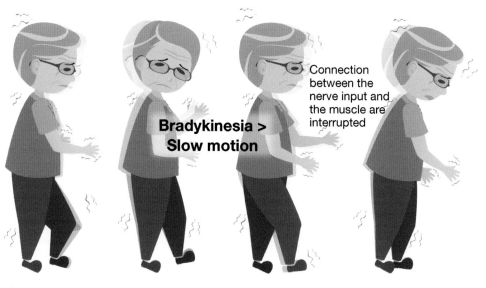

Bradykinesia >
Slow motion

Connection
between the
nerve input and
the muscle are
interrupted

Figure 6.12

- **Proprioception** (**pro**-pre-oh-**cep**-shun) > the ability to know where a limb is in space without looking. Our skeletal muscles have special sensors, the **muscle spindle**. These sense the stretch of the muscle. The fibrous capsule in the joints has similar sense fibers.

    – A proprioceptive or balance exercise using a **wobble board** after an ankle sprain is depicted by Figure 6.13.

    – Proprioception is lost in the feet with diabetes and vascular diseases causing patients to look down when walking.

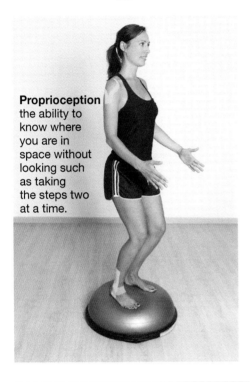

Proprioception the ability to know where you are in space without looking such as taking the steps two at a time.

Figure 6.13

Kitchen lab

1) While looking at your feet, walk heel to toe for 5 feet. Now look up and do it again. Did you hit heel to toe? Or were you off balance?

2) With arms out, touch index finger to your nose, alternating right and left hand. Now close your eyes and do it again. Did you find your nose?

6.18

- **Ataxia** (aa-**tak**-see-ah) > 'no order', the inability to coordinate muscle motion. This term is frequently used for description of walking, our gait.

6.19
These terms are seen with trauma or

- **Asterixis** (as-tur-**ik**-is) > 'no fixed position', involuntary jerking movements. This is seen in the hands and overall posture during metabolic or toxic encephalopathy, disease inside the brain.

- **Clonus** (**cloy**-nus) > 'a tumult', rapid contractions and relaxation of the muscles. Cerebral palsy and seizure activities often present with clonus.

Clonus > a tumult

Rapid contraction and relaxation of the muscles, associated with seizures.

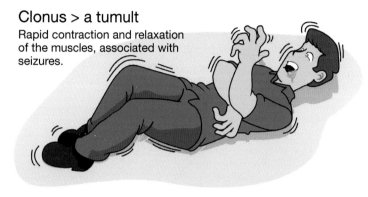

Figure 6.14

- **Tetany** (**tet**-ah-knee) > sustained muscle contraction. Essentially the muscle is stuck in a full contraction, it hurts! It may start with incomplete tetany: twitches, cramps, and spasms. A 'charlie-horse' is a brief moment of tetany in the foot or calf.

- **Tonic** (tohn-ik) > continuous unremitting action > associated with seizures and encephalopathy.

- **Spasticity** (spas-**tis**-i-tee) > increased muscle tone > this will produce hyperactive tendon reflexes. Spasticity is seen with cerebral palsy, stroke, multiple sclerosis, and spinal cord injuries.

- **Torticollis** (**tor**-tea-**kol**-lis) > spasmodic neck muscle contraction. Torticollis occurs with damage to cranial nerve 11, trauma, or neck lymphadenopathy. Synonym: wryneck or twisted neck.

- **Extrapyramidal symptoms** (**ek**-stra-peer-**am**-ee-dal) > abnormal involuntary movements. This may present with lip smacking, pill rolling (fingers doing repetitive motion), or tics. These are noted with Parkinsonism, meningitis, and medication use particularly antipsychotics and some antiemetics (against vomiting).

- **Akathisia** (ak-ah-**thiz**-ee-ah) > unable to maintain sitting posture.

illness causing brain or spinal cord changes. There is interruption of the nerve–muscle interaction or the reverse, hyperactivity to cause muscle spasms.

Tics > habitual contraction of a specific muscle. You can induce a tic (particularly of the eyelid) thinking about it. Medications can induce tics as well.

Muscle cells do not reproduce themselves on a daily basis as the skin or skeletal cells do. They are only minimally replaced with injury or illness. Muscle can grow larger, shrink, or scar. The suffix -trophy > development – is used extensively to describe muscles.

- Atrophy (**at**-row-fee) > no development or less development > when the muscle is injured or not used due to the loss of nervous stimulation it wastes. There is loss of cellular volume; it gets smaller. Amyotrophic (a-**my**-oh-**trow**-fik) lateralizing sclerosis (**ALS**), quadriplegia, and protein malnutrition are examples of this level of muscle loss.
  - Immobilizing a joint for long periods of time (six or more weeks) will lead to a level of atrophy of the involved muscles from disuse. PT and exercise usually improve the muscle tone and strength over time.
  - Damage to brain or peripheral nerves can cause specific muscle atrophy due to loss of neurological signals. A spinal injury causing paralysis of limbs is an example.
    - o Quadriplegia (**qwa**-dree-**play**-gee-ah) > all four limbs are paralyzed
    - o Hemiplegia (**hem**-ee-**play**-gee-ah) > ipsilateral, both the arm and leg are paralyzed
    - o Paraplegia (**pair**-ah-**play**-gee-ah) > both legs are paralyzed

- Hyper**trophy** (**hi**-purr-**trow**-fee) > overdevelopment > muscle cells can enlarge or bulk up. Anything which causes the heart to labor against resistance will result in hypertrophy of the heart, cardiomegaly (**kar**-dee-oh-**meg**-a-lee).
  - Left ventricular hypertrophy (**LVH**) > enlargement of the left ventricle of the heart. As with any muscle which enlarges, it becomes flabby over time. It becomes weak and less effective leading to congestive heart failure (**CHF**).

- Dys**trophy** (dis-**trow**-fee) > difficult or bad development > when the muscle cells do not develop as designed due to muscle protein dysfunction.
  - Muscular dystrophy (**MD**) > genetic lack of the muscle protein dystrophin. **Dystrophin** is one of the rate limiters to the sarcomere, the functional unit of muscle. It keeps the sarcomere from contracting to the point of breaking. MD is characterized by sarcomere breakage leading to progressive muscle weakness.
  - There are viral illnesses that may cause dystrophy – poliomyelitis (**poy**-lee-oh-my-eh-**lie**-tis) is an example. It produces muscle weakness and atrophy in an ascending pattern, from the feet up.

6.20
Anabolic steroids: These medications increase growth and metabolism of muscle cells, similar in function to testosterone. Illegal use may cause significant side effects including heart disease, kidney failure, and stroke.

Troph/o is the word root

-trophy is the suffix indicating the quality of development or growth

6.21
Muscle testing includes strength testing bilaterally, electrodynamometer.

An **EMG**, electromyogram will reveal if the neurological stimulus is making a muscle react.

- **Myasthenia gravis** (**my**-as-**thee**-knee-ah **gra**-vis) **(MG)** > autoimmune disease attack muscle cells leading to loss of tone and strength.

- **Convulsions** (**kon**-vul-shuns) > abnormal, uncoordinated muscle contractions. Convulsions are usually caused by a brain or spine disruption.

- **Fibrillation** (**fib**-ri-**lay**-shun) > muscle fibers contract rapidly, irregularly, or randomly. When the heart fibrillates it cannot pump blood efficiently and death may occur.

Laboratory tests include:

CK > creatine kinase > a waste product of muscle use or injury.

CK–MB > CK muscle–brain is used to check for cardiac muscle loss.

✓ The Mr. Universe event is an elite body-building competition promoting 'increased muscle size'. The medical term is _____ .

6.22 hypertrophy or hypermyotrophy

✓ Knowing where your feet are without looking is part of this sensory term.

6.23 Proprioception

✓ Construct the medical term for 'slow to motion'.

6.24 Bradykinesia

---

cpt® AND LTC*

An enormous amount of healthcare takes place outside hospitals and their attached rehabilitation facilities. The current procedural terminology (*cpt®*) coding process was developed to capture all this care – be it in an office, home, or even at a school. The recovery time and skills in caring for musculoskeletal injuries typically extend past the acute care of an operating room and/or the two weeks at the rehabilitation facility. Long-term care facilities such as skilled nursing facility or home care provide treatment to all ages when there is a need. The *cpt®* list over 50 sites of care from an Assisted Living Facility (LTC) to Hospice to mass immunization centers.

Mrs. Kya is living in the Alzheimer's unit of a skilled nursing care facility. She is being seen by the visiting physical therapist for carpel tunnel syndrome therapy (Figure 6.15).

The *cpt®* code for the location of care would be 31, indicating skilled nursing care and the initial PT visit is coded with 97001. Physical therapy often includes equipment (the dumbbell) and therapy modalities such as electrical stimulation (Figure 6.16); this is coded 97014 or paraffin bath (97016).

Patients in skilled nursing facilities are most likely to have co-morbidities requiring any number of professionals. Stroke survivors will utilize PT to help restore muscle

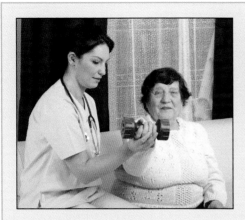

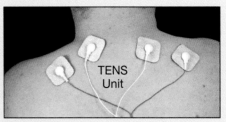

TENS
Unit

Figure 6.16

Figure 6.15

strength and balance if possible. Occupational therapy (OT) will contribute by helping with special tools to help a stroke survivor with fine motor activities such as buttoning a shirt. The SLP will help with speech recovery. Most facilities contract this work out and the *cpt*® provides codes for the activities, time spent, and return visits. This tracking is key to reimbursement and it is assessed by OSHA, NIH, and other agencies for disease and injury prevalence and consequences. Documentation with proper use of medical terminology remains the basis for providing continuity of care and the efforts to improve quality care for all populations.

★ IMPORTANT NOTE: The reader is notified that these examples are from an online search of the *cpt*®. The information may no longer be valid. Do not use these codes for patient care episodes; look up new ones!

MUSCLE INJURY AND ILLNESS

Shin splints, tennis elbow, groin pull, and low back pain are all terms heard on the sports report and they are all represent overuse of the musculoskeletal system.

- **Muscle sprains** are the most frequent. These occur when the muscle fibers are torn due to over-stretching. The sprain may be mild with only the micro-anatomy breaking at points (Grade 1). It may also pull so hard on the tendon there are both microtears and marked inflammation, tendinitis (Grade 2). The tendon can pull a chip off the bone, an avulsion fracture (Grade 3). Finally, the muscle belly can tear (also a Grade 3). The more fibers involved – the more pain, bleeding, and time to heal (Figure 6.17).

6.25

Myalgia > muscle pain

Myasthenia > muscle weakness

-sthenia > strength

Myatonia > abnormal muscle tone

Myobradia > slow muscle reaction time

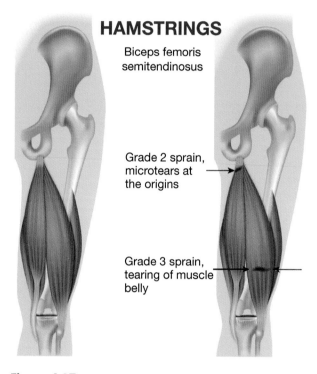

HAMSTRINGS

Biceps femoris
semitendinosus

Grade 2 sprain,
microtears at
the origins

Grade 3 sprain,
tearing of muscle
belly

Figure 6.17

- **Rotator cuff** tears > Supraspinatus, infraspinatus, teres major, and subscapularis. These tend to tear at the tendon insertions. **SITS** is the acronym for the four rotator cuff muscles: note that three have location names.
  o Supra > over the spine of the scapula
  o Infra > under the spine of the scapula
  o Sub > under the scapula (anterior side)
- **Back pain** usually concerns the neck (cervical) and lower back (lumbar.) Low back pain is a regular occupational injury. **OSHA** (Occupational Safety and Health Administration) and all insurance companies promote training in **ergonomics** (ur-go-**no**-miks) to help avoid injury.
  o **Lumbago** is the older term for lower back pain. The numerous back muscles are collectively referred to as the paravertebrals (around the vertebrae).
  o **Neck pain** > trapezius and occipital strap muscles.

Erg/o > work
Ergonomics is the science of workplace, tools, and equipment. These professionals use ergonomics to improve safety and decrease work-related injuries.

- Tendinitis and Fasciitis are both functions of repetitive use of the muscles and inflammation of their attached tendons or fascia. These injuries may be called repetitive motion disorders, **RMD**.
    - **Tennis elbow** > epicondylitis (**ep**-ee-kon-dee-**lie**-tis) > inflammation on the condyle. Overuse is from grasping anything which pulls on the extensor tendons at their origin on the epicondyle of the elbow.
    - **Plantar fasciitis** (**fash**-ee-**eye**-tis) > inflammation of the aponeurosis on the bottom of the foot. High-impact sports on hard surfaces tighten the sheath.
    - **Carpal tunnel syndrome** > repetitive motion such as typing, knitting, or using a tool cause swelling around the retinaculum, compressing the median nerve of the hand.
    - **Gamer's thumb** > abductor pollicis longus and brevis > repetitive motion of the thumb. The eponym is De Quervain's tenosynovitis (**ten**-oh-sin-oh-**vie**-tis).

- **Shin splints** are properly called periosteitis (**pear**-eh-**os**-tea-**eye**-tis) > inflammation of the periosteum. The anterior tibia has only skin and thick periosteum protecting it. Overuse from jogging or running creates inflammation of the tight, board tendinous connection. This translates to swelling in an area where there is little space for edema (Figure 6.18). There will be pain with every step until it is rested.

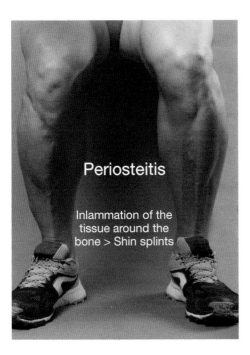

Periosteitis

Inlammation of the tissue around the bone > Shin splints

Figure 6.18

6.26
Evaluation of tendonitis, fasciitis, synovitis, and muscle pain includes a physical exam looking for heat, crepitus, swelling, edema, hematomas, adequate circulation, and range of motion.

Ultrasound (**US**), **CT** scans, and **MRI** can be used to evaluate for more serious injuries such as tears. MRI is best for looking at soft tissues.

6.27
Treatment of most of these overuse conditions starts with **RICE**: rest, ice, compression, and elevation.

- **Compartment syndrome (CS)** > occurs when intense pressure builds up inside an enclosed space in the body. The distal extremities are most vulnerable to blunt trauma. The swelling and hematoma of the injury tighten the compartment. The perilously high pressure in the muscle compartment impedes the flow of blood to and from the affected muscle fascicles. It is a limb emergency, requiring surgery to prevent permanent injury to the nerve and blood supply.

  – Compartment syndromes can occur anywhere in the body. A subdural hematoma (bleeding under the dura mater of the brain) is a CS. The blood and swelling is trapped with nowhere to go except to compress structures.

6.28
An emergency fasciotomy is required to save the limb.

Fasciotomy > to cut into the fascia (surrounding the muscle)

✓ Construct a word meaning 'suturing of the muscle'.

6.29
Myorrhaphy

✓ Leo has been hammering nails all day while constructing a home. Now, even opening the door to the car hurts up at his elbow. He has _____ . (proper medical term please)

6.30
epicondylitis

✓ The initial set LTC stands for _____ .
_____

6.31
long-term care

Word building

 *Using the word roots **with the linking vowel to build as many valid terms with the suffixes given.** Please define each term.*

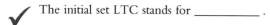

Muscul/o   Nucle/o   Erg/o

-ar -lytic -graph -gram -meter -ic

6.32
The instructor has the list!

Muscle pain > myalgia > occurs with injury but our muscles can ache with systemic infections such as the influenza too. Pulled or sprained muscles are often stiff as well but they tend to work out with a little activity. There are two conditions causing pain and actual muscle tenderness (hurts to touch).

- **Fibromyalgia** (**fie**-brow-my-**al**-gee-ah) > a painful muscle condition without weakness. It is associated with trigger points, sleep disturbances, and fatigue. Serum CK and ESR are normal as is the EMG testing and muscle biopsy. The cause is unknown.

- **Polymyalgia rheumatica** (**pol**-ee-my-**al**-gee-ah ru-**mat**-ee-ka) > painful and stiff muscles. It may be linked with an autoimmune disorder. It will have a positive ESR but negative CK, EMG, and muscle biopsy.

6.33

CK > creatine kinase (also seen as CPK > creatine phosphokinase)

ESR or **Sed Rate** > Erythrocyte sedimentation rate (indicates a problem but does not define it)

Muscle weakness > myasthenia > specific to skeletal muscle myopathies. There are intermittent weakness conditions which come and go with the availability of the neurotransmitter, acetylcholine, or the fuel of the sarcomeres: glucose and oxygen.

- **Myasthenia gravis** > inadequate ACh flow at the neuromuscular junction (NMJ). Testing includes Anti-AChR radioimmunoassay, repetitive nerve stimulation (the muscle will tire), EMG, and Tensilon test.

- **Botulism (boch**-U-lizm) > blocks the release of the ACh at the synapse (NMJ).

- **Multiple sclerosis (**sklar-**oh**-sis)**(MS)** > loss of myelin slows muscle reaction resulting in intermittent weakness.

- **Medications** which potentially cause a rhabdomyolysis include cyclosporine, any of the 'statin' anticholesterol medications, and several street drugs: cocaine, amphetamines, ecstasy, and LSD.

Many muscle disorders cause persistent weakness such as

- Poliomyelitis > enterovirus causing muscle paralysis which progresses up the ascending motor nerves.

- Polymyositis (**pol**-ee-**my**-oh-**sigh**-tis) > inflammation of several voluntary muscles simultaneously; the weakness tends to be more proximal.

- Muscular dystrophies > 25 hereditary, progressive muscular dystrophies defined currently by genotype. Proximal muscles are affected more than distal muscles. All MD conditions will have elevated **CK** and abnormal **EMG** results. Most will have normal nerve conduction studies (**NCS**) because it is a defective muscle function.
  - Duchenne's (**DMD**) is an X-linked recessive disorder. Defective dystrophin leads to girdle muscle weakness.
  - Becker's is also X-linked, with a defect in dystrophin.

Both Duchenne's and Becker's lead to respiratory collapse in the 3rd to 4th decade of life.

Myositis > inflammation of the muscle > often used for severe infection of the muscle secondary bacteria, virus, or parasites as listed here:

- Influenza (viral) > **in**-flew-**en**-zah.

- Dengue fever (viral) > **den**-gay.

- Coxsackievirus B (viral) > kok-**sak**-ee-**vie**-rus.

- Trichinellosis (parasite) > **trik**-ee-**nell**-oh-sis (condition of).

6.34

The Tensilon test uses the drug edrophonium. It inhibits the breaking down of the ACh, providing more stimulus to the muscle. A patient with myasthenia gravis will have stronger muscles after being injected with edrophonium.

LIKE ALERT!

Myel/o > spinal cord or bone marrow

My/o > muscle

They can sound alike.

6.35

Did You Know?

Human-bite wounds become infected more often than any other animal bite with both aerobic and anaerobic bacteria.

- Toxoplasmosis (parasite) > **tox**-oh-plaz-**moe**-sis (condition of).

- *Staphylococcus aureus* (bacterium) > **staf**-ee-low-**kock**-us aw-**re**-us.

- *Streptococcus pyogenes* (bacterium) > **strep**-toe-**kock**-us pie-**oh**-jenes.

- *Clostridium perfringens* (anaerobic bacterium) > klos-**trid**-ee-um purr-**frin**-jens.

The muscles provide a deep, warm, moist environment where infections propagate quickly especially with penetrating wounds. This may set up a condition called **gas gangrene** (**gan**-green). The fermentation of the bacteria releases gas, which takes up space and destroys muscle and other tissues (Figure 6.19). This is **myonecrosis** (**my**-oh-neh-**krow**-sis) > abnormal condition of muscle death.

A closed fist punctured by teeth is the most likely to be infected setting up cellulitis, compartment syndromes, and myositis.

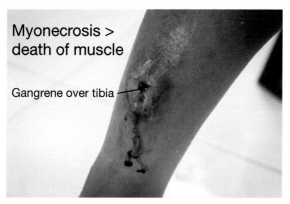

Myonecrosis > death of muscle

Gangrene over tibia

Figure 6.19

Restless leg syndrome (RLS) > sensorimotor disorder of unknown origin. It is characterized by dysesthesias deep in the muscles making the person want to move their limbs. Dysesthesias (**dis**-es-**thee**-zee-ahs) > bad sensations.

Periodic limb movement disorder (PLMD) or nocturnal myoclonus > random muscle fiber trigger causing motion. It is interrelated with **NREM** (non-rapid eye motion) sleep but it is not well understood.

6.36
Myoclonus > one or series of muscle contractions

Esthesi/o > Greek for sensation, perception of

✓ The proper term for shin splints is _____ .

✓ The science of making work safe is _____ .

✓ An emergency _____ will relieve the pressure of a compartment syndrome in the lower leg.

6.37
periosteitis or periostitis
6.38
ergonomics
6.39
fasciotomy

PHARMACY CORNER: MUSCLE MEDICATIONS*

Muscle relaxers, as we understand them, are really muscle action blockers. Figure 6.20 depicts the trigger–response process of each and every move we make. It begins with the brain neurons and a decision to move.

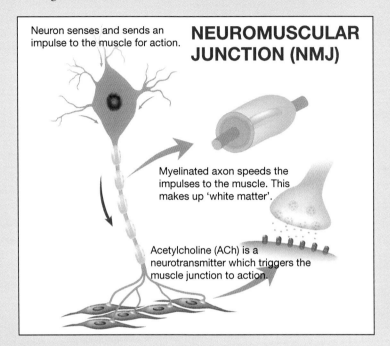

NEUROMUSCULAR JUNCTION (NMJ)

Neuron senses and sends an impulse to the muscle for action.

Myelinated axon speeds the impulses to the muscle. This makes up 'white matter'.

Acetylcholine (ACh) is a neurotransmitter which triggers the muscle junction to action.

Figure 6.20

The neurons in charge of your leg muscles send a signal down myelinated nerve fibers (axons). The myelin coat speeds the nerve impulse to the synapse, which is full of vesicles of **acetylcholine** (**ACh**), a neurotransmitter. The ACh is released into the **neuromuscular junction** (**NMJ**) triggering the sarcomeres to contract.

Medications such as **succinylcholine** are used to relax the skeletal muscles during surgery by blocking the muscle receptor sites for the ACh. It is like a parking meter being unable to accept a coin. Given enough, the muscles can be paralyzed completely. Curare functions in the same way. During anesthesia, succinylcholine is given in amounts to stop muscle twitching so the surgeon does not have to hit a moving target ☺.

The toxins produced by the bacterium *Clostridium botulinum* create a **tetanus** (no motion) because these block the release of ACh at the synapse (NMJ). No ACh, no trigger = no motion. A tetanus vaccination is recommended every ten years to avoid wound botulism. However, the toxin is used as a pharmacotherapeutic to control bladder hyperactivity, chronic headaches, and upper limb spasticity – onabotulinumtoxinA – Botox.

Antispasmodic medications work by inhibiting activity at the neuron or brain level. They reduce the level of excitation, though their ability to stop spasm (spasmolytic) may have more to do with sedation then the actual slowing of the signals. Antispasmodics include 'muscle relaxers', which are utilized to treat low back pain, neck pain, fibromyalgia, and tension headaches:

- Cyclobenzaprine (Flexeril®)
- Metaxalone (Skelaxin®)
- Methocarbamol (Robaxin®)

An overdose of any of these medications can stop respiration and potentially all muscle action leading to death. As with all medications, *they should be taken or administered as prescribed.*

* IMPORTANT NOTE: Medicine is always in evolution. Do <u>not</u> use this information for patient care.

UNIT SUMMARY

1   The elastic qualities of muscle tissue are distinctive to three types: skeletal, smooth, and cardiac. The skeletal (rhabd/o) muscles move our skeleton, generate heat, and bind and cushion our body. The smooth muscles (lei/o) move the contents of our visceral organs down their respective tracts. The cardiac (cardi/o) muscle's sole responsibility is pumping blood to or from the heart through the closed highway of arteries and veins.

2   Skeletal muscles number approximately 640 and function to maintain our posture against gravity. Muscles move our blood, our respirations, allow speech and swallowing, and even reactions to annoying flies. Skeletal muscle tissues work to give us strength, endurance, and a constant tone. They also store myoglobin, an emergency reserve of oxygen and fuel to be recruited when needed.

3   Descriptives define the form and function of the skeletal muscle by the arrangement of fascicles, the muscle fibers. Convergent, spiral, and multipennate are large, strong muscles anchored centrally and inserted to a common point to tug the skeleton into position. Parallel, fusiform, and pennate muscles tend to be long and streamlined and are found in tiny places such as the finger and large places such as the quadriceps of the leg. Circular muscles round up the mouth, eye orbits, and all the sphincters in and outside the body.

4   The muscle nomenclature has several facets including the general shape or size of the muscle, the location of the muscle on the skeleton, the

number of origins of the muscle, and the direction the muscle moves the body. Some names are based on the function of the muscle or even the type of person who uses a particular muscle most often.

5   Rehabilitation facilities and long-term care programs (both inpatient and outpatient) utilize a variety of professionals to get a patient back on their feet. All three muscle types need to be reconditioned to help patients reach maximum recovery. No matter the age of the patient PT, OT, RT, Pharmacy, and TR work together to prevent further illness or injury and add to strength, balance, and flexibility.

6   Motion is an intricate dance between the brain, skeleton, muscles, circulation, and even some hormones. Safe motion depends on proprioceptive receptors in the muscles, joints, and ear to keep us on balance. Terms of movement include kinesiology, kinesalgia, dyskinesia, and bradykinesia.

7   Disease and injury interrupt the function of healthy muscles no matter their type. Symptoms include descriptives such as atrophy, dystrophy, clonus, tetany, tonic, spasticity, torticollis, and akathisia.

8   Injury includes the sprains, partial tears, bruising, hematomas, and full ruptures of the muscle and/or tendons. Compartment syndrome and myositis are both serious conditions threatening limb and life. Hereditary diseases include 25 types of muscular dystrophy, causing a steady decline in strength and mobility.

UNIT WORD PARTS

Word roots with linking vowel		
Cardi/o > heart	Cephal/o > head	Condyl/o > condyle
Electr/o > impulse, electrical	Ergo/o > work	Esthesi/o > sensation
Fasci/o > band, fascia	Kines/o; Kinesi/o > movement	Lei/o > smooth
Muscul/o; My/o; Myos/o > muscle	Myel/o > spinal cord or bone marrow	Neur/o > nerve
Oste/o; Osse/o > bone	Pyr/o > heat, temperature	Rhabd/o > striated, skeletal
Sarc/o > flesh	Scler/o > hardening	Skelet/o > dried up (bones)
Tendin/o; Ten/o; Tend/o > tendon	Ton/o > tone, stretch	Viscer/o > body organs

Prefixes: attached to the front of the word root to change meaning		
A- or An- > no, not, absent, without	Apo- > derived from	Auto- > self
Bi- or Di- > outside, outer, external, away from	Brady- > slow	Dys- > poor, difficult
Epi- > upon, over	Hemi- > half	Hyper- > increased, more than, more of
Iso- > equal, same	Multi- > many	Peri- > around
Polio- > gray	Poly- > many	Quadri- > four

Suffixes change the meaning of the word, linking vowel is usually 'o' with consonants		
-algia or -dynia > pain	-cele > herniation	-centesis > remove fluid with surgical needle
-ectasia > dilatation	-globin > protein type	-gram > record
-graphy > instrument to record	-itis > inflammation	-ity > quality
-lysis > destroy, break	-oma > tumor	-plasty > repair of
-plegia > paralysis	-poiesis > to create	-rrhaphy > suture
-scope > instrument	-spasm > muscle contraction	-sthenia > strength
-tomy > cut into	-trophy > development	

Acronyms, abbreviations, and initial sets		
ACh > Acetylcholine	ADLs > activities of daily living	ALS > amyotrophic lateralizing sclerosis
CHF > congestive heart failure	CK > creatine kinase or CPK > creatine phosphokinase	CK-MB > creatine kinase muscle–brain
CPAP > continuous positive airway pressure	cpt® > current procedural terminology coding system	CS > compartment syndrome (in this setting)
CT or CAT scan > computerized tomography	DMD > Duchenne's muscular dystrophy	EMG > electromyogram
ESR > erythrocytes sedimentation rate (sed rate)	HTN > hypertension	LTC > long-term care
LVH > left ventricular hypertrophy	MG > myasthenia gravis	MRI > magnetic resonance imaging

Acronyms, abbreviations, and initial sets*		
MS > multiple sclerosis	NIH > National Institute of Health	NMJ > neuromuscular junction
NREM > non-rapid eye motion	OSHA > Occupational Safety and Health Administration	OT > occupational therapy
PEM > protein energy malnutrition	PLMD > periodic limb movement disorder	PT > physical therapy
RICE > rest, ice, compression, elevation	RLS > restless leg syndrome	RT > respiratory therapy
SCM > sterno-cleidomastoid muscle	SITS > supraspinatus, infraspinatus, teres major, and subscapularis	SLP > speech and language pathology
TENS > transcutaneous electrical nerve stimulation	THR > target heart rate	TR > therapeutic recreation

 UNIT WORKSHEETS

Building terms: Use the proper prefix/word root/linking vowel/suffix as appropriate.

Example: to cut into the stomach > gastr/o/tomy

a) Muscle herniation > _____

b) No tone > _____

c) Difficult movement > _____

d) Abnormal condition of muscle death > _____

e) Repair of a tendon > _____

f) Pain of the fibers and muscles > _____

g) Excessive development > _____

h) Tiny muscle fibers > _____

Know your acronyms and initial sets! For the acronym or initial set given, spell it out correctly.

a) LTC _____

b) SCM _____

c) ADLs _____

* **The use of any acronyms, abbreviations, or initial sets depends on the context of the note. RT, PT, OT, etc., all have different meanings in other settings. When in doubt, spell it out.**

d) CK   _____

e) EMG   _____

f) NMJ   _____

g) ALS   _____

h) OSHA   _____

Best choice: Pick the most appropriate answer.

1 This is a storage protein found in the muscle tissues.

   a) Actin   c) Tropomyosin

   b) Titin   d) Myoglobin

2 A leiomyoma is a tumor affecting the _____ muscle.

   a) Cardiac   c) Skeletal

   b) Smooth   d) Mixed

3 The skeletal muscle responsible for breathing is the

   a) SCM   c) Diaphragm

   b) Intercostal   d) External oblique

4 The configuration of these muscles is important for sphincter control.

   a) Spiral   c) Convergent

   b) Parallel   d) Circular

5 The functional unit of the muscle is the

   a) Osteon   c) Sarcomere

   b) Alveoli   d) Myocytes

6 Which of the following conditions blocks ACh at the NMJ, causing paralysis?

   a) Poliomyelitis   c) Fibromyalgia

   b) Influenza myositis   d) Botulism

Name the muscle condition! Based on the description and/or function name the muscle condition.

a) Inflammation of the tendon _____

b) While testing a muscle against resistance it 'stutters' _____

c) Knowing where your hand or foot is in space _____

d) Ipsilateral paralysis of the arm and leg _____

e) Viral infection destroying the ascending motor neurons; its prefix means 'gray'. It causes _____

f) A tear in one or more of SITS muscles/tendons is called a _____ tear.

Multiple correct: Select ALL the correct answers to the question or statement given.

1 Mark all the correct functions of skeletal muscle.

   a) Body heat   d)   Peristalsis

   b) Bind and cushion   e)   Posture

   c) Pushes circulation   f)   Respiration

2 Which of the following concern the arrangement of muscle fibers?

   a) Triceps   d)   Location

   b) Circular   e)   Bipennate

   c) Parallel   f)   Fusiform

3 Which of the following are a 'size' naming term for muscles?

   a) longissimus   d)   adductor

   b) vastus   e)   quad

   c) latissimus   f)   brevis

Spelling challenge! Circle the correct spelling based on the definition given.

1 'No muscle development'

          Amyotophic   Enmyotrophic   Amyotrophic   Imyotophic

2 'Inflammation of the tendon and synovium'

          Tenosynovitis   Tendiosynoveitis   Sinovoteniitis   Tenesynoviitis

---

Define the term: Spelling *does* count in your definition too.

1 Myasthenia >   _____

2 Kinesiologist >   _____

3 Rhabdomyosarcoma > _____

4 Cardiomyopathy >   _____

5 Myorrhaphy >   _____

6 Myatonia >   _____

7 Tenomyoplasty >   _____

8 Syncytium >   _____

Find it! Using the words in the table – match the definition given or answer the statement. Some may not be used. It is recommended you know all the choices.

leiomyoma	antispasmodic	myalgia	hyperkinesia	quadriplegia
myoglobin	dystrophy	endomysium	myogram	rhabdomyolysis
hypertrophy	tetanus	fibroma	myorrhaphy	tendinous
amyotonic	myocyte	ataxia	neuromuscular	bradykinesia

1 _____ Pain of the muscle

2 _____ Loss of the skeletal muscle

3 _____ Suture the muscle

4 _____ Excessive motion

5 _____ No motion due to toxin

6 _____ Abnormal development

7 _____ Tumor of the fibers

8 _____ Muscle cells

9 _____ Record of the muscle

10 _____ Paralysis of all four limbs

Matching: Some will not be used.

	Letter	Defined as
Ataxia		a) inflammation of muscle
Kinesalgia		b) a tumult, rapid contraction
Epicondylitis		c) oxygen-rich muscle protein
Myoglobin		d) no motion, poor gait
Clonus		e) inflammation around the bone
Gas gangrene		f) inflammation above the condyle
Myositis		g) pain in many muscles
Periosteitis		h) inadequate acetylcholine
		i) fermentation of a bacterial wound
		j) pain with motion

An essay: Explain how the various muscle relaxers work in the muscle to slow, stop, or relax motion in your own words.

Note challenge: This is a combination note for home care. You may need to look up a few terms. Answer the questions that follow.

3–14–14 Physical therapy

S. 54 yo woman S/P sarcoma <u>excision</u> with skin graft, Right ankle. Hospital × 1 week. 1st full day home. Alert and cooperative.

O. Right ankle with full dressing in place and it appears dry. She is able to wiggle her toes. The right ankle <u>dorsiflexion</u> is 15% (same as in hospital). <u>Plantar flexion</u> is not allowed yet. She is able to lever up out of the chair and use the scooter we brought today.

A. S/P Ankle surgery with graft. Appropriate progress and able to move around house on scooter.

3–14–14 Occupational therapy

S. Single 54 yo woman S/P right ankle surgery. Mostly sedentary with scooter for bathroom privileges. No showering yet. Since she is single and alone, goal is to make sure she can easily access <u>BR</u> and kitchen.

O. Easy-chair is appropriate for rest and close to BR and kitchen. Moved key elements in kitchen to counter level. Reaching tool demonstrated. Water dispenser place near chair. Removed loose rugs.

A. S/P ankle surgery with graft. <u>ADLs</u> are met as long as patient takes her time and uses scooter, reaching tool, and water source.

3–15–14 Nursing

S. 54 yo woman S/P excision of <u>sarcoma</u>, Right ankle with graft. Alert and moving well on scooter in the living and kitchen area. Complains of some pain at ankle and graft donor site.

O. Vital signs good, 114/74, 68, 98.6. Wound dressing removed. Graft appears intact with no evidence of marked <u>inflammation</u> or <u>exudates</u>. Graft is tight, allowed 5 degrees plantar flexion today per MD and PT. Wound packed with loose Kerlix and ace wrapped. Pulses equal. Right <u>proximal</u>, anterior thigh donor graft site <u>exudative</u> but not infected. Wound cleaned and redressed.

A. SP Ankle surgery, wounds clean and dressed. FU tomorrow. Continue non-weight bearing and elevation 40 min/hr.

Questions:

1 Translate all the acronyms/initial sets and give meaning to the words which are underlined in the note.

2 What information do you need to code this care? Use the chart below to assign appropriate codes★. There may be more than one correct code per column. Do your best. We are not trying to make you a coder but we do want you to think about how the medical terminology impacts care and coding.

3 Why is the patient being seen by both PT and OT? What is the difference in their functions?

ICD-10-CM*	cpt®: location	cpt® visit type	cpt® therapy
Z42.8 Encounter for other plastic and reconstructive surgery following medical procedure or healing wound.	04 Homeless shelter	99024 RN postoperative follow-up visit	97597 Active wound care
Z01.8 Encounter for other specified special examination	11 Office	99509 Home visit for assistance with ADLs and personal care	97602 Debridement
Z48.00 Encounter for change or removal of nonsurgical wound dressing	12 Home	97001 PT evaluation	97110 Therapeutic procedure
Z48.01 Encounter for change or removal of surgical wound dressing	15 Mobile Unit	97003 OT evaluation	97116 Gait training
Z52.1 Skin donor		97006 AT reevaluation	97533 Adaptive training
Z60.2 Problems with living alone			97035 Ultrasound therapy

★ **IMPORTANT NOTE: The reader is notified that these examples are from an online search done in 2016. Do <u>not</u> use these codes for patient care episodes; look up new ones!**

Unit 7

Nervous system and psychiatry

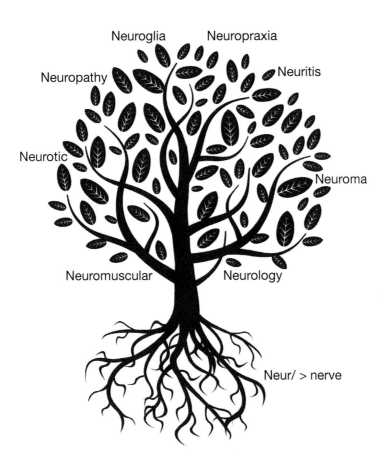

Neuroglia

Neuropraxia

Neuropathy

Neuritis

Neurotic

Neuroma

Neuromuscular

Neurology

Neur/ > nerve

TARGETED LEARNING

1   Recognize word parts and assemble medical terms related to the anatomy of the nervous system and psychiatry.

2   Correctly construct, define, pronounce, and spell medical terms.

3   Relate neurological diseases and injury with appropriate diagnostic evaluation and pharmacotherapeutics.

4   Explore the impact of medical documents on medical research via a review of Alzheimer's.

5   Associate accidental and intentional overdoses with psychiatric medication and the ICD Table of Drugs and Chemicals.

KEY WORD PARTS

Word roots with linking vowel	Prefixes	Suffixes
Astr/o > star	Auto-	-algia
Cephal/o > brain, toward the head	Epi-	-asthenia
Cerebell/o > cerebellum	Hypo-	-cele
Cerebr/o > cerebrum, brain cortex	Mal-	-esthenia
Crani/o > skull	Micro-	-glia
Dendr/o > branching	Oligo-	-megaly
Myel/o > spinal cord or bone marrow	Para-	-phagia
Neur/o > nerve, neuron	Peri-	-phasia
Psych/o > mind, soul	Poly-	-plegia
Radic/o or Radicul/o > root	Sub-	-praxia
Vertebr/o; Rachi/o > spine, back bone	Sym-, Syn-	-thymia

THE MIND AND SOUL

Aristotle, a Greek, addressed the dichotomy of the mind and soul in his treatise on the 'nature of life'. The discussion or debate has been going on since that time. Are we body or mind or soul or all three? How does a three-pound mass of tissue, chemicals, and hormones produce learning, love, hope, sadness, faith, joy, tears, and smiles? How does the tangible which science continues to define yield the intangibles in each of us with our infinite diversity?

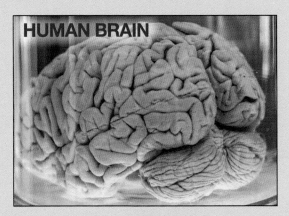

Figure 7.2

The medical terminology of the brain addresses both the physical anatomy and the emotional anatomy. There is real chemistry traveling to and from the billions of neurons. Sodium, potassium, and calcium are running a perpetual race translating electrical impulses to the neurotransmitters. The neurotransmitters in turn trigger a hand or a foot to move or an eye to blink. Hormones work alongside the neural impulses to manage the intricate dance we call homeostasis. We can track the emotions, hunger, anger, joy, and more via PET scans. To date we still do not understand how thinking and emotions truly function. Perhaps, you will be one of the medical researchers who will unlock the secrets of the 'nature of life'.

THE NEURONS AND SUPPORT NEUROGLIA

Neurons are the most unique of the four major tissue types. The epidermal, connective, and muscle tissues come in a variety of types. Neurons are neurons. Other than minor changes in configuration, all neurons will have the dendrites, the body of the neuron, an axon, and terminals (Figure 7.3). There are an estimated 86 billion densely packed neurons in the protective shell of the cranium. The spinal cord adds another 1 billion neurons.

7.1

Suffixes

–cyte > cell

–lemma > covering

–glia > glue

–blast > embryonic

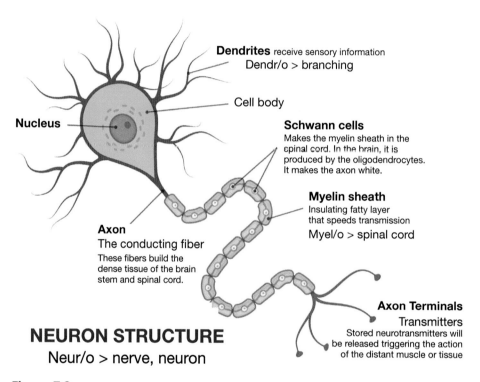

Dendrites receive sensory information
Dendr/o > branching

Cell body

Nucleus

Schwann cells
Makes the myelin sheath in the spinal cord. In the brain, it is produced by the oligodendrocytes. It makes the axon white.

Myelin sheath
Insulating fatty layer that speeds transmission
Myel/o > spinal cord

Axon
The conducting fiber
These fibers build the dense tissue of the brain stem and spinal cord.

Axon Terminals
Transmitters
Stored neurotransmitters will be released triggering the action of the distant muscle or tissue

NEURON STRUCTURE
Neur/o > nerve, neuron

Figure 7.3

- **Neur/o** > neuron (**nur**-on), nerve tissue. The neuron is the functional unit of the nervous system.
  - Neurology (nur-**ol**-oh-gee) > study of the nervous system.
  - Neuropathy (**nur**-oh-**nop**-ah-thee) > disease of the nerve/neurons.
  - Neuritis (**nur**-eye-tis) > inflammation of the nerves.
  - Neurosis (nur-**oh**-sis) > an abnormal psychological disorder.

–algia > pain

–praxia > action, movement

–fibril > little fiber

–itis > inflammation

- **Dendr/o** > branching > dendrites (**den**-drits) are the densely packed branches which provide an enormous surface area for receiving input.

- **Axon** (**aks**-on) > impulse-generating and conduction pathway, like an extension cord. One neuron = one axon, these are the nerve fibers. They can be very short or up to a meter long.

- **Axon terminal** > the signal arrives and a neurotransmitter is released. Synonyms: synapsis, boutons, synaptic knobs or podocytes.

  - **Syn**apsis > together + to clasp > functional membrane to membrane contact between nerve cells.

There are up to 600 billion more cells making up the brain. Their collective name is **neuroglial** (nur-**oh**-glee-al) **cells**. These are the specialized support cells maintaining the milieu for the neurons. They manage the homeostasis of the brain. **Gli/o** > glue.

- **Astrocytes** (**as**-tro-sites) > 'star' cells. These are the most abundant neuroglial cell, outnumbering the neurons approximately 3 to 1. Astrocytes are responsible for what we call the blood–brain barrier (**BBB**) (Figure 7.4).

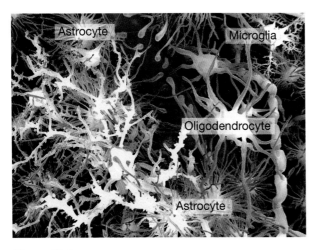

Figure 7.4

Did You Know?

Neurons are amitotic, unable to replicate. However, for a cell, they have extreme longevity – optimally 100 years! They have a high metabolic rate and run on two elements in abundance: **glucose** and **oxygen**.

7.2

Did You Know?

At birth, it is estimated only 1% of our neurons are mature. As we grow, so does our number of effective neurons. This is why it takes time for brain, bones, muscles, etc. . . . to manage all the tasks of life. The brain is considered mature around age 25.

- **Oligodendrocytes** (ol-ee-go-**den**-dro-sites) > scant branching cells. These cells extend short branches to the axons and excrete myelin, wrapping the axons (Figure 7.5). The myelin will increase the rate of the electrical conduction from about 0.5 m/s (meters per second) to 150 m/s. The coating makes the axons appear white versus the gray of unmyelinated fibers.

7.3
Oligo- > scant
Dendr/o > branching
Myel/o > spinal cord or bone marrow
Oligodendrocytes are unique to the brain. In the peripheral nervous system (the spinal cord) the **Schwann cells** will do the same work.

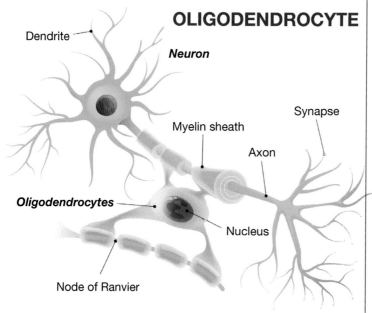

OLIGODENDROCYTE

Dendrite
Neuron
Synapse
Myelin sheath
Axon
Oligodendrocytes
Nucleus
Node of Ranvier

Figure 7.5

- **Microglia** (my-**krow**-glee-ah) > small glue. These tiny support cells act as the white blood cells of the nervous system (Figure 7.4). They have the cleanup duty for excess fluids and damaged tissues. Microglia are phagocytes; they 'eat' pathogens.

7.4
Micro- > tiny
-glia > glue
Phag/o > to eat
Path/o > disease

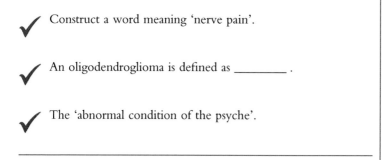

Construct a word meaning 'nerve pain'.

7.5
Neuralgia

An oligodendroglioma is defined as _____ .

7.6
a tumor involving the oligodendrocytes

The 'abnormal condition of the psyche'.

7.7
Neurosis

Word building

Using the word roots with the linking vowel to build as many valid terms with the suffixes given. Please define them too.

Neur/o Dendr/o Myel/o

-cyte –dynia –ology –praxia –plasty –blast
–itis –plegia –osis –pathy

7.8
The instructor has the list!

Neurons have three basic directions – the way stimulation flows.

- **Afferent** (af-air-ent) > to bring to, moving to the center. These axons move UP the tract heading to the brain. They carry the information of the moment from temperature, wind, sound, sights, smells, and sensations. Some afferent nerves will stop in the spine and others will go directly to the brain.

- **Efferent** (ef-air-ent) > to bring out, moving away from the center. These neurons with their axons move information DOWN the tract. They impact the cells to act such as the muscles in the eyes to read this sentence. Some will stop in the spine and others will travel all the way to the tips of the fingers.

7.9
The term, afferent is used for the blood vessels as well. **Afferent** arteries carry blood into the filtering units of the kidneys. The **efferent** arteries will carry it away from the filtering units (glomeruli).

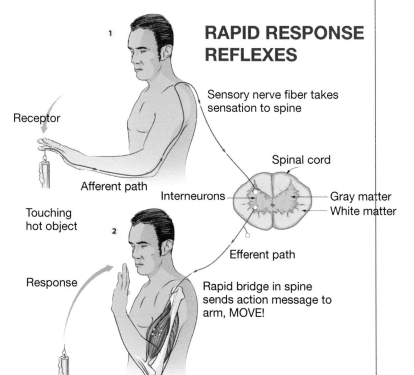

Figure 7.6

- **Interneurons** (**in**-tur-**nur**-ons) > in-between the neurons. Found only in the spine and brain, these are like quick turn-arounds on the highway. An afferent neuron sends the impulse directly to the action efferent neuron for an immediate reaction. These are the reflexes from blinking our eyes to keep dust out to pulling a hand away from a flame (Figure 7.6). It is an ultra-rapid response.

- **Poly**synaptic reflexes (**pohl**-ee-sin-**ap**-tik) > more complex and we do these every day as well. An example – walking barefoot across the room when the right foot steps on a tack. It coordinates balancing, lifting the foot off the ground and saying ouch!

Reflexes are survival oriented. The spine can respond rapidly to move the hand away from harm, and the slight lag time before OUCH is heard is the time it takes for the sensation to be perceived by the brain.

Kitchen lab

 You will need a newborn baby (0–4 months old) to demonstrate these reflexes. Or you may remember your children doing these:

7.10

Withdrawal reflex: Suddenly coming close to the baby's face > the baby turns his/her head away to avoid a collision. This remains for our lifetime.

Rooting reflex: Stroking the baby's cheek with a finger > she/he turns and begins sucking. This is a pure survival drive.

Tongue-thrust reflex: Touch a baby spoon to the tip of his/her tongue > the tongue will push it away protecting the airway from foreign bodies. This is why solid food should not be offered during 0–6 months of age.

Can you think of other protection reflexes in infants or adults? Discuss it with your instructor.

✓ Protective reflexes are more likely to be controlled by which of the following pathways?

Afferent   Interneuron   Efferent

7.11
Interneuron

✓ The proper term for neuroglial cells acting like WBCs in the brain.

7.12
Microglia

Neurotransmitters (**nur**-oh-**trans**-mit-turs) > specific chemical agents of the nervous system (Figure 7.7). The axon's impulse triggers the release of neurotransmitters 'across' the synaptic cleft. Most of the neurotransmitters trigger a reaction OR inhibit a response, which maintains homeostasis.

- **Excitatory** (ek-**sigh**-tah-tor-ee) > the act of increasing the rapidity or intensity.

- **Inhibitory** (in-**hib**-ee-tor-ee) > the act of depressing or stopping a function.

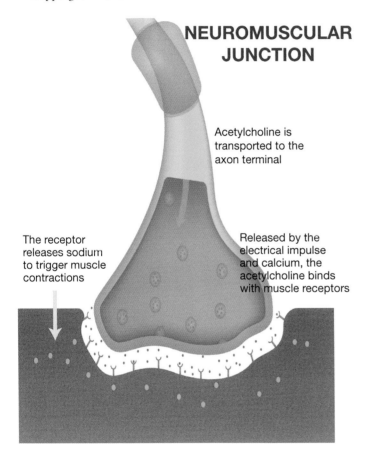

NEUROMUSCULAR JUNCTION

Acetylcholine is transported to the axon terminal

The receptor releases sodium to trigger muscle contractions

Released by the electrical impulse and calcium, the acetylcholine binds with muscle receptors

Figure 7.7

- **Acetylcholine** (**as**-ee-til-**ko**-lene) (**ACh**) > effects the neuromuscular junctions (**NMJ**), several glands, and many parts of the brain.
  - Acetylcholinesterase (**as**-ee-til-**ko**-lin-**es**-tur-ace) (**AChE**) > the enzyme breaks down any **ACh** left floating in the synaptic cleft. It is a rate-limiter.

7.13
The electrolyte required for triggering the release of neurotransmitters is **calcium** (Ca^{++}). Across the synapsis, the receptor cells' major electrolyte is **sodium** (Na^{++}).

Dopamine is found primarily in the brain.

Many medications used for psychiatric care inhibit or enhance neurotransmitters.

-ase > enzyme will break down the chemical it is attached to, such as

Lipase > breaking down fat

- **Catecholamines** (**kat**-ee-**kol**-ah-meanz) > a class of neurotransmitters, this is part of our fight-or-flight response.

  - **Epinephrine** (**ep**-ee-**nef**-rin) > generally excitatory to fight or flee. Abbreviation: Epi > **ep**-ee

  - **Norepinephrine** (nor-**ep**-ee-**nef**-rin) > primarily excitatory and part of emotional response. Abbreviation: Norepi > nor-**ep**-ee

  - **Dopamine** (**doe**-pah-mean) > strongly inhibitory, regulating mood and motor control (motion).

  - **Hypocretin** (**hi**-poe-**crey**-tin) > helps manage arousal, wakefulness, and appetite at the limbic system and pineal gland.

- **Serotonin** (**ser**-oh-**toe**-nin) > found primarily in the brain and gastrointestinal tract. In the brain, it is linked to supporting mood balance. In the GI tract, it excites the smooth muscle to promote peristalsis during sleep to process nutrients.

- **Histamine** (**his**-tah-mean) > intensely excitatory, this is found in the majority of cells. In the brain, histamine is part of body water and temperature control. Histamine is liberated with injury, triggering the inflammation reaction and repair.

- **Enkephalins** (en-**kef**-ah-lins) and **Endorphins** (en-**door**-fins) > found in the brain, retina of the eyes, and intestinal tract. These are our natural painkillers; they act like opiates covering pain receptors.

7.14
SSRI > selective serotonin reuptake inhibitors are medications used to treat depression and anxiety. By disallowing the recycling of the serotonin left in the synaptic clefts, there is more available to balance the mood.

WHEN THE MIND FAILS

In 1906, Dr. Alois Alzheimer was the first physician to note the physical changes of the brain as being associated with overwhelming memory loss and deteriorating psychological changes. At autopsy, the brain had shriveled and there were atypical deposits in and around the neurons. Thus, the research on Alzheimer's began. It was a slow start. The electron microscope was not used regularly for medical research until after WWII. While studies were conducted, any disease causing dementia was termed organic brain syndrome (**OBS**) or senility. Dementia (deh-**men**-she-ah), the progressive loss of cognitive intelligence was expected in aging people.

It was not until the 1970s when scientists, providers, and families began noting an increase in OBS. It seemed to have a very specific pathway and microscopic changes. It was also evident that while Alzheimer's is definitely seen in the elderly, it does

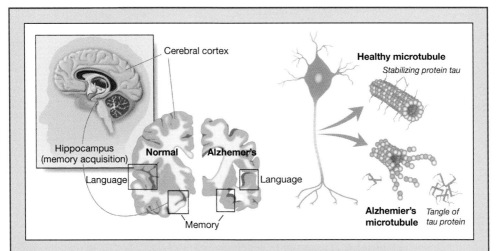

Cerebral cortex

Healthy microtubule
Stabilizing protein tau

Hippocampus
(memory acquisition)

Normal **Alzhemer's**

Language

Language

**Alzhemier's
microtubule** *Tangle of
tau protein*

Memory

Figure 7.8

occur in younger people as well. The epidemiologists and medical researchers began to comb thousands of medical records in an effort to define numbers and similarities with this disease.

In 1984 and 1986 respectively, two proteins normally seen in the brain were found to be involved in the disease, beta-amyloid (**bey**-tah **am**-ee-loyd) and the tau (tohw) protein. Like all the proteins of the body, production of healthy amyloid and tau depends on the DNA and RNA translation for correct reproduction. In Alzheimer's, something is triggering these two proteins to 'misfold' becoming tangles in the brain matrix (Figure 7.8). The brain does depend on a certain amount of organization. These tangles are called 'neurofibrillary tangles', **NFT**s. A distorted protein will NOT repair or do the work of the brain. The first gene associated with early Alzheimer's was defined in adults with Down syndrome.

Medical researchers include neurophysiologists, neuropathologists, biochemists, neuro-geneticists, and clinical practitioners. They study the aftermath via autopsy but before this, they study medical records. The medical records enable this research by finding the patients with the right set of symptom progression – memory loss, confusion, short attention span, poor direction sense, and finally personality changes. The terminology used, the pattern of symptoms, the timing of the progression, and other exposures are all part of the language you are learning.

CENTRAL NERVOUS SYSTEM

The **nervous system** is much like a computer, an intricate network, which involves a hard drive and lots of software. The nervous system does not work on 0011100011 . . . but on sodium, potassium, calcium, hormones, and neurotransmitters. There are many word roots associated with the brain.

- **Cephal/o** > brain or head > generally used to discuss the entire head.
  - Cephalad (**sef**-ah-lad) > a direction toward the head.

- **Encephal/o** > inside the head, the brain > linking form for the brain itself.
  - Encephalitis (en-**sef**-ah-**lie**-tis) > inflammation of the brain.
  - Encephalogram (en-**sef**-ah-**low**-gram) > the record obtained of brain electrical activity.
  - Encephalomalacia (en-**sef**-ah-**low**-oh-mah-**lay**-she-ah) > softening of the brain.

- **Cerebr/o** > cerebrum (**ser**-eh-brum) > specifically refers to the cortex of both hemispheres and basal ganglia of the brain. It is interchanged with cephal/o but cerebral is specific to the brain cortex with its convolutions (gyri), fissures, and sulci (Figure 7.9).
  - Cerebritis (**ser**-eh-**bry**-tis) > inflammation of the brain tissues.
  - Cerebrospinal (**ser**-eh-bro-**spy**-nal) > pertaining to the brain and spine.

7.15
Suffixes

-algia > pain

-edema > swelling

-cele > herniation

-ic or -al > pertaining to

-itis > inflammation

-centesis > removal of fluid

-dynia > pain

-gram > record

-malacia > softening

-megaly > enlargement

-meter > measurement

-motor > movement of

-osis > abnormal condition of

-pathy > disease of

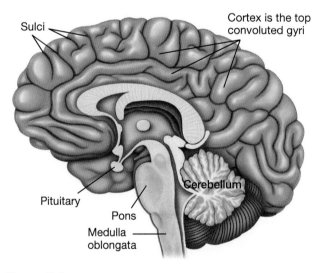

Figure 7.9

- The **cortex** > outer portion of an organ > the cortex of the brain is composed of 6 layers, each with millions of neurons and their axon terminals linked to millions of dendrites. It is composed almost exclusively of gray matter, which sits on the deeper structures of the brain (white matter) like a thick blanket.

- **Ventricul/o** > chamber > ventricles of the brain are fluid-filled with cerebral spinal fluid (**CSF**). The brain has two lateral ventricles and the 3rd ventricle, which bathes the mid-brain. The 4th ventricle bathes the cerebellum. It circulates around the brain and spinal cord as seen in Figure 7.10.

  – Ventricular (ven-**trik**-U-lar) > pertaining to the ventricle(s).

7.16

Cortex, cortices > kor-teks or kor-tea-sez. The kidneys and adrenal glands have anatomy termed 'cortex' as well.

Ventricle is a chamber no matter where it is found, such as the two ventricles of the heart.

Cerebrospinal fluid (CSF)

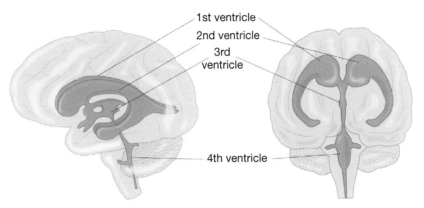

1st ventricle
2nd ventricle
3rd ventricle
4th ventricle

CSF is produced by the ependymal cells in the ventricles.

Figure 7.10

- **Cerebell/o** > small brain > specifically refers to the smaller mass of brain tissue behind (posterior to) the pons and medulla. It functions as a fine tuner for all motion.

  – **Cerebellar** (ser-eh-**bel**-lar) speech > explosive utterance with slurring (loss of the fine tuning).

  – **Cerebellar gait** > loss of the fine tuning creates a wide, stuttering gait. Synonym: cerebellar ataxia.

- **Thalam/o** > Greek for 'bedroom' > a large, ovoid body of compact gray matter in the diencephalon (mid-brain).

  – **Thalamotomy** (thal-ah-**mot**-oh-me) > to cut into the thalamus. In this case, a procedure to destroy a selected area to relieve pain, epilepsy, or involuntary movements.

– **Hypothalamus** (**hi**-poe-**thal**-ah-mus) > below the thalamus. This area contains several structures which have a huge impact on the body's homeostasis. It forms the floor of the 3rd ventricle of the brain.

THE HYPOTHALAMUS

Hypo- > under, less than, decreased. In this reference under the thalamus

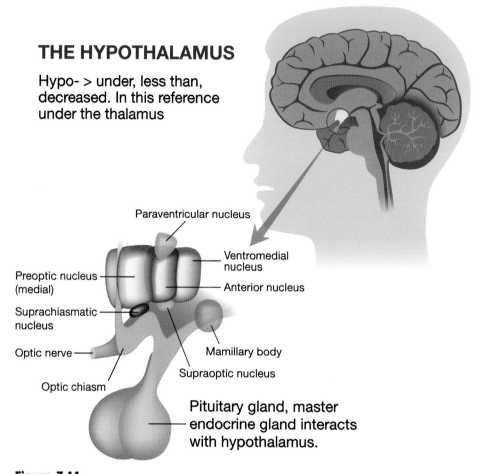

Paraventricular nucleus

Ventromedial nucleus

Preoptic nucleus (medial)

Anterior nucleus

Suprachiasmatic nucleus

Optic nerve

Mamillary body

Supraoptic nucleus

Optic chiasm

Pituitary gland, master endocrine gland interacts with hypothalamus.

Figure 7.11

Kitchen lab

Neuroplasticity describes the brain's ability to learn new things. Try this, with your non-dominant hand, write your signature. If you are like most people, it will look terrible. Repeat the effort and within 50 tries it will improve. You have trained your brain. A new pathway has been created. If you practice regularly, the signature will be permanent. This is how we learn to play instruments or drive a car.

7.17

✓ Construct a word meaning 'headache'.

✓ Construct a word meaning 'softened cerebrum'.

✓ Construct the medical term for 'to cut into the thalamus'.
_____ / ___ / _____ .

Word building

Using the word roots with the linking vowel to build as many valid terms with the suffixes given. Please define them too.

Crani/o Cephal/o Encephal/o

–itis –malacia –pathy –tomy –ic –megaly
–edema –algia –cele

The areas of the brain have their own specific names but it is important to remember all these areas are highly interactive and part of an extremely dense cell matrix. These 'designations' are used to denote areas of function as noted in Figure 7.12.

- Diencephalon (**die**-en-**sef**-a-lon) > through + inside the brain > is deep to the cortex of the brain – in the middle, between the cerebrum. This area includes the structures coordinating many of our body functions: the thalamus, hypothalamus, the optic chiasm, and pineal gland. It is surrounded by the limbic system.

- **Frontal** > largest, most anterior lobes of the cerebral cortex. In the past this area was considered the 'smart' part of our brain where learning, math, music, etc. . . . was processed. Today, the entire cortex (including the frontal lobe) is thought to be the end point of the **reticular activating system (RAS)** and it is all part of 'thinking'.

- **Parietal** (pah-**rye**-eh-tal) > wall > found in many systems, but in the brain it is the lobe of the brain immediately behind the central fissure. It does 'wall off' the deeper ventricles and mid-brain. This part of the cortex is a huge section of the body awareness and motion with the sensory association area – it is our **cognitive area**.

- **Temporal** (**tem**-pore-al) > pertaining to time > lateral and inferior to the frontal and parietal lobes. This area of the cortex seems to be most involved in the sensory inputs from sound, speech, memory, and visual perceptions. It also houses the distinct areas of the limbic system, amygdala, and hippocampus, which are involved with emotional responses and speech.

7.18 Cephalgia
Cephalodynia

7.19
Cerebromalacia

7.20
Thalam/o/tomy

7.21
The instructor has the list!

7.22
Di- > two, twice, between, or through

Hypo- > under, less than, less, decreased

The four lobes of the brain are protected by the bones of the cranium by the same names.

Did You Know?

Each neuron of the cortex can interact with up to 250,000 other neurons at any moment in time.

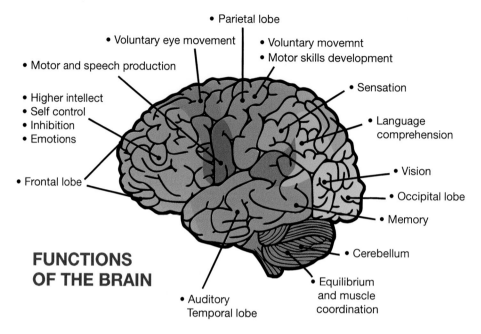

- Parietal lobe
- Voluntary eye movement
- Voluntary movemnt
- Motor skills development
- Motor and speech production
- Sensation
- Higher intellect
- Self control
- Inhibition
- Emotions
- Language comprehension
- Vision
- Frontal lobe
- Occipital lobe
- Memory
- Cerebellum
- Equilibrium and muscle coordination
- Auditory
Temporal lobe

FUNCTIONS OF THE BRAIN

Figure 7.12

- **Occipital** (ock-**sip**-ee-tall) > back of the head, pyramidal > most posterior lobe of the cerebrum and directly above the cerebellum. It functions to recognize and process vision and is a large part of proprioception, cognition when awake, and balance.

- **Insula** (**in**-sue-la) > island > hidden section of the frontal cortex deep within the lateral sulcus. It is an area involved with consciousness. These functions include recognition, cognitive learning, insight or intuition, self-awareness, and interactive relationships. This area is associated with psychopathy (**sigh**-ko-**pah**-thee) > diseases of the emotion or mentation or psyche.

The structures of the **limbic** (**lim**-bik) **system** have always been a bit vague as is the alternate name, the emotional brain. This region gives us a sense of 'experience' such as anger, hunger, fear, sadness, happiness, joy, pleasure, satisfaction, etc. The wrap-around configuration of the mid-brain explains why the smell of popcorn reminds us of a good movie or the sight of a sunset warms our heart.

- **Hippocampus** (**hip**-oh-**kam**-pus) > Greek for 'seahorse' > named for its shape, not its function. Associated with forming, organizing, and storing new **memories** with their emotional responses.

7.23
The limbic system interacts with the thalamus, hypothalamus, several cranial nerves, and the **RAS** via the corpus callosum. Without the modification of the cortex (our rationale), the limbic

THE LIMBIC SYSTEM

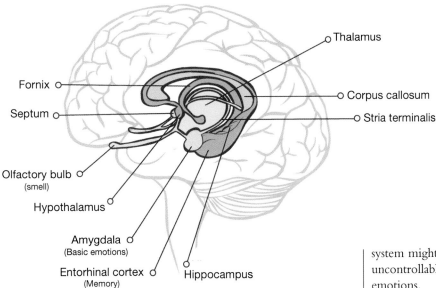

Thalamus

Fornix

Corpus callosum

Septum

Stria terminalis

Olfactory bulb
(smell)

Hypothalamus

Amygdala
(Basic emotions)

Entorhinal cortex
(Memory)

Hippocampus

Figure 7.13

- **Amygdala** (a-**mig**-da-la) > resembling an 'almond' > concentration of nuclei related to our emotions and motivation when interacting with others. It is felt to be involved with **autistic** responses or lack thereof.

✓ The medical term meaning 'to grasp together'.

✓ The area of the brain covered by the parietal bone is most active with which activities?

✓ The initial set for the blood–brain barrier.

The **brain stem** is the area of the brain which is 'unpaired' versus the cerebrum, which has a right and left. Ten of 12 of the cranial nerves will emerge on either side of the brain stem (Unit 8). The brain stem (by convention) begins with the mid-brain and ends as it passes through the magnum foramen to be called the spinal cord. It is continuous (Figure 7.14).

system might create uncontrollable emotions.

The cellular changes noted with **Alzheimer's** consistently begin in the temporal area of the limbic system.

7.24
Synapsis

7.25
Cognition of aware-ness and motion

7.26
BBB

7.27

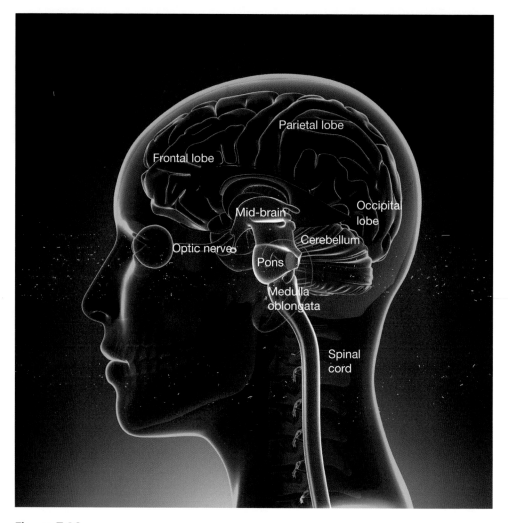

Figure 7.14

- The **mid-brain** > between the diencephalon and pons. It is composed of mixed sensory, motor, and reflexive nerves coordinating eye movement, pupillary reflex, muffling loud noises, and muscle control.
  - Part of the mid-brain is the **substantia nigra** (sub-**stan**-she-ah **nigh**-gra) > black substance > which is implicated in Parkinsonism and Huntington's disease.
- **Pons** > bridge > responsible for integrating the reflexes of the face, eyes, hearing, and the all-important respiratory rate.

Did You Know?

The clear **CSF** is produced by the choroid plexus of the brain ventricles and it is circulated by pulse of the blood flow and the movement of the microvilli of the ependymal cells.

- **Medulla oblongata** (meh-**due**-lah ob-long-**gah**-ta) > much the same configuration of the spinal cord with the white and gray matter tracts coming and going from the brain.

- It is a reflex center for breathing, heart rate, blood vessel dilatation/contraction (blood pressure), vomiting (**emesis**), cough, sneezing, and swallowing.

We make about 500 ml of **CSF** each day but it is recycled, so there is about 1/2 cup or 120 ml moving around all the time.

The **spinal cord** is the extension of brain, officially beginning at the magnum foramen and ending at about L1–2 in most people, about 17 inches long (45 cm). The cord itself is about 0.5 inches wide (1 to 1.5 cm) and much like putty, soft and pliable. It is protected anteriorly and posteriorly by the vertebrae (spinal column) (Figure 7.15). The spinal nerves exit to the body and back again in 31 segments. The cord tapers off to the **conus medullaris** (**ko**-nus med-U-**lahr**-ris) in the region of L1, then the spinal nerves form the **cauda equina**.

7.28

SPINAL CORD (CROSS SECTION)

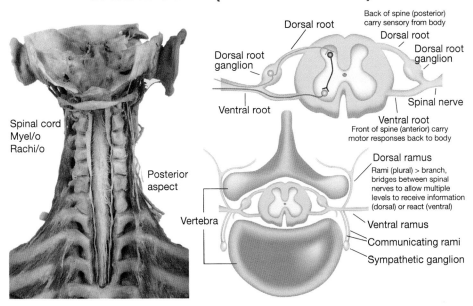

Figure 7.15

- **Myel/o** > spinal cord > this linking form indicates the medulla oblongata, spinal cord, AND bone marrow due to their consistency.
  - **Myelitis** (**my**-eh-**lie**-tis) > inflammation of the spinal cord
  - **Myelomalacia** (**my**-eh-low-mah-**lah**-she-a) > softening of the spinal cord

- **Radic/o, Radicul/o** > root, primary or beginning point of a nerve. Synonym: rhiz/o = root, rhizotomy, to cut into the nerve root.
  - **Dorsal** > these nerve bundles enter the backside (posterior) spinal column carrying mostly afferent or sensory information.
  - **Ventral** > these nerve bundles enter the front (anterior) spinal columns or tracts carrying mostly efferent or motor instructions.
  - **Radiculitis** (rah-**dik**-U-**lie**-tis) > inflammation of the nerve root.
  - **Radiculoneuropathy** (rah-**dik**-U-low-nur-**op**-ath-ee) > disease of the spinal nerve roots and nerves.
- **Ganglia** (**gang**-klee-ah) > swelling or knot > collection of neurons located in the peripheral nervous system (**PNS**). Ganglia is plural, ganglion is singular.
  - **Gangliocytoma** (**gang**-klee-oh-sigh-**toe**-ma) > rare tumor of a peripheral neuronal node.
  - **Ganglion cyst** (**gang**-klee-on sist) > usually benign tumor in the hand or foot ganglion.

Did You Know?

The blood circulation in the **CNS** is moving about 1.7 pints (1 liter) *a minute!* The blood vessels are configured like a traffic circle called the **Circle of Willis**. With the many communicating rami, the brain and spinal tissues are supplied with two vital elements: oxygen and glucose. The snug junctions of the cell walls of the **CNS** capillaries are part of the **BBB**, protecting the brain from large foreign bodies and infections.

Rachicentesis is another name for a **lumbar puncture** > to remove fluid by puncture.

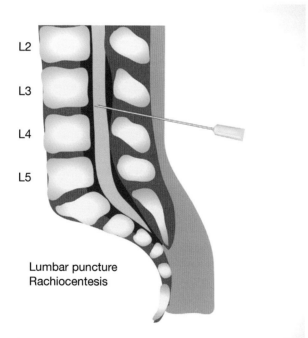

L2

L3

L4

L5

Lumbar puncture
Rachiocentesis

LUMBAR PUNCTURE

Figure 7.16

- **Rami** (plural), **Ramus** (**ray**-my or **ray**-mus) > branch > a nerve division branching out for motor control from the ventral root or ganglia.

The spinal cord with its **CSF** and relatively easy access is used to evaluate the wellness of the **CNS**. The spinal fluid should be clear and colorless. When an infection is suspected, a **lumbar puncture** (**LP**) or spinal tap can be performed by inserting a needle between lumbar vertebrae and into the subarachnoid space (Figure 7.16).

- Presence of low glucose indicates infection (bacteria are consuming the **CSF** glucose).

- Increased **CSF** pressure indicates intracranial pressure (**ICP**) from a bleed, mass effect, or hydrocephalus > condition of fluid in the brain.

Nerves are not neurons. They are bundles of peripheral nerve fibers (axons). As seen with muscle fibers, nerve fibers are held together by fascia (Figure 7.17).

ANATOMY OF A NERVE

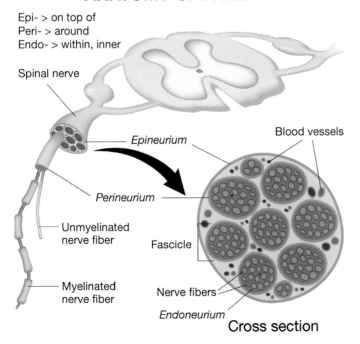

Epi- > on top of
Peri- > around
Endo- > within, inner

Spinal nerve

Epineurium

Blood vessels

Perineurium

Unmyelinated
nerve fiber

Fascicle

Myelinated
nerve fiber

Nerve fibers

Endoneurium

Cross section

Figure 7.17

7.29

Did You Know?

If you took all the neurons and nerves together and lined them up, they would make a 90,000-mile track – compared to the blood vessels with all the capillaries of nearly 600,000 miles.

Plexus is used both as singular and plural, though **plexuses** is also correct for the plural.

Nerves in the peripheral nervous system (**PNS**) are picking up sensory information and giving motor instruction in response to the brain – these are mixed nerves. When the nerves enter the spinal cord, these are called **tracts**. The white tracts (myelinated) form the white **columns**. The gray tracts (unmyelinated) form the gray columns surrounding the central canal, which contains the circulating **CSF**.

As the large spinal nerves leave the spine they form four major **plexuses** (**pleks**-us), grouped networks of nerves branching off to specific areas.

- The cervical plexus serves the head, neck, diaphragm, and arms.

- The thoracic covers the chest and abdominal muscles.

- The lumbar plexus covers the legs.

- The sacral plexus covers the bowel, bladder, and sexual functions.

The meninges (meh-**nin**-jez) of the brain and spinal cord protect, contain, and help bathe the central nervous system in **CSF**. The brain is just a little bit smaller than the cranium; the meninges and **CSF** essentially float the brain, which cushions the dense tissue and helps nourish all areas.

- **Mening/o** > membrane, covering > three layers of connective tissue covering and protecting the brain and spinal cord (Figure 7.18).
  - Meningitis (**men**-in-**ji**-tis) > inflammation of the meninges.
  - Meningioma (meh-**nin**-jee-**oh**-ma) > tumor of the meninges.
  - Meningocele (meh-**ning**-oh-seal) > herniation of the meninges. Note, the hard 'g' sound with the linking vowel 'o'.

- **Dura mater** (**dur**-ah **mah**-tur) > hard, tough matter. Dura mater is the thick, tough connective tissue which is also part of the inner periosteum of the cranial bones.

- **Arachnoid mater** (ah-**rak**-noyd **mah**-tur) > spider web matter. It is the fine but tough web acting as the middle layer of the meninges. It is related to the rich capillary bed of the meninges. Lumbar puncture pierces this layer to test the **CSF**.

- **Pia mater** (**pee**-ah **mah**-tur) > tender, delicate matter. It is the fine mesh adhering to every nook and cranny of the cortex of the brain and spinal cord.

7.30

Meninx is the singular > men-inks

Meninges is the plural > men-in-gees

Kitchen lab

Look around your environment: home, car, school, and work for items functioning like the meninges, protecting in layers. For instance, how is a quilt like the meninges?

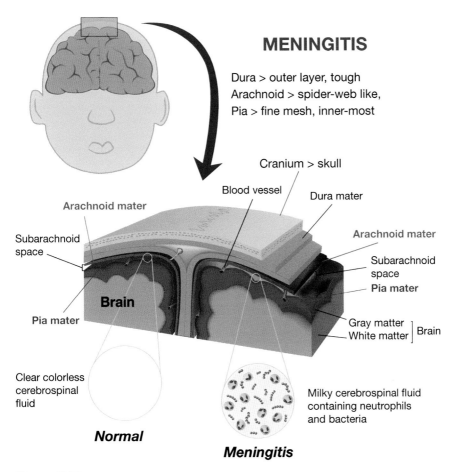

MENINGITIS

Dura > outer layer, tough
Arachnoid > spider-web like,
Pia > fine mesh, inner-most

Cranium > skull

Blood vessel

Dura mater

Arachnoid mater

Subarachnoid space

Arachnoid mater

Subarachnoid space

Pia mater

Brain

Gray matter ⎤ Brain
White matter ⎦

Pia mater

Clear colorless cerebrospinal fluid

Milky cerebrospinal fluid containing neutrophils and bacteria

Normal

Meningitis

Figure 7.18

✓ Construct a word meaning 'inflammation of the spinal cord and its meninges'.

7.31
Meningomyelitis

✓ A myelogram is ordered for James. What is a myelogram?

7.32
A record of the spinal cord. An X-ray procedure.

Word building

Using the word roots with the linking vowel to build as many valid terms with the suffixes given. Please define them too.

Mening/o Psych/o Cerebr/o

–itis –malacia –oma –ectomy –logy –meter –cele

7.33
The instructor has the list!

CONSCIOUSNESS

Psychiatry, psychologists, counselors, and other professionals are concerned with our consciousness and our subconscious. Why do we cry during a good movie but never at the loss of a loved one? Is there life after physical death? Why do I hear voices or have to wash my hands all the time? These and so many more questions are the fabric of life and our brain. Psychiatry is the study of the mind, the soul, the self. *The Diagnostic and Statistical Manual of Mental Disorders* (DSM-5) is the criterion for all things concerning the intangibles of our emotions. There are terms used regularly and others will need to be looked up, particularly all the 'phobias', the fear of XXX. Here are a few of those terms:

- Coprolalia (**kop**-row-**lah**-lee-a) > compulsive use of obscene words.
- Agoraphobia (**ag**-or-ah-**foe**-bee-ah) > fear of being in public places.
- Megalomania (**meg**-al-oh-**may**-knee-ah) > extravagant self-importance.
- Dyslexia (dis-**lek**-see-a) > difficult reading.
- Anxiety (ang-**zi**-eh-tea) > feeling of worry, uneasiness, dread.
- Dysthymia (dis-**thigh**-me-ah) > long-term sense of unhappiness, sadness, and hopelessness.
- Schizophrenia (**skiz**-oh-**fre**-knee-ah) > chronic psychosis, which includes bizarre behavior, delusions, or sudden catatonic states.

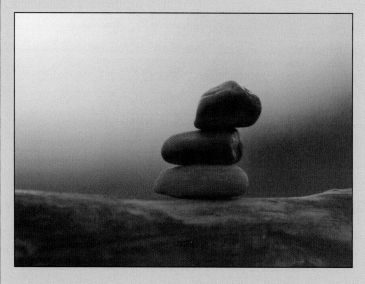

Figure 7.19

Today, research is ongoing as to why some people have more depression or attention deficit disorder or autism or panic disorder than other people. Researchers are sure the neurotransmitters are involved but there must be other triggers in our environment and/or in the structure of the brain setting one patient on an antisocial pathway versus a simple anxiety.

EVALUATION OF THE CNS AND DISEASE

The 31 segments of the spinal nerves permit a physical examination to evaluate the cord's wellness or injury at any of these levels. The levels of innervation are called the **dermatomes**. In this case, it is cutting the body into skin sensory areas (Figure 7.20).

- **Herpes zoster (VZV)** > Shingles > viral remnant of the chickenpox, which will sit in a nerve root for decades before erupting again. The painful, raised papules and vesicles will follow the spinal nerve dermatome. The infected dermatome shown in Figure 7.21 involves the right-hand T10 dermatome.

7.34
When a clinician checks the presence of CNS function they check most of the dermatomes with:

Soft touch

Sharp/dull touch

Temperature

Vibratory touch

Discrimination from one location to another.

LIKE ALERT!
Dermatome is also the instrument to slice or cut skin.

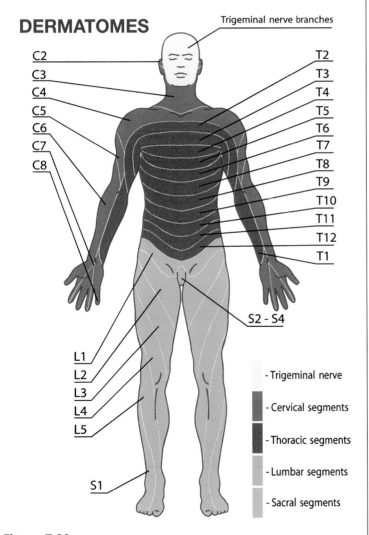

Figure 7.20

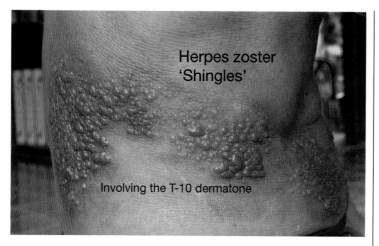

Herpes zoster 'Shingles'

Involving the T-10 dermatone

Figure 7.21

The **Glasgow Coma scale (GCS)** > rapid examination of the eye, verbal, and motor responses. It is used to objectively evaluate a patient's consciousness level. An initial assessment is made and then it is repeated to determine progress of treatment. The range is from 3 – the very worst to 15 – which is normal (Figure 7.22).

7.35
A neurological exam includes:

Appearance and general behavior

Mood and Effect

Cranial nerve testing

Sensation

Strength

Reflexes

Balance (cerebellum)

Gait

Mental status exam

Behaviour	Response
Eye Opening Response	4. Spontaneously 3. To speech 2. To pain 1. No response **Glasgow Coma Score (GCS)**
Verbal Response	5. Oriented to time, person, and place 4. Confused 3. Inappropriate words 2. Incomprehensible sounds 1. No response
Motor Response	6. Obeys command 6. Moves to localized pain 4. Flex to withdraw from pain 3. Abnormal flexion 2. Abnormal extension 1. No response

Figure 7.22

The **mental status examination (MSE)** can help differentiate between structural damage versus mental health changes. The scoring is similar to the GCS, helping the provider establish a baseline and the value of subsequent testing. 0 is poor, 30 is best, and 20 is average. Injury, illness, and psychiatric conditions will present with different findings.

- Alzheimer's patients will have difficulty with the memory sections.

- Schizophrenia may present with expansive speech, stream of ideas, and an inability to stay on task.

Imaging the brain and spinal cord is done by different types of computerized tomography. Tomography is many cuts organized into 3-D images by a computer. These examinations have essentially replaced the radiographic myelogram and even arteriograms.

CT scan was the first computerized evaluation tool; it uses X-ray (radiation). It is utilized to evaluate masses, bleeding, and infections.

Magnetic Resonance Imaging (MRI) uses magnetic energy to illuminate the brain and cord. It is excellent for defining the soft tissue distinctions of the dense mass. Because MRI does not radiate the patient, it is good for repeated examinations to track progress.

Positron emission tomography (PET) utilizes nuclear medicine to track structural changes via the blood flow. A radiographic tracer is injected into the bloodstream. It is utilized to check the brain's basic functions, look for cancers, and to evaluate some mental disorders.

Single-photon emission computed tomography (SPECT) is similar to PET. Again, the tracer is designed to track the perfusion of the brain or spinal area in this case. It is helpful in mental health disorders and some organic changes.

Evoked potential studies (EP) is a process of measuring the brain waves in response to a smell, sight, noise, or touch. **EP** is not a type of tomography.

7.36
Evaluation of mental health, organic brain, or cord changes always begins with a thorough physical exam as above, and then the imaging studics follow. To define a lesion or condition, a biopsy is still the gold standard for evaluation. Confirmed Alzheimer's, for instance, is not established until the autopsy in 90% of cases.

 The 'GCS' is the initial set for? What does it check?

 What is a 'dermatome' in reference to the CNS?

7.37
Glasgow Coma Scale; level of consciousness.
7.38
The spinal roots affect a specific sensory area of the skin.

✓ What is the initial set for the imaging study which is best for distinguishing soft tissues without radiation?

7.39
MRI

From shaken baby syndrome to football concussions, head injuries occur all too frequently. The cranium does protect but it is also a hard shell for the brain to bang against. These are closed head injuries.

- **Coma (ko-**mah) > profound loss of consciousness (**LOC**). Coma may be initiated by trauma, metabolic or hormonal changes, infections, or toxins.

- **Concussion (kon-kush-**un) > damage of the brain tissue with edema – diffuse axonal injury. An abrupt stop (deceleration) such as shaking a baby or a sudden stop in a vehicle can result in concussion (Figure 7.23).

- **Sub**dural hema**toma** > blood is trapped UNDER (sub) the dura mater and presses on the brain tissue (Figure 7.24).

7.40
Sport teams are collaborating on research to help prevent, identify, and treat the effects of repeated small concussions. Some individuals will progress to advanced brain degeneration, termed chronic traumatic encephalopathy (**CTE**).

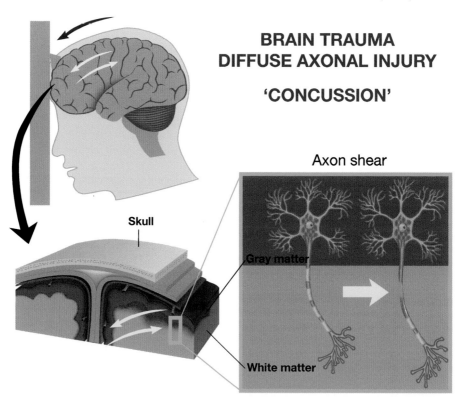

BRAIN TRAUMA
DIFFUSE AXONAL INJURY

'CONCUSSION'

Axon shear

Skull

Gray matter

White matter

Figure 7.23

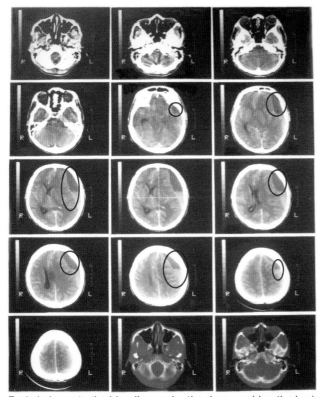

Red circles note the bleeding under the dura crushing the brain

SUBDURAL HEMATOMA

Figure 7.24

- Epidural hematoma > blood is trapped between the cranium and the dura mater. Epi- > upon, on top of

Head injuries of any type can cause permanent damage to the brain. The loss of a few neurons may not seem like much in the face of billions of cells, but over time memory and emotions may be affected. Accident prevention and smart sports play is vital to decrease the risk of these injuries.

Open skull injuries involve blows or projectiles which break into the cranium such as gunshots, knifes, shrapnel, and blunt-force trauma. Assuming a person lives, the debris and fluids must be evacuated and the cranium repaired.

- **Craniotomy (kray**-knee-**ot**-oh-me) > to cut into the skull. Trephination (**tref**-i-**na**-shun) is an alternate term, which is used when fluid/blood is evacuated via a drill hole.

7.41
Suffixes
-malacia > softening

-metry > measuring

-pathy > disease

-cele > herniation

- **Craniectomy** (**kray**-knee-**ek**-toe-me) > to surgically remove part of the skull bone.

- **Craniofenestria** (**kray**-knee-oh-feh-**nes**-tree-a) > to surgically create a window in the skull.

The brain itself has no 'sensory' endings – meaning it does not feel pain during surgery. Headaches are a result of vascular spasm, pressure on the meninges, or a change in **CSF** levels – too low or too high.

-plasty > repair

-schisis > split

-sclerosis > hardening

Spinal injuries from contusions to complete transection occur often too. An **incomplete** injury is the term used when motor function is preserved. **Complete** is the loss of all motor and sensory functions.

- **Spinal contusion** > bruising of the spine. A contusion can cause temporary paralysis due to the edema and microbleeding. Recovery may or may not be complete.

- **Partial** or **Complete** transection (across the section) is the most serious injury and the hardest to recover from. A high spinal cord injury in the C1–4 region is typically fatal because the swelling communicates to the brain stem stopping those cardiac and respiratory reflexes.

  - **Quad**riplegia (**qwa**-dree-**play**-gee-ah) > all four limbs are paralyzed.

  - Hemiplegia (hem-ee-**play**-gee-ah) > ipsilateral, both the arm and leg are paralyzed.

  - Paraplegia (pair-ah-**play**-gee-ah) > both legs are paralyzed.

  - **Paresis** (pah-**ree**-sis) > partial or incomplete paralysis.

7.42
An MRI is usually used to evaluate a spinal injury. Treatment is stabilization and decreasing swelling as quickly as possible. The swelling compresses the spine even in the absence of obvious structural damage.

Cervical injury patients will require respiratory support. Paraplegic patients will be reasonably independent from T1 or below.

Primary brain tumors begin within the brain. Metastatic cancers arrive in the brain, migrating from other areas via the bloodstream. MRI is the choice for evaluation of brain masses.

- **Glial tumors** occur at a rate of approximately 60%, and of those 80% tend to be aggressively malignant.

  - **Astrocytoma** (**as**-tro-sigh-**toe**-ma) > begins with the astrocytes.

- **Glioblastoma** (**glee**-oh-blas-**toe**-ma) > high-grade, very aggressive astrocytoma, which involves other glial cells (Figure 7.25).

- **Benign tumors** may be a bit of a misnomer. They are not malignant but they can cause trouble by taking up space in the dense tissues of the brain or spinal cord.

7.43
Liver, lung, prostate, breast, and colon cancers can metastasize to the brain. There are many types of brain tumor.

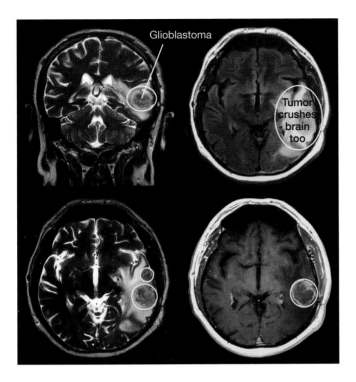

Glioblastoma

Tumor crushes brain too

Figure 7.25

— **Pituitary** (pi-**tu**-i-ter-ee) > usually microadenomas (small tumors of the glands). Most are non-functioning (not putting out hormones). The first sign of this growth is typically a change in vision due to the proximity of the optic chiasm.

✓ Construct the term for 'repair of the cranium'.
_____/__/_____ .

7.44
Crani/o/plasty

✓ If blood is trapped under the dura mater, it is termed a
_____ .

7.45
subdural hematoma

✓ Mia was horseback riding when she fell and severed her spine at T10. What kind of paralysis is she likely to have?

7.46
Paraplegia

Word building

Using the word roots with the linking vowel to build as many valid terms with the suffixes given. Please define them too.

Rachi/o Hemat/o Radicul/o or Radic/o
-itis -oma -ectomy -ic -meter -dynia -ar

7.47
The instructor has the answers!

Diseases of Motion occur at the **CNS** level; they are all neurodegenerative diseases. After Alzheimer's, they are the most common diseases of the elderly.

- **Parkinson's disease** > degeneration of the dopamine neurons in the substantia nigra. Patients can develop this disease as young as 20 years old. Symptoms include

  - Bradykinesia (**braid**-ee-ki-knee-**see**-ah) > slow to motion.

  - Resting tremor > repetitive, oscillatory movement at rest.

PARKINSON'S DISEASE

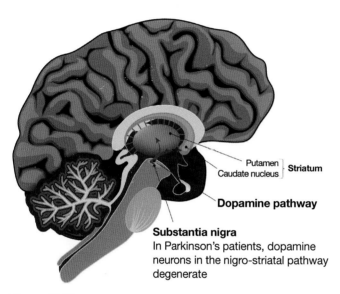

Putamen
Caudate nucleus } **Striatum**

Dopamine pathway

Substantia nigra
In Parkinson's patients, dopamine neurons in the nigro-striatal pathway degenerate

Figure 7.26

- Stroke, liver failure, infections, tumor, and drugs can induce a Parkinson-type motion loss as well.

- **Huntington's disease (HD),** also known as Huntington's chorea. It is a progressive and fatal disorder with un-patterned, semipurposeful, and involuntary motion.

- **Tourette's** (**tur**-ets) **syndrome** > multiple tics with vocalization.

  - Echolalia (**ek**-hoe-la-**lee**-ah) > repeating other people's words.

  - Palilalia (pal-i-la-**lee**-ah) > repeating one's own words.

- **Tardive dyskinesia** (**tahr**-div **dis**-key-**knee**-zee-ah) **(TD)** > characteristic symptoms include repetitive choreiform actions such as lip-smacking, pill-rolling (hands busy moving imaginary

7.48
Treatment for **CNS** motion disorders includes levodopa, replacing dopamine. The use of dopamine agonists such as pramipexole enhances the effect of dopamine.

Echolalia, palilalia, and coprolalia are seen with schizophrenic patients as well.

Athetosis (ath-eh-toe-sis) > slow, writhing, involuntary motion
Ataxia > inability to control muscle motion, balance is off

Cataplexy (kat-ah-pleks-ee) > sudden loss of muscle tone

pills), and tongue motions. Medications associated with this disorder are antipsychotics and metoclopramide. Treatment is to stop the medications. Synonym: Extrapyramidal side-effects (**EPSE**).

- Cerebral palsy > motor loss or palsy (paralysis) associated with brain damage. Injury may occur in utero, at birth, or after birth (at any age). It is distinguished by both mental and physical incapacities, contractures, and spasticity.

Epilepsy and seizures are caused by sudden and unexpected, excessive and hypersynchronous firing of the neurons. This creates a variety of symptoms. The body's reaction ranges from a stillness or almost zombie state to marked convulsions with loss of bowel and urine control.

Focal seizures tend to be in an isolated area of one hemisphere (Figure 7.27).

- **Generalized seizures** arise from one of the hemispheres but spread rapidly to involve both sides completely.
  - Absence (ab-**sonce**)> brief lapse in consciousness, loss of time without collapse.
  - Tonic–clonic (**tohn**-ik **kloh**-nik) > sudden contraction of the muscles followed by muscle flaccidity (flabbiness).
  - Atonic (a-**toh**-nik) > sudden loss of muscle tone.
  - Myoclonic (**my**-oh-**cloy**-nik) > sudden muscle jerking of one or more muscles.

Evaluation of seizure activity includes an **EEG**, electroencephalo-gram. Seizures may be treated with an assortment of medication or by selective surgery called **ablation** (ab-**lay**-shun) > to destroy the function.

Neuropathies occur in the brain, the spinal cord, and the peripheral nervous system (**PNS**) – a sample:

- **Alcoholic neuropathy** > parasympathetic system slowly grinds to a halt including the GI tract, liver functions, cardiac and respiratory rates.

- **Guillain–Barre** (geh-ah-an bah-ray **sin**-drum) **Syndrome** (**GBS**) > result of a virus usually, this can be fatal due to cardiac arrhythmias and blood pressure (**BP**) fluctuations.

- **Bell's palsy** > CN 7 weakness on one side of the face, a palsy (Figure 7.28). It tends to be temporary, lasting 3–6 months.

7.49

Did You Know?

Epilepsy and seizures are reflected on the **EEG** as a change in the amplitude of the neuronal reactions, not the speed.

The term **post-ictal** refers to the slight confusion or disorientation of the person after the seizure. **Ictal** is Latin for stroke.

7.50

LIKE ALERT!

GBS is also used for Group B *Streptococcus* infection.

Suffixes
–pathy > disease
–esthesia > condition of sensation

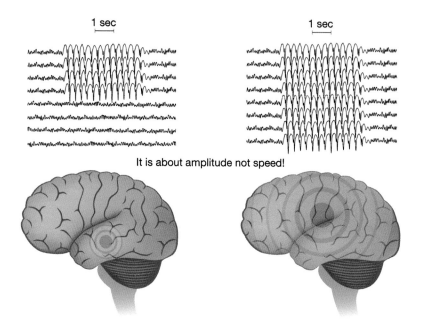

It is about amplitude not speed!

Partial seizure   Generalized seizure

Figure 7.27

BELL'S PALSY

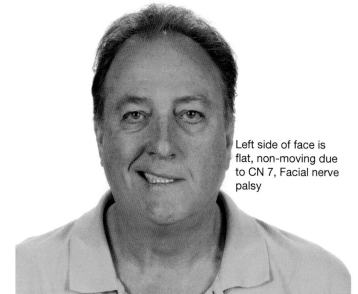

Left side of face is flat, non-moving due to CN 7, Facial nerve palsy

Figure 7.28

- **Carpal tunnel syndrome (CTS)** > compression of the median nerve of the wrist. This can also be termed a radiculopathy. **Sciatica** is another specific or mononeuropathy at the hip > single disease of the nerve.

- **Diabetic neuropathy** > hyperglycemia over time breaks the tiny capillaries. Lack of blood supply no longer maintains the nerve endings. Smoking increases the risk of neuropathy as well. The paresthesias are painful, irritating, and tingling, beginning in the feet and spreading up the peripheral nervous system.
  - **Dysesthesia** (**dis**-es-**thee**-zee-ah) > painful, disagreeable sensation.
  - **Paresthesia** (**pear**-es-**thee**-zee-ah) > numbness, tingling.
  - **Hyperesthesia** (**hi**-pur-es-**thee**-zee-ah) > abnormal sensitivity to touch, pain, or other stimulus.

-asthenia > condition of weakness

-osis > abnormal condition

-phasia > condition of speech

-plagia > condition of eating and swallowing

-plegia > condition of paralysis

Brady- > slow

Tachy- > fast

Multiple sclerosis (**mul**-tea-pel **sklar**-oh-sis) **(MS)** > demyelinating disease slowly eroding the myelin sheath from the axons both in the **CNS** and peripheral nerves slowing or stopping motor responses.

AUTOIMMUNE DISEASE
Multiple sclerosis > condition of hardening

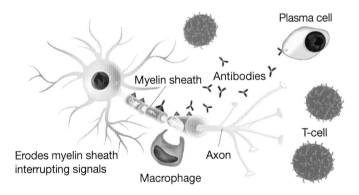

Plasma cell

Myelin sheath   Antibodies

T-cell

Erodes myelin sheath interrupting signals

Axon

Macrophage

Figure 7.29

- Triggers include viral illness, autoreactive T-lymphocytes, and environmental exposures, which may include the use of sunscreens – setting up an autoimmune response.

Amyotrophic lateral sclerosis (ALS) (a-**my**-oh-**trow**-fik) > progressive motor neuron degeneration. Muscle control is lost until the respiratory muscles stop.

7.51
All of these autoimmune diseases take time to diagnose as their symptoms tend to come and go initially and appear in random, seemingly unrelated areas. The average time to diagnosis is 5 years.

Diagnostics include:

Antibody testing

Anticholinesterase testing

Evoked potentials

CFS study

Biopsy

- Triggers include viral illnesses, structural lesions, autoimmune reactions, lead poisoning, medications, and metabolic disorders.

Myasthenia Gravis (**my**-as-**thee**-knee-ah **gra**-vis) (**MG**) > disruption of the NMJ with decreased ACh receptor sites. My/asthenia > muscle weakness.

- This autoimmune disease typically presents with diplopia, myasthenias, fatigue, eyelid **ptosis** (drooping), loss of muscle strength, and respiratory functions.

Infections of the CNS and spinal cord are many. Unlike many infections in other areas of the body, **CNS** infections can leave significant sequelae (seh-**qwell**-ay) – residual seizures, hearing loss, motor control issues, and memory impairment.

- **Meningitis** > bacterial or viral infection of the brain and cord meninges. It is characterized by an extreme headache, fever, and extreme pain with neck movement because the inflamed meninges are moving. This pain and reluctance to move the neck is called **nuchal rigidity**.
  - Nearly 50% of cases are due to Streptococcus pneumoniae.
  - Neisseria meningitidis has decreased with the availability of a vaccination. It is recommended for all college-age students.

- **Viral encephalitis** > inflammation of the brain > similar to meningitis with fever, milder headache, and a change in consciousness. Confusion, anxiety, hallucinations, and psychotic breaks are seen with this condition. Causes include:
  - West Nile Virus (**WNV**) from mosquitoes.
  - St. Louis encephalitis virus.
  - Herpes Simplex Virus (**HSV**).

- There are **many infectious diseases** causing **CNS** symptoms and mimic other **CNS** disorders. They are part of the possibilities for everything discussed in this Unit.
  - Rocky Mountain Spotted Fever (tick-borne).
  - Lyme's disease (tick-borne).
  - Botulism.
  - Herpes Zoster virus (**VZV**).
  - Cytomegaly virus (**CMV**).
  - Epstein–Barr virus (**EBV**).
  - Coccidiomycosis (fungus) > kok-**sid**-ee-**oy**-doe-my-**ko**-sis.
  - Toxoplasmosis (**tok**-so-plaz-**moe**-sis) is a parasite.
  - Poliomyelitis (**poy**-lee-oh-my-eh-**lie**-tis) > inflammation of the gray matter of the spine.

7.52
Diagnostics begin with blood and **CSF** evaluation and cultures. West Nile Virus (**WNV**) and other viral antigens may be examined. **MRI** or **CT** with **EEG** is also part of the evaluation. Biopsy is not done unless absolutely necessary.

Treatment for infections depends on the type of pathogen. Antibiotics for the bacteria. Antifungals for the fungal infections.

Antivirals to slow the viral infections.

Chronic inflammation can cause meningitis too, such as systemic lupus erythematosus (**SLE**) and sarcoidosis.

Polio- > gray

- **Prion diseases** (**pry**-on) involve infectious proteins which cause degeneration of the brain and spinal cord, e.g., **CJD**, Creutzfeldt–Jacob disease, which is thought to be caused by eating meat of an infected animal. These are rare.

✓ Echolalia means _____ _____

7.53
repeating other people's words

✓ Which of the following initial sets can cause a meningitis and is transmitted by mosquito?

        CMV   HSV   WNV   VZV

7.54
WNV

✓ Parkinsonism and Huntington's are examples of

      Synonyms   Eponyms   Abbreviations   Acronyms

7.55
Eponyms

PHARMACY CORNER*

Honestly, there is probably not a medication or herb on the planet which cannot harm the CNS in high enough doses. Even simple over-the-counter medications such acetaminophen and diphenhydramine are all too often used as suicide drugs. Yet, in the United States, we tend to believe the bumper-sticker, MEDICATE ME. We take a pill to calm our anxiety and treat our headache and other pills to treat the depression which the other two may be causing.

True, some medications do not make it past the blood–brain barrier. If there is damage to the liver due to alcohol or other medications, the liver's lack of function can soon put the brain out of commission. Any organ failure affects the glucose and oxygen levels needed to keep the brain alert and working. There are several medication groups which function at the brain level.

- **Sedatives**: Opiates such as morphine, tramadol, and Dilaudid can cause sedation and may stop respirations in high doses. No oxygen, no brain.

- **Anti**depressants: sertraline, amitriptyline, duloxetine, bupropion, selegiline; each represent a different class of medication modifying our mood. They all work by changing the brain chemistry – primarily the neurotransmitters.

- **Anxiolytics** (**ang**-zee-oh-**lit**-iks): These are all benzodiazepines but one, such as diazepam, lorazepam, and chlordiazepoxide. Sedation occurs and some can cause confusion with delirium, especially in the elderly.

- **Bipolar medications**: lithium, valproic acid, carbamazepine, and lamotrigine are all used as mood stabilizers. Recurrent side effects include rash, nausea, and in some cases hepatotoxicity (liver failure).

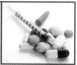

- Antipsychotics (**an**-teh-sigh-**kot**-iks) are used for schizophrenia, severe depression, and even in Alzheimer's: thorazine, loxapine, haloperidol, clozapine, risperidone, aripiprazole, and lurasidone. These are all well known for causing **EPSE**s, dry mouth, weight gain, and some sedation.

- **Stimulants and Non-stimulants**: Used for ADHD, ADD, and narcolepsy: amphetamine, dextroamphetamine, and methylphenidate are the stimulants. Atomoxetine, clonidine, and guanfacine are non-stimulants. These are all designed to improve concentration and impulse control. The side-effect profiles are high, which range from over-sedation to frankly wired for action.

- Antiepileptics (**an**-teh-ep-i-**lep**-tik): phenytoin, carbamazepine, and valproic acid are the older medications used for decades for seizure and chronic headache. Other medications have been used with some success such as gabapentin, lamotrigine, topiramate, clonazepam, and phenobarbital.

This is a short list of medications which impact the brain both mechanically and emotionally. Like all medications, the side-effect profile and drug–drug/drug–food interactions must be considered. Medical documentation of the symptoms of the disease process, the medications, and their effects inform all the providers as to the status of the patient. Precision and clarity are vital to the continuity of care and patient safety.

* IMPORTANT NOTE: Medicine is always in evolution. Do <u>not</u> use this information for patient care.

PSYCHIATRIC ILLNESS

Psychiatric illnesses are many and come with many variations and opinions as to cause and treatments. Psychiatric illnesses have many potential causes but genetics, environmental exposure, head trauma, medication influences, and infections top the list.

- **Autism** (**ah**-tizm) > delays or abnormal functions in social interactions. Something, likely in our environment, has driven this condition from rare to common in the last 4 decades. Many large-scale analyses have ruled out vaccinations but the jury is still out on the trigger of this condition.

- **Schizophrenia** > Greek for 'split mind'. This chronic condition is characterized by abnormal perceptions of life, hallucinations, stream of thought, and withdrawal from the world. The causes are under investigation but both autism and schizophrenia may have a prenatal viral infection trigger.

7.56
Dementia (deh-**men**-she-ah) >
A cognitive impairment which tends to progress

Delusion (deh-**lew**-shun-al) >
false or incorrect judgment

- **Anxiety** > sense of dread or uncomfortable sensations. The majority of people have some anxiety at some time in their life; like most mental disorders, symptoms persisting longer than two weeks may be labeled anxiety. A **panic attack** is severe anxiety which can suddenly stop all useful activity.

- **Depression** > sense of sadness, a reduction in functioning. Seen frequently, almost all individuals will have an acute, or chronic major depressive condition. Post-traumatic stress disorder (**PTSD**) is a depressive disorder secondary to extreme traumatic or a personal threat episode or set of episodes.

Hallucination (hal-**lew**-si-**nah**-shun) > Visual, auditory, tactile, olfactory perception of an object or event that is not real.

- **Phobic** (foe-bik) **disorders** > marked or persistent fear of objects or situations. Since there are literally thousands, here is a small sample.
  - Hippopotomonstrosesquippedaliophobia > fear of long words (really ☺).
  - Alektorophobia > fear of chickens.
  - Metathesiophobia > fear of change.
  - Koumpounophobia > fear of buttons.
  - Chaetophobia > fear of hair.

- **Bipolar** > unpredictable swing in moods, in two different directions.
  - Mania is characterized by excessive psychomotor activity, effusive social interactions, impulse control issues, and impaired judgment.
  - The depressive side can range from crying to catatonia.

7.57
Catatonic > down + tone > periods of rigidity (non-motion), stupor, or negativism

---

- **Attention Deficit Disorder (ADD)** > adults or children > inability to stay on task.

- **Attention Deficit Hyperactivity Disorder (ADHD)** > adults or children > inability to slow down and attend to a task.

- **Fetal alcohol syndrome (FAS)** > physical and mental alteration associated with hyperactivity, growth deficiency, and learning disability (Figure 7.30).

Like autism, these disorders seem to have exploded over the last four decades. The diagnosis should not be based on one episode of evaluation, especially in children.

7.58
The cause of ADD and ADHD is unknown though research is ongoing. Researchers are looking at genetic change or environmental triggers such as lead poisoning and prenatal exposure to tobacco, alcohol, and specific drugs.

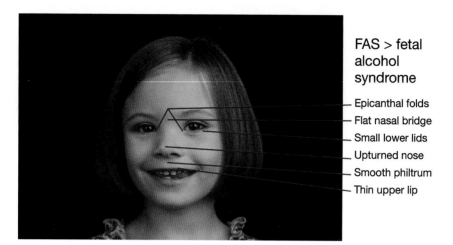

FAS > fetal alcohol syndrome

— Epicanthal folds
— Flat nasal bridge
— Small lower lids
— Upturned nose
— Smooth philtrum
— Thin upper lip

Figure 7.30

- **Learning disabilities** are numerous including many genetic and structural causes of mental retardation.

    – Dyslexia > impaired reading.

    – Dysgraphia (dis-**graf**-ee-ah) > impaired writing skills.

    – Dyscalculia (**dis**-kal-**Q**-lee-ah) > impaired math skills.

    – Dyspraxia (dis-**prak**-zee-ah) > difficulty in performing motor tasks, a sensory integration disorder.

    – Central auditory processing disorder (**CAPD**) > difficulty processing sounds.

    – Visual processing disorder > difficulty processing visuals.

7.59
Disabilities are classified by developmental or intellectual and/or physical challenges.

✓ Construct a word meaning 'disease of many nerves'.
_____

7.60
Polyneuropathy

✓ 'An *anencephalic* child was born today'.
Define anencephalic.

7.61
No brain

✓ Construct the word meaning 'protrusion of the spinal cord and meninges'. _____ /__ /____ /___ /____

7.62
Mening/o/myel/o – /cele

CODING: TABLE OF DRUGS AND CHEMICALS*

All medications whether they are over-the-counter, used in anesthesia, street drugs, chemotherapy, oral, or IV have the potential for inappropriate use. The medications associated with the treatment of neurologic and psychiatric conditions are no different. In the ICD Table of Drugs and Chemicals there are six columns with every current chemical and medication with room for more.

- **Poisoning, accidental (unintentionally)**. This is an 'accident' common in children and the elderly. Children because they think the medication might be candy and elders because they may forget they have already taken a medication.

- **Poisoning, intentional self-harm**. From the CDC statistics there were 41,000 completed suicides in the United States in 2013. A good number of these completed and attempted suicides involved the use of medication.

- **Poisoning, assault**. When does an overdose become a murder? It is beyond his text to address this huge question; however, as an example: If someone decides to kill a junkie with an extra dose of crack or a caregiver deliberately adds extra morphine to a hospice patient's medications – it is considered an assault.

- **Poisoning, undetermined**. Did the young adult intend to attempt suicide during his/her 21st birthday alcoholic binge? Probably not, but if the event is unclear, this is the coding column to use.

- **Adverse effects**. All medications can cause adverse effects even at normal dosing. The newer sedatives which are used for chronic pain may cause sleep-eating, sleep-walking, and even sleep-driving. Some medications designed to help with psychiatric diagnoses may actually increase suicidal ideation.

- **Underdosing**. This occurs more habitually than we probably realize as an individual may only take their medications when they are in the mood. If this is the case, perhaps their cholesterol or hypertension is affected. If the underdosing is a chemotherapy because an unethical person is cutting the dose to save money, then the effects are an untreated cancer and the result can be death.

Medical terminology, the medical documentation of the effects and intent of medication is vital to the care of the patient. Knowing when, where, how much, intent, and other co-morbid conditions determines immediate life-saving care and chronic care. The EHR must be correct as these statistics are used to improve the wellness of the entire population. What you record, correct spelling, and how you describe it does have an impact.

* **IMPORTANT NOTE: The reader is notified that these examples are from an online search done in 2016. Do <u>not</u> use the codes for patient care episodes; look up new ones!**

UNIT SUMMARY

1 The central nervous system includes the brain (encephal/o) and spinal cord (myel/o). The brain is housed in the cranium. The brain is a dense matrix of neurons and four support cells called the neuroglia (neuron glue). It weighs about three pounds and floats in a bath of cerebral spinal fluid (**CSF**).

2 While science and medicine continue to make advances in the understanding of the structures, chemistry, and hormones of the brain, we are still unclear how the mechanics give us consciousness, learning, and emotions. The neurotransmitters are numerous, some work globally and others work in specific locations. Acetylcholine, dopamine, epinephrine, and endorphins are examples of those working throughout the body.

3 The brain is composed of the cortex (outer layer) and a myriad of deeper structures integrating all our sensory perceptions, mood, urgency, and actions via the reticular activating system after passing through the thalamus and hypothalamus.

4 The lobes of the brain mirror the bone of the cranium by name: the frontal, parietal, temporal, and occipital lobes. The insula lobe is deep to the frontal cortex and the cerebellum rounds out the major sections of the brain. The limbic system is a collection of structures in the mid-brain area housing and processing our memory, learning, thoughts, and emotions.

5 The brain stem (medulla oblongata) and spinal cord have much the same configuration and texture, thus the linking form myel/o is used for both. The spinal cord is the extension of the brain with specific nerve tracts of white (myelinated) and gray (non-myelinated) axons.

6 The meninges are the protective coverings of the brain and spinal cord. They contain, protect, and help with bringing nutrients and capillary flow to the structures.

7 Evaluation of changes within the brain includes a number of computerized examinations such as **CT** scans, **MRI**, **EEG**, and evoked potentials (**EP**). To evaluate the effect of illness or injury from psychiatric or organic changes to the brain, the clinician does a sequence of examinations.

8 Head injuries can do real and lasting damage. Closed head injuries include hematomas involving the meninges such as a subdural hematoma.

9 Disease processes of the **CNS** and **PNS** are numerous as well, ranging from carcinoma to infections. The brain does have a blood–brain barrier but opportunistic infections can make a home via the bloodstream.

10 Psychiatric illnesses are outlined in the DSM-5 and include anxiety, depression, schizophrenia, and neuroses. There are many medications for the treatment of both psychiatric and organic conditions such as Alzheimer's. These medications can be quite effective but they also have larger side-effect profiles than other medications and are easily abused.

11 Medical researchers pore over medical records and the language of medicine to learn what the first symptoms are for disease processes such as Alzheimer's, Parkinsonism, schizophrenia, and autism. Their research looks at the progression of symptoms in relationship to genetics, exposures, and the chemistry of the brain in search of solutions.

UNIT WORD PARTS

Word roots with linking vowel		
Astr/o > star	Cephal/o > head	Cerebell/o > cerebellum
Cerebr/o > cerebrum, cortex	Cervic/o > neck	Copr/o > foul, filth, feces
Crani/o > skull, cranium	Dendr/o > branching	Encephal/o > brain
Mening/o > coverings, membrane	Myel/o > spinal cord or bone marrow	Neur/o > nerve
Phag/o > eating, swallowing	Phas/o > speech	Psych/o > mind, soul
Radic/o; Radicul/o > root	Schiz/o > split	Thalam/o > thalamus
Ventricul/o > chamber, ventricle	Vertebr/o; Rachi/o; Spondyl/o > back bone, spine	

Prefixes: attached to the front of the word root to change meaning		
A-, An- > no, not, absent	Ab- > away from center, away from normal	Bi- > two
Brady- > slow	Di- > two, through	Dys- > poor, difficult, painful
Endo- > inside, inner	Epi- > upon, on top of	Hemi- > half
Hypo- > below, under, less than	Inter- > between	Micro- > smallest, tiny
Multi- > many	Oligo- > scant, too few	Para- > near, departure from normal
Peri- > around	Poly- > many	Quadri- > four
Tachy- > fast	Uni- > one, single	

Suffixes change the meaning of the word, linking vowel is usually 'o' with consonants		
-algia or -dynia> pain	-ase > enzyme will break down the chemical	-asthenia > condition of weakness
-blast > embryonic cell, developing	-cele > herniation	-centesis > removal of fluid via needle/syringe
-cyte > cell	-edema > swelling	-esthesia > sensation, feeling
-fibril > small fiber	-gram > record of	-graphia > writing
-lemma > covering	-lexia > reading	-malacia > softening
-megaly > enlargement	-motor > movement, action	-osis > condition (abnormal)
-paresis > partial paralysis	-pathy > disease	-phagia > eating, swallowing
-phasia > speech	-plegia > paralysis	-praxia > action, motion

Acronyms, abbreviations, and initial sets		
ACh > acetylcholine	AChE > acetylcholin-esterase	ADD > attention deficit disorder
ADHD > attention deficit hyperactivity disorder	ANN > autoimmune autonomic neuropathy	BBB > blood–brain barrier
BP > blood pressure	CJD > Creutzfeldt-Jacob disease	CMV > cytomegaly virus
CNS > central nervous system	CSF > cerebral spinal fluid	CT > computerized tomography
CTE > chronic traumatic encephalopathy	CTS > carpal tunnel syndrome	EBV > Epstein–Barr virus
EEG > electroencephalo-gram	EP > evoked potential	Epi > epinephrine
EPSE > extra-pyramidal side-effects	FAS > fetal alcohol syndrome	GABA > γ (gamma)–aminobutyric acid
GBS > Guillain-Barre syndrome	GCS > Glasgow coma scale	ICP > intracranial pressure
LOC > loss of consciousness	LP > lumbar puncture	MG > myasthenia gravis
MRI > magnetic resonance imaging	MS > multiple sclerosis	NFT > neurofibrillatory tangles
Norepi > norepinephrine	OCD > obsessive compulsion disorder	PET > positron emission tomography
PNS> peripheral nervous system	PTSD > post-traumatic stress disorder	RAS > reticular activating system
SBS > shaken baby syndrome	SPECT > single Photon emission computed tomography	SSRI > selective serotonin reuptake inhibitors
TD > tardive dyskinesia	WNV > West Nile virus	VZV > varicella zoster virus

UNIT WORKSHEETS

Building terms: Use the proper prefix/word root/linking vowel/suffix as appropriate.

Example: to cut into the stomach > gastr/o/tomy

a) Softening of the spinal cord > _____

b) Blood collection under the dura (two words) > _____

c) Slow to motion > _____

d) To cut into the skull > _____

e) Using foul language > _____

f) Inflammation of the brain (inside the brain) > _____

g) Below the thalamus > _____

h) Scant 'branching' cells > _____

Know your acronyms and initial sets! For the acronym or initial set given, spell it out correctly.

a) ADHD   d) MS   g) ACh

b) CTS   e) EEG   h) PTSD

c) LP   f) NMJ

Best choice: Pick the most appropriate answer.

1 This linking form is most commonly used to indicate a direction 'toward the head'.

   a) Myel/o   c) Cerebr/o

   b) Cephal/o   d) Encephal/o

2 This suffix indicates a 'partial paralysis'.

   a) –pathy   c) –paresis

   b) –phasia   d) –phagia

3 These abundant neuroglial cells make up part of the blood–brain barrier.

   a) ependymal   c) Schwann cells

   b) microglia   d) astrocytes

4 This neurotransmitter affects all the neuromuscular junctions.

   a) Serotonin   c) Endorphins

   b) Dopamine   d) Acetylcholine

5 The functional unit of the brain is the

   a) Osteon   c) Neuron
   b) Alveoli   d) Glomeruli

Name the brain/mind term! Based on the description and/or function name the neurological or psychological term.

a) Impaired reading _____

b) Medications which 'destroy anxiety' _____

c) To surgically remove part of the skull _____

d) Inflammation of the spinal cord membranes _____

e) The state of being aware of self and the external environment _____

f) The fear of water _____

g) The specialist who studies and treats disease of the CNS _____

h) Disease of the mind or psyche _____

Multiple correct: Select ALL the correct answers to the question or statement given.

1 Mark all the correct viral infections causing a brain or cord infection.

   a) Toxoplasmosis   d) Botulism
   b) Cytomegaly   e) Herpes zoster
   c) Epstein–Barr   f) Lyme's

2 Which of the following are specialized support cells of the CNS?

   a) Microglia   d) Ependymal
   b) Oligodendrocytes   e) Astrocytes
   c) Goblet   f) Oocytes

Spelling challenge! Circle the correct spelling based on the definition given.

1 'Painful, disagreeable sensations'

              Disasthenia Anesthescia Dysesthesia Akiniesia

2 'No muscle development'

              Amyotophic Enmyotrophic Amyotrophic Imyotophic

3 'Softening of the brain'

         Endocephalacele Encephalomalacia Ensephalomelacia Endocephalomsia

Define the term: Spelling *does* count in your definition too!

1 Cephalodynia > _____

2 Astrocytoma > _____

3 Meningoencephalocele > _____

4 Poliomyelitis > _____

5 Polysynaptic > _____

6 Cephalohematoma > _____

7 Trephination > _____

8 Anesthesia > _____

Find it! Using the words in the table – match the definition given or answer the statement. Some may not be used. It is recommended you know all the choices.

hyperesthesia	narcolepsy	microglia	epineurium	meningitis
neurosis	dysgraphia	diencephalon	multipolar	craniofenestria
meningocele	myelination	hemiplegia	radiculitis	cerebritis
cephalometrics	gangliocytoma	myoclonic	amyloid	neurosis

1 _____ 'smallest glue'

2 _____ inflammation of brain cortex

3 _____ difficult writing

4 _____ opening in the skull

5 _____ inflammation of the nerve root

6 _____ brain protein

7 _____ excessive or painful sensations

8 _____ paralysis of one side

9 _____ outer wrapping of the nerve

10 _____ abnormal condition of the 'nerves'

Matching: Some will not be used.

	Letter	**Defined as**
Anxiety		a) Breaks down ACh at the NMJ synapsis
Thalamus		b) Area of the brain associated with emotions
Acetylcholinesterase		c) Loss of cognitive intelligence
Limbic		d) Compact gray matter in the diencephalon
Coma		e) Loss of the myelin sheath, slows reactions
Insomnia		f) X-linked recessive disorder of muscles
Dementia		g) Feeling of worry, uneasiness, dread
Multiple sclerosis		h) Characteristic of slowing or stopping an action
		i) Profound LOC
		j) Loss or interruption of sleep

Suffix challenge: Define the suffix and explain how it is used.

1 -lalia

2 -phasia

3 -plegia

4 -lexia

5 -cele

6 -phobia

7 -plagia

8 -asthenia

An essay: Explain the medications which may be used for suicide and how they might be coded in ICD.

Note challenge: This is a combination note on home care. You may need to look up a few terms. Answer the questions which follow.

S. Ms. Tie is an 83-yo woman with a history of <u>Alzheimer's</u>, diabetes, <u>HTN</u>, and breast cancer (terminal). She has been treated in the last week for a viral pneumonia. This morning she was found <u>unconscious</u> with respirations of 4 per minute. Daughter reports she was coughing a lot last night and she might have gotten up for medication. Inspection of her medications revealed a full bottle of guaifenesin but an empty bottle of morphine sulphate. All of her other medications appear to be in appropriate amounts.

O. 83-yo woman unconscious with a GCS of 5. There is no evidence of <u>fasciculations</u> or myoclonic activity. There is no <u>cyanosis</u>. Lungs are with <u>crackles</u> and slow rate. Heart: regular rhythm but rate is 53/min, <u>bradycardia</u>. Abdomen is soft and nontender. Active bowel sounds. 2+ pitting <u>edema</u> of the anterior tibia. Pulses are weak.

A. Respiratory depression > <u>bradypnea</u>
Possible morphine overdose
Comorbidities: HTN, Alzheimer's, Breast Cancer (terminal), DM

P. NARCAN (naloxone) 0.4 mg IV now

Questions:

1 Translate all the acronyms/initial sets and give meaning to the words which are *underlined* in the note.

2 Based on Ms. Tie's PMH which of the conditions might lead to her mistaking her medications?

3 What part of the ICD would you look up the overdose? Which of the six columns would be most appropriately coded?

4 Can the presence of breast cancer have the potential to make Ms. Tie's Alzheimer's worse? Why?

Unit 8

Special senses

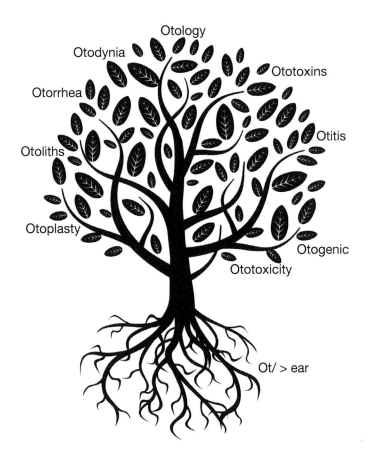

Otology

Otodynia

Ototoxins

Otorrhea

Otoliths

Otitis

Otoplasty

Otogenic

Ototoxicity

Ot/ > ear

TARGETED LEARNING

1 Recognize word parts and assemble medical terms related to the special senses: skin, eyes, ears, nose, and throat, with the associated cranial nerves.

2 Correctly construct, define, pronounce, and spell medical terms.

3 Relate special senses and cranial nerves illness and injury with appropriate diagnostic evaluation and pharmacotherapeutics.

4 Associate special senses disease and injury with the use of the ICD Tabular List of Diseases.

KEY WORD PARTS

Word roots with linking vowel	Prefixes	Suffixes
Audi/o; Acous/o > hearing	A-, An-	-cele
Blephar/o or Palpebr/o > eyelid	Ab-	-clysis
Conjunctiv/o > mucous membrane of the eye	Amblyo-	-cusis
Corne/o or Kerat/o > horny layers, clear portion of eye	Aniso-	-dynia
Dacry/o or Lacrim/o > tears	Diplo-	-lith
Gloss/o or Lingua > tongue	Dys-	-megaly
Irid/o or Ir/o > iris	Eso-	-meter
Myring/o or Tympan/o > drum	Exo-	-opia
Nas/o or Rhin/o > nose	Macro-	-osis
Opthalm/o or Opt/o or Ocul/o > eye	Mio-	-ptosis
Osm/o > smell, concentration of solution	Mydro-	-rrhaphy
Ot/o or Aur/o or Auricul/o > ear	Nyct-, nocto-	-rrhea
Pupill/o or Cor/o > pupil	Presby-	-sclerosis
Retin/o > retina, inner layer of eye	Scoto-	-trichia
Vitre/o > glassy	Xero-	-tropia

MAKING SENSE OF THE SENSES

For the person who exhorts, 'You are on my last nerve', he or she clearly does not understand how many nerve endings we have in our skin – billions. Human senses include sight, smell, hearing, taste, and touch (Figure 8.2). These neurological gifts bring the environment to us moment to moment. They are at once protective and mysterious.

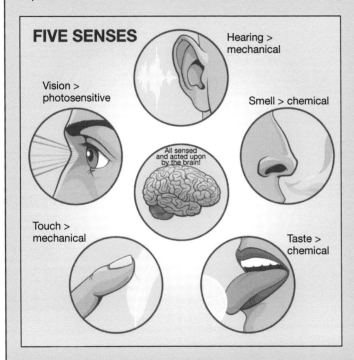

FIVE SENSES

Vision > photosensitive

Hearing > mechanical

Smell > chemical

All sensed and acted upon by the brain!

Touch > mechanical

Taste > chemical

Figure 8.2

Pain, for instance, is generated. This pain can be tracked up the afferent pathway to the brain. It is not understood why one person has an extreme reaction to pain and another appears to have minimal pain. We do know the smell of popcorn will make most of us remember a good movie. A sunset may warm our emotions. A stiff, cold wind may send us finding protection. This is what the senses are for, survival! We turn away from obnoxious odors or tastes. We sneeze and cough out irritants. We move our hand away from heat or blink fiercely to keep blowing dust out of the eyes. We need our senses to examine and interact with the environment and there are plenty of nerves to serve us.

RECEPTORS

From our skin with several types of nerve ends to pick up heat, cold, soft, and sharp touch to our complex eyes and ears, humans gather information at every turn. Our senses work via a set of 'receptors' > to receive stimulation.

- **Mechanoreceptors** (**mek**-ah-no-reh-**sep**-tours) > triggered with 'deforming' of the area – touch! Something mechanical is changing – sound waves pushing on the ear drum, pressure on a blood vessel, or a fly landing on the skin.

- **Chemoreceptors** (**key**-moe-reh-**sep**-tours) > activated with the detection of a chemical – taste and smell! The aerosols of odors and chemistries of foods run by this process.

- **Thermoreceptors** (**ther**-moe-reh-**sep**-tours) > sparked via changes in temperature – this is touch, smell, and taste! There is hot to taste and hot to touch with hot soup. Inhaling cold air hurts.

- **Nociceptors** (**no**-see-**sep**-tours) > generated by injury such as surgery, burn, chemical irritant, pressure, loud sounds, or intense light. Damage = pain.

- **Photoreceptors** (**foe**-toe-reh-**sep**-tours) > produced by light only – this is our eyes, vision specifically!

- **Osmoreceptors** (**oz**-moe-reh-**sep**-tours) > caused by chemical or the shift of fluid balance of the body. This is a function of the hypothalamus to maintain homeostasis.

Kitchen lab

While nerve endings are abundant throughout the epidermis and dermis, some areas are endowed with MANY tactile endings. To test this you need a paperclip, bend it in a 'U'. Have a partner close his/her eyes. Now, gently but firmly place the tips on the skin of the arm at the same time. Ask your partner if they feel one prick or two (Figure 8.3). Check the finger tips, dorsum of the foot and hand, leg and arms, and face. If your partner says, '2 points', move the points closer together until they report only 1 point. Record your findings. How close do the tips become to get a 1 point answer? Discuss your findings with the instructor. This is called 'two-point discrimination'. It is an important test for patients with neuropathy from diseases such as diabetes.

8.1

Exter/o > outside

Viscer/o > internal organ

Mechan/o > mechanical

Chem/o > chemical

Therm/o > temperature

Phot/o > light

Noc/i > hurt, pain

Osm/o > concentration of solution or smell

Dendr/o > branching

8.2

Did You Know?

When you smell a great meal cooking, your mouth waters and your tummy grumbles. Yet, very quickly you do not notice the odors as much. **This is adaption.** Sensations which are not associated with danger adapt

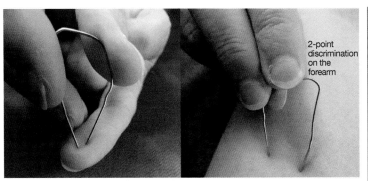

2-point
discrimination
on the
forearm

2-point discrimination test relates the density of
nerve endings. It changes with disease or injury.

quickly, such as
walking barefoot.
Painful or noxious
sensations are
SLOW to adapt.

Figure 8.3

Peripheral neuropathy (**nur**-oh-**nop**-ah-thee) > disease of the
nerve/neurons. The skin receptors are sensitive to damage and the
loss of blood supply. Tobacco and diabetes are two principal causes
of capillary loss in the extremities. The loss of the capillaries leads to
the loss of the nerve endings, the receptors! No receptors, no
sensations.

- **Diabetic neuropathy** sets a patient up for unseen and un-felt
  damage to the feet in particular. Because of the loss of sensation a
  person with diabetes can walk on a rock in their shoe for days.
  Unless the person looks at their feet the injury can go from a
  puncture to an ulcer, and at its worse, cause gangrene leading to
  amputation. Figure 8.4 demonstrates the use of a monofilament
  to check sensation on the bottom of the foot.

8.3
Tobacco has no
redeeming value. It
causes vascular
disease by itself
AND makes other
diseases such as
diabetes worse.

Neur/o > nerve

-pathy > quality
of disease.

Neuropathy is used
to indicate painful
sensations >
dysesthesias.

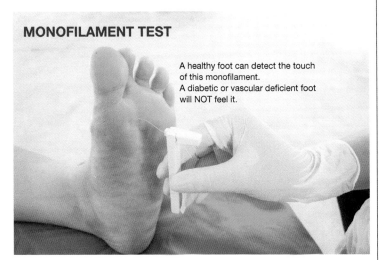

MONOFILAMENT TEST

A healthy foot can detect the touch
of this monofilament.
A diabetic or vascular deficient foot
will NOT feel it.

Figure 8.4

- Early onset neuropathy feels like tingling (the irritating kind) or burning pain. This is termed 'dysesthesia' (**dis**-es-**thee**-zee-ah) > Bad or painful sensations.

- Other peripheral neuropathies occur due to compression (temporary or permanent) of the local nerve, such as carpal tunnel syndrome or hitting the 'funny bone'. It can also occur due to infections such as herpes zoster (shingles).

✓ The sound-waves at the concert were quite intense. Sound waves on the ear drum are (circle the correct answer).

Chemoreceptors Nociceptors Mechanoreceptors Osmoreceptors

| **8.4** |
| Mechanoreceptors |

✓ Which of our senses use photoreceptors?

| **8.5** |
| Eyes |

✓ What is the linking form for 'temperature'?

| **8.6** |
| Therm/o |

PHARMACY CORNER*

Nerve pain, neuropathy, dysesthesia, lancinating pain, ants crawling, shooting pain, painful tingling, and burning pain are descriptions of the pain generated by injured nerves, both large and small. There are several classes of medications utilized to improve chronic neuropathy. Most work by adjusting the function of one or more of the neurotransmitters in the brain and spinal cord (Figure 8.5).

- **Tricyclic antidepressants** inhibit the uptake of norepinephrine and serotonin. This calms the mind, adding to the ability to rest. Rest relieves pain. These have a good safety profile and were the first medications used to impact neuropathy.

- **Serotonin-norepinephrine reuptake inhibitors** (**SNRIs**) actively increase the availability of serotonin. This quietens the brain, providing a mental balance which reduces pain. The side-effect profile is higher and they may induce insomnia (Figure 8.5).

- **Anti-seizure** medications have been shown to help with neuropathy. These work by slowing down the nerve signals transmitting the pain. A protracted signal equals less pain. These medications adjust many signals and their effects from patient to patient can be quite different. They come with very specific warnings including suicidal ideation and severe skin consequences.

- **Opioids** are the gold standards for effecting pain. Morphine, in particular, is very useful for severe pain because it is similar to our natural enkephalins and endorphins. The 'mu' receptors block the pain. They also block bowel motion – so constipation is a real problem. Opioids are also addictive. Use with care.

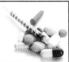

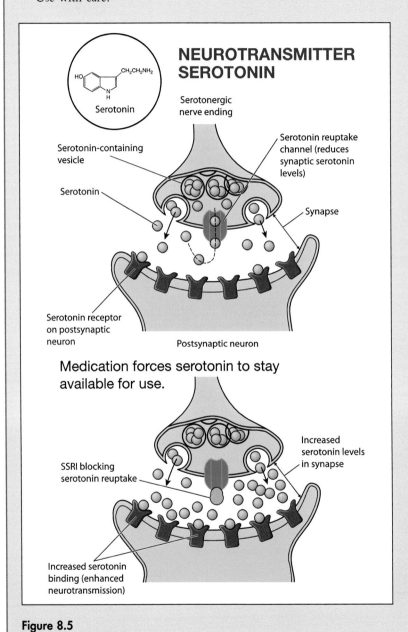

NEUROTRANSMITTER SEROTONIN

Serotonin

Serotonergic nerve ending

Serotonin-containing vesicle

Serotonin

Serotonin reuptake channel (reduces synaptic serotonin levels)

Synapse

Serotonin receptor on postsynaptic neuron

Postsynaptic neuron

Medication forces serotonin to stay available for use.

SSRI blocking serotonin reuptake

Increased serotonin levels in synapse

Increased serotonin binding (enhanced neurotransmission)

Figure 8.5

★ **IMPORTANT NOTE: Medicine is always in evolution. Do <u>not</u> use this information for patient care.**

THE NOSE AND PARANASAL SINUSES

It is said the sense of smell is the most primitive of our senses. It is properly called **olfaction** (ol-**fak**-shun). Chemoreceptors are at play with cranial nerve 1 (CN I or CN 1) running the process (Figure 8.6). It is also the only CN with direct access to the sensory environment, the nose. The dendrites come through the cribriform plate of the ethmoid bone to the basal cell layer of the superior turbinate. Because the dendrites are exposed to the environment, they are reproduced by the basal cell epithelium daily.

- **Olfactory** (ohl-**fak**-tor-ee) **>** Latin, ol > face and factus > to smell. Only two terms are seen regularly: olfactory and olfaction. **Osm/o** is the linking form for smell. It is also the linking form representing the balance of chemicals maintaining our fluid balance.
  - **Anosmia** (an-**oz**-me-ah) > condition of the inability to smell.
  - **Cacosmia** (kah-**koz**-me-ah) > condition of 'bad odors'. This is a subjective perception of a noxious odor.
- **Rhin/o** > Greek for nose. It is generally used to describe disease or injury of the nose.
  - **Rhinitis** (rye-**nigh**-tis) > inflammation of the nose.
  - **Rhinoantritis** (**rye**-no-an-**try**-tis) > inflammation of the nose and one or both maxillary sinuses.

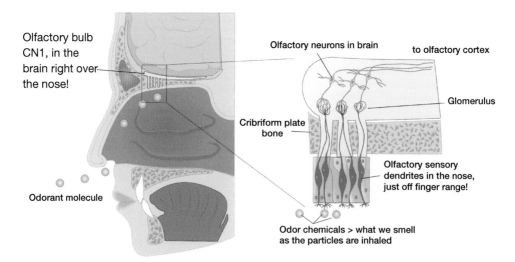

Olfactory bulb CN1, in the brain right over the nose!

Odorant molecule

Olfactory neurons in brain

to olfactory cortex

Glomerulus

Cribriform plate bone

Olfactory sensory dendrites in the nose, just off finger range!

Odor chemicals > what we smell as the particles are inhaled

Figure 8.6

Cranial nerve 1 > CN 1
Olfactory nerve > smell

- **Nas/o** > Latin for nose. Nasal (**nay**-zal) > pertaining to the nose. Nasal is often used to describe anatomy location such as a nasal polyp or nasal cavity or nasal bone.
  - **Nasogastric** (**nay**-zo-**gas**-trik) > pertaining to the nasal passage to the stomach.
  - **Nasopharynx** (**nay**-zo-**fair**-inks) > part of the pharynx (throat) above the soft palate. It opens anteriorly to the nasal cavity. This is why you can snort fluids out of your nose! ☺

The nose does have several functions: to consolidate odors for identification, warm incoming air, and protect from foreign bodies (Figure 8.7).

- **Turbinate** > Latin for 'shaped like a top'. Bilaterally, there are three bony turbinates covered by mucus-producing tissue which filter and warm the air on the way to the lungs. An alternate term for turbinate is **concha** (**kong**-ka) > shell-shape.
  - **Turbinectomy** (**tur**-bi-**nek**-toe-me) > surgical removal of the turbinate bone.
  - **Turbinotomy** (**tur**-bi-**not**-oh-me) > surgical incision into the turbinate bone.

Rhin/o > nose has many appropriate suffixes:

-itis > inflammation

-rrhea > discharge from

-cele > herniation

-metry > measurement

-dynia > pain

-edema > swelling

-lith > stone

-logy > knowledge of

-plasty > repair of

-rrhaphy > suturing

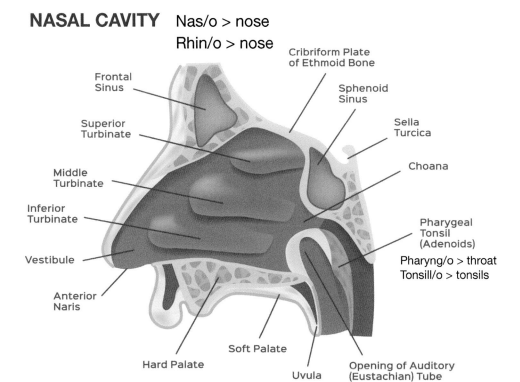

NASAL CAVITY Nas/o > nose

Rhin/o > nose

Frontal Sinus

Superior Turbinate

Middle Turbinate

Inferior Turbinate

Vestibule

Anterior Naris

Hard Palate

Soft Palate

Uvula

Cribriform Plate of Ethmoid Bone

Sphenoid Sinus

Sella Turcica

Choana

Pharygeal Tonsil (Adenoids)

Pharyng/o > throat
Tonsill/o > tonsils

Opening of Auditory (Eustachian) Tube

Figure 8.7

- **Nasal hairs** or **nose hairs** > **vibrissae** (vie-**bris**-ay) is the proper term. Vibrissae function to capture foreign particles from entering the nasal cavity and gathering ambient moisture.

- **Nasal cilia** (**see**-lee-ah) > microscopic equivalent of nasal hair. It is part of the mucus production floating debris up and out.

8.8

Meat/o > passage

Meatus is both singular and plural

There are several anatomical meatuses:

Urethral meatus

Auditory (ear) meatus, both external and internal

Concha is the singular, Conchae (**kong**-key) is the plural.

Vibrissa is the singular.

Working with the nose are the **para**nasal (**pear**-ah-**nay**-zal) **sinuses** which function to warm and moisturize air flow (Figure 8.8). The word 'sinus' is a cavity or hollow. The term is not unique to the nose or face and it has no specific linking form. Sinus is both singular and plural but 'sinuses' is also correct.

8.9

These linking forms are used almost exclusively for the convenience of anatomy designation.

Front/o > front

Maxill/o > maxillary

Sphen/o > wedge shaped

Ethm/o > sieve

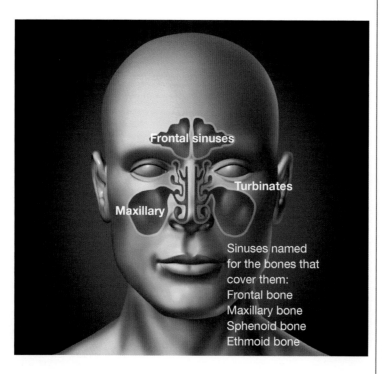

Frontal sinuses

Turbinates

Maxillary

Sinuses named for the bones that cover them:
Frontal bone
Maxillary bone
Sphenoid bone
Ethmoid bone

Figure 8.8

- Antr/o > any almost closed cavity, Greek for cave. This word root is used in reference to the maxillary sinuses.
  - Antronasal (**an**-trow-**na**-zal) > pertaining to the maxillary sinus and nose.

- **Sinusitis** (**sigh**-nu-**sigh**-tis) **>** inflammation of the paranasal sinuses.

- Designated by location: frontal, ethmoid, maxillary, or sphenoid.

Disease and injury to the nose and sinuses is common. The ability to smell diminishes with aging. This can set the elder up for missing important signals of danger such as smoke in a kitchen or not noticing a body odor.

- Brain trauma is a cause of anosmia.

- A broken nose can disrupt the cribriform plate of the ethmoid bone and create an anosmia as well.

- Brain tumors and systemic disease can cause a dysosmia. Recent research has shown dysosmia and anosmia may be an early change of Alzheimer's and Parkinsonism.

- A viral upper respiratory infection (a cold) blocks the turbinate drainage. The sinus mucus cannot drain effectively and it becomes a warm, wet, dark place for more virus, bacteria, or even fungus to grow.

- Despite the fact that most sinus infections are caused by viruses, sinusitis is the 5th most frequent infection treated by antibiotics.

- Plain X-rays can show air–fluid levels in the sinuses. A CT or MRI can be used with more precision as needed.

8.10
There are many conditions which block the sinuses or nasal passages.

Foreign bodies

Nasal or sinus polyps

Tumors

Barotrauma (diving or altitude changes)

Allergic rhinitis

URI > upper respiratory infections

 Construct a medical term for 'inflammation of the nose'.

 A nasopharyngolaryngoscopy is?

8.11
Rhinitis
8.12
An instrument to look up the nose, pharynx, and larynx.

Word building

 Using the word roots with the linking vowel to build as many valid terms with the suffixes given. Please define them too.

Rhin/o Therm/o

–itis –ology –cyte –meter –ic –al –tomy –rrhea

8.13
The instructor has the list!

The **tongue** brings the sense of taste – the proper term is gustatory (**gus**-tah-tor-ee). Taste is more than enjoying a good meal; it is also an important survival sense designed to avoid eating rotten food or ingesting dangerous chemicals. The tongue is also an essential part of our eating and swallowing process and vital to speech (Figure 8.9). Smell and taste are required to capture flavors. It takes three cranial nerves to manage taste and another one for motion.

- **CN 7 > Facial** (**fay**-shal) nerve. CN VII gives taste and pain reception to the anterior two-thirds of the tongue. It is also the nerve of funny faces, moving the superficial muscles of the face and scalp. CN 7 innervates the salivary glands (saliva) and lacrimal glands (tears). These are both vital to taste and protection.

- **CN 9 > Glossopharyngeal.** CN IX gives taste and pain reception to the posterior one-third of the tongue. It is key to the muscles of swallowing and the secretion of saliva.

- **CN 10 > Vagus** (**vay**-gus). CN X is the only CN to leave the cranium and is active with the heart, pharynx, larynx, and the GI tract. It gives a scant taste sensation to the back of the tongue

8.14

Did You Know?

There are four identified tastes: sour, bitter, sweet, and salty. There are two less defined sensations: Umami (**u**-mah-me) > Japanese for savory. The other is fatty tastes. Both can be tracked with a PET scan but their perception is unique to each individual.

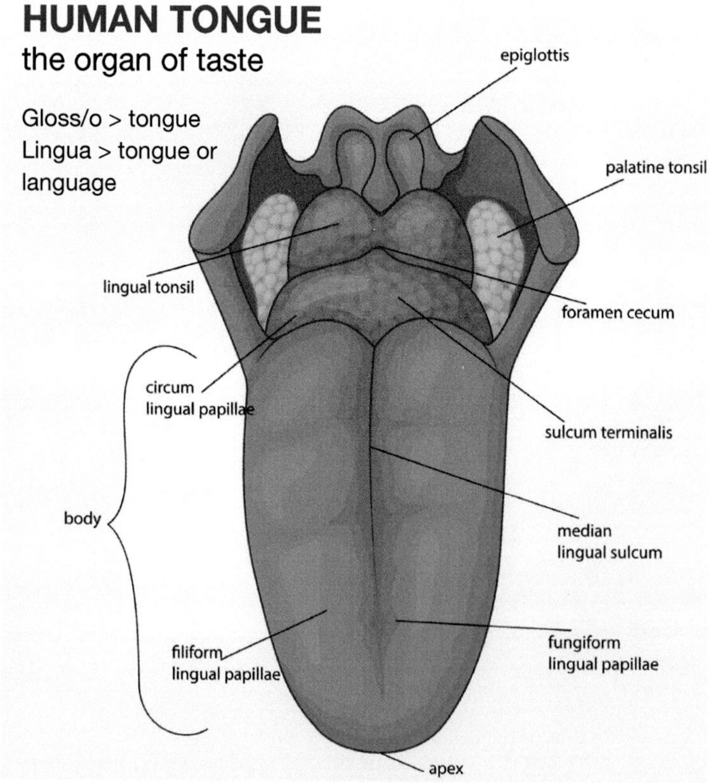

HUMAN TONGUE
the organ of taste

Gloss/o > tongue
Lingua > tongue or language

epiglottis

palatine tonsil

lingual tonsil

foramen cecum

circum lingual papillae

sulcum terminalis

body

median lingual sulcum

filiform lingual papillae

fungiform lingual papillae

apex

Figure 8.9

and the walls of the oral pharynx. It also provides safety sensations to close the epiglottis when swallowing (gag reflex).

- **CN 12 > Hypoglossal (hi**-poe-**glos**-sal). CN XII does not provide any taste sensation but it does provide the proprioceptive sense to the tongue. This is protective most of the time. It keeps us from biting our tongue when we are chewing and aids in speech.

The tongue, of course, is only part of our mouth. All the structures of the mouth, like those associated with the nose, enable the function of tasting and swallowing, and speech (Figure 8.10).

- **Gloss/o** > Greek for tongue. The tongue is a strong and very active muscle held firmly in place posteriorly. The **frenulum (fren**-U-lum) is the movement 'tether' of the tongue. Being 'tongue tied' actually refers to a tight frenulum which severely restricts tongue action. A **frenuloplasty** is performed to help improve speech.

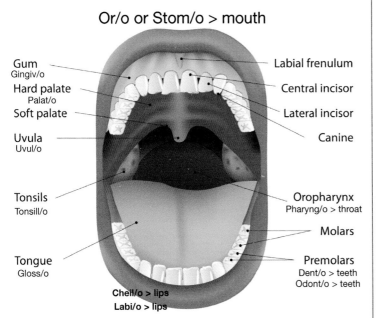

Or/o or Stom/o > mouth

Gum — Gingiv/o
Hard palate — Palat/o
Soft palate
Uvula — Uvul/o
Tonsils — Tonsill/o
Tongue — Gloss/o

Labial frenulum
Central incisor
Lateral incisor
Canine
Oropharynx — Pharyng/o > throat
Molars
Premolars — Dent/o > teeth / Odont/o > teeth

Cheil/o > lips
Labi/o > lips

Figure 8.10

- Macroglossia (**mak**-roe-**glos**-ee-ah) > enlarged tongue.

- Microglossia (**mik**-roe-**glos**-ee-ah) > small tongue is also called **atrophy**. This is associated with vitamin B$_{12}$ deficiency, xerostomia (dry mouth), and iron-deficiency anemia.

- Glossotrichia (**glos**-oh-**trik**-ee-ah) > hairy tongue. This is also called 'hairy leukoplakia', associated with a number of disease processes including **AIDS**, the use of smokeless tobacco, and lymphomas.

- **Lingua** (**ling**-gwa) is singular; linguae (**ling**-gway) is the plural > Latin for tongue.

✓ Construct the proper name of CN 9 (IX)?
_____ /__ /_____ /____

8.16
Gloss/o/pharyng/eal

✓ What is the definition of the word parts of the term 'hypoglossal'?

8.17
Pertaining to under (hypo) the tongue (gloss/o)

Word building

Using the word roots with the linking vowel to build as many valid terms with the suffixes given. Please define them too.

Gloss/o Nas/o Stomat/o (or Stom/o)

-al -itis -tomy -scopy -plasty -rrhaphy -dynia

8.18
The instructor has the list!

ENT PROFESSIONALS AND NOTES*

The initial set, ENT, is shorthand for the professionals or the examination of the **e**ar, **n**ose, and **t**hroat. An otolaryngologist studies, evaluates, and treats disease and injury of the ear, nose, and throat. The throat includes the nasopharynx, oropharynx, and laryngopharynx. This means they cover anything from an earache to vocal cord polyps and everything in between. As professionals they share the mouth (oral cavity) with dentists and oromaxillary surgeons. Additionally, audiologists specialize in hearing conditions of the ear versus a neurologist who may evaluate balance issues with ear involvement. Suffice to say, the head and neck includes many of our systems: gastrointestinal, respiratory, neurological, immunity, endocrine, and major vessels.

An examination of the head and neck may include the following terminology, which of course translates to creating a diagnosis with coding implications. This is a basic history and physical set excluding the full dental exam:

- **Ears**: *History*: Hearing loss? Change in hearing? Earache (otalgia or otodynia)? Tinnitus (ringing in the ears)? Ear discharge (otorrhea)? Balance issues? Dizziness?

- *Physical*: Pinna – are there piercings, edema, erythema, or skin lesions? External meatus: cerumen impaction, edema, erythema, foreign body. Tympanic membrane (**TM**): intact, good landmarks, edema, fluid line, erythema, motion with Valsalva maneuver. CN 8 grossly intact (hearing).

- **Nose**: *History*: nasal pain, change in smell, rhinorrhea, epistaxis (bloody nose), congestion, sinus pain? *Physical*: External nose: symmetrical, skin lesions, open to air flow. Internal exam: nasal mucosa pink and moist versus erythema, edema, or exudates? Nasal septum intact? Foreign bodies or polyps. Sinuses non-tender, and transillumination clear. CN 1 grossly intact (smell).

- **Throat**: *History*: throat pain (pharyngodynia, pharyngalgia, or sore-throat), drainage? Painful swallowing (dysphagia)? Change in voice (dysphonia)? *Physical*: tongue without edema, erythema, or coatings. Tongue has full range of motion (**FROM**). Teeth intact, any damage? Uvula rises in the midline, no edema or erythema. Oropharynx mucosa is pink and moist without drainage or exudates. Tonsils present without enlargement, erythema, or exudates. CN 7, 9, 10 are grossly intact (taste, tongue motion, uvula motion, and voice clear).

★ IMPORTANT NOTE: Medicine is always in evolution. Do **not** use this information for patient care.

THE EAR

The ability to hear the noise of our environment is a critical survival element of our sensory system. The external ear gathers sound waves. The mechanical sound waves hit the tympanic membrane (**TM**), where they are amplified and conveyed to the inner ear. They ripple across the fluid-filled spaces like a wave. There, the mechanical wave is converted by the cochlear structures to nerve energy. CN 8 is the vestibulocochlear nerve, which runs a pathway to the auditory interpreter of the temporal lobe (Figure 8.11).

The linking forms associated with the ear are many and they are frequently inappropriately interchanged:

- Ot/o > ear, used for entire structure of the ear.
  - Otic (**oh**-tik) > pertaining to the ear.
  - Otomycosis (**oh**-toe-my-**ko**-sis) > abnormal condition of ear fungus.
  - Otodynia (**oh**-toe-**dine**-ee-ah) > earache, ear pain.
    -otia > suffix meaning 'condition of the ear'.

8.19

Did You Know?

Owls have the best hearing in the animal kingdom. Bats and dolphins have the best sonic location skills.

As young people, hearing range is between 20–20,000 Hz. As elders, it will be between 50–8,000 Hz.

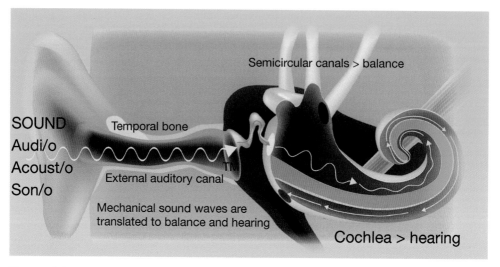

Figure 8.11

- **Auricul/o**; aur/i > ear, used for the outer ear, the auricle (**awr**-i-kel) or pinna (**pin**-ah). The auricle has many named curves and fossae but none involve word roots.

- **Audi/o**; audit/o > hearing, specific to the sound the ear perceives.
  - Audiometer (**aw**-dee-**om**-ee-tur) > measure of received sound.

- **Acous/o** > hearing, perception of sound, specific to sound and the passage of sound.
  - Acoustic (ah-**kus**-tik) injury > sustained or sudden loud noises such as loud concerts or jackhammers.
  - -acusis or -cusis > suffixes taken from this word root > hearing
    o Hyperacusis (**hi**-purr-ah-**kyu**-sis) > hypersensitivity to sounds.
    o Presbycusis (**prez**-bee-**kyu**-sis) > 'old hearing'. This term is used for the normal hearing changes of aging.

- Son/o > sound. The sonar is a process of tracking sound under water or a fluid medium. In medicine, it is used for ultrasound examinations of fluid environments such as the uterus during pregnancy or the evaluation of the bladder.

Related suffixes
–logist > specialist
–dynia > pain
–pathy > disease of
–algia > pain
–rrhea > discharge from
–toxic > poison
–scopy > process of looking
–sclerosis > abnormal hardening
Hz > hertz, is a unit of sound

The **anatomical structures** of the ear are divided by three distinct areas (Figure 8.12).

- The external ear is easily examined: the pinna and the external acoustic auditory canal.

The middle ear is evaluated by how the tympanic (tim-**pan**-ik) membrane looks.

- **Tympan/o**; tympan/i > Greek, 'stretched like a drum'.
  - Tympanometry (**tim**-pah-**nom**-ee-tree) > this is a specific measurement of the compliance of the drum. It checks for movement. It is NOT a hearing test.
  - Tympanocentesis (**tim**-pah-no-sen-**tea**-sis) > surgical puncture of the TM with a needle to aspirate fluid.
- **Myring/o** > Latin for drum. Myrinx (mir-ingks) > singular for tympanic membrane.
  - Myringoplasty (mi-**ring**-go-**plaz**-tea) > surgical repair of the ear drum.

8.20
Suffixes
-itis > inflammation
-ectomy > surgical removal
-tomy > to cut into
-centesis > surgical puncture to remove fluid
-plasty > surgical repair
-rrhea > discharge from
-osis > abnormal condition of
-scope > instrument to look
-ic > related to

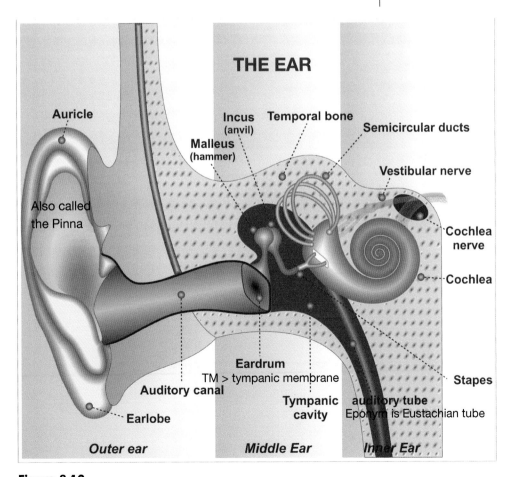

Figure 8.12

- **Oss/i** > small bones. The middle ear has the three smallest bones of the body, collectively called the ossicles.

  - **Malleus** (**mal**-ee-us) > hammer, it is actually more like a club. It the largest of the three and firmly attached to the backside of the **TM**.

  - **Incus** (**ing**-kus) > anvil, it is the middle bone, through which the sound vibration will pass. It cannot be seen via the TM unless the drum is severely retracted.

  - **Stapes** (**stay**-pees) > stirrup, it is the last and smallest of the set. Its foot-base connects firmly with the oval window, which is a small membrane between the middle and inner ear.

    o Stapedotomy (**stay**-peh-**dot**-**oh**-me) > surgical procedure to help with hearing loss due to otosclerosis (hardening of the ear).

- **Eustachian** (yu-**stay**-she-an) tube or auditory tube > middle ear structure allows the normal fluid of the area to drain to the pharynx. Eustachian is an eponym, named after the sixteenth-century anatomist Bartolomeo Eustachi.

- The middle ear has two *muscles*: the **tensor tympani** (**tim**-pah-knee) attached to the handle of the malleus. It tenses to protect the TM from too much motion during loud sounds. The **stapedius** (stay-**pee**-dee-us) muscle does the same at the oval window.

The **inner ear** has two distinct areas which correspond to the two CN roots (Figure 8.13).

- **Vestibul/o** > small chamber or entry area. The sound waves are transmitted via the oval window and the energy is communicated to the vestibular apparatus AND the cochlear apparatus.

  - Semicircular canals > balance side of the inner ear, a bony labyrinth (maze).

  - Otoliths > ear stones > tiny crystals sitting on the gel-like membranes of the inner ear. They dampen down the motion.

- **Cochle/o** > cochlea (**kok**-lee-ah) is the singular and cochleae (plural). It looks like a snail shell; the mechanical sound wave will end deep in the shell at the Organ of Corti, the cochlear nerve.

ANATOMY OF THE COCHLEA

VESTIBULAR SYSTEM

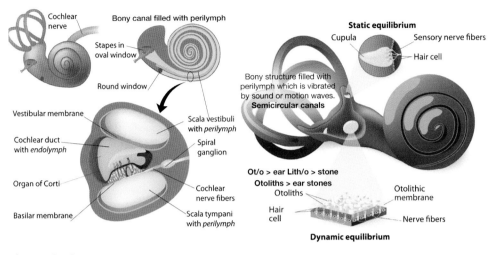

Figure 8.13

✓ What are the medical terms for each of the ossicles?

8.22
Malleus, incus, stapes

✓ Construct the medical term for 'ear scope'.
___ / __ / ____

8.23
Ot/o/scope

✓ Construct the medical term for 'inflammation of the tympanic membrane' (two terms possible). _____ / ___

8.24
Tympanitis
Myringitis

Word building

Using the word roots with the linking vowel to build as many valid terms with the suffixes given. Please define them too.

Ot/o Myring/o Audi/o

–itis –ology –meter –ic –tomy –rrhea –centesis –sclerosis

8.25
The instructor has the list!

Illness and injury of the ear

The external ear is most susceptible to injury (Figure 8.14). The auricle (pinna) is skin and cartilage, easily pulled and folded. Trauma to the ear can lead to auricular cellulitis (sell-U-lie-tis) or a perichondritis (pear-ee-kon-dry-tis).

- Tearing of the lobe, pinna from piercings being pulled out.

- Fight induced: bites, tears, contusions, cuts, and burns.

TYPES OF OTITIS

External otitis
Otitis externa > OE

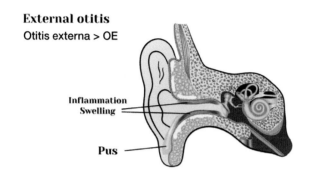

Average otitis
Otitis media > OA

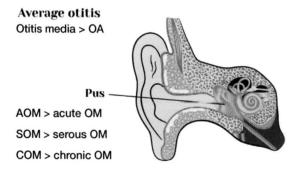

AOM > acute OM

SOM > serous OM

COM > chronic OM

Internal otitis
More commonly called
inner ear dysfunction

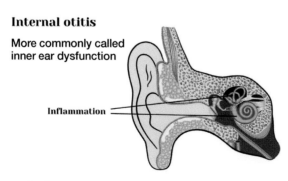

Figure 8.14

8.26

The external ear and canal are not prone to tumors. They are a site for skin cancers due to sun exposure.

Otitis externa is quite painful as the space is limited. Like the skin over the shin, there is no room for swelling. The nociceptors of stretch react actively. Heat from a flashlight can calm the pain.

The acoustic canal (ear canal) is protected by a coat of cerumen (seh-**rue**-men) > earwax. When it gets too wet (swimmer's ear), the skin can become macerated which sets the area up for an infection. This is called **otitis externa** (oh-**tie**-tis eks-**tur**-nah) (**OE**).

- The acoustic canal is also frequently visited by flying insects! Foreign bodies include insects, rocks, jelly-beans, dirt, and whatever a two-year-old can put in the ear ☺. Foreign bodies, cerumen impaction, and insects are removed by warm irrigation > -clysis.

The **middle ear** has three common conditions:

- **Otitis media** (oh-**tie**-tis **me**-dee-ah) (**OM**) > inflammation of the middle ear (Figure 8.14). The chamber is small and it gets populated by viruses when the nose is blown. Otodynia (otalgia), TM erythema, and fever are characteristic.
  - **AOM** > Acute otitis media
  - **SOM** > Serous otitis media > fluid without infection
  - **PET** > Pressure-equalizing tubes > used to provide middle ear a drainage pathway. **LIKE ALERT!** PET is also a nuclear medicine scan.
- **Cholesteatoma** (ko-leh-steh-ah-**toe**-ma) > a mass occurring in the middle ear. It is characterized by a foul-smelling otorrhea and is associated with patients who have had TM perforations.

8.27
Testing options include:

Tympanogram (**tim** pan **oh** gram) > record of the movement of the TM. Mobile is good. Immobile indicates inflammation and/or fluid behind the drum.

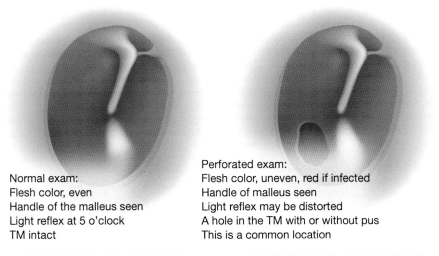

Normal exam:
Flesh color, even
Handle of the malleus seen
Light reflex at 5 o'clock
TM intact

Perforated exam:
Flesh color, uneven, red if infected
Handle of malleus seen
Light reflex may be distorted
A hole in the TM with or without pus
This is a common location

NORMAL EARDRUM   **RUPTURED EARDRUM**

Figure 8.15

- **Tympanic membrane perforations** occur with trauma and infection (Figure 8.15). This opens the middle ear to the environment. Hemorrhea (**hem**-oh-ree-ah) is bloody discharge from the ear. Trauma includes being clapped over the ear, barotrauma, Q-tips, and other things used to scratch the canal, and OM releasing its exudates the hard way.

- Otosclerosis (oh-toe-skleh-**roe**-sis) > hardening of the ossicles. Less vibration reaches the inner ear and hearing loss and/or tinnitus is the result.

Audiogram > record for checking hearing

Tuning forks > a simple way to check conduction loss versus sensorineural hearing loss

Otoscope > instrument to look at the ear

The **inner ear** can suffer tumors and changes from any number of conditions including hypertension and diabetes. Tobacco use adds to hearing loss because of the loss of capillaries.

- **Hearing loss** is divided into two types. Both can occur at the same time.
  - **Sensorineural** (**sen**-soar-ee-**nur**-al) > caused by injury or disease of the cochlea.
  - **Conductive** (kon-**duk**-tive) hearing loss > caused by something blocking the sound wave, such as a cerumen impaction or otosclerosis.

- **Tinnitus** (**tin**-knee-tus) > noise in the ears: ringing, wind noise, booming, buzzing, clicking, or whistling. This can be caused by anything disrupting the fine hair cells in the cochlea. Causes include Meniere's disease, otosclerosis, chronic otitis media, and labyrinthitis.

- **Benign positional vertigo** (**vur**-tea-go) (**BPV**) > sensation of spinning. Sometimes the patient feels like they are spinning and others report the room spinning. BPV may be due to a viral infection of the labyrinth or the otoliths needing adjustment.

8.28
For otosclerosis, the stapes can be replaced with a prosthesis to set up the vibration pathway again.

Profound hearing loss can be improved in some with a **cochlear implant**. The microphone brings the sounds up the electrical connections directly into the malfunctioning cochlea.

✓ The initial set 'ETD' stands for eustachian tube dysfunction. What does 'dysfunction' mean?

✓ Construct the proper term for 'discharge from the ear'. ____ / __ / ____

✓ What does 'hemotympanum' mean?

8.29
Abnormal or bad functioning of the auditory tube

8.30
Ot/o/rrhea

8.31
The presence of blood in the middle ear.

ICD TABULAR LIST OF DISEASE*

Documentation of an illness or injury consists of many medical terms. How they are written, the description of an illness, the physical findings, laboratory, and imaging studies all add to the story of an earache or a Bell's palsy. The diagnoses and findings translate in the coding from the ICD. The Alphabetic Index of Disease is the first step.

Otitis Media, acute – H66.90. From here, the coder will go to the Tabular List of Disease. This area of the ICD is an arrangement of 21 body system classifications or the character of the injury or disease. The tabular list expands on the simple diagnosis of H66.90. This code could mean an acute inflammation, chronic suppurative, allergic, exudative . . . it is nonspecific. The Tabular List of Disease contains the differentiations or possible specific causes.

- **'H60 to H95'** section covers the Diseases of the Ear and Mastoid Process

- **'H66'** is Suppurative and unspecified otitis media. There are several directions to help the coder pick the correct code or additional codes:

  – *Use additional code for any associated perforated TM*

  – Use additional code to identify: exposure to tobacco smoke; exposure to tobacco smoking in the perinatal period; history of tobacco use; occupational exposure to tobacco smoke; tobacco dependence; or tobacco use.

You can see from the additional codes that tobacco smoke exposure is implicated in otitis media. This demonstrates the importance of the history of exposures, and allergies, and more. These codes are then tracked by infection control agencies and the CDC.

- **'H66.01'** is one of the many choices for a suppurative OM. The coder uses the SOAP note to determine the correct code. This is a short example of possibilities:

  – H66.011 Acute suppurative OM with spontaneous rupture of the ear drum, right

  – H66.012 Acute suppurative OM with spontaneous rupture of the ear drum, left

  – H66.013 Acute suppurative OM with spontaneous rupture of the ear drum, bilateral

If the SOAP note reports a ruptured TM, one of the codes above is correct. BUT, if the provider did not note which ear is impacted, the H66.017 code is used for unspecified ear. The coder cannot make up a code! A coder chooses the code matching most closely to the given diagnoses and findings within the given note. What is written, spelling, and language makes a difference in the continuity of care.

* IMPORTANT NOTE: The reader is notified that these examples are from an online search done in 2016. Do <u>not</u> use these codes for patient care episodes; look up new ones!

THE EYE

We are visual learners, more than half of our data and recall (memories) in the brain comes through our eyes! The complexity of the eye is reflected in the four cranial nerves running the eye itself and the myriad of connections they make with other cranial nerves and the brain. The optic nerve's (CN 2) sole activity is sensing light (Figure 8.16)! It contains more than 1,000,000 afferent nerve fibers.

- Opt/o; Optic/o; Ophthalm/o > Greek for eye.
  - Ophthalmology (of-thal-**mol**-oh-gee) > study of the eyes.
  - Optic (**op**-tik) > pertaining to the eye. This is used to describe anatomy: the optic nerve, the optic chiasm, optic ataxia . . .
- Ocul/o > Latin for eye. Oculodynia (ok-**yu**-low-**dine**-ee-ah) > eye pain.

The **extraocular** (eks-tra-**ock**-U-lar) **muscle (EOM) cranial nerves**:

- The **oculomotor** (ock-U-low-**moe**-tur) **CN 3** nerve > many responsibilities.
  - First the **intrinsic** muscles are the iris and ciliary muscles
    o Regulates the movement of the iris, which opens or closes the amount of light coming through the pupil like a camera shutter.

8.32
Ophthalm > eye is a typically misspelled word root and it is mispronounced too. The first 'h' is usually missing. Be aware.

Of-thal-**mol**-oh-gee AND **op**-thal-**mol**-oh-gee are both heard and accepted for pronunciation.

8.33
Extraocular palsies occur due to injuries to the eye muscles.

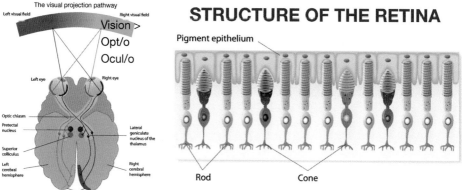

The visual projection pathway

Vision >
Opt/o
Ocul/o

STRUCTURE OF THE RETINA

The receptors of the eye are:
Rods — they pick up color — red, blue, and green
Cones — they pick up light and are only marginally active during day-light hours. At night they can pick up light literally millions of miles away, such as the stars at night. On earth we are limited by the curve of the earth. We can see headlights on a good night between 2 to 3 miles.

Figure 8.16

- Adjusts the shapes of the lens, the focusing apparatus of each eye.
- Second is the **extrinsic** muscles, the skeletal strap muscles: superior rectus, medial rectus, inferior rectus, and inferior oblique muscles (Figure 8.17).
- Elevate the eyelids (the levator palpebrae).

- The **trochlear** (tro-**klee**-ar) **CN 4** nerve > moves the eye in (nasally) and up.

- The **abducens** (ab-**due**-sens) **CN 6** nerve > moves the eye laterally, away from the nose, it **ab**ducts.

Trauma to the eye orbit can compress the nerve fibers or the muscle itself causing a paralysis.

Brain tumors can do the same by compressing the nerve.

Multiple sclerosis, diabetes, myasthenia gravis, and vascular disease can affect their function as well.

MUSCLES OF THE HUMAN EYE

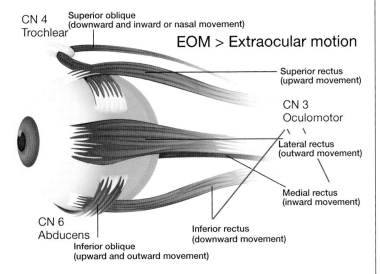

Figure 8.17

✓ Construct a word meaning 'instrument to look at eyes'.
_____/__/_____

✓ What is the function of the optic nerve?
_____

8.34
Ophthalm/o/scope

8.35
Vision, sensory only to light

The **external eye structures** generate many word roots from both the Latin and Greek. Refer to Figure 8.18 for their location.

- **Scler/o** > hardness. In this use, sclera is the white of our eyes. It is the tough, protective capsule which gives the eye its spherical shape.
  - Scleritis (**skler**-eye-tis) > inflammation of the sclera.

- **Corne/o** > Latin for 'horny or scaly'. In the eye, it is the absolutely translucent window in front of our pupil. It is avascular.
  - **Limbus** > margin or boundary between the sclera and cornea.

- **Kerat/o** > Greek for 'horny or scaly' because the cells of the surface are replaced daily just like the epidermis.
  - A corneal (**kor**-knee-al) abrasion > scratch or burn to the cornea.
  - Keratotomy (**ker**-ah-**tot**-oh-me) > a cut into the cornea.

- **Lacrim/o** > Latin for tears. It is used to refer to the anatomy of the lacrimal (**lak**-ri-mal) system: glands, puncti, and ducts.

- **Dacry/o** > Greek for tears. It is used to describe conditions.
  - Dacryolith (**dak**-ree-oh-lith) > tear duct stone.

- **Palpebr/o** > Latin for eyelid. It is used to refer to the anatomy of the eyelid such as palpebral fissure (**pal**-peh-bral).

8.36
Suffixes

-itis > inflammation

-rrhea > discharge from

-cele > herniation

-lith > stone

-osis > abnormal condition

-plasty > surgical repair of

-ectomy > surgical removal

-ostomy > surgical creation of new opening

-ptosis > prolapse, sinking down

-tropia > to turn

LIKE ALERT!

Dacry/o > tears

Dactyl/o > digits

Documenting Abbreviation

PERRLA > Pupils equally round and reactive to light and accommodation

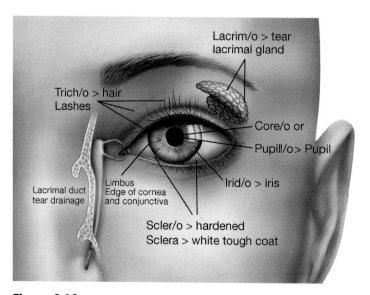

Figure 8.18

- Blephar/o > Greek for eyelid. It is used to describe conditions.
  - Blepharitis (**blef**-ah-**rye**-tis) > inflammation of the eyelid.
  - Blepharoplasty (**blef**-ah-roe-**plaz**-tea) > surgical repair of the eyelid.
- Conjunctiv/o > transparent mucus membrane covering the inner eyelids and sclera of the eye (Figure 8.19) > Latin for 'to bind together'.
  - Conjunctivitis (kon-**junk**-tea-**vigh**-tis) > inflammation of the inner lid area. It is characterized by redness, edema, and exudates, the lower lid may droop (blepharoptosis > **blef**-ah-rope-**toe**-sis). This is also known as 'pink eye'.

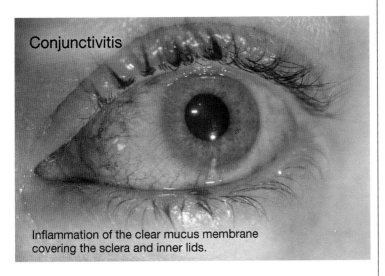

Conjunctivitis

Inflammation of the clear mucus membrane covering the sclera and inner lids.

Figure 8.19

The eye lashes and brows are part of our protective mechanisms. They catch dust and debris.

- En**trop**ion (en-**trow**-pee-on) > lashes turn into the eyeball, which can damage structures.
- Ec**trop**ion (ek-**trow**-pee-on) > lid and lashes roll outward.

The **internal structures of the eye** are packed into 0.9 inches (2.28 cm) of spherical globe as seen in Figure 8.20.

- Pupill/o > Latin for pupil. The pupil is the open hole formed by the iris. If the cornea was not in the way anything could fly in.
- Cor/o; Core/o > Greek for pupil.
  - Corectopia (**kor**-ek-**toe**-pee-ah) > condition of the pupil not being in the center of the iris.
  - Anisocoria (an-**ee**-so-**kor**-ee-ah) > condition of unequal pupils (side to side).

8.37
Prefixes
Aniso- > unequal
Hyper- > excessive
Nyct- > night
Photo- > light
Scoto- > night
Mydro- > widen, enlarge

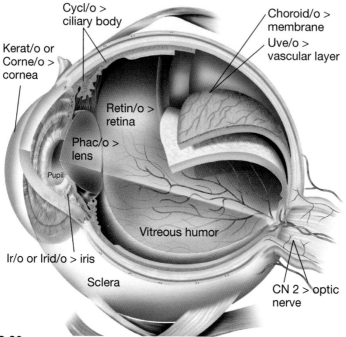

Cycl/o > ciliary body

Choroid/o > membrane

Uve/o > vascular layer

Kerat/o or Corne/o > cornea

Retin/o > retina

Phac/o > lens

Pupil

Vitreous humor

Ir/o or Irid/o > iris

Sclera

CN 2 > optic nerve

Figure 8.20

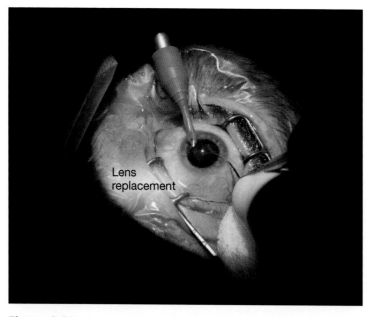

Lens replacement

Figure 8.21

- **Ir/o** or Irid/o > Greek meaning 'rainbow' or the iris. Its color comes from the melanic cells ranging from golden to deep browns. It changes the size and diameter of the pupil via the ciliary muscles innervated by CN III.
  - **Iritis** (eye-**rye**-tis) > inflammation of the iris. This is an extremely painful condition because any light makes the iris move and movement hurts.
  - **Irid**oplegia (ir-e-doe-**pleh**-jee-ah) > condition of paralysis of the iris.
- **Phac/o** or Phak/o > shaped like a lens or lentil bean.
  - Phacoemulsification (**fak**-oh-ee-mul-see-fi-**kay**-shun) > procedure to emulsify and aspirate the lens. This is done to correct cataracts; a new lens is implanted (Figure 8.21).

- **Cycl/o** > Greek for circle. It is used to refer to the ciliary body, muscles, and suspensory ligaments which move the iris and lens (Figure 8.20).
  - **Cycl**oplegia (**sigh**-klo-**pleh**-jee-ah) > condition of paralysis of the ciliary muscle. Medication will cause a temporary cycloplegia to allow examination and surgical interventions.
- **Retin/o** > Latin for 'net'. The retina is the incomplete inner surface of the posterior eye. It is the sensory net which receives light energy (Figure 8.22). It gets its orange-ish glow from the blood vessels of the choroid layer beneath the retina.
  - **Macula** retina > small spot or depression. For the eye, this site has the maximum number of color receptors.
  - **Fovea** (**foe**-vee-ah) **centralis** > center of the macula retina. It is the point of most precise vision.
- **Vitre/o** > Latin for glassy. The vitreous body is the transparent jelly-like filling of the posterior section of the eyeball. It sits behind the lens and holds the retina in place. It is not a clear fluid but a fine-fine mesh or network (vitreous stroma).
  - **Vitre**ous (**vit**-ree-us) **floaters** are tiny collagen fibers of the stroma which are dislodged. In time, they dissolve.
- **Aque/o** > Latin for water. The aqueous humor is produced by actions of the ciliary body, which actively secretes the humor. It will flow behind the lens and into the anterior chamber of the eye bringing nourishment to the lens, iris, and interior surface of the cornea. Any blockage of this flow will cause glaucoma (glaw-**ko**-ma).

Mio- > smaller, constrict

Diplo- > double

Amblyo- > dull or dim

Xero- > dry

Did You Know?

Sneezing, squinting, and blinking fast are protective reflexes to close the eyes until the pupils can adjust to sudden bright light.

8.38 Evaluation of the eyes

Visual acuity is a simple check to see how well the eye focuses.

Visual field test checks central and peripheral vision. It can be done during a physical exam but today, a machine does a better job of finding field loss.

Ophthalmoscopy allows the clinician to see inside the eye. It is the only exam to check vessels without doing a cutdown or angiogram.

Slit lamp microscopy is also a hand-held instrument with a magnified view.

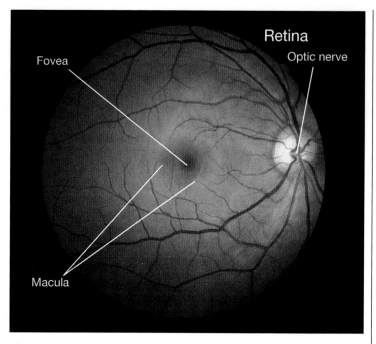

Fovea

Retina

Optic nerve

Macula

Figure 8.22

Retinal photographs are an easy exam to visualize the blood vessels.

Tonography records intraocular pressures.

✓ What is the word for 'inflammation of the ciliary body'?

8.39
cyclitis

✓ The corneal reflex is designed to protect the cornea from touch. A corneal abrasion makes it past this reflex. Which CN runs the reflex?

8.40
CN 5 trigeminal

Word building

Using the word roots with the linking vowel to build as many valid terms with the suffixes given. Please define them too.

Irid/o or Ir/o Blepar/o Conjunctiv/o

-al –itis –tomy –plasty –rrhaphy –dynia –pathy – osis

8.41
The instructor has the list!

External illness and injury of the eye

- **Corneal abrasions** are easily seen with **fluorescein** (floor-es-eh-cen) stain viewed through a cobalt-blue light. The lesion will shine yellow-green. A patch is applied to let the eye rest.

- **Subconjunctival hemorrhage** (sub-kon-**junk**-tie-val **hem**-or-ahj) > rupture of small vessels leaching in-between the layers of the sclera. These are usually quite benign despite how impressive they look (Figure 8.23).

- **Pinguecula** (ping-**qwek**-U-la) > white to yellow accumulation of protein on the bulbar conjunctiva. It does not encroach onto the limbus. A **pterygium** (tear-**i**-jee-um) encroaches past the limbus onto the cornea. Both are benign and only removed if vision is impacted.

- **Blepharitis** > inflammation of the eyelids. This is associated with seborrheic dermatitis and appears as greasy, crusted, and ulcerated.

  - A **stye** is properly called a **hordeolum** (hor-**deh**-oh-lum). It is caused by a staphylococcal infection of an eyelash.

  - treated with warm compresses and topical antibiotics.

  - A **chalazion** (kah-**lay**-zee-on) > deeper, chronic, inflammatory granuloma. It is also called a tarsal cyst and is seen in the lower lid. Surgery may be required (Figure 8.24).

8.42
Did You Know?

The red (pink) eye, swelling, and discharge may be caused by allergies, but the worry is it may be viral or bacterial infection.

Viral conjunctivitis is seen with a viral upper respiratory infection (URI). It is easily spread by children (and adults) because they rub their eyes and spread it to others.

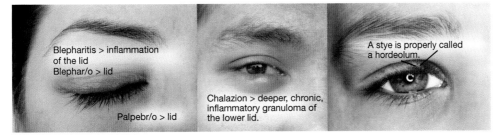

Subconjunctival hemorrhage, bleeding under the clear conjunctiva. It is impressive but seldom dangerous.

Pterygium crosses the limbus

Figure 8.23

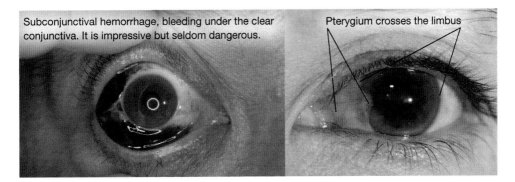

Blepharitis > inflammation of the lid
Blephar/o > lid

Palpebr/o > lid

Chalazion > deeper, chronic, inflammatory granuloma of the lower lid.

A stye is properly called a hordeolum.

Figure 8.24

Glaucoma (glaw-**ko**-ma) > a steadily, progressive optic neuropathy characterized by increased intraocular pressures. The chronic pressure inexorably damages the optic disc (Figure 8.25). Untreated, it will cause blindness. The World Health Organization (**WHO**) estimates 37 million cases of blindness are due to glaucoma. Treatment includes topical medications and laser surgery to open the pathway and decrease the pressure.

8.43
Glaucoma can be detected with the following:

Visual acuity testing

Visual field testing

Dilated eye exam

Tonometry > measurement of intraocular pressure

Pachymeter (pah-**kim**-ee-tur) > the measurement of the thickness of the cornea. Pachy > Greek for 'thick'.

GLAUCOMA

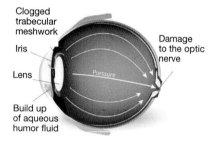

Clogged trabecular meshwork

Iris

Lens

Pressure

Build up of aqueous humor fluid

Damage to the optic nerve

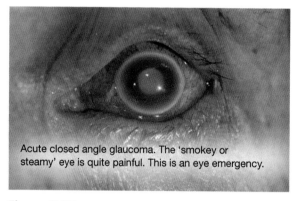

Acute closed angle glaucoma. The 'smokey or steamy' eye is quite painful. This is an eye emergency.

Figure 8.25

Loss of vision has many causes from an inflammation to tumors. The disease process interrupts the precious blood supply and/or the neural net of the retina and CN 2.

- **Amaurosis fugax** (**am**-awe-**row**-sis **foo**-gaks) > transient ischemic attack (**TIA**) of the retina, a temporary loss of blood flow.

- **Optic neuritis** (**op**-tik **nur**-eye-tis) > inflammation of the optic nerve (CN 2).

- **Papilledema** (**pap**-il-eh-**dee**-ma) > bilateral swelling of the optic discs. This is caused by temporary or chronic intracranial pressure from a brain mass or an elevated CSF pressure.

8.44
Amauros > Greek for 'dark or obscure'

Fugax > Latin for 'fleeting'

It is unusual to see the two languages mixed.

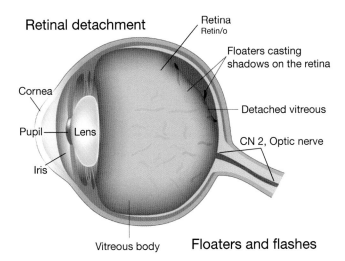

Retinal detachment

- Retina (Retin/o)
- Floaters casting shadows on the retina
- Cornea
- Detached vitreous
- Pupil — Lens
- CN 2, Optic nerve
- Iris
- Vitreous body
- **Floaters and flashes**

Figure 8.26

Opt/o > vision
Ocul/o > vision
Neur/o > nerve
Crani/o > head
Retin/o > retina (network)
Scler/o > hardened
Macul/o > small spot
-edema > swelling
-ic > pertaining to
-ar > pertaining to
-itis > inflammation
CSF > Cerebro-spinal fluid

- **Retinal detachment** (**ret**-i-nal) > loss of part of the retina from its layers. It bubbles up and away from the interior wall of the globe. This causes floaters, flashing lights, and scotomas (Figure 8.26).

- **Retinitis pigmentosa** > gradually progressive degeneration of the retina beginning in childhood.

- **Macular** (**mak**-U-lar) **degeneration** > slowly developing loss of the macula of the eye, the point of best central vision. This is usually a function of aging with thickening and separation of the retinal floor slowly changing the macula.

Retinopathy (**ret**-i-**nop**-ah-thee) > disease of the retina. This term is used for many conditions which disrupt the retina. Some of these are the results of uncontrolled systemic disease. By far the most common cause is diabetes.

8.45

Gluc/o > sugar
Capill/o > tiny vessels, capillaries
Vitre/o > glassy
Hem/o > blood
Vascul/o > vessels
Cyt/o > cell
Myc/o > fungus
Tox/o > poisonous
Plasm/o > living fluids
Hist/o > tissue
Immun/o > protector

- **Diabetic retinopathy** > because excess glucose molecules take up space in the tiny capillaries, the capillaries break. In the eyes, this causes vitreous hemorrhages, retinal detachment, and neovascular vessels. These all cause loss of vision in time (Figure 8.27).

- **Hypertensive retinopathy** > chronic blood vessel hypertension breaks the tiny capillaries of the eyes too. The blood vessels will have AV (arterial-venous) nicking from vessel torsion.

- **Infectious retinopathy** > infections in the posterior eye are usually opportunistic associated with immune-compromised patients:

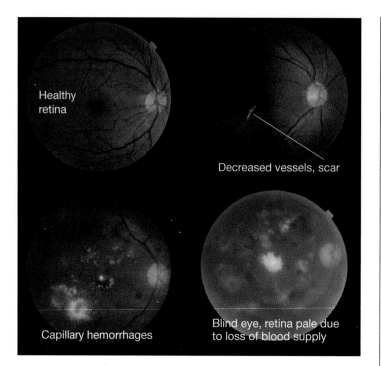

Healthy retina

Decreased vessels, scar

Capillary hemorrhages

Blind eye, retina pale due to loss of blood supply

DIABETIC RETINA SCREENING

Figure 8.27

- **Cytomegalovirus** (**sigh**-toe-**meg**-ah-low-**vigh**-rus) (**CMV**) > a group of herpes viruses.
- **Coccidioidomycosis** (kok-**sid**-eh-**oy**-doe-my-**ko**-sis) > abnormal condition of a systemic fungal infection which can invade the brain and eye.
- **Toxoplasmosis** (**tock**-so-plaz-**moe**-sis) > abnormal condition of a protozoan parasite which can cause a fatal encephalitis.
- **Histoplasmosis** (**his**-toe-plaz-**moe**-sis) > abnormal condition of these fungal spores. It can be fatal in the immunodeficient.

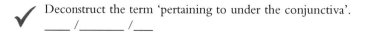

What is the term used to describe bilateral swelling of the optic disc?

8.46
Papilledema

The common term of this eyelid swelling is a stye. What is the proper medical name?

8.47
Hordeolum

Deconstruct the term 'pertaining to under the conjunctiva'.
____ /_____ /___

8.48
Sub/conjunctiv/al

Eye tumors can occur in any area of the external or interior eye. These tumors occur in the posterior eye and are associated with vision changes.

- **Melanoma** (**mel**-ah-**no**-ma) > the eye is populated with the pigment cells, melanocytes. Like the skin, excess UV exposure can set a person up for a melanoma of the sclera, iris, or retina (Figure 8.28). Ocular melanomas are often found late and can easily metastasize to the brain.

8.49

Melan/o > black

Blast/o > immature

Fibr/o > fiber, thread

EYE MELANOMAS

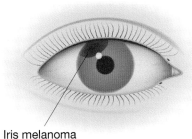
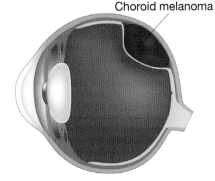

Choroid melanoma

Iris melanoma

Figure 8.28

- **Retinoblastoma** (**ret**-i-**noh**-blas-**toe**-ma) > tumor of the retina, blast/o is the linking form for immature cells, in this case the germ layer of the retina.

Eye descriptions and findings

- **Scotoma** (sko-**toe**-ma) > area in the visual field that is blank, empty, or muted. A blind spot. This occurs with retinal detachment.
- **Astigmatism** (ah-stig-mah-tizm) > lens of one eye has a slightly different refractivity (curvature) than the other.
- **Amblyopia** (am-blee-oh-pee-ah) > condition of dim vision, visual impairment.
- **Strabismus** (strah-biz-mus) > one eye is not parallel to the other (Figure 8.29). Caused by weak **EOM**. It is also called a 'wandering eye'. It can cause diplopia > double vision.
- **Esotropia** (**es**-oh-**trow**-pee-ah) > condition of one eye turning in.
- **Exotropia** (**eks**-oh-**trow**-pee-ah) > condition of one eye turning out.

8.50

Skotos > French for 'darkness'

Stigma > Greek for 'point'

Strabismos > Greek and French for 'squinting'

Fundus > bottom or lowest part of the eye in this unit

Accommodation > ability of the pupil to adjust and focus. It slows as we age.

STRABISMUS

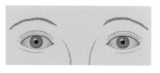
Normal

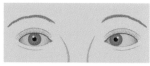
Esotropia – eye turns inward

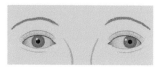
Exotropia – eye turns outward

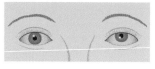
Hypertropia – eye turns upward

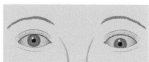
Hyportropia – eye turns downward

Figure 8.29

- **Hyper**tropia (**hi**-purr-**trow**-pee-ah) > condition of one eye turning up.
- **Hypo**tropia (**hi**-poe-**trow**-pee-ah) > condition of one eye turning down.
- **Hyper**opia (**hi**-purr-**oh**-pee-ah) > condition of farsightedness, vision is better at a distance because the light meets behind the retina.
- **My**opia (my-**oh**-pee-ah) > condition of nearsightedness, vision is better up close because the light joins in front of the retina.
- **Presby**opia (**prez**-bee-oh-pee-ah) > 'old eyes'. It refers to the condition of the loss of accommodation with aging.
- **Hemi**anopia (**hem**-ee-an-**oh**-pee-ah) > condition of loss of one half of the visual fields of one or both eyes.
- **Diopter** (die-**op**-tur) > unit of refraction power of the lens.

Ambly- > dim

Eso- > inward

Exo- > outward

Dipl- > double, twice

-tropia > abnormal turn or deviation

-opia > condition of vision

UNIT SUMMARY

1 The special senses are the extension of the central nervous system; they bring our environment into the brain for interpretation and action. The skin nerve endings bring us soft touch, pressure, stretch, hot, cold, and pain sensations.

2 Neuropathy means 'disease of the nerves' and it is used to describe the pain associated with the nervous system. Control of neuropathy is seldom complete but there are medications to diminish the pain for most patients.

3 The olfactory nerve (CN1) is the chemoreceptor for smell. It is the only CN to have receptors in contact with the environment. Humans can distinguish thousands of smells though the ability decreases slowly as we age. The nose has two linking forms, rhin/o and nas/o.

4 The facial sinuses concentrate odors as they rise to the superior turbinate. They also moisturize and warm air on the way to the lungs. The mucous production serves to trap dust and foreign debris.

5 Taste is a complex combination of three cranial nerves: 7, 9, and 10. Gloss/o is the linking form for the tongue which holds the chemoreceptor papillae, this is our gustatory sense. These and CN 12 contribute to our sensory net of pain (too hot or too cold) and the movement of the tongue to manage chewing, swallowing, and speech.

6 The vestibulocochlear nerve (CN 8) gives us hearing (audi/o) and balance (vestibul/o). Some anatomists consider this nerve as two because of their distinctly different functions in the same small space. There are many linking forms for the structures or functions of the external, middle, and internal ear: tympan/o, myring/o, acous/o, ot/o, oss/i, myring/o, auricul/o, audi/o, and son/o. -otia is the suffix of a condition pertaining to hearing.

7 Vision is the most complex of our special senses run by four cranial nerves. Vision is run by the CN 2, the optic nerve carrying the input of the rods and cones of the retina. CN 3, 4, and 6 run the extraocular muscles (EOMs), the lid motion, and motion of the iris. The linking forms for vision include: ophthalm/o, opt/o, and ocul/o. -opia is the suffix of a condition pertaining to vision.

8 The external eye includes many structures designed to protect the eyeball for the environment including the eyebrows, eyelashes, the conjunctiva, lacrimal glands with their moisturizing tears, and lacrimal ducts to drain those tears to the nose. The sclera (the whites of the eye) is the tough external coat of the eye giving it form and shape with the very specialized clear cornea in the front. Linking forms include: scler/o, corne/o, kerat/o, lacrim/o, dacry/o, palpebr/o, blephar/o, and conjunctiv/o.

9 The internal eye has several layers and structures all designed to focus light onto the retina. The pupil is the light opening, regulated by the size of the iris, and adjustments of the lens. The linking forms include: pupill/o, cor/o, core/o, ir/o, irid/o, phac/o, phak/o, cycl/o, choroid/o, retin/o, uve/i, vitre/o, aque/o, and fove/o.

10 The Tabular List of Diseases of the ICD is the 21 section area where coding is exactly defined. There are additional coding instructions to help coders expand their search and code all appropriate information. The documentation needs to be complete to cover location; changes such as a rupture or defect; and associated with things such as tobacco or injury.

UNIT WORD PARTS

Word roots with linking vowel		
Antr/o > almost closed cavity (sinuses)	Aque/o > water	Audi/o; Acous/o > hearing
Blephar/o; Palpebr/o > eyelid	Conjunctiv/o > mucous membrane of eye	Corne/o; Kerat/o > horny layers
Cycl/o > circle, ciliary body	Dacry/o; Lacrim/o > tear	Gloss/o; Lingu/o > tongue
Irid/o; Ir/o > iris	Laryng/o > voice box, larynx	Meat/o > passage
Mechan/o > mechanical, motion	Myring/o; Tympan/o > drum	Nas/o; Rhin/o > nose
Noc/i > hurt, pain	Ophthalm/o; Opt/o; Ocul/o > vision	Osm/o > smell, concentration of solution
Oss/i > small bones	Ot/o; Aur/o; Auricul/o > ear	Phac/o; Phak/o > lens
Pharyng/o > throat, pharynx	Pupillo/o; Cor/o > pupil	Retin/o > retina
Scler/o > eye sclera (hard)	Stom/o; Stomat/o; Or/o > mouth	Ton/o > sound, tone
Uve/i > middle layer of the eye, vascular	Vitre/o > glassy	

Prefixes: attached to the front of the word root to change meaning		
A-, An- > no, not, absent	Ab- > away from center, away from normal	Amblyo- > dull or dim
Aniso- > unequal	Diplo- > double, twice	Dys- > poor, difficult, painful
Eso- > inward, inner	Exo- > outward, outer	Hyper- > increase, above
Hypo- > below, under, less than	Macro- > large	Micro- > smallest, tiny
Mio- > smaller, constricted	Mydro- > widen, enlarge	Nyct-; nocto- > night
Presby- > old	Scoto- > dark, night	Xero- > dry

Suffixes change the meaning of the word, linking vowel is usually 'o' with consonants		
-algia, -dynia > pain	-cele > herniation	-centesis > removal of fluid via needle/syringe
-clysis > rinse out	-cusis > hearing	-cyte > cell
-lith > stone	-megaly > enlargement	-meter > measure
-oma > tumor	-opia > condition of vision	-osis > condition (abnormal)
-pathy > disease	-phagia > eating, swallowing	-plasty > surgical repair of
-ptosis > falling, drooping	-rrhaphy > suturing	-rrhea > discharge, flow
-sclerosis > condition of hardening	-trichia > hairy (condition of)	-tropia > condition of turning

Acronyms, abbreviations, and initial sets		
AIDS > autoimmune deficiency syndrome	AV nicking > arteriovenous crossing under torsion	BPV > benign positional vertigo
CN > cranial nerve	dB > decibels	DM > diabetes mellitus
EBV > Epstein-Barr virus	ENT or EENT > Ear, nose, throat or Eye, ear, nose, and throat	EOM > extraocular muscles or movement
HIV > human immune virus	HTN > hypertension	Hz > hertz, sound measure
NAD > no acute distress	OM (AOM) (SOM) > otitis media; acute otitis media; serous otitis media	PERRLA > pupils equally round and reactive to light and accommodation
PET > pressure-equalizing tubes or nuclear medicine scan	TM > tympanic membrane	URI > upper respiratory infection

UNIT WORKSHEETS

Building terms: Use the proper prefix/word root/linking vowel/suffix as appropriate.

   Example: to cut into the stomach > gastr/o/tomy

a) Inflammation of the iris > _____

b) Old eyes > _____

c) Abnormal sense of smell, poor > _____

d) Condition of a small tongue > _____

e) An instrument to look at the nose > _____

f) Pertaining to the tongue and pharynx (CN 9) > _____

g) An earache > _____

h) Pertaining to under the tongue (CN 12) > _____

Know your initial sets/acronyms! For the initial set or acronym given, spell it out correctly.

a) PERRLA   _____

b) SOM   _____

c) URI   _____

d) DM   _____

e) PET (both definitions) _____

f) AIDS   _____

g) Hz   _____

h) EOM   _____

Best choice: Pick the most appropriate answer.

1 Receptors responding to 'deforming' the area are called _____ .

   a) Photoreceptors

   b) Nociceptors

   c) Mechanoreceptors

   d) Chemoreceptors

2 The sense of taste is properly called _____ .

   a) Olfactory

   b) Tectorial

   c) Osmolar

   d) Gustatory

3 This is the center of our most precise vision.

   a) Organ of Corti

   b) Fovea centralis

   c) Canal of Schlemm

   d) Choroidal layer

4 If you move your eyes up and inward, which EOM cranial nerve is in use?

   a) Trigeminal

   b) Trochlear

   c) Abducens

   d) Optic

5 This muscle functions to protect our hearing.

   a) Erector pili

   b) Oculomotor

   c) Tensor tympani

   d) Abducens

Name the term! Based on the description and/or function name the term.

a) Abnormal condition of ear fungus _____

b) To cut into the cornea of the eye _____

c) Pertaining to the tongue and pharynx _____

d) Condition when the eye turns down _____

e) No sense of smell _____

f) Sensory receptors ability to adjust to stimuli _____

Multiple correct: Select ALL the correct answers to the question or statement given.

1 Mark all the correct initial set/acronyms associated otitis media?

   a) PET   d) SOM

   b) OM   e) PERRLA

   c) EOM   f) AOM

2 Which of the following prefixes are most appropriate to describe the 'turn' of the eye?

a) Eso-

b) Hypo-

c) Micro-

d) Exo-

e) Poly-

f) Hyper-

3 Which of the following are names of cranial nerves?

a) Facial

b) Temporal

c) Vestibulocochlear

d) Vagus

e) Occipital

f) Hypoglossal

Spelling challenge! Circle the correct spelling based on the definition given.

1 'An instrument to look at the eyes'

Opthalmoscope   Ophthmaskope   Ophthaloscope   Ophthalmoscope

2 'Hardening of the ear ossicles'

Ottosclarosis   Otosclerosis   Otosclarosis   Otosklerosis

3 'Surgical puncture of the TM'

Tympenocentisis   Tympanocentesis   Tynponosenesis   Typanocentesis

Define the term: Spelling *does* count in your definition too!

1 Hemotympanum > _____ _____

2 Mydriasis > _____

3 Esotropia > _____

4 Retinopathy > _____

5 Xerostomia > _____

6 Pharyngodynia > _____

7 Sialolith > _____

8 Blepharospasm > _____

Find it! Using the words in the table – match the definition given or answer the statement. Some may not be used. It is recommended you know all the choices.

otodynia	pinguecula	amblyopia	myopia	iridocele
glossotrichia	olfactory	presbycusis	retinopexy	decibels
strabismus	neuropathy	rhinitis	myringotomy	uveitis
ossiculectomy	scotoma	stomatomycosis	glaucoma	oropharyngeal

1 _____   Herniation of the iris

2 _____   Condition of a hairy tongue

3 _____   Earache

4 _____   Measurement unit of sound/loudness

5 _____   Abnormal condition of the mouth with fungus

6 _____   Old ears, hearing changes of aging

7 _____   Pertaining to the mouth and throat

8 _____   To cut into the drum

Matching: Some will not be used.

	Letter	Defined as	
Conjunctivitis		a)	a stye
Exotropia		b)	largest and first of the ear ossicles
Otitis externa		c)	pertaining to injuries caused by sound
Antritis		d)	inflammation of the inner lining of lower eye lid
Malleus		e)	inflammation of the maxillary sinuses
Tympanometry		f)	outward turning of the eye
Iridoplegia		g)	measuring the movement of the eardrum
Hordeolum		h)	old eyes, changes with aging
		i)	inflammation of the external ear
		j)	condition of paralysis of iris

An essay: Explain how the various medications used to treat neuropathy work to diminish pain or dysesthesias in your own words.

Note challenge: SOAP note from the ER. You may need to look up a few terms. Answer the questions which follow. Recall this is a limited SOAP note, it is not to be used for patient encounters.

S. Shanice is a 42-yo woman who was pouring household bleach into a cup when her cat jumped up, knocking the bleach out of her hand. The bleach splashed into both eyes. She had immediate pain and burning. She was able to call 911. The 911 operator had her rinse her eye with cool water. The

EMS have brought her to the ER for care. PMH: She has HTN treated with hydrochlorothiazide. No allergies. No tobacco use. No previous injury or eye issues.

O. 42-yo woman with distress. BP 156/96, P 85, R 16. Patient is having difficulty opening her eyes but she is receptive to light and there is a good red reflex bilaterally. Bulbar conjunctiva is bubbling with marked erythema. Limbus is sharp. Cornea under the slit lamp reveals many pocking lesions, they are not coalescing. None penetrate the thickness of the cornea. Puncta of both eyes with erythema and mild edema. Copious tears noted. Skin around the eye with mild erythema. Litmus test: pH 4. Remainder of exam is negative.

A. 1) Acute conjunctivitis

2) Corrosive burn of the cornea and conjunctiva, bilateral

3) HTN

P. Continue irrigation of the eyes until acid level has achieved normal

IV *NS* 0.9 NaCl *TKO*

Morphine sulfate 5 mg *IV* push for pain

Ophthalmologist consult

Vital signs q 30 minutes

Repeat eye exam and check acuity once pain is controlled

Questions:

1 Translate all the acronyms and give meaning to the words which are underlined in the note.

2 What information do you need to code this care? Use the chart below to assign appropriate codes from the various sections of the ICD★. There may be more than one correct code per column. Do your best. We are not trying to make you a coder but we do want you to think about how the medical terminology impacts care and coding.

3 What place would you choose for this incident?

4 What was the intent of the injury?

5 How does the documentation of this ER visit help or hinder your understanding of the incident and how it could be coded?

Alphabetic index	Tabular list of disease and injury	Injury, poisoning, and other external causes
Conjunctivitis H10.9	Acute toxic conjunctivitis (ATC) (chemical) H10.21 (Code first T51–65 to identify chemical and intent)	T26 Burn of Eye and Adnexa Use additional external cause to identify the source, place, and intent of burn (X00–X19, X75–77, X96–X98, Y92)
-acute H10.3	-ATC right eye H10.211 -ATC left eye H10.212 -ATC bilateral H10.213 -ATC unspecified H10.219	T26.4 Burn of eye and adnexa, part unspecified
-chemical H10.21 (see also Corrosion, cornea)	Exposure *keratoconjunctivitis* H16.211 -right eye H16.211 -left eye H16.212 -bilateral H16.213 -unspecified H10.219	T26.5 Corrosion of eyelid and periocular area -T26.51 right eye -T26.52 left eye
-serous H10.23		T26.6 Corrosion of cornea and conjunctival sac -T26.61 right eye -T26.62 left eye
-toxic H10.23		
Corrosion (injury) (acid) (caustic) (chemical) T30.4		
-cornea (and conjunctiva) T26.6		

⋆ IMPORTANT NOTE: The reader is notified that these examples are from an online search done in 2016. Do not use these codes for patient care episodes; look up new ones!

Unit 9

Immune and
endocrine systems

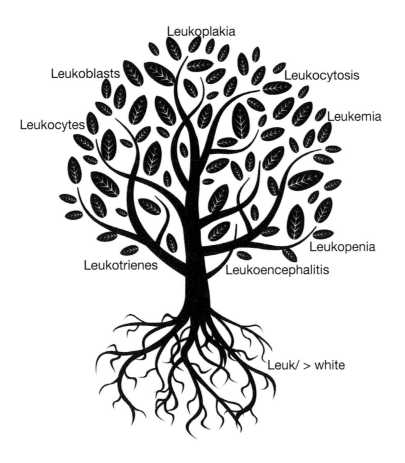

Leukoplakia

Leukoblasts

Leukocytosis

Leukocytes

Leukemia

Leukopenia

Leukotrienes

Leukoencephalitis

Leuk/ > white

TARGETED LEARNING

1 Recognize word parts and assemble medical terms related to the immune and endocrine systems.

2 Correctly construct, define, pronounce, and spell medical terms.

3 Identify immunizations (vaccinations) used to prevent infectious diseases and their consequences.

4 Relate immune and endocrine illness and injury with appropriate pharmacotherapeutics and other therapeutic options.

5 Define the function of medical documentation and coding for CDC and Epidemiology as related to tracking infectious disease.

KEY WORD PARTS

Word roots with linking vowel	Prefixes	Suffixes
Aden/o > gland	Allo-	-algia
Andr/o > man, male	Ana-	-cyte
Cortic/o or Cort/o > outer layer	Anti-	-dynia
Crin/o > secretion, to secrete	Auto-	-ectomy
Cyt/o > cell	Dia-	-emia
Globul/o or Globulin/o > protein	Endo-	-gram
Gluc/o or Glyc/o or Glycos/o > sugar, glucose	Exo-	-ism
Gyn/o or Gynec/o > female, woman Estr/o > female	Hyper-	-itis
Immun/o > protection	Hypo-	-lithiasis
Leuk/o > white	Macro-	-logy
Path/o > disease	Neo-	-megaly
Pituit/o > pituitary	Pan-	-oma
Splen/o > spleen	Para-	-osis
Thym/o > thymus	Peri-	-pathy
Thyr/o or Thyroid/o> thyroid	Poly-	-tropin

FINDING THE LEUKOCYTES

The act of drawing blood from a vein (phlebotomy) is not unique to modern medicine. However, it was not until the development of the microscope that men and women of knowledge discovered the whole cells of the blood. The white blood cells (leukocytes) were described as early as 1843. Later, it was Dr. Paul Ehrlich and Dr. Robert Koch who created stains illuminating the five different leukocytes and began to experiment to determine their impact on immunity. It was from this research that the first vaccination to prevent smallpox came into existence, with many vaccines to follow. Two centuries later, the World Health Organization (**WHO**) certified the global extermination of smallpox in 1979 (*WHO Factsheet*; Archived from the original on September 21, 2007).

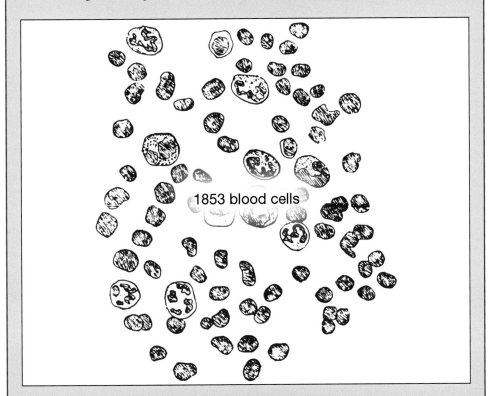

1853 blood cells

Figure 9.2

The use of an electron microscope and advancements in technology bring an understanding of the immune system's influence on the homeostasis. It is not just about infections such as smallpox or the Zika virus but about autoimmune diseases as well. Not to be unsung, the endocrine system helps preserve and spur immunity under stress, both systems affecting every function of the human's complex body.

IMMUNITY

The complexity of the immune (im-**mewn**) system is best illustrated in the layers of immunity it conveys. From the skin to the specificity of T-cell functions, the body has several lines of defense from the pathogens of life.

Pathogen > 'disease production' > any microorganism or foreign body causing disease.

The bugs or pathogens: viruses, bacteria, fungi, and parasites want in and the body's defenses are designed to keep them at bay. **The first level** includes:

- **Mechanical** > implies a solid or related 'blocking' protection.
  - **Skin** > dermat/o or derm/o > delivers a protective barrier to excess water, injury, insects, bacteria, fungi, and viruses.
  - **Mucous membranes** > muc/o or muc/i > protects via the carbohydrate-abundant glycoproteins capturing and floating away foreign bodies and toxins.

9.1

Immun/o > exempt or protected

Immunity > quality of protection

Immunocyte > cell capable of producing antibodies

Glyc/o > sugar, glucose

- **Chemical** defenses pertains to the molecules joined in a variety of compositions destroying the invading enemies of the body.
  - **Sweat, tears**, and **saliva** all contain a level of lysozymes to destroy surface bacteria and viruses.
- The **gastric mucosa** will produce hydrochloric (HCl) acid and pepsin to digest proteins while killing more opportunistic invaders.
- **Vaginal mucosa** is slightly acidic to stave off excess fungi, bacteria, and viruses.

9.2

Sialaden/o > salivary glands

Lys/o > to destroy, to dissolve

Gastr/o > stomach

Prote/o > proteins, major nutrient

-zymes > enzymes, fermentation

- **Automatic reflexes** expel invaders.
  - **Cough** > tuss/o > ejects irritants forcibly from the lungs and bronchial tree. An antitussive works 'against cough'.
  - **Sneezing** > ousts irritants from the nose and sinuses.
  - **Vomiting** > emesis > banishes irritants from the stomach.
  - **Diarrhea** > **dia-** is through; **-rrhea** is flow > fast-moving stool flowing through is a method to clear toxins from the gut.

9.3

Pulmon/o > lungs

Bronchi/o > airway tubes

Enter/o > small intestines

Col/o > colon

✓ What is the word for 'quality of self-protection'?

✓ What is the medical term for 'vomiting'?

✓ What is the proper medical term for a 'disease production'?

9.4 Autoimmunity

9.5 Emesis

9.6 Pathogen

The second level of shielding begins the journey into the bloodstream. This is nonspecific immunity – running on automatic!

- **Phagocytosis** (**fag**-oh-sigh-**toe**-sis) > condition of 'eating' cells. Specific white blood cells (leukocytes or WBCs) ingest and consume debris and pathogens. The **mono**cytes (**mon**-oh-sites) station themselves in various organs to lay-in-wait for the foreign invaders to cross their path. They are also termed **macro**cytes (**mak**-row-sites) > large cells or **macrophages** (**mak**-row-fahjs) (large eaters; Figure 9.3).

9.7
Phag/o > to eat
Pin/o > to drink
Leuk/o > white
Macro- > large
Mono- > single, one

CELL-MEDIATED IMMUNE RESPONSE

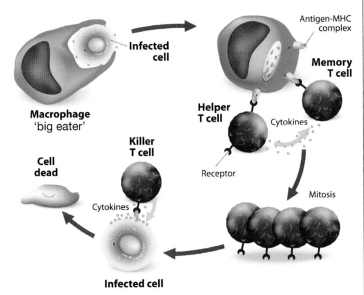

Figure 9.3

- **Pyrexia** (pie-**rek**-see-a) > condition of fever, fire, or heat > an elevation in body temperature is the body's attempt to burn out the pathogens. It also stimulates the phagocytosis. The response begins at the hypothalamus, a brain region interacting with the master gland, the pituitary gland. Together they regulate the release of a number of hormones (Figure 9.4). Synonym: Therm/o > temperature.

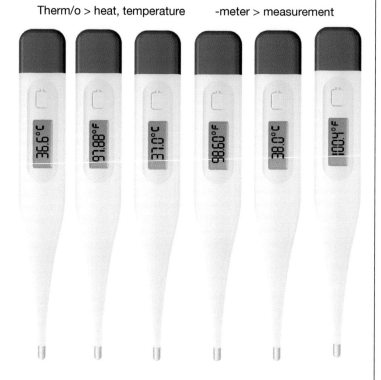

Therm/o > heat, temperature   -meter > measurement

Figure 9.4

- **Inflammation** (in-flam-**may**-shun) > 'in flames'. A set of intricate responses to injury. An essential reaction of the body to recognize and begin repair of injury typified by pain, redness, swelling, and heat generation.
  - When inflammation is caused by a pathogen it is called an infection (in-**fek**-shun) > to enter or to corrupt. An accumulation of bacteria and its debris is called pus > py/o.
  - Inflammation triggers the release of localized hormones or paracrines including histamine (**his**-tah-mean) and prostaglandin (pros-tah-**glan**-din).

9.8

LIKE ALERT!

Py/o > pus

Pyr/o > fire, heat, fever

Antipyretic > against fever > a medication or procedure to lower the temperature.

9.9

Did You Know?

Infection control is best begun with a thorough hand-washing regimen with warm, soapy water for 20–30 seconds. Avoid antibacterial soap, it helps build superbugs (Figure 9.5).

Py/o > pus or purulent discharge

Should take 30 seconds

WASH YOUR HANDS

Easiest and best way to avoid infections

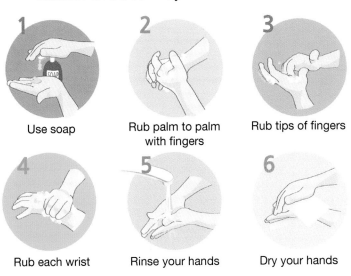

Use soap	Rub palm to palm with fingers	Rub tips of fingers
Rub each wrist	Rinse your hands	Dry your hands

Figure 9.5

- There are two classes of proteins guarding the body from within – the **interferons** (in-tur-**fear**-ons) and **complement** (kom-play-ment) proteins.
  - **Interferons** are produced by the T lymphocytes (lim-**foe**-sites), fibroblasts, and others in response to viral infections. Interferons inhibit viral growth and alert the phagocytes to get to work.
  - **Complement**, a set of 20 proteins sensitive to temperature in the presence of attacking bacteria (Figure 9.6). The cascade or domino-effect activates phagocytosis and antibody production.

9.10

Lymph/o > living fluid; 'spring water'

Fibr/o > fiber, thread

-blast > immature, developing

Bacterium > singular

Bacteria > plural

Virus > singular

Viruses > plural

- **Natural Killer (NK)** cells sound quite mysterious but they are a type of lymphocytes which mature and function from the lymph tissues such as the tonsils or the appendix.
  - They attach to microbes and certain cancer cells, destroying them before they can take hold.

9.11

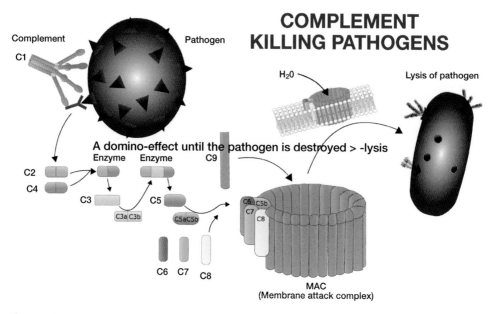

COMPLEMENT KILLING PATHOGENS

Figure 9.6

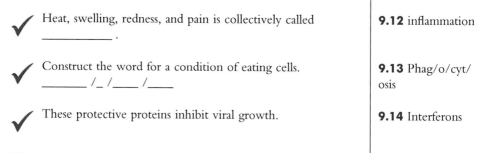

✓ Heat, swelling, redness, and pain is collectively called _____ .

9.12 inflammation

✓ Construct the word for a condition of eating cells.
_____ /_ /_____ /_____

9.13 Phag/o/cyt/osis

✓ These protective proteins inhibit viral growth.

9.14 Interferons

Word building

Using the word roots with the linking vowel to build as many valid terms with the suffixes given. Please define each term.

Immun/o Phag/o Cyt/o

–logy –osis –therapy –cyte –gen –genesis

9.15
The instructor has the list!

PHARMACY CORNER*

Inflammation occurs in the body literally moment to moment. The small cut or bruise on the skin is just the tip of the iceberg. Inflammation is a response to irritation from stress, pathogens, friction, radiation such as **UV** light, heat or cold, or chemicals eaten, touched, or inhaled. The release of the histamine and prostaglandin causes vasodilation, an enlargement of the vessel walls allowing them to leak fluid in and around the injured area. The swelling of the vessels also gives the **neutrophils** and **monocytes** the ability to sneak out of the vessel and start cleaning up the debris. This is called **diapedesis** (**dye**-ah-pee-**dee**-sis) (Figure 9.7). The histamine and other chemicals act as signals attracting the healing fluids, clotting factors, and leukocytes to the area of injury.

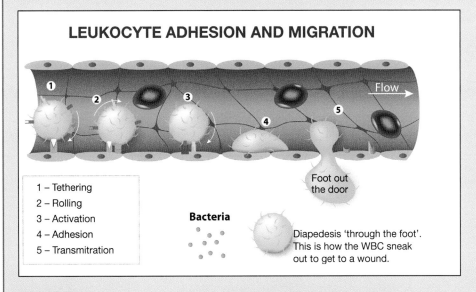

LEUKOCYTE ADHESION AND MIGRATION

1 – Tethering
2 – Rolling
3 – Activation
4 – Adhesion
5 – Transmitration

Bacteria

Foot out the door

Diapedesis 'through the foot'. This is how the WBC sneak out to get to a wound.

Figure 9.7

Medications are developed to limit this protective response. They modify the inflammation by blocking the histamine and/or the prostaglandin. Non-steroidal anti-inflammatory drugs (**NSAIDs**) such as ibuprofen and naproxen block prostaglandin and will lower a fever. Anti-histamines such as *diphenhydramine* cause vasoconstriction, preventing the release of fluids. Both of these decrease pain and swelling, reducing erythema (redness) and pyrogenesis (heat production). While NSAIDs diminish pain or fever, the science is still out on whether stalling a healing process is a good idea in the long run. This is especially true of prostaglandin interruption in the gastric mucosa; it may set a patient up for gastric carcinoma if the medications are used regularly.

* IMPORTANT NOTE: All discussions of medications are for basic education. A medical provider should be consulted on any medication options. Do <u>not</u> use this information for patient care.

THIRD LINE OF DEFENSE

Lymphocytes are one of the five WBC types produced by the bone marrow. These offer very precise protection – each time infection arrives, they mount a specific defense unique to each person and pathogen. There are two types of lymphocytes: T-cells and B-cells develop in the bone marrow and hang out in the lymph tissues of the body. Some T-lymphocytes develop in the thymus, lymph nodes, and spleen (Figure 9.8).

- **T-lymphocytes** are the soldiers of the immune system. They mature in the thymus and wander the circulation to attack pathogens directly. There are four types:

  - **Killer T-cells** kill by punching holes in the pathogen and inserting lymphokines (**lim**-foe-kins) essentially executing the infected cell.

  - **Helper T-cells** secrete a different lymphokine signaling for more T-cells and B-cells to join the battle.

  - **Memory T-cells** do no actual fighting but will remember the pathogen in the future, enabling a swift immune response next time.

9.16
Lymph is also the excess fluid leaking between cells. It is gathered by the lymphatic vessels to be cleansed and recycled. There are many terms regarding this system of the body (Unit 10). They are also part of the immune system.

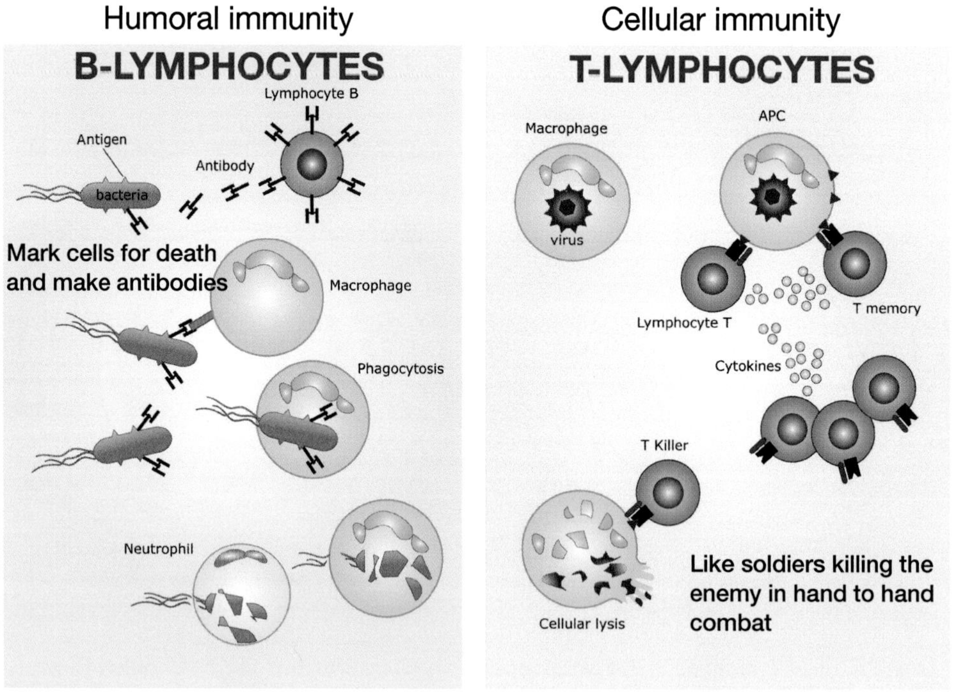

Humoral immunity

B-LYMPHOCYTES

Lymphocyte B

Antigen

Antibody

bacteria

Mark cells for death and make antibodies

Macrophage

Phagocytosis

Neutrophil

Cellular immunity

T-LYMPHOCYTES

APC

Macrophage

virus

Lymphocyte T

T memory

Cytokines

T Killer

Cellular lysis

Like soldiers killing the enemy in hand to hand combat

Figure 9.8

- **Suppressor T-cells** call the lymphocytes to rest when the infection or pathogen is defeated. They basically summon the soldiers back to base. If these suppressor T-cells are inhibited, an autoimmune condition can begin, the body destroying healthy tissue.

Did You Know?

CRISPR, **C**lustered **R**egularly **I**nterspaced **S**hort **P**alindromic **R**epeats – is the newest and most exciting genetic research. If it proves out, the hope is the T-lymphocytes will be specifically activated to target identified cancer cells only! There is anticipation it may also help with other genetic diseases such as muscular dystrophy.

- **B-lymphocytes** fight pathogens by marking them for death and creating millions of antibodies by hooking onto the pathogen. This gives the T-lymphocytes a ready target.

- **Plasma cells** secrete the antibodies in the millions (Figure 9.9). This takes about two weeks. This is why a vaccination takes time to protect.

PLASMA CELL
B-lymphocyte

Golgi apparatus

Antibody

Nucleus

Build antibodies in the millions to fight antigens.

Mitochondria

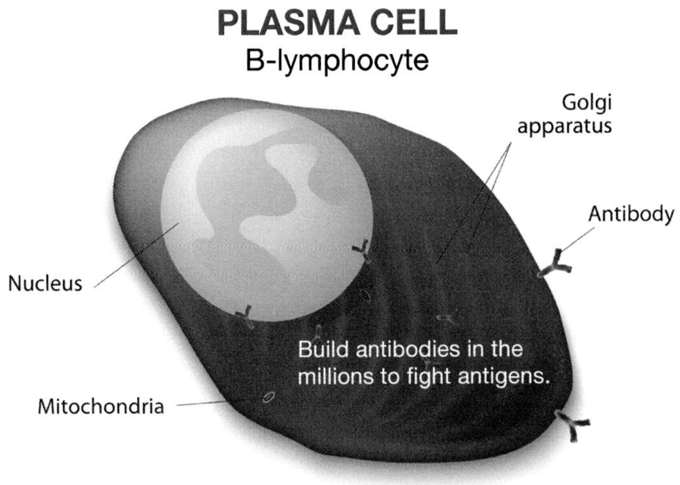

Figure 9.9

- **Memory B-cells** will remember the pathogen or antigen for life. This gives the patient immunity from this particular infection in the future.

- Anti**gen** > against production or beginnings > any substance creating an immune response. This is what the B-cells target, the bad guys.

- Anti**body** > an immunoglobulin (a protective protein) will link to a specific antigen, marking it for destruction by the immune system. This is the function of the B-lymphocytes.

9.17
Vaccinations encourage the development of the **antibodies**. There several types:

Live, attenuate vaccines

Inactive vaccines

Toxoid vaccines

Subunit vaccines

Conjugate vaccines

Kitchen lab

The study of infectious disease is a function of the clinical laboratory. Use the website or internet to look up the recipe to make your own agar plates and grow some of the bacteria from your home or work environment. After you do all the steps (it will take 4–5 days) answer the questions below:

1 Describe the bacteria colonies in your agar plates: what color are they? Small or large? Circular or more linear? Fuzzy?

2 After letting your cultures grow for a few days, how does one drop of household bleach change your plates?

3 What does the abbreviation set C&S stand for?

Share your findings with your instructor. Be sure to dispose of your plates properly (seal them up)!

IMMUNOLOGY

Immunology (im-**mew**-nol-**oh**-gee) > study of protection is done by specialists in autoimmune disease, immunodeficiency disease, organ transplants, and cancer. This section reviews key terms, acronyms, and initial sets (Figure 9.10).

- **Tox/o** > poison. Many infections produce **toxins** (**tok**-sins) causing damage. *Clostridium botulinum* is one of these – tetanus. Other toxins are poisons such as rattlesnake or bee venom. Other linking forms are toxic/o, tox-, tox/i.

- **Infection** > to enter into the body or invade and corrupt the body.

- **Anaphylaxis** (an-ah-**fee**-lax-is) > immediate immunologic reaction to a foreign body, an antigen such as poison ivy, peanut oil, or dust.

- **Chemotactic** (**key**-mo-**tak**-tik) factors > one or more biochemical elements attracting leukocytes to the area of inflammation.

- **Opsonin** (**op**-sew-nins) > specialized molecule paints the target on the pathogen making it easily found by the leukocytes.

- **Leukotrienes** (**lew**-ko-**try**-enz) > fatty molecules impart slow and steady vascular changes associated with inflammation. They last longer than the initial histamine release.

9.18
tox/o terms:

Toxemia > toxic substance in the blood

Toxicity > the state of being poisonous

Toxicogenic > caused by a poison

9.19
Type I reactions are associated with these active substances of inflammation:

Histamine

Bradykinin

Serotonin

Leukotrienes

WHITE BLOOD CELL
How each WBC provides immune response

Granulocytes

Neutrophil

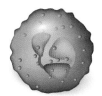

(phagocyting a bacteria
and other pathogens)

Eosinophil

(control mechanisms
associated with allergy)

Agranulocytes

Monocyte
(phagocytosis)

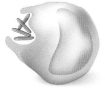

Lymphocyte
(secretion of antibodies)

Basophil
(contain
histamine
and heparin)

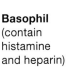

Histamine release
from the basophils

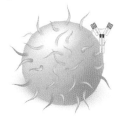

Figure 9.10

 Which of the lymphocytes will produce millions of antibodies in response to an infection?

 What is the definition of 'toxicosis'?

 What is the definition for 'immunologist'?

Word building

Using the word roots with the linking vowel to build as many valid terms with the suffixes given. Please define each term.

Tox/o Lymph/o Bacteri/o

–logy –osis –logist –genic –emia

9.20
B-lymphocytes

9.21
An abnormal
condition due to
toxins (poisons)

9.22
A specialist in the
study of the
immune system

9.23
The instructor has
the list!

TRACKING DISEASE*

Over 50 people became ill after eating at local restaurants. The bug (bacteria) in this case is *Escherichia coli* (*E.coli*). *E.coli* populates the bowels. However, given the opportunity and its ability to mutate, it becomes a pathogen. Genetics aid bacteriologists in being able to identify the exact strain, taking its DNA fingerprint, STEC 026, Shiga toxin-producing. This toxin disrupts protein production of the cells causing damage to or death of cells.

All the individual offices and facilities report these cases to the epidemiologists (**ep**-ee-dee-me-**ol**-oh-jist) at local health departments. When the **ICD** code B96.2 begins showing up in a defined population, the CDC (Centers for Disease Control and Prevention) begins the search for the source of the contamination. With 50+ people infected in the first outbreak, the role of the CDC is do the microbiology and genetic fingerprinting of the strain involved. They follow the food trail. Though an exact food is not identified; the investigation permits for destruction of remaining food stuffs and a clean-up – stopping the infection from spreading to others. This is the ultimate goal of the CDC to stop illness and injury when possible.

This pursuit is aided by a genetic/molecular test, the *Pulsed-Field Gel Electrophoresis* (**PFGE**); it looks for definitive DNA fragments denoting an infection or toxin. Eventually, the preliminary ICD code of B96.2 is updated to the more precise B96.21 Shiga toxin-producing *E. coli* found in the tabular list.

The use of the ICD to identify and track illness or injuries is a vital component to public health worldwide. The importance of adequate and accurate documentation of conditions and their diagnosis allows for rapid recognition and response to deadly threats. Infectious diseases in particular can travel the globe rapidly, such as HIV, H1N1, Zika virus, and Ebola. Coding is essential to the epidemiologist's work of tracking and the scientist's ability to develop vaccines or cures for these diseases.

* IMPORTANT NOTE: The reader is notified that these examples are from an online search done in 2016. Do _not_ use these codes for patient care episodes; look up new ones!

IMMUNOGLOBULINS AND IMMUNE DISEASE

Antibodies come in five forms, and these are **immunoglobulins** (**im**-mew-no-**glob**-u-lins) > protective proteins. They work with specificity: a lack of or absence of these antibodies leads to immune-deficient disease and/or autoimmune diseases.

- **IgA** > immunoglobulin A populates the orifice areas of the body: mouth, vagina, gastrointestinal tract, kidneys, ears, and eyes.

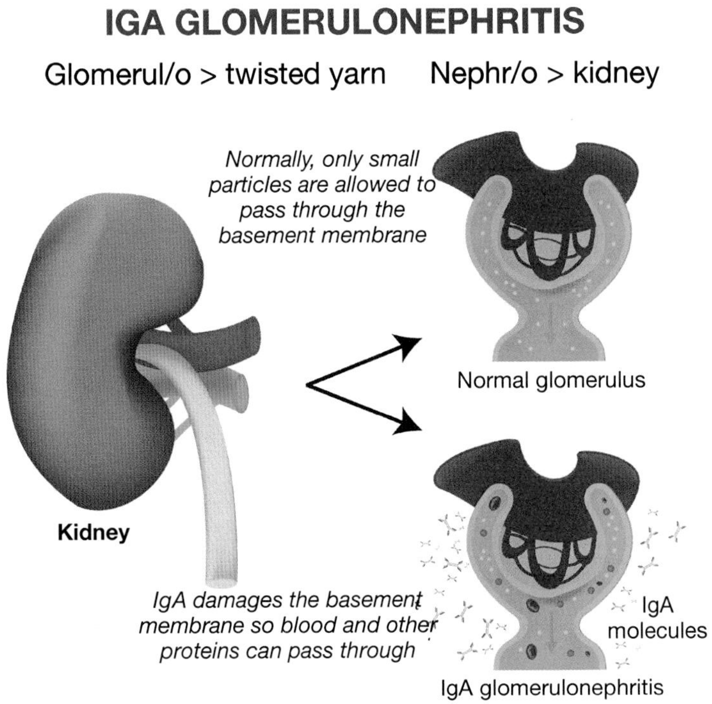

IGA GLOMERULONEPHRITIS

Glomerul/o > twisted yarn   Nephr/o > kidney

Normally, only small particles are allowed to pass through the basement membrane

Normal glomerulus

Kidney

IgA damages the basement membrane so blood and other proteins can pass through

IgA molecules

IgA glomerulonephritis

Figure 9.11

- **IgD** > immunoglobulin D is found in small numbers on the internal surfaces of the abdominal and thoracic regions.

- **IgE** > immunoglobulin E is found in the respiratory tract, skin, and mucous membranes and is associated with allergies and parasites.

- **IgG** > immunoglobulin G permeates all body fluids and is the only antibody type to cross the placenta to protect the fetus.

- **IgM** > immunoglobulin M is the first to respond to infection and is found in the blood and lymph tissue.

Hypersensitivity (**hi**-purr-**sen**-si-**tiv**-i-tea) > exaggerated response of the body to a foreign body or antigen.

- **Allergies** (al-ur-jeez) > immune reaction to an irritant. This is a consequence to environmental antigens or allergens such as pollen, animal dander, or inhalants (Figure 9.12).

- **Urticaria** (**ur**-tea-**kare**-ee-ah) > eruption of itchy wheals or welts usually associated with allergies, cold, or heat. Synonym: hives.

9.24
Laboratory testing for the identifiable level of antibodies helps providers define:

– Allergies

– Autoimmune disease (Figure 9.11)

– Cancers such as multiple myeloma

– Re-occurring infections

– Response to immunizations and rejection medications

One of these is an **ASO** > antistreptolysin O, to determine whether the patient has been exposed to group A *Streptococcus*

9.25

- **Pruritus** (pru-**ree**-tus) > itching, used in relationship to the intense itchy-reaction of allergies.

- **Bronchial asthma** (**bron**-key-al **az**-mah) > marked narrowing of the bronchial tubes, edema of the mucosa, and inflammation which can be life threatening. This occurs due to the sudden release of histamines, leukotrienes, and prostaglandins.

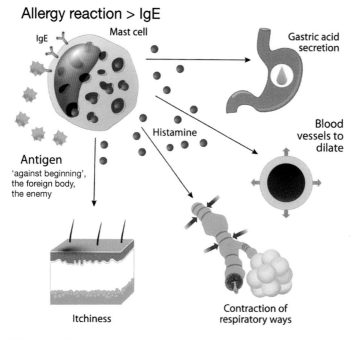

Allergy reaction > IgE

Figure 9.12

Did You Know?

There are four types of hypersensitivity:

Type 1: IgE-mediated hayfever

Type 2: tissue-specific drug reactions causing hemolysis (blood breakdown)

Type 3: immune complex kicks in such as with gluten allergies

Type 4: Cell-level reactions such as poison ivy

Immunodeficient Diseases are grouped in primary and secondary causes. Autoimmune implies an interference with the suppressor T-cells to send the lymphocytes to rest at the appropriate time and place, or a genetic mutation. Secondary causes include infections such as Human Immunodeficiency Virus (**HIV**).

- **B-cell (lymphocytes)** defects seem to involve defective switches for IgA and IgG and overproduction of IgM. The effect is fewer cells targeting the antigens.

- **T-cell (lymphocytes)** defects slow or stop the maturation of the T-cells blocking the ability kill antigens, particularly fungi.

- There are several genetic mutations disrupting both B- and T-cells from a lack of leukocyte formation to abnormal B- and T-cell activity and an absence of IgA.

9.26
As the science of genetics has progressed, more and more single gene defects are being identified. These tend to be erratic and are not inherited. Many appear in individuals with known allergies, eczema, and other dermatoses.

- Defects in the complement and phagocytic mechanisms disrupt function permitting pathogens to get the upper hand.

 IgA and IgE are properly called

_____

 What is the medical term for intensely 'itchy'?

 What are the two linking forms for 'cells'?

9.27
immunoglobulins

9.28 Pruritus

9.29
Cyt/o and cellul/o

Autoimmune **diseases** can be found in all systems and tend to influence several areas of the body simultaneously. The endocrine system leads the way in demonstrating how integrated the two systems are in sustaining homeostasis.

- **Hyperthyroidism** (**hi**-purr-**thigh**-royd-izm) > hypermetabolic state associated with weight loss, tremors, and exophthalmos. Eponym: Graves' disease.

- **Myxedema** (mix-i-**deem**-ah) > waxy, thick, non-pitting swelling associated with hypothyroidism (hi-**poe**-thigh-**royd**-izm).

9.30

WORD OPPOSITES

Hyper- > more, many, elevated, increased

Hypo- > less, decreased, lower

These are close in sound and spelling AND the differences in the symptoms of conditions such as thyroidism are huge. Be careful to use them properly.

Glyc/o or Gluc/o or Glycos/o > glucose or sugar

Myx/o > mucus from the Greek

Thyr/o or Thyroid/o > thyroid

Ren/o or Nephr/o> kidney

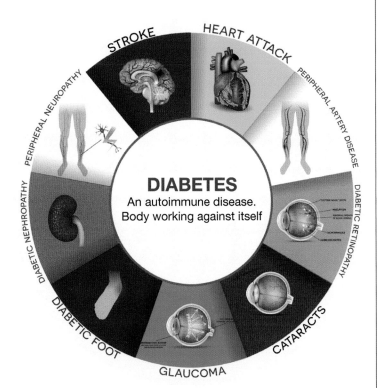

Figure 9.13

- **Insulin-dependent diabetes mellitus (IDDM)** > caused by the lack of insulin production at the islet cells of the pancreas. Uncontrolled, this causes hyperglycemia (hi-**purr**-gleye-**see**-me-ah) and eventual organ failure (Figure 9.13).

- **Chronic adrenocortical insufficiency** > relative or complete loss of the adrenal gland to produce the stress hormones. Eponym: Addison's disease.

- **Gonad deficiencies** > these conditions cause ovarian or testicular failure.

The **gastrointestinal (GI) system** has many autoimmune diseases:

- Gluten-sensitive enteropathy. Eponym: Celiac disease.

- Ulcerative colitis (**ul**-sir-a-tiv **koh**-lie-tis) (**UC**).

- Crohn's (kronz) disease (an eponym).

- Atrophic gastritis (at-**row**-fik gas-**try**-tis).

Neuromuscular tissues are at risk as well:

- Multiple sclerosis (**sklar**-oh-sis) (**MS**).

- Myasthenia gravis (**my**-as-**thee**-knee-ah **gra**-vis) (**MG**).

- Rheumatic fever (roo-**mat**-ick **fee**-vur) (**RF**).

- Cardiomyopathy (**kar**-dee-oh-**my**-op-ah-thee).

- Postinfectious encephalitis (en-**sef**-ah-lie-tis).

Connective tissue autoimmune diseases include:

- Rheumatoid arthritis (**roo**-mah-**toyd** are-**thri**-tis) (**RA**).

- Systemic lupus erythematosus (sis-**tem**-ik **lew**-pus er-**rith**-eh-mah-**toe**-sus) (**SLE**).

- Polyarteritis nodosa vasculitis (polly-**ahr**-tur-eye-tis no-**doe**-sah **vas**-Q-**lie**-tis).

- Scleroderma (**sklar**-oh-**dur**-mah).

- Ankylosing spondylitis (**ang**-key-los-ing **spon**-di-**lie**-tis).

Alloimmune (al-low-im-mewn) diseases occur as well. Allo- > from another or away from normal.

- Tissue and organ transplant from other people, such as the heart, seen in Figure 9.14.

- Gammaglobulin reactions such as using horse serum to fight the toxins of a rattlesnake bite.

9.31
Laboratory

ESR or Sed Rate > erythrocyte sedimentation rate

ANA > antinuclear antibody

RF > rheumatoid factor

All used as preliminary immune disease evaluation

9.32

Auto- > self

Allo- > from another

Neo- > new

A or An- > no, not, or absent

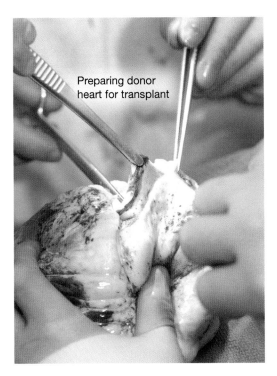
Preparing donor heart for transplant

Figure 9.14

- Neonatal hemolytic (**he**-moe-**lit**-ik) disease when the Rh of mom and infant do not agree.

Causes of **Secondary immune deficiencies** are abundant: really anything promoting illness or injury can slow down the immune response.

- The extremes of age > newborns have less developed immunity and the elderly have an aging immunity setting both up for more infections. Pregnancy can also stress the immunity.

- Psychological stress > emotional trauma and eating disorders.

- Physical stress > lack of sleep, anesthesia, surgery, burns, and fractures.

- Poor diet > inadequate proteins, insufficient nutrients such as the B vitamins, iron, or zinc.

- Environmental exposures > **UV** light (sun burns), chemical exposures (tobacco, insecticides, etc. . . .), radiation exposure, and chronic hypoxia.

- Infections > **HIV**, cytomegalovirus (**CMV**), and hepatitis B.

Nat/o > birth

Xen/o- > other species

Hem/o > blood

Globul/o > protein

Prote/o > protein

Esthesi/o > sensation, feeling

Psych/o > mind, mental

Physi/o > natural, function

Oxi/o or Ox/o > oxygen

KILLER INFECTIOUS DISEASES

There are many ancient diseases known to have killed and maimed millions over the millennium. Today, many of these are controlled with development and administration of vaccinations. Some of these diseases include:

- Tetanus (**tet**-ah-nus) > caused by a bacterium found in the soil, dust, and manure. The bacterium is *Clostridium botulinum* and it causes 'lockjaw', a paralysis of the muscles. There is no cure and it is deadly.

- Diphtheria (dif-**thear**-ee-ah) > another bacterium found readily in the environment. It is quite contagious causing a severe sore throat, lymphadenopathy, fever, and weakness.

- Pertussis (purr-**tus**-is) > also known as whooping cough. It is caused by a bacterium leading to a dangerous level of coughing. It is especially perilous in infants because it can close the trachea and bronchial tubes, resulting in suffocation.

- Mumps > viral illness causing encephalitis (inflammation of the brain), meningitis (inflammation of the brain/spinal cord coverings), and deafness.

- Measles (**me**-zuls) > contagious viral illness and one of the leading causes of death in young children under age 5 worldwide, even today.

- Rubella (ruw-**bell**-ah) > also known as German measles, is a contagious viral illness. While the disease itself is mild in most people, it is especially dangerous to pregnant women. It can cause birth defects or spontaneous miscarriage.

The first vaccination for smallpox occurred around 1796 in Europe. The term 'vaccination' comes from the Latin for 'cows > vaca' because cowpox lesions were used to prevent human smallpox. The **DTaP** (diphtheria, tetanus, and pertussis) and **MMR** (measles, mumps, and rubella) vaccinations we use today to protect children and adults were developed as late as the 1980s. New vaccinations for diseases such as HIV, Zika, and Ebola are under development. They will give immunity to these killer diseases.

ENDOCRINE SYSTEM

Like the immune system, the endocrine system can be hard to visualize because it also works via the bloodstream. Endocrine hormones are secreted by a variety of organs and tissues in one location and affect cell and tissues at distant locations. Hormones are chemical messengers traveling the circulation. There are seven major endocrine organs and several 'paracrines' > localized hormones interacting with all systems (Figure 9.15).

- **Endocrine** (en-doe-krin) > body system whose specialized tissues (glands) secrete hormones into the bloodstream to affect tissues elsewhere in the body.

- **Exocrine** (ek-so-krine) > gland secreting to the outside via a duct such as the bile duct and pancreatic duct, excreting digestive enzymes into the duodenum.
  - Duct (duk-t) > Latin, 'to lead'

9.33

Endo- > within, inside

Exo- > outside, outer

Para- > near

Crin/o > secretions

WORD ALERT!

Hormon/o > hormone

Home/o > same, alike

Hormones help provide homeostasis. They sound similar.

ENDOCRINE SYSTEM

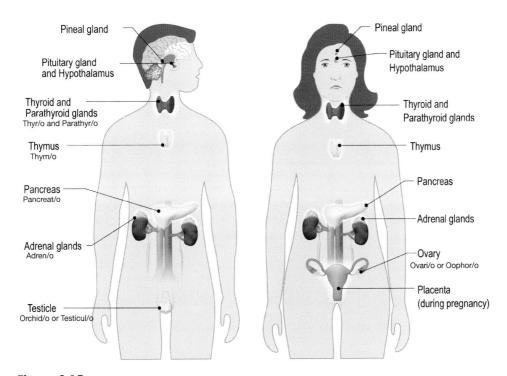

Pineal gland

Pituitary gland and Hypothalamus

Thyroid and Parathyroid glands
Thyr/o and Parathyr/o

Thymus
Thym/o

Pancreas
Pancreat/o

Adrenal glands
Adren/o

Testicle
Orchid/o or Testicul/o

Pineal gland

Pituitary gland and Hypothalamus

Thyroid and Parathyroid glands

Thymus

Pancreas

Adrenal glands

Ovary
Ovari/o or Oophor/o

Placenta
(during pregnancy)

Figure 9.15

Pituitary (pi-**tu**-i-ter-ee) **gland** > master gland of the body! It is about the size of a large pea. It interacts with the hypothalamus of the brain and produces nine hormones (Figure 9.16):

- **Pituit/o** > **Anterior pituitary** will produce
  - **Growth hormone** (**GH**) > affecting bones and muscles growth and repair.
  - **Thyroid** (**thigh**-royd)-**stimulating hormone** (**TSH**) > triggers the thyroid in the anterior neck.
  - **Luteinizing** (**lew**-tin-i-zing) **hormone** (**LH**) > activates the gonads: testicles and ovaries.
  - **Follicle-stimulating** (**fol**-ee-kal) **hormone** (**FSH**) > prompts the gonads to generate gametes (sex cells).
  - **Prolactin** (pro-**lak**-tin) (**PRL**) > travels to the breast to stimulate milk production.

THE PITUITARY GLAND HORMONES

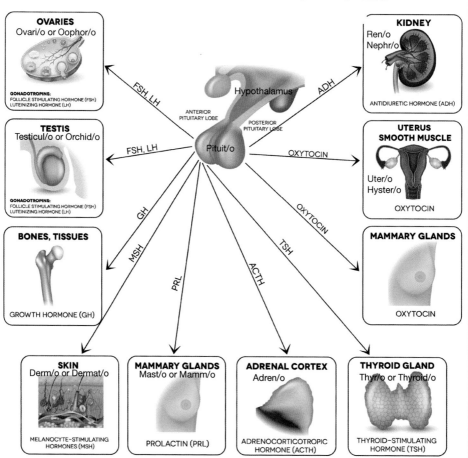

Figure 9.16

- **Melanocyte-stimulating** (**mel**-ah-no-sites) **hormone** (**MSH**) > triggers melanocytes of the skin, eyes, and mucus membranes providing darker skin tones and UV protection.
- **Adrenocorticotropic** (a-**dre**-no-**kor**-tea-ko-trow-pik) **hormone** (**ACTH**) > stimulates the adrenal glands.

The **Posterior pituitary** has the interactive, portal vascular system with the hypothalamus allowing a broad-reaching feedback loop to adjust water and blood pressure at all times (Figure 9.17).

- **Antidiuretic hormone** (**ADH**) travels to the kidney and blood vessels. It is also called vasopressin, and it raises blood pressure.

- **Oxytocin** (**ock**-see-**toe**-sin) travels to the uterus to begin contractions of birth and the breast to let milk down for the infant. Toc/o > Greek for 'child birth'.

- Pituitary adenoma (ah-**den**-oh-ma) > condition of the pituitary gland. It is usually a benign tumor; it does not disrupt hormone secretion in most patients. It causes trouble as it enlarges – crowding the optic nerves.

Together they only weigh about 110 grams out of the 70,000 grams of the average adult, yet they affect every cell day to day.

9.35
The pituitary portal vascular system connects the neuron control of the hypothalamus to the posterior pituitary, sending the two vital hormones directly into the bloodstream. This also called the neurohypophysis. The anterior pituitary is called the adenohypophysis.

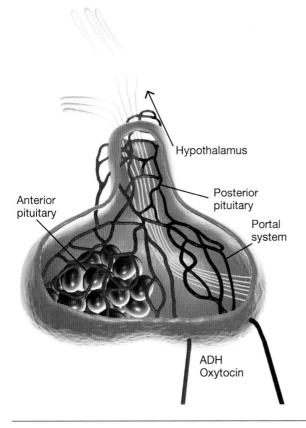

Hypothalamus

Anterior pituitary

Posterior pituitary

Portal system

ADH
Oxytocin

Figure 9.17

Build three words using endo-, exo-, and para- with the word root meaning 'secrete'.

9.36 Endocrine, Exocrine, Paracrine

 Measles can cause 'inflammation of the brain'. What is the proper medical term?

9.37 Encephalitis

 This term is used to describe a 'chemical messenger secreted in one place and effects tissues or cells in other areas'.

9.38 Hormones

Word building

*Using the word roots **with the linking vowel to build as many valid terms with the suffixes given.** Please define each term.*

Pituit/o Crin/o Glyc/o
(use a prefix as desired)

-ary -itis -oid -gen -oma -ectomy

9.39
The instructor has the list!

The thyroid gland is the largest of the endocrine organs and is found at the base of the neck, a bow-tie over the trachea (Figure 9.18).

- Thyr/o or Thyroid/o > thyroid responds to **TSH** and produces

  - **Triiodothyronine** (try-**eye**-oh-doe-**thigh**-roe-neen) > **T3**, the metabolically active hormone that is produced from the **T4**. It touches every physiological process including growth, neurologic development, body temperature, heart rate, and energy and oxygen consumption.

  - **Thyroxine** (thigh-**rok**-zeen) > **T4**, the active iodine compound which becomes the active T3.

  - **Calcitonin** (**kal**-see-**toe**-nin) > decreases blood calcium levels of blood and tissues. It works with the parathyroid glands to manage calcium.

Thyroid carcinoma (**kar**-sin-**oh**-ma) > seen in women more than in men and comes in four types. Risk factors include the genetics noted earlier and radiation exposure.

- **Goiter** (**goy**-tur) > specific term for chronic thyromegaly associated with iodine insufficiency. Iodine is added to all refined table salt (sodium chloride) to ensure adequate intake.

- **Thyroiditis** (**thigh**-royd-**eye**-tis) > inflammation of the thyroid occurs in a variety of settings, Hashimoto's thyroiditis, an autoimmune hypothyroidism is seen most often.

9.40
Suffixes
-ectomy > surgical removal
-oid > like, similar
-itis > inflammation
-oma > tumor
-ism > condition of (multiple symptoms)
-megaly > enlargement
-toxic > extreme excess
TFS > thyroid function studies
FNA > fine needle aspiration is used to biopsy thyroid lesions

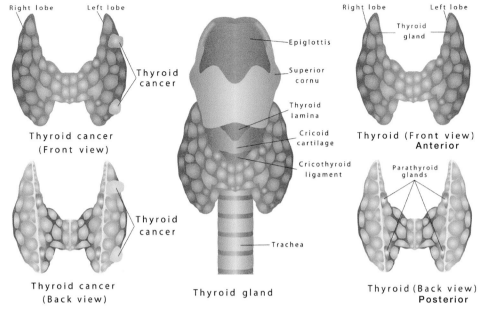

Right lobe   Left lobe

Thyroid
cancer

Thyroid cancer
(Front view)

Thyroid
cancer

Thyroid cancer
(Back view)

Right lobe   Left lobe

Epiglottis

Superior
cornu

Thyroid
lamina

Cricoid
cartilage

Cricothyroid
ligament

Trachea

Thyroid gland

Right lobe   Left lobe

Thyroid
gland

Thyroid (Front view)
Anterior

Parathyroid
glands

Thyroid (Back view)
Posterior

ANATOMY OF THYROID GLAND

Figure 9.18

Nuclear medicine iodine exam > traces radioactive iodine to the thyroid to illuminate lesions.

CT or **MRI** may be used as well.

Hashimoto's > an eponym for a specific form of hypothyroidism.

The Parathyroid (**pair**-ah-**thigh**-royd) **glands** are four tiny glands attached to the posterior thyroid, as seen on Figure 9.18. These produce parathyroid hormone (**PTH**) > designed to increase calcium in the bloodstream. **PTH** also regulates other minerals such as magnesium and phosphate. It acts on the bone, the gut (to absorb calcium or not), and the kidneys (to retain calcium or not).

- Increased **PTH** stimulates the **osteoclasts** (**os**-tea-oh-klasts) > bone carvers, these bone cells are phagocytes to release bone calcium into the bloodstream.

- Increased calcitonin (from the thyroid) stimulate the **osteoblasts** (**os**-tea-oh-blasts) > immature cells are the bone builders. These take excess calcium out of the bloodstream to build and recycle bone.

- **Hyperparathyroidism** > associated with muscle weakness, myalgia, osteoporosis, polyuria, nephrolithiasis, anorexia, and arthralgias.

9.41

Prefixes

Eu- > good, normal (euthyroid)

Hyper- > more, increased

Hypo- > less, decreased

Associated words:

Hypocalcemia

Hypercalcemia

Hypermagnesemia

Hypomagnesemia

-emia > condition related to the blood

- **Hypoparathyroidism** > linked with hyperreflexia, tonic–clonic seizures, and laryngeal spasm, alopecia, and bone deformities.

Investigation includes laboratory studies, nuclear medicine scans, neurological testing, and CT or MRI scans.

✓ Build a medical term for 'multiple symptomatic condition due to decreased thyroid function'.

9.42 Hypo-thyroidism

✓ What is the abbreviation for 'thyroxin'.

9.43 T4

✓ Gary is having double vision and a CT scan reveals an enlargement of the pituitary gland. What is the medical term for a 'gland tumor'?

9.44 Adenoma

The **thymus** (**thigh**-mus) > typically forgotten endocrine gland because until the last half-century science thought it was an organ of infancy only (Figure 9.19). It is located in the superior mediastinum and is largest during infancy and slowly starts to atrophy during adulthood. It slows down but does not stop.

9.45

Thym/o > thymus

–cyte > cell

–genic > condition of beginning, development

Aplasia > no development

Atrophy > wasting of tissues (no development)

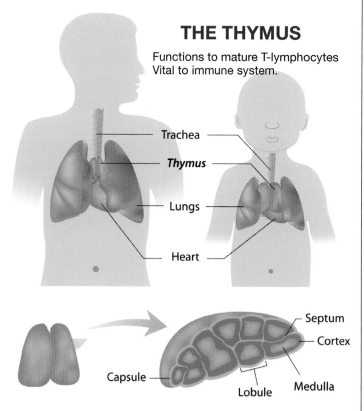

THE THYMUS

Functions to mature T-lymphocytes Vital to immune system.

Trachea

Thymus

Lungs

Heart

Septum

Cortex

Capsule

Lobule

Medulla

Figure 9.19

- Thymosin (**thigh**-moe-zin) > hormone produced by the thymus to mature T-lymphocytes.

- Disease of the thymus will cause some level of immune deficiency.
  - **DeGeorge syndrome** (eponym) is a genetic disorder causing aplasia (a-**play**-ze-ya) of the thymus. It is also associated with other endocrine deficiencies.

The pancreas (**pan**-kree-as) > both an exocrine and endocrine organ vital to the digestion and use of all the major nutrients: carbohydrates, proteins, and fats (lipids) (Figure 9.20).

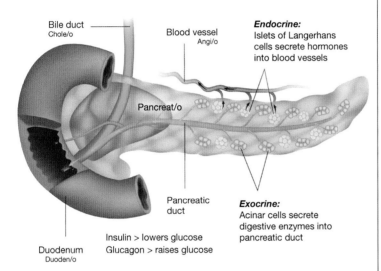

Bile duct
Chole/o

Blood vessel
Angi/o

Endocrine:
Islets of Langerhans
cells secrete hormones
into blood vessels

Pancreat/o

Pancreatic
duct

Exocrine:
Acinar cells secrete
digestive enzymes into
pancreatic duct

Duodenum
Duoden/o

Insulin > lowers glucose
Glucagon > raises glucose

Figure 9.20

There are several word roots related to the pancreas and its functions:

- **Pancreat/o** > pancreas. Lies deep to the stomach in the LUQ.

- **Gluc/o** or **Glyc/o** or **Glycos**/o > glucose > the functional 'sugar' which fuels all cell activity.
  - **Gluc**agon (glue-**ka**-gone) > one of the endocrine hormones secreted by the pancreas. It increases the level of glucose in the blood to maintain homeostasis when food is not available.
  - **Gluc**oneogenesis (glue-**ko**-knee-oh-**jen**-eh-sis) > metabolic process when the body converts lipids or proteins to glucose for cell use via the liver.

9.46
Did You Know?

Pancreas has a plural term:

Pancreata > Greek meaning 'all flesh' or 'sweet bread'

Early scientists thought the pancreas was essentially a large packing-peanut for the stomach due to its rubbery consistency, until the 1850s.

Other 'glucose' terms**:

Glycogenesis > converting stores to active glucose

Glycolysis > breaking down glucose

Glycosidase > an enzyme breaks up carbohydrates

- **Insulin/o** > insulin (in-**sue**-lin) > one of the endocrine hormones secreted by the pancreas. It reduces the level of glucose in the blood. Insulin is required to help circulating glucose into the cells. Glucose is required as the energy (the fuel) to run all cell activity; it will be converted to **ATP**, adenosine triphosphate.

  - **Insulinoma** (in-**sue**-lin-**oh**-ma) > insulin tumor.

  - **Insulinemia** (in-**sue**-li-**knee**-me-a) > excessive insulin in circulating blood.

There are four other pancreatic endocrine hormones:

- **Somatostatin** (**sew**-mah-toe-**stat**-in) > seems to be a bioregulator specific to the pancreas. It is connected with the nutrient absorption process for carbohydrates, proteins, and lipids.

- **Gastrin** (**gas**-trine) > pancreatic gastrin may help control the production of the glucagon.

- **Grehlin** (**greh**-lin) > this poorly understood hormone seems to stimulate growth hormones in children, controls appetite, and may play a role in insulin use by the body.

- **Pancreatic polypeptide** is a paracrine (a local hormone) responding to hypoglycemia. In the presence of a protein-rich meal it signals 'satisfaction' or 'fullness'.

9.47
These hormones are found in other areas of the body, thus the designation of 'pancreatic gastrin' or 'pancreatic grehlin'. While these appear to be paracrines localized to the pancreas, the effects are felt in several systems.

- **Diabetes mellitus** (die-ah-**bee**-tis **mel**-li-tus) (**DM**) > dysfunction of carbohydrate metabolism. It is not a single disease, it has several manifestations.

  - **Type I** is due to an absolute lack of insulin production from the pancreas, known as insulin-dependent DM (**IDDM**). It is thought to be an autoimmune disease associated with environmental and genetic factors.

  - **Type II** is the so-called **NIDDM**, non-insulin-dependent diabetes mellitus. The name can be misleading because some Type II patients do need insulin replacement. There is some insulin production as seen in Figure 9.21, or it might be normal but resistance is evident – glucose is not getting into the cells and there is too much in the bloodstream.

  - **Gestational** (jes-**tay**-shun-al) > **GDM** is glucose intolerance with decreased insulin production in pregnant women. This is seen with obese mothers or a mother with a family history of DM.

9.48
Diabetes > Greek for 'through a siphon' due to the polyuria associated with diabetes. The 'mellitus' means honey-sweet.

Diabetes insipidus does not involve insulin but the inadequate secretion of vasopressin (**ADH**) by the pituitary gland, increasing urine production.

DKA > diabetic ketoacidosis

Figure 9.21

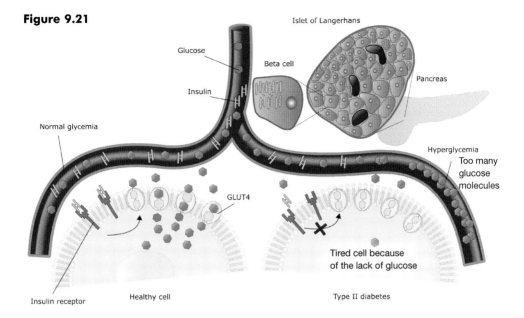

- Drug-induced, infection (pancreatitis), cancers, and other endocrine abnormalities may trigger a DM.
- Symptoms associated with DM include several medical terms:
  - **Polyuria** (**pol**-ee-**yur**-ee-ah) > excessive urination; this includes **nocturia** (nok-**tur**-ee-ah) > urinating at night.
  - **Polydipsia** (**pol**-ee-**dip**-see-ah) > excessive thirst, drinking.
  - **Polyphagia** (**pol**-ee-**fay**-jee-ah) > excessive eating, hunger.
  - **Fatigue** (fa-**teeg**) > the sensation of being tired, less capacity to do normal activities or weariness.
  - **Cachexia** (ka-**kek**-see-ah) > weight loss and wasting due to chronic illness. Despite eating more (polyphagia) with no insulin to push the glucose into the cells for use, weight and energy are lost.
- The complications of uncontrolled diabetes include:
  - **Neuropathy** (**nur**-oh-**nop**-ah-thee) > nerve disease, loss of peripheral nerves due to capillary bed loss leading to paresthesias (**pair**-es-**thee**-zee-ahs) > loss of feeling leads to the ulcer seen in Figure 9.22.
  - **Retinopathy** (**ret**-i-**nop**-ah-thee) > retinal disease, loss of vision due to capillary bed loss and hemorrhage.
  - **Nephropathy** (neh-**frop**-ah-thee) > renal disease, loss of renal function due to capillary bed loss.
  - **Vascular disease** > loss of capillary beds can eventually lead to gangrene and the need for limb amputation.

Associated laboratory

Gl > glucose

FBG > fasting blood glucose

An FBG of 126 mg/dl is diagnostic of diabetes

GTT or **OGTT** > oral glucose tolerance test

HgbA₁C > glycosylated hemoglobin gives a measure of overall glucose utilization over a three-month period.

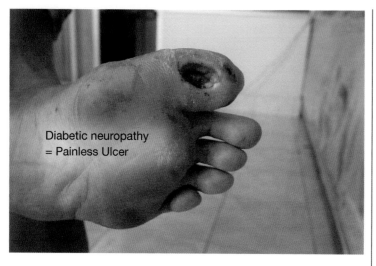

Diabetic neuropathy
= Painless Ulcer

Figure 9.22

- **Pancreatic cancer** > currently the 4th leading cause of death in the United States. Because of the lack of an organ capsule, its deep location (retroperitoneal) and absence of early symptoms, death occurs within 12 months for nearly 95% of patients after discovery. Most are adenocarcinoma (from the exocrine side of the pancreas). Tobacco use is a risk factor.

- **Pancreatitis** (**pan**-kree-ah-**tie**-tis) > inflammation of the pancreas occurs from a variety of causes (Figure 9.23).
    - Obstruction of the bile or pancreatic ducts by stones > choleliths (bile stones)
    - Alcoholism
    - Trauma, burns, and severe stress reaction

9.49

Chole/o > bile

Nephr/o > kidney

Neur/o > nerves

Retin/o > retina of the eyes

Capill/o > vascular bed

Hem/o > blood

-itis > inflammation

-ectomy > removal

-algia > pain

-dynia > pain

-graphy > process of recording

-lithiasis > condition of infestation (stones)

PANCREATITIS

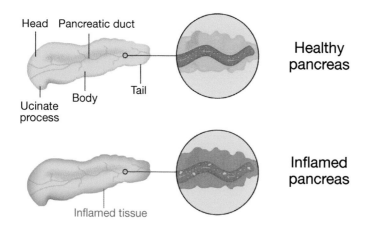

Head   Pancreatic duct

Ucinate process

Body   Tail

Healthy pancreas

Inflamed tissue

Inflamed pancreas

Figure 9.23

✓ This endocrine gland is found in the mediastinum. What is the gland and where is the mediastinum?

9.50 Thymus; Middle of the chest (thorax)

✓ Build the word meaning 'surgical removal of the pancreas'.

9.51 Pancreat-ectomy

✓ What is the initial set for an oral glucose tolerance test?

9.52 OGTT

Word building

Using the word roots with the linking vowel to build as many valid terms with the suffixes given. Please define each term.

Pancreat/o Thym/o Parathyr/o
(use a prefix as desired)

–itis –megaly –oma –ectomy –dynia –graph

9.53
The instructor has the list!

The adrenal (ad-**ree**-nul) **gland** is a mighty, yet tiny, endocrine gland sitting atop the kidneys (renal). If the pituitary gland is the master-gland, these are the back-up masters (Figure 9.24).

9.54

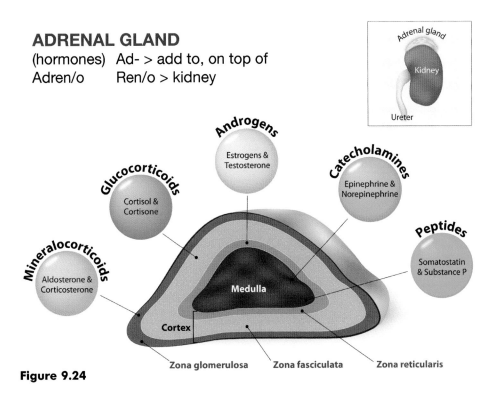

ADRENAL GLAND
(hormones)   Ad- > add to, on top of
Adren/o   Ren/o > kidney

Adrenal gland
Kidney
Ureter

Androgens
Estrogens & Testosterone

Catecholamines
Epinephrine & Norepinephrine

Glucocorticoids
Cortisol & Cortisone

Peptides
Somatostatin & Substance P

Mineralocorticoids
Aldosterone & Corticosterone

Medulla

Cortex

Zona glomerulosa   Zona fasciculata   Zona reticularis

Figure 9.24

- The **cortex** of the adrenal gland makes up 80% of its mass and it receives the **ACTH** from the pituitary gland. It has three identifiable cell types and produces several hormones:

  - **Cortisol** (**kor**-ti-sol) > long-term stress hormone, it tends to reduce the inflammatory and immune responses. It modifies the reaction to injury to maintain homeostasis.

  - **Aldosterone** (al-**doss**-tur-own) > potent mineralocorticoid which promotes retention of sodium at cellular level. Where salt is, water follows; aldosterone works with the **ACTH** of the pituitary to protect the water stores during stressful times.

  - **Androgens** (an-**drow**-jens) > Testosterone and estrogens > while minimal from this location. Are in a feedback loop with ACTH, not the gonads. Their exact actions are not well understood.

- The **medulla** (meh-**due**-lah) of the adrenal gland is the middle core producing the immediate fight-or-flight hormones. These are the hormones of action for the sympathetic nervous system.

  - **Epinephrine** (ep-ee-**nef**-rin) > stronger of the two, it will last seconds to minutes depending on the target cells. Like all catecholamines (**kat**-ee-**kol**-ah-meanz) it increases brain blood flow via increased heart rate and blood pressure, bronchodilatation to increase oxygen intake during respirations, and enhanced muscle response.

  - **Norepinephrine** (nor-**ep**-ee-**nef**-rin) > seems to be involved with conditions which tend to develop slowly such as hypoxia or pressure injury.

Kitchen lab

 All of us have been startled or scared silly. This sensation, from waking suddenly to smashing a finger in the door, engaged your fight-or-flight response.

Think back to one of these episodes – describe the physical changes: did you feel your pulse in the neck, breathing increased, assume a protective posture? How long did it take to calm down?

Tell your instructor about your experience of the catecholamines.

Endocrine functions are checked in three blood tests:

RIA > Radio-immunoassay

ELISA > Enzyme-linked immuno-sorbent assay

Bioassay > uses graded doses of hormone

The gonads (go-**nadz**) are responsible for the species survival: for the production of a new human. The term is inclusive of both sets of endocrine glands, male and female.

- Gonad/o > seed > both gonad sets are stimulated by the pituitary **FSH** and **LH**.
  - Gonadotropin (go-**nad**-oh-**trow**-pin) > utilized for any hormone effecting or reacting with the testicles or ovaries.
- Testicul/o or test/i > the testicles (**tes**-ti-kuls) are found in the scrotal sac of men > Latin, associated with the male anatomy.
  - Orchid/o or Orchi/o > Greek for testicles. It is used to express testicular disease or injury.
  - **Testosterone** (tes-**tos**-tur-ohn) > hormone triggers the secondary sexual features at puberty in the nervous system, bone, muscles, skin and hair, and the penis.
- Ovari/o or Oophor/o > ovaries are found in the pelvic cavity in women in close proximity to the uterus (Figure 9.25).
  - **Estrogen** (**es**-trow-jen) > hormone triggers the secondary sexual features at puberty (**pew**-bur-tea) and helps regulate the menstrual cycle.
  - **Progesterone** (pro-**jes**-tur-ohn) > hormone is released by the ovary after an ovum (**oh**-vum), the egg, is released. It prepares the uterus to accept a zygote (**zeye**-goat), the fertilized egg.

9.55
More on the many terms of the reproductive system is found in Unit 15.

O/o > egg or seed

Oophor/o > ovary

'phor' is to carry; the ovary carries the eggs. Oophor/o is used to describe ovarian injury or disease.

Andr/o > man

Gyn/o or Gynec/o > woman

Trop/o > to turn, reaction, change

Gest/o > to carry, to bear

Progesterone means a hormone which 'prepares to carry'

Uter/o > uterus

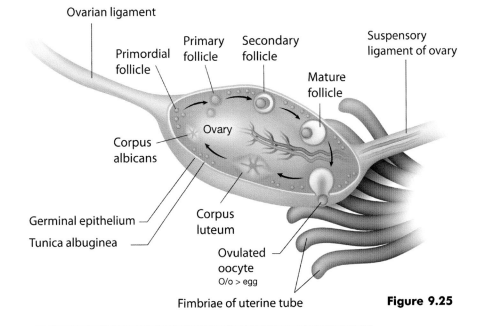

Figure 9.25

Ovarian ligament
Primordial follicle
Primary follicle
Secondary follicle
Mature follicle
Suspensory ligament of ovary
Ovary
Corpus albicans
Germinal epithelium
Tunica albuginea
Corpus luteum
Ovulated oocyte
O/o > egg
Fimbriae of uterine tube

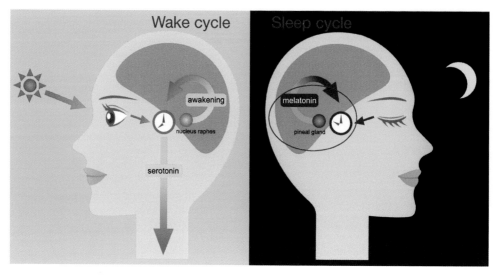

Figure 9.26

The pineal (**pie**-kneel) **gland** > another brain endocrine gland (Figure 9.26). The name is from its shape, a tiny, flattened pinecone. It is found between the two superior colliculi (**ko**-lic-Q-lie) of the mid-brain. It produces the hormone, **melatonin** (mel-ah-**tone**-in), associated with maintaining the sleep cycle.

Paracrines > 'near secretions' are found throughout the body; here are a few:

- **Erythropoietin** (eh-**rith**-row-**poe**-eh-tin) **(EPO)** > kidneys secrete this in response to the need for more RBC. It stimulates the bones to produce blood cells.

- **Somatostatin** > produced by a variety of tissues (GI, nervous, and muscles), it tends to inhibit the effects of other hormones.

- **Gastrin** > stomach hormone triggers the release of HCl and pepsin and stimulates the reabsorption of bile and other elements in the GI tract.

- **Grehlin** > produced in the GI tract, pancreas, and possibly the brain, it promotes hunger and secretion of growth hormone.

- **Prostaglandin** > found in almost all cells; associated with several inflammatory and repair reactions.

9.56
While a warm glass of milk at bedtime is reported to help with sleep, it has only trace amounts of melatonin and tryptophan.

9.57
Paracrines are called 'localized' but in reality they affect tissues at a distance, too, like their 'gland'-specific tissues. Some are found in almost all tissue areas as part of the inflammatory reaction. All are vital to homeostasis.

- **Leukotrienes** > found in many cells, these modify inflammation and the allergic response.

- **Atrial natriuretic factor (ANF)** > heart secretes this; affects blood vessels, kidneys, and adrenal glands.

- **B-type natriuretic peptide (BNP)** > elevated in the presence of heart failure.

- **40+ Neurotransmitters** are the chemical triggers of the nervous system: dopamine, acetylcholine, nitric oxide, serotonin, GABA, melatonin, and more.

UNIT SUMMARY

1   The immune system is a broad-ranging defense scheme the body employs to protect and maintain homeostasis: From mechanical barriers such as the skin, to the ability to build antibodies to protect the body from antigens. An antigen (against life) includes foreign bodies such as bacteria, viruses, fungi, and parasites.

2   There are three lines of defense including the mechanical and chemical responses of the skin and gastrointestinal systems to keep pathogens out. When injury or illness occurs inflammation begins by recognizing the danger, responding, and then cleaning up the mess.

3   Immunoglobulins are antibodies; there are five protein types: IgA, IgD, IgE, IgG, and IgM. These protein-based antibodies are involved with any number of inflammatory reactions including environmental allergies, gluten intolerance, hemolysis, and cell-mediated reactions.

4   The bone marrow is the source of all blood cell production including the white blood cells, the leukocytes. From these come the cell-mediated lymphocytes fighting infection. The T-lymphocytes take on invaders one-on-one and the B-lymphocytes target antigens, create millions of antibodies, and remember the enemy in the future.

5   Autoimmune diseases occur when the body's protective mechanism of the cellularly active lymphocytes actually turns on healthy tissues. Many endocrine, gastrointestinal, and neuromuscular conditions are related to this disruption of immunity.

6   Tracking the ICD codes of infectious disease, inflammatory reactions, and autoimmune disease allows science, public health, and medicine to develop ways to maintain homeostasis. Antibiotics, immunotherapies, genetic therapies, and anti-inflammatory medications relieve or control many of these conditions.

7   The endocrine system is a collection of very small glands impacting all the functions of the entire body via hormones. Hormones are chemical messengers sent from one location which impact areas quite distant.

8   The pituitary gland is the master gland found deep in the skull surrounded by the optic chiasm. The anterior pituitary will provide seven hormone triggers: GH, FSH, LH, TSH, MSH, PRL, and ACTH. The posterior pituitary interacts directly with the hypothalamus producing ADH and oxytocin.

9   The nine pituitary hormones affect the next endocrine gland or specific tissues. The pituitary is the master gland, coordinating with all the endocrine organs, hypothalamus, and the entire nervous system.

10 The thyroid, parathyroid, adrenal, pancreas, and gonads all produce specific hormones affecting everything including metabolism, stress reactions, nutrient use, and reproduction of the species.

UNIT WORD PARTS

Word roots with linking vowel		
Aden/o > gland	Andr/o > man, male	Bacteri/o > bacteria
Cortic/o > outer layer	Crin/o > to secrete	Cyt/o or Cellul/o > cells
Derm/o or Dermat/o > skin	Gen/o > beginning, genesis	Globul/o > protein
Gluc/o; Glyc/o; Glycos/o > glucose, sugar	Gyn/o; Gynec/o or Estr/o> woman, female	Hem/o or Hemat/o > blood
Immun/o > protective	Leuk/o > white	Path/o > disease
Phag/o > to eat	Pin/o > to drink	Pituitar/o > pituitary
Py/o > pus	Pyr/o > heat, fever	Ren/o or Nephr/o > kidney
Splen/o > spleen	Thalam/o > thalamus	Thym/o > thymus
Thyr/o or Thyroid/o > thyroid	Tox/o > poison	Vir/o > virus

Prefixes: attached to the front of the word root to change meaning		
A-; An- > no, not, absent	Ad- > toward, add to	Allo- > other, differing
Ana- > up, toward, apart	Auto- > self, of self	Dia- > through
Endo- > within, inside	Eu- > good, normal	Exo- > outside, outer
Hyper- > more, increased, elevated	Hypo- > less, decreased, below	Macro- > large, larger
Neo- > new, recent	Pan- > all, entire	Para- > near, departure from normal
Peri- > around, about, near	Poly-> many, plural	Tri- > Three

Suffixes change the meaning of the word, linking vowel is usually 'o' with consonants		
-algia, -dynia > pain	-cyte > cell	-ectomy > surgical removal
-emia > condition in blood	-gram > a record	-graphy > process of recording
-ism > collection of symptoms	-itis > inflammation	-lithiasis > infestation of stones
-logy > study of	-megaly > enlargement	-oma > tumor
-osis > abnormal condition	-pathy > disease of	-tropin > turning toward, having affinity

Acronyms, abbreviations, and initial sets		
ACTH > adreno-corticotropin hormone	AIDS > autoimmune deficiency syndrome	ANA > antinuclear factor
ANF > atrial natriuretic factor	APC > antigen-presenting cells	ASO > antistreptolysin O
ATP > adenosine 5′ triphosphate	B-cells > B-lymphocyte	CAM > cellular adhesive molecules
CBC > complete blood cell count	CMV > cytomegalovirus	C&S > culture and sensitivity
DM > diabetes mellitus	DMARD > disease-modifying antirheumatic drug	ELISA > enzyme-linked immunosorbent assay
EPO > erythropoietin	FBG > fasting blood glucose	FBS > fasting blood sugar
FNA > fine needle aspirate (a biopsy)	FSH > follicle-stimulating hormone	GDM > gestational diabetes mellitus

GH > growth hormone	GI > glucose	HgbA1C > glycosylated hemoglobin
HIV > human immuno-deficiency virus	IDDM > insulin-dependent diabetes mellitus	LFS > liver function studies
LH > luteinizing hormone	MG > myesthesia gravis	MS > multiple sclerosis
MSH > melanocyte-stimulating hormone	NIDDM > non-insulin-dependent diabetes mellitus	OGTT or GTT > oral glucose tolerance test
PAMP > pathogen-associated molecular pattern	PMN > polymorphonuclear neutrophil	PRL > prolactin
PRR > pattern recognition receptor	PTH > parathyroid hormone	RA > rheumatoid arthritis
RF > rheumatoid fever or rheumatoid factor (lab)	RIA > radio-immunoassay	SLE > systemic lupus erythematosus
TLR > Toll-like receptor	TSH > thyroid-stimulating hormone	T-cell > T-lymphocyte
UC > ulcerative colitis	UV > ultraviolet	

UNIT WORKSHEETS

Building terms: Use the proper prefix/word root/linking vowel/suffix as appropriate.

   Example: to cut into the stomach > gastr/o/tomy

a) Inflammation of the pancreas > _____

b) Black cells > _____

c) The study of women > _____

d) An abnormal condition of white cells (WBCs) > _____

e) A specialist who studies disease > _____

f) Surgical removal of the thymus > _____

g) Protective proteins > _____

h) Loss of feeling > _____

Know your initial sets/acronyms! For the initial set or acronym given, spell it out correctly.

a) LH   _____

b) ANA   _____

c) CBC   _____

d) HgbA1C   _____

e) RIA   _____

f) TSH   _____

g) ACTH   _____

h) IDDM   _____

Best choice: Pick the most appropriate answer.

1 Immunoglobulin _____ is the only one crossing the placenta to the fetus.

    a) IgA

    b) IgD

    c) IgG

    d) IgM

2 The optic chiasm (cranial nerve II crossing) will be effected by this endocrine tumor.

    a) Thymoma

    b) Sarcoma

    c) Glioblastoma

    d) Pituitary adenoma

3 Which of the following provides first-level immune protection?

    a) Skin

    b) T-lymphocytes

    c) Complement proteins

    d) Inflammation

4 These T-cells do their job by punching holes in the pathogen and disabling the infected cell.

    a) Suppressor

    b) Memory

    c) Helper

    d) Killer

5 Endocrine gland manages our sleep with melatonin.

   a) Pancreas

   b) Pituitary

   c) Thyroid

   d) Pineal

6 Insulin and glucagon are part of the _____ functions of the pancreas.

   a) Exocrine

   b) Endocrine

   c) Paracrine

   d) Epicrine

Name the condition or term! Based on the description and/or function.

a) Associated with myalgias, osteoporosis, polyuria, and nephrolithiasis _____

b) Weight loss, polyuria, polydipsia, capillary loss, and fatigue _____

c) Inflammation of the thyroid _____

d) Presence of heat, pain, redness, and swelling _____

e) Hypermetabolic state with weight loss, tremors, and exophthalmos _____

f) Caused by the toxin of *Clostridium botulinum*, known as 'lockjaw' _____

g) Intense itchiness _____

h) Thyromegaly associated with iodine-insufficiency _____

Multiple correct: Select ALL the correct answers to the question or statement given.

1 Mark all the correct hormones produced by the anterior pituitary?

   a) Growth hormone   d) Thyroid-stimulating hormone

   b) Testosterone   e) Luteinizing hormone

   c) Melatonin   f) Prostaglandin

2 Which of the following hormones is associated with the adrenal cortex?

   a) Epinephrine   d) Androgens

   b) Thyroxine   e) Calcitonin

   c) Aldosterone   f) Cortisol

3 Which of the following are 'bacterial' pathogens known to cause significant illness or death?

   a) Diphtheria   d) Pertussis

   b) HIV   e) Measles

   c) Tetanus   f) Mumps

Spelling challenge! Circle the correct spelling based on the definition given.

1 'Immediate, severe reaction to an antigen'

Annaphilaxis   Anephylaxis   Anaphylaxis   Anephylexis

2 'Pertaining to the outer layer of the adrenal gland'

Adrenocortical   Adenocartical   Adrencortical   Adrinocortikal

3 'Making new sugars'

Glyconewgenesis   Gluconeogenesis   Glycosineogenesis   Gluconeogenisis

---

Define the term: Spelling *does* count in your definition too!

1 Urticaria > _____

2 Myxedema > _____

3 Pyrexia > _____

4 Prostaglandin > _____

5 Antibody > _____

6 Polydipsia > _____

7 Toxigenic > _____

8 Retinopathy > _____

Find it! Using the words in the table – match the definition given or answer the statement. Some may not be used. It is recommended you know all the choices.

pyosis	leukocytosis	phagocytes	viremia	monocyte
bacteriology	pathophysiology	autoimmune	androgens	exocrine
thymoma	paracrine	glycosuria	orchiectomy	aldosterone
allograph	adenomegaly	euthyroid	endocrine	melatonin

1 _____   Good thyroid

2 _____   Surgical removal of the testicle

3 _____   The study of bacteria

4 _____   Virus in the bloodstream

5 _____   Sugar in the urine

6 _____   Outside secretion

7 _____   Tumor of the thymus

8 _____   The study of disease function

9 _____   Abnormal condition of pus

10 _____   Eating cell

Matching: Some will not be used.

	Letter	Defined as
Pancreatitis		a) cell and neurotransmitter associated with inflammation
Pituitary adenoma		b) largest leukocytes, a phagocyte
Myxedema		c) condition of fever
Hemoglobulin		d) severe pain because it has no capsule when inflamed
Pyrexia		e) waxy, thick edema, non-pitting
Gluconeogenesis		f) *Clostridium botulinum* will cause 'lockjaw'
Tetanus		g) deep bruising associated with inflammation
Histamine		h) tumor of the pituitary gland
		i) literally, 'blood protein'
		j) the liver can make 'new sugar'

An essay: Explain the function of 'inflammation' and how medications can modify this protective mechanism.

Note challenge: SOAP note from the ER. You may need to look up a few terms. Answer the questions which follow. Recall this is a limited SOAP note, it is not to be used for patient encounters.

S. 26 y/o male is found in his home in a semicomatose state. His roommate states he has been a little confused for the last two days. He has had polyuria and polydipsia for over a week. He stopped doing his usual workout 2 weeks ago but is losing weight too. He has had a bad cold for the last week. He has an old prescription for Sulfonylurea at the back of the medicine cabinet. He is a smoker.

O. 26 y/o male who responds to deep pain stimuli only. Eyes are PERRLA and funduscopic exam reveals some recent retinal hemorrhages bilaterally. Thyroid without lesions or enlargement. Lungs: rales in the RLL. Heart: 96 rate, faint, weak. Abdomen: soft, nontender, no masses effect, no hepatosplenomegaly. CVAs nontender. Lower legs with +1/5 pitting edema. Pulses equal. Blood Gl is 417 mg/dl. Positive for ketonuria. WBC is elevated at 24,100 microliter. HgbA1C is 15.6%. CXR with infiltrate in RLL.

A. DKA
   NIDDM uncontrolled
   Diabetic retinopathy
   RLL Pneumonia
   Tobacco abuse

Questions:

1 Translate all the acronyms and give meaning to the words which are underlined in the note.

2 What does HgbA1C stand for? Does level indicate lack of medication use? Why?

3 Using the *DRAFT ICD* codes below, code the assessment list. Do not use for patient encounters.

Alphabetic index
Diabetes, diabetic (mellitus, sugar) E11.9
Circulation complication NEC E11.59
Kidney complication NEC E11.29
Retinopathy E11.319
Due to underlying condition E08.9
Hypoglycemia E08.649
Ketoacidosis E08.10
Specific type NEC E13.9
Type 1 E10.9
Type 2 E11.9

Unit 10

Blood and lymphatics

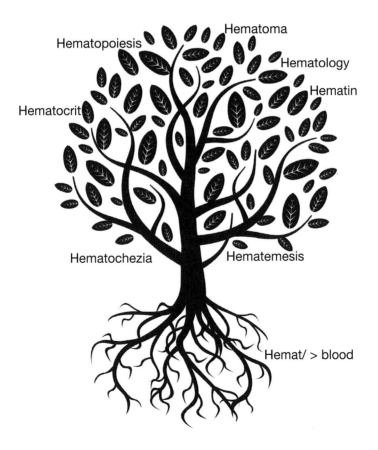

Hematopoiesis

Hematoma

Hematology

Hematin

Hematocrit

Hematochezia

Hematemesis

Hemat/ > blood

TARGETED LEARNING

1   Recognize word parts and assemble medical terms related to the blood and lymphatics.

2   Correctly construct, define, pronounce, and spell medical terms.

3   Relate blood and lymphatic illness and injury with appropriate pharmacotherapeutics and other therapeutic options.

4   Explore the many hematological laboratory assessments and how they are coded in **cpt** and **HCPCS**.

KEY WORD PARTS

Word roots with linking vowel	Suffixes	Abbreviations
Angi/o; Vas/o; Vascul/o > vessels	-blast	ANA
Arteri/o > artery	-cyte	BUN
Cyt/o > cell	-ectomy	CBC
Eosin/o > pink, orange	-emia	Chem 6 or BMP
Erythr/o or Eryth- > red	-gen	CMP
Hem/o or Hemat/o > blood	-lytic, -lysis	ESR or sed rate
Leuk/o > white	-penia	HCG
Mon/o > one, single	-phage	Hct
Myel/o > bone marrow or spinal cord	-philia	Hgb
Nucle/o or Kary/o > nucleus, center	-plastic, -plasia	MCH
Phleb/o or Ven/o > vein	-poiesis	MCHC
Ser/o > serum, fluid	-oma	MCV
Splen/o > spleen	-osis	PCR
Thromb/o or Coagul/o > clot, solid	-rrhexis	PMN
Thym/o > thymus	-stasis	PT and PTT

LIFE BLOOD

Serving size: 5.5 liters per adult (160 ounces)
1 ml = 5 million erythrocytes, 10,000 leukocytes, 3,000 platelets

Ingredients: Water, red blood cells (erythrocytes), white blood cells (leukocytes), platelets (thrombocytes), albumin, gamma globulin, anti-hemophilic factor, clotting factors, sodium, potassium, magnesium, calcium, phosphorus, iron, oxygen, hydrogen, nitrogen, carbon, glucose, lipids, hormones, and vitamins with trace minerals such as iodine, zinc, manganese, copper, fluoride, chromium, and selenium.

Life blood circulates in the closed system of a pump and thousands of miles of pipes. The pump is the heart and the pipes the arteries and veins down to the tiniest capillary level. For millennia humans have understood the importance of blood to life, but it is only in the last three centuries that science began to define all the components of the liquid termed 'blood'. The first human to human transfusion was reportedly in 1818, and in the 1940s science started to define how blood cells are formed and their many functions. Today, a single liter of donated blood can be used to save several patients by using its many individual components. Donating blood is the gift which keeps on giving.

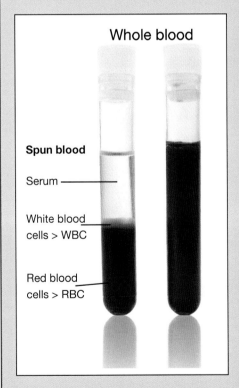

Whole blood

Spun blood

Serum

White blood
cells > WBC

Red blood
cells > RBC

Figure 10.2

HEMATOLOGY AND ERYTHROCYTES

The study of blood, hematology (he-mah-**tohl**-oh-jee) begins in an unlikely source, the bones. Deep in the core of the long bones in particular, is the red bone marrow; this is the site of hematopoiesis (he-mah-toe-poy-**ee**-sis) – blood production. From the bone marrow, all the cells begin as hemopoietic stem cells (Figure 10.3).

- **Hem/o; Hemat/o;** and **Heme-** > blood, specifically whole blood with all its dissolved elements and solid cells.

  - -poiesis > to produce, to form.

  - -plastic > pertaining to development or formation.

  - -lysis > destruction, dissolution, break apart.

  - -oma > tumor, a **hematoma** is specifically a collection of blood trapped, creating a mass effect.

  - -stasis > to stop or control, **hemostasis** is to stop bleeding.

- **Myel/o** > bone marrow (and spinal cord).

Bone marrow

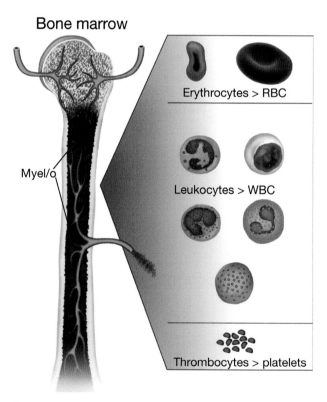

Erythrocytes > RBC

Leukocytes > WBC

Thrombocytes > platelets

Figure 10.3

10.1

LIKE ALERT!

To the early Greek anatomist (pre-microscope) the tissues of the bone marrow and the spinal cord resembled each other – thus both were given the term: myel/o. Myel/o means two different areas of the body **and** sounds similar to my/o > muscle and myl/o > molar tooth. Make sure you are using each in the correct context.

- –proliferative > unusual and excessive production of the bone marrow's initial stem cells.
- –genesis > beginning of, development.
- –suppression > unusual reduction in bone marrow cell production.

Erythrocytes (eh-**rith**-row-sites) > RBC, red blood cells are the only cell type in the body without a nucleus when mature. It is forced out by the heme, the protein built of the iron (**Fe**) carrying millions of oxygen (**O**) molecules each to the billions of body cells.

- Erythr/o > red, specifically, red blood cells; the bone marrow will produce 200+ trillion new RBCs daily in healthy adults. There are several laboratory values used to define RBC health.
  - **Hemoglobin** (**Hgb, Hb**) (**he**-moe-**glow**-bin) > Laboratory: the red respiratory protein within the RBCs. About 4% heme (iron) and 96% globin (protein) (Figure 10.4).

HUMAN HEMOGLOBIN

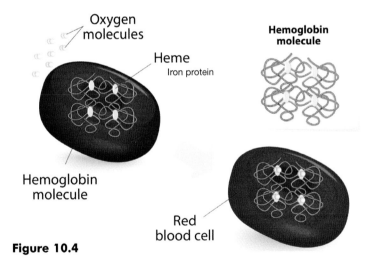

Figure 10.4

- **Hematocrit (Hct)** (**he**-mat-**oh**-krit) > percentage of the volume of the blood taken up by the whole cells. The majority, 96% are erythrocytes. An increased **Hct** may indicate **polycythemia** (**pol**-ee-sigh-**thee**-me-ah) > too many red blood cells.
- **Reticulocytes** (re-**tik**-U-low-site) > actual number or percentage of young erythrocytes. Reticul/o > Latin for small net. An elevated retic count indicates stress to make more RBC such as a sudden blood loss. Abbreviation: retics

- **MCV** > mean corpuscular (kor-**pus**-q-lar) volume refers to the size of the RBC 'body (corpus)'.
- Smaller than normal is called **microcytic**; larger than normal is called **macrocytic**.
- **MCH** > mean corpuscular hemoglobin denotes the actual content of each erythrocyte.
- **MCHC** > mean corpuscular hemoglobin concentration, the average concentration in a given volume of packed RBCs. Packed red blood cells (**PRBC**) are administered to improve vascular volume and oxygen carrying capacity to those with blood loss.
- **Ferritin** (**fair**-i-tin) > indirect measure of stored iron via the RBCs, it is the complex protein containing about 23% iron.
- **TIBC** > total iron binding capacity, measures the transferrin (trans-**fair**-in). Transferrin is the glycoprotein part of heme; it permits the iron and oxygen (oxyhemoglobin) to function together.

LIKE ALERT!

Eryth- > (no extra 'r') also means red and redness. It is used to describe skin and other lesions > erythema

 Construct a word meaning 'beginnings of bone marrow'.

 What does the initial set MCHC stand for?

 The scientist who studies blood is properly called a
_____ .

10.3 Myelogenic or myelopoiesis

10.4 Mean corpuscular hemoglobin concentration

10.5 hematologist

Word building

 *Using the word roots **with the linking vowel to build as many valid terms with the suffixes given.** Please define each term.*

Hem/o or Hemat/o Erythr/o Myel/o

–logy –osis –cyte –lysis –genesis –pathy

10.6
The instructor has the list!

Erythrocyte abnormalities are listed as an anemia (a-**knee**-me-a) > relative lack of blood due to injury, diet, or illness. Literally, without (an-) blood (-emia) as seen in Figure 10.5.

- **Iron-deficiency anemia** > seen worldwide, low serum iron due to poor diet and/or recurrent bleeding such as heavy menses in women or slow GI bleeding. It is defined by a hypochromic (**hi**-poe-**krow**-mic) > low color and microcytic RBC, and an elevated **TIBC**. Correcting the deficiency or ending the chronic bleeding treats this condition.

- **Pernicious** (purr-**nish**-us) **anemia** > due to inadequate intake or absorption of vitamin B$_{12}$. There are many causes including some medication side effects, poor diet, alcohol abuse, and genetics. It is distinguished by macrocytic erythrocytes. Vitamin B$_{12}$ may be increased by diet, injection, nasal spray, or sublingual pathways.

- **Aplastic** (a-**plaz**-tik) **anemia** > markedly decreased production of all cells from the bone marrow or **pancytopenia**. They are fragile and break easily. Synonym: hemolytic anemia. Exposure to toxic chemicals, radiation, and chemotherapies may cause the bone marrow to stop making cells. Autoimmune disease and some viruses have been implicated as well.

- **Hereditary** or **congenital** anemias > abnormal shape of the erythrocytes leading to excessive RBC destruction or hemolysis.
  - **Sickle (sik-el) cell** > abnormality of hemoglobin S (protein) makes the cells resemble a 'C' or sickle.
  - **Thalassemia** (**thal**-ah-**see**-me-ah) > genetic condition, thalassemia major is associated with severe anemia, weakness, and splenomegaly. Thalassemia minor is typified by a lower **Hgb** and microcytic anemia.

10.7

A-, an- > no, none, without, absent

Micro- > small, smallest

Macro- > large, larger

Hypo- > less, lower, decreased, low

Hyper- > more, high, increased, above

Pan- > all, everything

Poly- > many

Pernicious > Latin for destructive, dangerous, or harmful. The term is used for conditions which develop slowly, chronically, or sneak up on the individual.

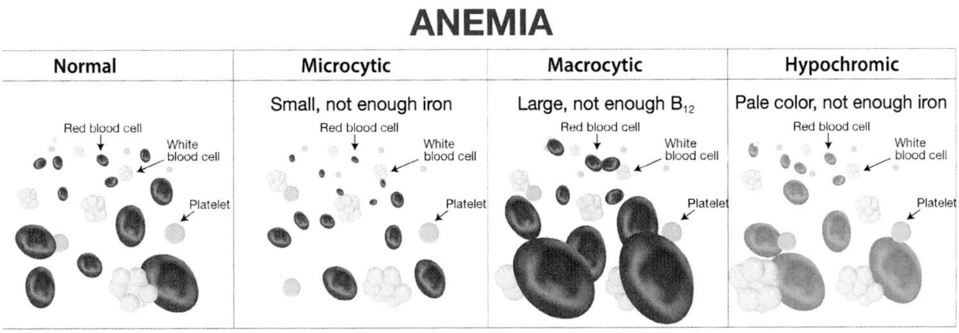

ANEMIA

Normal	Microcytic	Macrocytic	Hypochromic
	Small, not enough iron	Large, not enough B$_{12}$	Pale color, not enough iron

Figure 10.5

COLORS OF INJURY

A bruise by any other name! The skin gets some of its color and tones from the erythrocytes casting their red or pink hues. When the skin is damaged by leaking or a contusion (kon-**two**-zun), blood vessels are broken releasing blood under the skin (subdermal). All released blood changes color as the heme and bilirubin are reabsorbed – from purple, red, blueish, greenish, yellow, and gone. This collection of blood has a variety of names!

- **Ecchymosis** (ek-key-**moe**-sis) > Condition of blood under the skin, usually quite purple due to a spontaneous bleed. Commonly used for larger lesions which may be caused by leukemia, renal failure, cancers, or liver dysfunction. *ICD★: R23.3 Spontaneous ecchymosis*

- **Bruise** (brews) > Diffuse extravasation of the blood under the skin, usually a flat lesion, purple/red due to breaking capillaries from trauma. Most bruises take five to seven days to dissipate. Longer depending on the depth and width of the injury. *ICD: T14.8, also see contusion*

- **Purpura** (**purr**-purr-ah) > Hemorrhage under the skin starts out red, becomes dark purple. Several smaller, deep, flat lesions due to systemic issues such as chemotherapy, HIV, steroid use, cancer, or some medications. *ICD: D69, 14 varieties listed*

- **Petechiae** (peh-tea-**key**-ah) > Tiny, pinpoint hemorrhages under the skin begin red, become dark purple and will not blanch when pressed. This can occur from strain such as sneezing or coughing too hard, medications such as warfarin, acetaminophen, and NSAIDs, and several infections such as strep throat, CMV, and mononucleosis. *ICD: same as Ecchymosis, R23.3*

- **Hematoma** (he-mah-**toe**-ma) > A collection of blood under the skin. The bleeding is contained or walled-off in a specific location frequently in the soft tissue or even muscle. It creates a mass-effect which is why it has the suffix, –oma > tumor. *ICD too many to list here, found under Hematoma (traumatic)(skin surface intact)*

Contusion and bruise tend to be interchangeable in medical documentation. The location, size, color, depth, and pain associated help differentiate the possibilities as the ICD demonstrates. Injuries such as contusions or bruises are also coded for location at the time of injury, activity, and method of injury.

★ **IMPORTANT NOTE: The reader is notified that these examples are from an online search done in 2016. Do <u>not</u> use these codes for patient care episodes; look up new ones!**

LEUKOCYTES

Leukocytes (**lew**-koh-sites) > group of white blood cells (WBCs). The leukocytes are a critical component of the immune system. There are five types described by a variety of terms.

10.8

- Granulocytes (**gran**-U-low-sites) > when mature these leukocytes present with a 'grainy' appearance – like sand suspended in the cytoplasm. There are three such cell types:

  - Basophils (**bay**-sew-fil) > get their name from the color they take from 'basic' staining, they 'like' the stain > -phil. Take on a blueish tinge. Typically seen in low numbers, these cells contain heparin and histamine parahormones stimulating inflammatory reactions (Figure 10.6). Abbreviation: **Baso.**

BASOPHIL

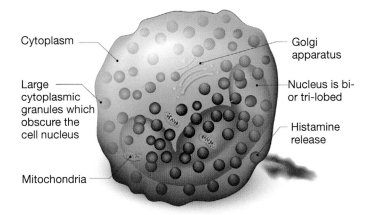

Cytoplasm

Golgi apparatus

Large cytoplasmic granules which obscure the cell nucleus

Nucleus is bi- or tri-lobed

Histamine release

Mitochondria

Appear in inflammatory reactions and allergic symptoms. Contain heparin and histamine

Figure 10.6

  - Neutrophils (**new**-trow-fils) > so called due to their 'neutral' dye staining, these are the most abundant leukocytes. Also called polymorphonuclear neutrophils (**PMNs**) or **segs**. Circulating in the bloodstream and 'eating' debris, bacteria, viruses, and more. The neutrophils are phagocytes (Figure 10.7).

NEUTROPHIL

Phag/o > to eat, very mobile

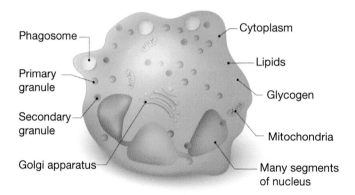

Phagocyting a bacteria
and other pathogens

Figure 10.7

- Eosinophils (ee-oh-sin-oh-fils) > denoted by 'rosy/pink or orange' coloration the staining dye imparts. These have a large, two-lobed nucleus; they favor 'eating' parasites and reacting to allergies (Figure 10.8). Abbreviation: **Eos.**

EOSINOPHIL

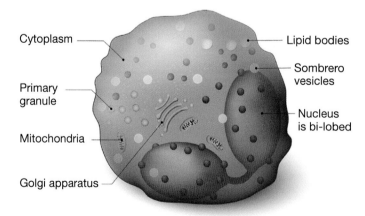

Control mechanisms
associated with allergy

Figure 10.8

Kitchen lab

Histopathology, the study of tissues has utilized a variety of 'stains' to illuminate the structures of the tissues and cells.

Wright's staining is used on WBCs.

You can duplicate the differences with food dye. Use one color (blue or red). Then place one equal-sized drop on a variety of foods: bread, rice, a cracker, noodle, etc.

Note the difference in the single color – it will change depending on the chemistry of each item. Let your instructor know your results.

• **Agranul**ocytes (a-**gran**-U-low-sites) > no granules are seen in the cytoplasm of these two leukocyte types.

– **Mon**ocytes (**mon**-oh-sites) > one kidney-shaped nucleus, another phagocyte. They respond to inflammation 10–12 hours after injury for cleanup duty. They can also paint the pathogens with opsonizing proteins to allow antibodies or complement to react (Figure 10.9). Synonym: Macrocytes (large cells) – they are the largest of the leukocytes. They are also called Macrophages (large eaters). Abbreviation: **Mono.**

10.9
Mono- > single, one or Mon/o > single or one. 'Mono' is one of the few prefixes acting as both prefix and root word. There are lots of root words and suffixes such as cyt/o and –cyte > cell.

MONOCYTE

Mono- > single and also called Macrocyte

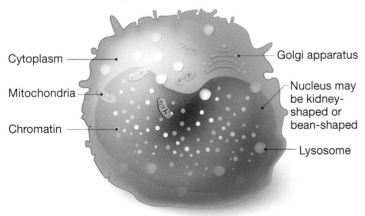

Cytoplasm

Mitochondria

Chromatin

Golgi apparatus

Nucleus may be kidney-shaped or bean-shaped

Lysosome

Monocytes engage in phagocytosis

Figure 10.9

LYMPOCYTE

B-cells: memory and antibodies

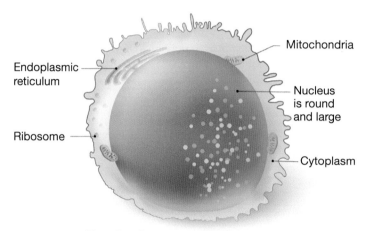

Endoplasmic reticulum

Ribosome

Mitochondria

Nucleus is round and large

Cytoplasm

T-cells: fight cells one-on-one

Figure 10.10

- **Lymphocytes** (lim-**foe**-sites) > one large nucleus, part of the specific immune response to infections with special T-cells and B-cells. They are produced in the bone marrow (myel/o) but also in limited numbers in the spleen, lymph nodes, tonsils, thymus, and Peyer's patches in the abdominal and pelvic regions. They mature in the thymus as well (Figure 10.10). Abbreviation: **Lymph, B-cells, and T-cells**.

The **CBC with differential**: complete blood count is **THE** laboratory study ordered most often in medicine. It can give a wealth of information on the wellness status of an individual. It includes the RBC indices discussed above and levels of the individual WBCs. This is called the **differential** part of the CBC, or the **diff**.

- **Neutrophilia** (**new**-trow-**fil**-ee-ah) or an 'elevated segs' > tend to indicate bacterial infections, marked inflammation, and even a heart attack. The bone marrow sends them out early; they are not mature yet.

- **Neutropenia** (**new**-trow-**pee**-knee-ah) > decreased number of circulating neutrophils. This is caused by severe infections (the body has run out of segs), some medication overdoses, or aplastic anemia (a-**plaz**-tik a-**knee**-me-a) to name a few.

10.10

Word parts

Bacteri/o > bacteria

Vir/o > virus

Immun/o > protective

Fung/i > fungus

Vascul/o > vessels

–osis > abnormal condition

–phil or –philia > condition of liking, affinity

- **Lymphocytosis** (**lim**-foe-sigh-**toe**-sis) > abnormal condition of the lymph cells > unusually elevated in viral infection, leukemias, and lymphoma.

- **Lymphocytopenia** (**lim**-foe-**sigh**-toe-**pee**-knee-ah) > low number of lymphocytes occurring with autoimmune diseases and associated with viral infections, bone marrow loss, or immune deficiency.

- **Monocytosis** (**moan**-oh-**sigh**-toe-sis) > occurs with chronic infections such as tuberculosis (**TB**) or fungal infections, vascular disease, and leukemias, which elevate the numbers of monocytes.

- **Monocytopenia** (**moan**-oh-sigh-toe-**pee**-knee-ah) > rare; if present repeatedly may indicate bone marrow injury.

- **Eosinophilia** (**ee**-oh-sin-oh-**fil**-ee-ah) > noted in patients with asthma, allergies, inflammatory reactions, and parasitic infections.

- **Basophilia** (**bay**-sew-**fil**-ee-ah) > rare, may be associated with autoimmune disease, some allergic reactions, and some leukemias.

✓ Name the granulocytes?

✓ Construct the word for a condition of 'too few lymph cells' _____ /_ /____ /_ / ____ .

✓ What is another name for PMN's?

Word building

Using the word roots with the linking vowel to build as many valid terms with the suffixes given. Please define each term.

Leuk/o Lymph/o Mon/o
(as prefix or root word)

-logy -osis -phil -cyte -lysis -genesis

-penia > less than, shortage

-oma > tumor

Lab units
Blood cell measurement are done in percent (%) or in absolute numbers 0/mcL (microliter)

Example
Monocytes 2–10%

0.8×10^3/mcL

Many blood tests are measured in mg/dl = milligram per deciliter

10.11 Neutrophils, Basophils, Eosinophils

10.12 Lymph/o/cyt/o/penia

10.13 Neutrophils or segs or granulocyte

10.14 The instructor has the list!

Leukocyte abnormalities are demonstrated by a proliferation of WBCs crowding out other cell activities and diminishing immunity. The general term for these conditions is **leukemia** (lew-**key**-me-ah).

- **Myelocytic** (**my-ee-low-sit**-ik) **leukemia** > overproduction of the immature granulocytes (myeloblasts). It first crowds the bone marrow and then the bloodstream. There are two types:
  - **Acute myelocytic leukemia (AML)** > consists of mostly the immature granulocytes in the marrow.
  - **Chronic myelocytic leukemia (CML)** involves of a mixture of the immature and mature granulocytes; in adults, there are some good long-term therapies.

- **Lymphocytic** (**lim**-foe-**sit**-ik) **leukemia** > proliferation of the lymphoblasts > immature lymphocytes appear in two types:
  - **Acute lymphocytic leukemia (ALL)** > typified by the sudden proliferation of the lymphoblasts in children and teens.
  - **Chronic lymphocytic leukemia (CLL)** > abnormal number of relatively mature lymphocytes in the bone marrow, spleen, and lymph nodes noted in the elderly.

10.15
Leukemia of any type is considered a malignant cancer. The overcrowding diminishes the numbers and function of the erythrocytes and platelets. This sets the patient up for anemias and bleeding disorders as well as an increased risk of deadly infections.

-blast > immature cell type

-emia > blood condition

 Review the CBC below and answer the questions. The **cpt** code for this exam is **8502**: Complete automated with differential WBC count.

Lab results CBC W DIFF 03/01/2016 09:33			
Patient	% range	Absolute numbers	Patient/range
BASO 0.8	0–2 BASO	ABS 0.10	0.0–0.2
EOS 4.0	0–7 EOS	ABS 0.20	0.0–0.8
HCT 48.3	**H** 37.0–47.0		
HGB 16.1 H	12.0–16.0		
LYMPH 27.8 1	9–48 LYMPH	ABS 1.70	0.9–5.2
MCH 29.3	27.0–37.0		
MCHC 33.3	33.0–36.0		
MCV 87.9	83.0–97.0		
MONO 8.3	3–9	ABS 0.50	0.1–1.0
MPV 9.6	7.2–11.1		
PLATELET 191	130–400		
PLATELETS: NO PLATELET CLUMPS SEEN ON SMEAR REVIEW			
RBC 5.50	**H** 4.20–5.40	RDW 12.8	11.5–14.5
SEG 59.1	40–74 SEG	ABS 3.50	1.9–8.0
WBC 5.9	4.8–10.1		

✓ 1 Explain the initial sets and define the terms as appropriate.
    Example: CBC, complete blood count reviews RBC, WBCs, and platelets.

✓ 2 There are two laboratory values elevated on this CBC. What do the abbreviations mean? Is there a disease process for 'too many RBCs'?

✓ 3 What are the other names for the WBC noted as 'SEG' on this report?

PLATELETS AND CLOTTING DISORDERS

The **platelets** (**playt**-lets) > the other solid elements of the blood. They are not cells but fragments of cells.

• **Megakaryocytes** (**meg**-ah-**kar**-ee-oh-sites) > derived from the same myeloid stem cell as the erythrocytes. As the name implies, they are large > mega-; nucleus > kary/o; cells > -cytes. The platelets or thrombocytes are fragments of these cells.

  – **Thromb/o** > clot, clotting is vital to homeostasis as it stops bleeding. As with all processes in the body, it must clot to stop the bleeding but not so much that the blood coagulates completely. Alternate word root: coagul/o.

The clotting process involves these sticky fragments > platelets or **thromb**ocytes (Figure 10.11), first they

• **Aggregate** (**ag**-ree-gate) > uniting, coming together, clustering. They release or cause the release of . . .

• **12 clotting factors** come into play to various degrees, most produced in the liver. They rely on vitamin K to function.

THROMBUS
Thromb/o > platelets

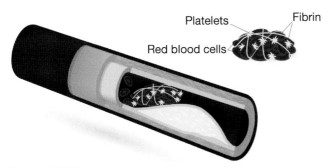

Platelets   Fibrin
Red blood cells

Figure 10.11

10.16
Did You Know?

Like cars on the highway, the blood cells get a lot of wear and tear. They have a finite lifespan.

Erythrocytes live 100–120 days and are recycled by the liver and spleen.

Neutrophils only have 6–48 hours to live.

Eosinophils live 8–12 days.

Basophils come out for inflammation lasting 5 hours to 5 days.

Lymphocytes, both T-cells and B-cells live a long time, 26 weeks to 1 year.

Monocytes hang out in the spleen until needed up to 6 months.

- **Fibrinogen** (fie-**bree**-no-jen) > blood plasma protein converts to fibrin to tie up or lock the blood clot in place after it is activated by thrombin.

  - **Prothrombin** (pro-**thrawm**-bin) > another blood protein formed in the liver, it will work with calcium to produce the thrombin to seal the wound.

  - **Thromboplastin** (**thrawm**-bow-plaz-tin) > substance found in tissues, leukocytes, and thrombocytes required for coagulation of the blood.

- **Fibrin** (**fie**-brin) > elastic-like, thin protein fibers or threads – it essentially helps tie up the platelets to form the scab or clot.

- **Thrombus** (**thrawn**-bus) > blood clot. In a healthy situation it stops bleeding from a laceration or bruise. Abnormal clotting within a blood vessel can cause damage or death by occluding the blood vessel, as seen in Figures 10.11 and 10.12.

  - Rate limiter, **heparin** (**hep**-are-rin) released by the basophils acts as an **ANTI**-coagulant to stop the clot forming at the appropriate time.

Thrombocytes (platelets) last between 9 and 12 days.

- Laboratory exams include a basic platelet count on the CBC and

  - **PT** > prothrombin time, the assay evaluates the cascade of coagulation. It is also called a Protime or **PT/INR**.

  - **PTT** > partial thromboplastin time is used to evaluate excessive bleeding or clotting disorders.

- **D-dimer**, a blood test, when positive indicates excessive heparin and anti-coagulant levels. This indicates a large clot or thrombus the body is trying to clear.

10.17
INR > International normalized ratio > a standard calculation based on the PT results. Used to monitor the level of anti-coagulant medication.

Clotting disorders or **dyscrasia** (dis-**kray**-zee-ah) > 'bad mixing', a general term used for a variety of blood disorders.

Hypercoagulable (hi-purr-ko-**ag**-U-la-bel) > used for any condition increasing the tendency for blood to clot leading to injury or death. There are several possibilities:

- Gene mutations and deficiencies such as **protein C** and **protein S** can cause the erythrocytes to have unusual shapes. These abnormal cells cause more damage to the inside of the capillaries and create traffic jams leading to thrombus formation.

- Elevated levels of homocysteine may increase thrombus formation. It is a waste product of protein use in the body. Genetically, elevated homocysteine is linked to premature vascular disease.

10.18
While used interchangeably there is a difference between a thrombus and an embolism (**em**-bowl-izm) > to insert in.

A thrombus is a blood clot whether it is forming a scab on the skin or blocking a vein or artery. An embolism travels in the

DEEP VEIN THROMBOSIS

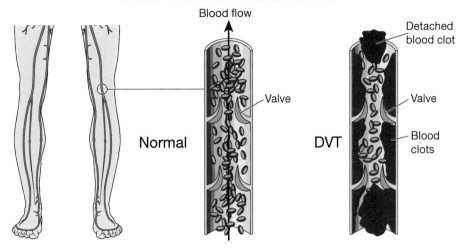

Figure 10.12

- Elevated levels of factor VIII is genetic and linked to deep venous thromboembolism (**VTE** or **DVT**) (Figure 10.12). When there is a factor VIII deficiency, excessive bleeding occurs; this is **hemophilia A**, a genetic disorder.

- Disseminated intravascular coagulation (**DIC**) may occur with cancer, sepsis (blood-borne infection), medication overdose, and occasionally with pregnancy and childbirth. This is widespread capillary level thrombus formation causing organ damage and, because it uses up the available clotting elements, leads to excessive bleeding and death.

bloodstream until it blocks a vessel. This can be a fat, air, or a foreign body embolism, or a blood thrombus breaking off in one place and traveling to another.

 What are the two linking forms for 'clot or blood clot'?

10.19 Thromb/o coagul/o

 John is going to the lab for a blood test to check his blood's clotting ability. What is the test called and what is its abbreviation?

10.20 Prothrombin PT or PT/INR

 Construct a word meaning 'white blood cell condition'. _____ /_____

10.21 Leukemia Leukosis (less common)

Word building

In this word building, spell out and define all the abbreviations given.

PTT CBC WBC PMN DIC DVT MCV Seg Eos

10.22 The instructor has the answers.

PHARMACY CORNER*

There are many medications making changes to our blood cells. Some are used intentionally to prevent thrombus formation or to treat an anemia. Others are unwanted side effects; patients need to be aware of these when utilizing a medication.

- Ibuprofen and aspirin are both anti-inflammatory over-the-counter (**OTC**) medications. Using low-dose aspirin makes the platelets less sticky, decreasing the risk of clotting. It can prevent a heart attack (myocardial infarction). Ibuprofen on the other hand has been associated with increased risk of stroke and heart attack. Both of these medications can cause bleeding in the gastrointestinal tract.

- Acetaminophen is another OTC pain medication. In excessive doses it can damage the liver and its ability to produce clotting factors. This can lead to an irreversible DIC.

- Hormone therapy such as birth control, post-menopausal medications, or steroids used for allergic reactions is linked to an increased risk of **DVT** or stroke. These tend to be rare but are more likely to occur at higher doses.

- Post-chemotherapy medications such as erythropoietin (**EPO**) are designed to stimulate the bone marrow to produce more erythrocytes, replacing those lost to chronic renal disease or chemotherapies. Neulasta can do the same for the leukocytes to help protect the immune-deficient patient regain protective strength.

- Blood thinners such as warfarin are used to decrease the likelihood of DVT, stroke, and heart attack. These require regular laboratory monitoring and can cause excessive bleeding.

These are but a few of the many medications affecting the 'blood'. Providers utilize medication to balance the homeostasis of an individual. It is essential that medication instructions are followed and any side effects are reported to avoid adverse reactions.

* IMPORTANT NOTE: All discussions of medications are for basic education. A medical provider should be consulted on any medication options. Do <u>not</u> use this information for patient care.

BLOOD CHEMISTRIES

A sample of human blood can give the scientist thousands of bits of information. Tissue and blood genetic tests number over 1,200 alone. **Phlebotomy** (fleh-**bot**-oh-me) > 'to cut into vein' > the process of drawing blood for laboratory study. Synonym: venipuncture (**ven**-ee-**punkt**-shur). The colorful-topped tubes are used to draw a myriad of tests. These are sent to various areas of the laboratory (Figure 10.13).

10.23
Blood evaluations
CBC
Chem 6 or Basic Metabolic Panel (**BMP**) checks Na,

Blood tubes

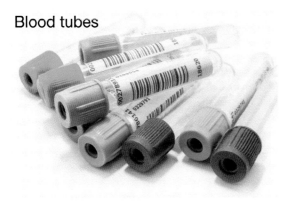

Figure 10.13

- **Hematology** > tests the whole or solid portions of the blood: erythrocytes, leukocytes, and thrombocytes, starting with the **CBC**.
  - **PTT**, **PT**, Coagulation studies, **INR**, D-Dimer, and Protein C & S.
  - **Hgb**, **Hct**, **WBC** with diff, T&B cell counts, **HgbA1C**, Platelets, and **ESR** (erythrocyte sedimentation rate), also abbreviated as 'sed rate'.

- **Chemistries** > use the serum of the blood to measure the balance of many electrolytes, hormones, vitamins, and more.
  - Therapeutic drugs and antibiotic levels, alcohol levels.
  - Lipids, glucose, liver function tests (**LFT**), cardiac enzymes, thyroid function studies (**TFS**), iron studies, protein assays, pregnancy tests (**βHCG**), C-reactive protein (**CRP**), vitamin levels, hormone levels, and electrolytes such as Na^{++}, K^+, Mg^{++}, Ca^{++}, and CO_2 to name a few.
  - Trace metals including zinc, selenium, copper, arsenic, lead, cadmium, and cobalt.

K, BUN, Glucose, Creatinine, CO_2

Chem 14 or Complete Metabolic Panel (**CMP**), depending on the facility, includes the basics with liver and renal functions

Hormone levels such as **TSH**, **FSH**, **HCG**, Estrogen or Testosterone

HIV, **RPR**, **ESR**, and **T&C**.

- **Serology** (sair-**ol**-oh-gee) > study of the immune response observed in the blood, in the serum, the liquid portion of the blood.
  - **PCR**, polymerase chain reaction > analyzes minute quantities of **DNA** and **RNA**. It allows DNA fingerprinting, bacterial and viral progression, and diagnosis of genetic disease.
  - Antibody surveys such as Hepatitis A, B, and C, **RF** (rheumatoid factor), **HIV**, **ANA** (anti-nuclear antibodies), syphilis, and viral antibodies.

10.24

Ser/o > denotes liquid portion of blood, fluid, whey

Prote/o > protein

Electr/o > power, electricity

Gen/o > beginning, genetic

Ven/o > vein

- Cytogenetics, molecular chemistries, and blood banking are also part of the many tasks of laboratory tests with blood.

Word building

 Using the word roots with the linking vowel to build as many valid terms with the suffixes given. Please define each term.

Ser/o Phleb/o Thromb/o

–logy –ous –logist –oma –emia

10.25
The instructor has the list!

LABORATORY AND cpt® AND HCPCS*

The current procedural terminology (**cpt**®) provides a five-numeric number for a huge number of procedures including the laboratory testing done to blood and tissues. Indeed, there are so many new procedures that it is updated monthly by the AMA (American Medical Association) as a vital part of the coding for the CMS (Centers of Medicare and Medicaid Services). It is the level 1 book encompassing everything from Hospital Inpatient Services to Newborn Care Services. Categories for Pathology and Laboratory include (incomplete list):

- Organ and Disease-Oriented Panels with drug assays
- Therapeutic drug assays
- Evocative and Suppression testing
- Urinalysis
- Molecular Pathology
- Genomic Sequencing Procedures and Multianalyte assays
- Chemistry
- Hematology and Coagulation
- Immunology
- Transfusion medicine
- Microbiology
- Cytopathology and Cytogenetics

All of these categories can involve the evaluation of the blood and lymph! Urine is checked for erythrocytes and leukocytes which may indicate renal dysfunction. Blood cultures (microbiology) can help define a blood-borne infection from bacteria, viruses, or fungi.

As with all coding activities, documentation is vital to discern the correct coding of laboratory procedures. There are some codes denoting several individual tests such as the **80050**, General Health Panel: *Complete metabolic panel, CBC with diff, and a TSH.* As a bundle, this code will cover all three. The provider/coder may not add these as individual tests, no double coding! With rare exceptions, many individual tests are also available such as a K$^+$ (potassium) versus doing entire BMP or an individual 'H&H', hematocrit and hemoglobin versus a CBC.

HCPCS, Health Care Common Procedure Coding System is the level II book. It was initially developed for coding services for Medicare patients in all possible outpatient settings. It is an alphanumeric with five digits. While some laboratory testing is covered, it tends to cover the durable medical equipment and supplies involved drawing blood or delivering PRBCs: the syringes, the needles, the tubes, the procedures of running a test.

All coding of durable materials, tests, and procedures need to be supported by the documentation of the SOAP note or other note types such as the Surgical report, Radiology report, or Pathology note to name a few.

★ **IMPORTANT NOTE: cpt and HCPCS are produced under the American Medical Association and approved by the CMS. Any codes noted here are from a 2016 online search. Do <u>not</u> use these for patient care encounters or coding.**

LYMPHATICS

The **lymphatic** (lim-**fat**-ik) **system** is the third vascular system of the body. It is similar to a vacuum cleaner collecting the leftovers of fluids (lymph), proteins, dead bacteria, and more to clean and recycle products into the venous circulation (Figure 10.14). This fluid is **interstitial** (**in**-tur-**stish**-al) **fluid** > fluid between the tissue cells.

10.26

- Lymph (limf) > fluid of life. In the same way that the WBCs sneak through the dilated vessels (diapedesis) to respond to inflammation, so does the fluid (serum) floating them out. It is also called 'serous' fluid when it oozes out of a wound; a clear yellowish fluid.

- Lymph **vessels** > specialized conduits siphon up the leftover serum (lymph), debris, and foreign bodies for a journey of cleanup and recycling (Figure 10.15).

  - Lymph/o > fluid of life, serum made up of water, WBCs, and proteins. **LIKE ALERT!** Lymph is used both for the fluid and solids siphoned up and recycled AND the lymphocytes, agranular WBCs. They are interactive but should not be confused.

  - Angi/o > vessel of any type, usually defined by the adjoined word root as seen here. Other word roots include vas/o and vascul/o

LYMPHATIC SYSTEM

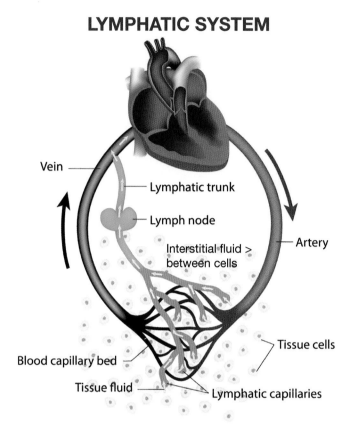

- Vein
- Lymphatic trunk
- Lymph node
- Interstitial fluid > between cells
- Artery
- Tissue cells
- Blood capillary bed
- Tissue fluid
- Lymphatic capillaries

Figure 10.14

- o Lymphangiitis (lim-**fan**-ji-tis) > inflammation of the lymph vessels.

- o Lymphangioma (lim-**fan**-gee-**oh**-ma) > tumor of the lymph vessels.

- o Lymphangiophlebitis (lim-**fan**-gee-oh-fleh-**by**-tis) > inflammation of the lymph vessels and veins.

Kitchen lab

You can create a lymphatic vessel siphoning effect in two ways: make two glasses with 1 cup of water in each and red or blue food coloring. 1) Take a large paper towel, roll it tightly into a ribbon; tie it with thread. Place one tip into one of the glasses and watch how far the dye travels up the towel. 2) With the second glass, cut a 6-inch piece of celery and place it in the glass. In the morning you will see the siphon columns in the celery. This is how our lymph vessels work to clean up the leftovers.

LYMPHATIC VESSEL

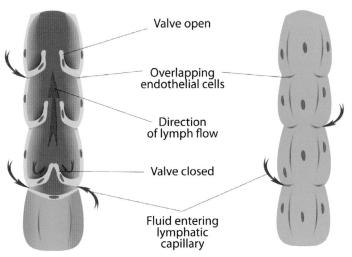

Valve open

Overlapping endothelial cells

Direction of lymph flow

Valve closed

Fluid entering lymphatic capillary

Longitudinal section

Siphons like a straw

Figure 10.15

- Lymph nodes are the way-stations on the path back to the heart; they can be likened to a washing machine. There are several of these at most joint areas such as the elbow (5–6), axillary (20–25), ankle, knee, groin (20–25), the neck (10–20), the clavicles and many internally (Figure 10.16). They capture debris and filter fluids.

- **Aden/o** > gland, used throughout the body for gland, it is associated with 'lymph'.
  - **Lymphaden**opathy (lim-**fad**-en-**nop**-ah-thee) > disease of the lymph nodes. When the body is fighting a hand infection, the elbow and axillary nodes will enlarge as they clean up debris.
  - **Lymphaden**ography (lim-**fad**-en-**nog**-raf-ee) > process of taking a radiographic picture of the movement of dye in the lymph vessels and nodes.
  - **Lymph**oma (lim-**foe**-mah) > tumor begins with an infection – fighting lymphocytes in the lymph nodes of the chest or abdomen. It is associated with weight loss, anemia, night sweats, cough, dyspnea, and swollen lymph nodes.

10.27
Common suffixes

–pathy > disease

–osis > abnormal condition

–megaly > enlargement

–itis > inflammation

–ectomy > surgical removal

–tomy > to cut into

–plasty > to repair

–pexy > to fix in place

Afferent means to 'bring into' or toward the center. It is used to denote fluid motion in vessels and organs.

Efferent is the opposite, 'to carry away'.

LYMPH NODE

Afferent pathway into the node

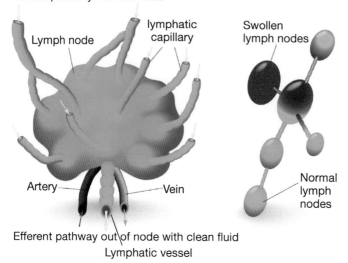

Lymph node

lymphatic capillary

Swollen lymph nodes

Artery

Vein

Normal lymph nodes

Efferent pathway out of node with clean fluid

Lymphatic vessel

Figure 10.16

✓ Construct a word meaning an 'enlarged gland'.

_____/__/_____

10.28 Adenomegaly

✓ Levon cut his foot on a dirty piece of glass. He now has streaks going up the leg and his posterior knee lymph nodes are enlarged. The best term for this is _____ .

10.29 lymphangiitis

✓ What cell types are usually found in a CBC?

_____

10.30 RBCs, WBCs, platelets

Word building

Using the word roots with the linking vowel to build as many valid terms with the suffixes given. Please define each term.

Angi/o Lymph/o Aden/o (Mix and match with two word roots too)

-logy –itis –megaly –oma –ectomy

10.31
The instructor has the list!

SPLEEN ANATOMY
Splen/o

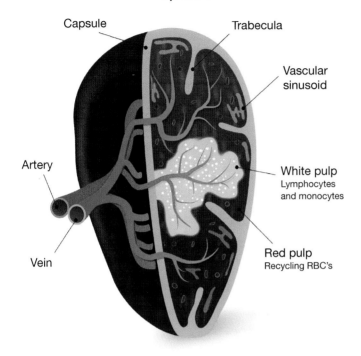

Capsule

Trabecula

Vascular sinusoid

Artery

White pulp
Lymphocytes and monocytes

Red pulp
Recycling RBC's

Vein

Figure 10.17

The **spleen** is the largest lymphatic organ of the body. It has several diverse functions including recycling spent RBCs (hematology), producing and maturing lymphocytes (immunity), and acting like a lymph node to filter the incoming blood for pathogens and foreign bodies (lymphatic). It is the first to initiate lymphocyte actions with blood-borne infections (Figure 10.17).

- **Splen/o** > spleen, second largest immune system organ (the bones are the largest). It is most susceptible to infectious disease.

    - **Splenomegaly** (**sple**-no-**meg**-ah-lee) > enlargement of the spleen. Mononucleosis is the usual viral cause.

    - **Splenorrhagia** (**sple**-nor-**ah**-je-ah) > hemorrhage (bleeding) from a ruptured spleen due to blunt trauma.

    - **Splenectomy** (sple-**nek**-toe-me) > surgical removal of the spleen.

    - **Asplenia** (a-**sple**-knee-ah) > without a spleen. When a patient is asplenic they are at risk for more infectious diseases due to the loss of function.

10.32
Did You Know?

The liver, kidneys, and the spleen are each protected and encased by a hard capsule. They are encapsulated. When they swell from infection, cancer, or other conditions, they cause significant pain from stretching of the capsule. Enlargement of any of these organs makes them more prone to blunt trauma rupture.

The **thymus** is considered part of the immune, endocrine, and lymphatic systems because it can produce and mature active lymphocytes (Figure 10.18).

THE THYMUS GLAND
Thym/o

Front view
Tucked in anterior mediastinum.
Matures T-lymphocytes

Structure

Capsule

Thymic corpuscle

Interlobular septum

Cortex

Medulla

Both lymphatic and endocrine

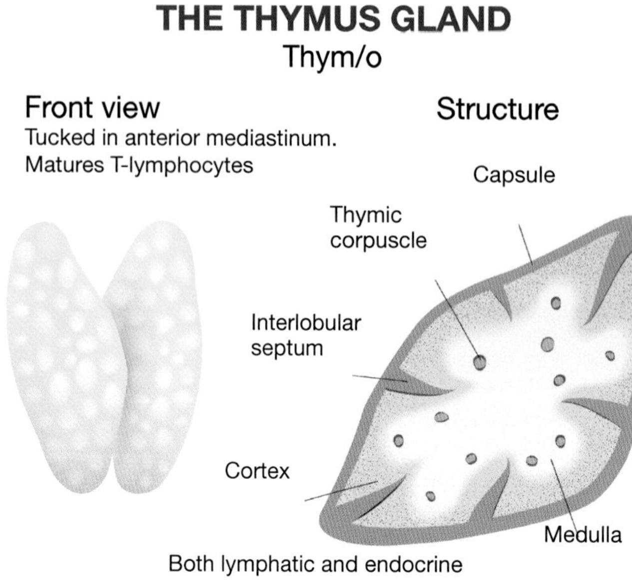

Figure 10.18

- Thym/o > Greek for 'wart'. This small organ resides in the upper mediastinum of the chest. It is larger at birth. Vital to maturation of the T-cell lymphocytes, the thymus is active throughout our lifespan fighting infections.
  - **Thymosin** (**thigh**-moe-sin) > the hormone it secretes to trigger T-cell function.
  - **Thymoma** (**thigh**-oh-ma) > tumor of the thymus.

Lymph **tissues** and pathways include a variety of structures found all over the body. They act as sentries for pathogens.

- **Tonsill/o** > tonsils (**tohn**-seals) are found in the posterior pharynx. They enlarge in the presence of viral, bacterial, or fungal infections.
  - Tonsillitis (**tohn**-si-**lie**-tis) > inflammation of the tonsils.
- **Adenoiditis** (**ad**-eh-noyd-**eye**-tis) > the adenoids surround the tonsils and function as lymph nodes in the nasopharyngeal region.
- **Peyer's** (**pie**-yhers) patches > collections of lymphoid tissue help protect the small intestines. They populate the mucosal (inner) lining of the intestines.

10.33
The thymus does have a thin capsule to protect it. It is the consistency of an eraser and feels 'bumpy' (wart-like).

10.34
-oid > like

Adenoid > to be like a gland or node

Lymphoid > to be like lymph

- **Thoracic duct** (thor-**as**-ik dukt) > lymph passage from the cisterna chyli region up into the chest that delivers the filtered lymph into the left brachiocephalic vein. It receives all the lymph from the lower body, left arm, chest, and head and neck.

- **Lacteals** (**lak**-teels) > specialized lymph vessels found in abundance in the intestines. They function to protect and carry the absorbed lipids from nutrition to the circulation via the thoracic duct (Figure 10.19).

INTESTINAL VILLI

Lymphatic lacteal (intestinal villi) absorbs fat and excess fluids

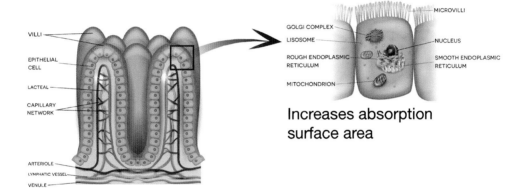

Figure 10.19

- Chyle (kiyl) > fatty, white to yellow lymph.
- **Cisterna** (sis-**tur**-nah) **chyli** > reservoir for chyle found near the superior abdominal aorta. It is on the pathway to the thoracic duct.

- Append/**o** or Appendic/**o** > 'to hang down; the abdominal appendix is lymph tissue hanging from the cecum of the ascending colon. The first lookout for the feces passage.
  - Appendicitis (a-**pen**-di-**sigh**-tis) > inflammation of the appendix.
  - Appendectomy (a-**pen**-deck-**toe**-me) > surgical removal of the appendix.

Cancer metastasis (**meh**-tah-**stay**-sis) utilizes the function of the lymphatics to spread to distant locations (Figure 10.20). Breast cancer begins in the tissues of the breast but spreads via the chest, clavicular, and axillary lymph nodes.

10.35

Meta- > beyond or change

-stasis > to stop or halt

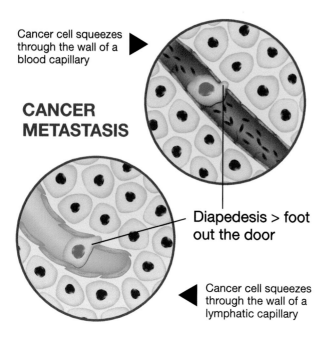

Cancer cell squeezes through the wall of a blood capillary

CANCER METASTASIS

Diapedesis > foot out the door

Cancer cell squeezes through the wall of a lymphatic capillary

Figure 10.20

Metastasis > beyond stopping

Cancer of all types kills approximately 120 people per 100,000 worldwide each year. Prevention strategies such as not smoking and a healthy diet and early detection are vital to decrease these numbers.

In the ICD *Table of Neoplasms, the primary site is noted first (as below) and then metastatic sites. These locations are most likely seeded by flow of the lymphatic system and bloodstream.

- Breast primary (C79.81) > bone, brain, liver, and lung

- Colon primary (C18.9) > lung, liver, and peritoneum

- Kidney primary (C64.9) > bone, brain, adrenal gland, liver, and lung

- Lung primary (C34.90) > bone, liver, brain, adrenal gland, and the other lung

- Ovary primary (C56.9) > lung, liver, and peritoneum

- Prostate primary (C61) > bone, liver, lung, and adrenal gland

- Thyroid primary (C73) > liver, bone, and lungs

---

* IMPORTANT NOTE: The reader is notified that these examples are from an online search done in 2016. Do <u>not</u> use these codes for patient care episodes; look up new ones!

✓ These groups of lymph tissue dot the intestinal mucosa.

10.36 Peyer's patch

✓ Construct a word meaning 'removal of the tonsils'.
_____ / _____ .

10.37
Tonsill/ectomy

✓ Mononucleosis is a viral infection which causes 'enlargement of the spleen'. What is the medical term?

10.38 Splenomegaly

Word building

Using the word roots with the linking vowel to build as many valid terms with the suffixes given. Please define each term.

Splen/o Thym/o Lymph/o (Use a prefix as desired)

–itis –oid –tomy –oma –ectomy

10.39
The instructor has the list!

UNIT SUMMARY

1 Hematology is the study of blood. Blood is a fluid consisting of several solid cell types and the serum with its water, nutrients, electrolytes, vitamins, minerals, clotting factors, and hormones.

2 The bone marrow is the place of a lifetime of hemopoiesis with the stem cells making several lines of cells including erythrocytes, leukocytes, and megakaryocytes. Megakaryocytes will lend their pieces as platelets (thrombocytes).

3 The red blood cells, erythrocytes, are the most abundant of the solid blood cells. When mature, they have no nucleus making room for each iron-heme protein to carry millions of oxygen molecules. This oxygen is vital to all cell life. A CBC will check the erythrocyte indices: hemoglobin, hematocrit, reticulocytes, MCV, MHC, and MCHC.

4 The white blood cells, leukocytes, are vital to the protective mechanisms of the body's immunity. Each of the five types of leukocytes serves to protect the systems from bacteria, viruses, fungi, and foreign bodies.

• Neutrophils > the most active by circulating in the bloodstream, these are the active phagocytes, eating debris. Also called segs, granulocytes, and PMNs.

• Eosinophils > A large bi-lobed nucleus quite active in allergy reactions and parasite phagocytosis.

- Basophils > secrete the parahormones heparin and histamine to stimulate the inflammatory reaction in response to injury.

- Monocytes > agranulocytes, these are the longest lived and largest of the leukocytes. They are the second line of cleanup and can mark pathogens for antibody or complement reactions. Also called macrocytes or macrophages.

- Lymphocytes > come in two types, the T-cells are the warriors of the specific defense to pathogens and the B-cells, the markers, produce antibodies and maintain memory.

5   The thrombocytes (platelets) are sticky pieces of the megakaryocytes circulating to begin the clotting process needed post-injury. Too many platelets, thrombus (blood clots) occurs. Too few platelets, excessive bleeding can occur.

6   The story of the blood and all its components is evaluated by a large number of laboratory tests including over 1,200 genetics tests, drug assays, chemistries, microbiology, hematology, and immunology. All of these are coded via the cpt® or HCPCS manuals.

7   Blood dyscrasias range from the anemias involving a change in erythrocytes to the leukemias which indicate leukocyte dysfunction. Medication, radiation, chemotherapy, slow blood loss, and immune deficiency can all cause significant and negative impact on the blood.

8   Like the blood, the lymphatic system is part of serology, immunology, and hematology. The lymph, the fluid of life is the serum lost to the work of the day and it is collected by the lymphatic vessels. The lymph nodes (lymphaden/o) are way-stations cleaning the serum and sending it progressively up into the chest to drop back into the venous circulation near the heart.

9   The spleen and thymus are organs of the lymphatic system AND the immune system. The spleen filters blood to remove spent erythrocytes, to trap and kill pathogens, and produces and houses a number of lymphocytes prepared to do battle. The thymus is vital to the production and maturation of the T-lymphocytes throughout life.

UNIT WORD PARTS

Word roots with linking vowel		
Angi/o; Vas/o; Vascul/o > vessels	Arteri/o > artery	Bacteri/o > bacteria (plural) bacterium (singular)
Bas/o > basic (staining)	Capill/o > capillary	Cyt/o > cell
Eosin/o > pink, rosy, orange	Erythr/o or Eryth- > red	Fibr/o > fiber, thread
Fung/i > fungus (singular) fungi (plural)	Gen/o > beginning, genes	Granul/o > sand-like
Hem/o or Hemat/o > blood	Immun/o > protective	Leuk/o > white
Lymph/o > living fluid	Mon/o > one, single	Myel/o > bone marrow or spinal cord
Neutr/o > neutral (staining)	Nucle/o or Kary/o > nucleus or center	Phleb/o or Ven/o > vein
Reticul/o > small web	Ser/o > serum, fluid	Spher/o > round, sphere
Splen/o > spleen	Thromb/o or Coagul/o > clot, solid	Thym/o > thymus

Prefixes: attached to the front of the word root to change meaning		
A-, An- > no, not, absent	Hyper- > more, increased, elevated	Hypo- > less, decreased, lower
Macro- > large	Mega- > enlarge, big	Micro- > small, tiny
Pan- > all, total	Poly- > many	Pro- > before, ahead of

Suffixes change the meaning of the word, linking vowel is usually 'o' with consonants		
-blast > immature, developing	-cyte > cell	-ectomy > removal, cut out
-emia > blood condition	-gen > beginning, developing	-itis > inflammation
-lytic or -lysis > destruction	-megaly > enlargement	-penia > fewer, less than
-oid > like, similar	-oma > tumor	-osis > abnormal condition of
-pathy > disease	-phage > to eat	-phil or -philia > like, to like
-plasty > to repair	-poiesis > making, developing	-rrhagia > excessive flow
-rrhexia > rupture	-stasis > to stop, halt	-tomy > to cut into

Acronyms, abbreviations, and initial sets		
ANA > antinuclear antibody	BUN > blood urea nitrogen	CBC > complete blood count
Chem 6 or BMP > basic metabolic panel	CMP > complete metabolic panel (Chem 14 or 16)	ESR > erythrocyte sedimentation rate (sed rate)
HCG > human chorionic gonadotropin (pregnancy test)	Hct > hematocrit	Hgb or Hb > hemoglobin
HgbA1C > glucose utilization measure	INR > international ratio, bleeding measure	MCH > mean corpuscular hemoglobin
MCHC > mean corpuscular hemoglobin concentration	MCV > mean corpuscular volume	PCR > polymerase chain reaction (genetic testing)
PMN > polymorphonuclear neutrophils	PRBC > packed red blood cells	PT or PTT > protime and partial thrombin time
RBC > red blood cells	RPR > rapid plasma reagin, syphilis test	TIBC > total iron binding capacity
TSH > thyroid-stimulating hormone	T&C > type and cross-match	WBC > white blood cells

UNIT WORKSHEETS

Building terms: Use the proper prefix/word root/linking vowel/suffix as appropriate.

Example: to cut into the stomach > gastr/o/tomy

a) Inflammation of the spleen > _____

b) The study of blood > _____

c) An abnormal condition of white cells (WBCs) > _____

d) A specialist who studies lymph > _____

e) Blood proteins > _____

f) Blood clot > _____

g) All cells are low > _____

h) Condition of no or less blood > _____

Know your initial sets/acronyms! For the initial set or acronym given, spell it out correctly.

a) PT   _____

b) MCV   _____

c) TIBC   _____

d) LFT   _____

e) Hgb   _____

f) INR   _____

g) CMP   _____

h) T&C   _____

Best choice: Pick the most appropriate answer.

1 The 'liquid' part of the blood is best called the

    a) Whole cells   c) Platelets

    b) Leukocytes   d) Serum

2 Myelosuppression means a reduction in

    a) Muscle action   c) Dentin production

    b) Glial action   d) Bone marrow production

3 This is the percentage of volume of the blood taken up by the solid cells.

    a) Partial prothrombin time   c) Hematocrit

    b) Hemoglobin   d) MCH

4 This anemia is characterized by a hypochromic and microcytic erythrocytes.

    a) Pernicious   c) Aplastic

    b) Iron deficiency   d) Thalessemia

5 These leukocytes are most reactive with allergic reactions and parasites.

    a) Neutrophils   c) Basophils

    b) Eosinophils   d) Lymphocytes

6 Asplenia

    a) Lack of red blood cells   c) No edema

    b) No spleen   d) Lack of white blood cells

Name the condition or term! Based on the description and/or function.

a) Carry heme-iron protein to transport oxygen to all body cells _____

b) A single large kidney-sharped nucleus, a phagocyte _____

c) Severe condition excessive clotting _____

d) Medication stimulating red blood cell production _____

e) General term for tests using serum to measure electrolytes, hormones, and more

_____

f) Inflammation of the lymph vessels _____

g) Tumor of the thymus _____

h) Inflammation of the bone marrow _____

Multiple correct: Select ALL the correct answers to the question or statement given.

1 Mark all the names or abbreviations for the leukocyte type which is most abundant?

   a) Basophil   d)   Thrombocytes
   b) segs   e)   PMN
   c) Neutrophil   f)   Granulocytes

2 Which of these leukocytes types are agranulocytes?

   a) Eosinophils   d)   Thrombocytes
   b) Lymphocytes   e)   Monocytes
   c) Neutrophils   f)   Megakaryocytes

3 Which of the following are laboratory tests used for evaluating thrombocytes?

   a) TSH   d)   Pertussis
   b) D-dimer   e)   INR
   c) PTT   f)   PT

Spelling challenge! Circle the correct spelling based on the definition given.

1 'Abnormal condition of round cells'

                Roundocytosis   Spearocytosis   Sferocytosis   Spherocytosis

2 'To cut into a vein'

                Flebotomy   Phebootomy   Phlebotomy   Phlibotomy

3 'Fluid between tissues'

                Introstitchial   Interstitial   Endrostictial   Ectostitial

---

Define the term: Spelling *does* count in your definition too!

1 Leukemia >   _____

2 Eosinophilia >   _____

3 Pancytopenia >   _____

4 Metastasis >   _____

5 Myelogenesis > _____

6 Osteomyelitis > _____

7 Pernicious > _____

8 Ecchymosis > _____

Find it! Using the words in the table – match the definition given or answer the statement. Some may not be used. It is recommended you know all the choices.

lymphocytosis	leukoplakia	lymphadenopathy	prothrombin
asplenic	myelocytic	hypochromic	thrombosis
intravascular	adenoiditis	basocytic	appendicitis
cytogenetics	phlebotomy	mononucleosis	macrocytic

1 _____ Abnormal condition of single nucleus

2 _____ Pertaining to large cell

3 _____ Disease of the lymph node

4 _____ No spleen

5 _____ Pertaining to cell beginnings

6 _____ Inflammation of node like

7 _____ To cut into the vein

8 _____ Pertaining to within the vessels

Matching: Some will not be used.

	Letter	Defined as	
Agranulocytes		a)	when elevated this indicates iron-deficiency anemia
Thrombolysis		b)	pertaining to the 'fluid of life' cells
Venipuncture		c)	specialist in studying serum
TIBC		d)	no granules are seen in the cytoplasm
Neutropenia		e)	tumor of a vessel
Heparin		f)	to cut into the vein
Lymphocytic		g)	decreased number of circulating 'segs'
Serologist		h)	to stop bleeding
		i)	natural anti-coagulant
		j)	destruction of platelets

An essay: Research the blood bank in your area: how many units do they need on an average day and how many donors can meet the need. What products do they prepare?

Note challenge: Translate the short note below: Note the meaning of the terms (underlined) Use your dictionary or appendix to look up words as needed. *A reminder, these case studies are developed to provide context for your learning. They are incomplete and should not be considered standard of care!*

S. 32-year-old woman in for a visit complaining of chest pain, dyspnea, and intermittent diarrhea. She reports weight loss, anorexia, and night sweats for the last two months. Normal menstrual period. No tobacco use. No nausea or vomiting. No hematochezia. No regular medications.

O. 32-year-old woman in no acute distress. Thin but no cachexia. No jaundice or cyanosis. Respiratory rate 22, a little labored. Lungs dull to percussion over the mediastinum with distant air flow. Heart 64, muffled and distant over the R mediastinum. Abdomen: soft, nontender, no masses. Positive lymphadenopathy R groin.

CBC: lymphopenia, anemia, with a neutrophilia

CXR: mass effect surrounding the great vessels and bronchi of the mediastinum

A. Lymphoma, presumptive diagnosis

Questions:

1 Translate all the acronyms and give meaning to the words that are underlined in the note.

2 The biopsy revealed a Stage III Lymphoma, Primary Source: R thoracic lymph nodes. Where in the ICD would this diagnosis be found?

3 What is the difference between a lymphoma versus leukemia?

Unit 11

Cardiovascular system

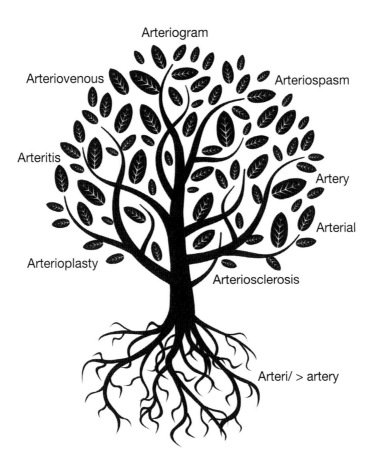

Arteriogram

Arteriovenous

Arteriospasm

Arteritis

Artery

Arterial

Arterioplasty

Arteriosclerosis

Arteri/ > artery

TARGETED LEARNING

1   Recognize word parts and assemble medical terms related to the cardiovascular system.

2   Correctly construct, define, pronounce, and spell medical terms.

3   Link vascular and cardiac illness and injury with appropriate pharmacotherapeutics and other therapeutic options.

4   Relate how documentation of a surgical note allows procedure coding.

KEY WORD PARTS

Word roots with linking vowel	Prefixes	Suffixes
Angi/o; Vas/o; Vascul/o > vessels	A-, an-	-ase
Aort/o > aorta	Anti-	-centesis
Arteri/o > artery	Bi- and Tri-	-clysis
Ather/o > fatty plaque, porridge	Brady-	-ectasias
Atri/o > atrium, chamber	Dys-	-gram, -graphy
Capill/o > hair-like tube, capillary	Endo-	-ism
Cardi/o > heart	Extra-	-lysis
Coron/o > crown, surround	Hyper-	-megaly
My/o, Muscul/o > muscle	Peri-	-pathy
Phleb/o or Ven/o > vein	Tachy-	-sclerosis
Ventricul/o > chamber, ventricle	Trans-	-stasis

THE HEART OF THE MATTER

Many philosophers, poets, and anatomists have written volumes on the small, muscular, and hollow organ, the heart. This circulation pump has over the centuries been endowed not only with the ability to move our life blood throughout the body but also it seems to be the center of our emotions, the sense of love, courage, and moral correctness. There are countless expressions illustrating the importance of the heart such as, 'take it to heart', 'an aching heart', 'a heart of gold', 'it does the heart good', and to have 'a change of heart' reflects perhaps a better decision.

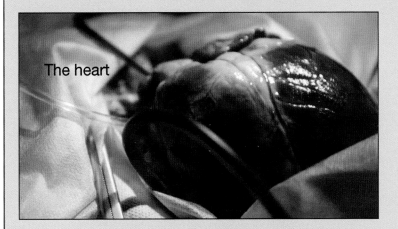

The heart

Figure 11.2

In fact, the heart weighs less than a pound (1.6 kg) and pumps blood over approximately 60,000 miles of blood vessels (Figure 11.2). The arteries and veins act as the roadways for the oxygen, nutrients, and hormones. The heart's steady beat (eurhythmia) allows for functions from brain to toes and will calm an infant hugged to a parent's chest. Working from the fourth week of gestation to the end of life in an unremitting rhythm, its power and importance cannot be measured by physiology or philosophers.

THE PIPES, THE VESSELS

Circulation of the human body is much like the many pipes beneath a city. Arteries and veins form a closed circuit where blood flows like water and waste flows through the pipes. Blood with its serum and solid elements is carried on the miles of vessels; there are three word roots for vessels.

- **Angi/o** > vessel or enclosure > describes disease processes of the vessels alone or in conjunction with other structures. Angi/o is also used for lymph vessels.

- **Angioedema** (**an**-gee-oh-eh-**dee**-ma) > swelling of a large area of capillaries and tissues, associated with allergic reactions.
    - **Angioscotoma** (**an**-gee-sko-**toe**-ma) > visual field defect caused by damage to retinal vessels.

- **Vas/o** > vessel > describes the action of the vessels such as
    - **Vasodilation** (**vay**-so-die-**lay**-shun) > an increase in the diameter or caliber of the vessel.
    - **Vasoactive** (**vay**-so-**ak**-tiv) > influencing the size and tone of the vessels.

- **Vascul/o** > vessels > anatomy designator such as vascular system or vascular ring.

Arteries are the larger of the two types of blood vessels (Figure 11.3). They are stronger and bear more pressure, like water pipes in homes. They begin as the ascending aorta exits the heart. Arteries always carry oxygenated blood away from the heart and get smaller on the way out to the tissues, with one exception. The pulmonary arteries (2) take deoxygenated blood to the lungs to get oxygen.

Arteri/o or **Arter/o** > artery or pipe > lined with smooth muscle which can contract or dilate as needed. They will decrease in luminal (opening) size to arterioles (little arteries) and finally miles and miles of capillary beds.

- **Arteriosclerosis** (ahr-**tier**-ee-oh-**sklar**-oh-sis) > hardening of the arteries. The walls actually calcify (become rock-like) and lose their flexibility.

- **Arteriogram** (ahr-**tier**-ee-oh-gram) > radiographic recording of dye as it flows through an artery. It can reveal blockage or kinks.

- **Arteriorrhexis** (ar-**tier**-ee-or-**rek**-is) > rupture of the artery such as an abdominal aortic aneurysm (**AAA**).

11.1

LIKE ALERT!

Vasodilatation and Vasodilation both mean an increase in vessel diameter.

Angi/o suffixes:

–itis > inflammation

–pathy > disease

–al > pertaining to

–gram > record of

–lith > stone

–oma > tumor

–lysis > destruction of

11.2

LIKE ALERT!

Arteriosclerosis > hardening of the artery

and

Atherosclerosis > hardening of the plaque

While these can occur at the same time, they are caused by different mechanisms.

Suffixes

–rrhage > flow

–rrhaphy > suture

–plasty > repair of

ARTERY

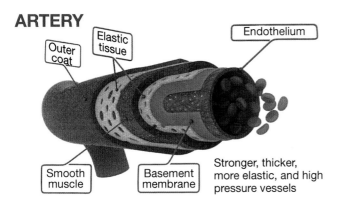

Endothelium

Elastic tissue

Outer coat

Smooth muscle

Basement membrane

Stronger, thicker, more elastic, and high pressure vessels

-pressor > raises BP

-ole > smaller

-graphy > process of recording

-gram or -graph > the record of or the machine making the record

-tomy > to cut into

Figure 11.3

- **Peripheral Arterial Disease (PAD)** > generalized condition of fatty plaque buildup in the larger arteries and arterioles of the legs and abdomen. This causes ischemia (loss of blood flow) – stopping a patient in their tracks due to muscle cramps (Figure 11.4). Synonym: peripheral vascular disease (**PVD**).

LEG ARTERY DISEASE
Atherosclerosis and blood clot

Ather/o > porridge   Scler/o > hardened   Condition of hardened cholesterol plaque

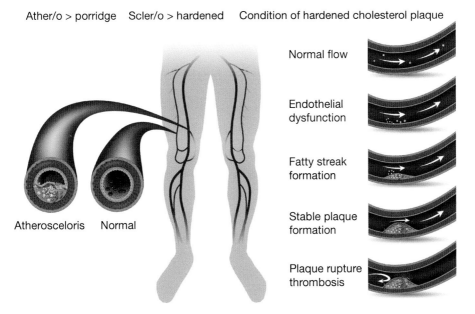

Normal flow

Endothelial dysfunction

Fatty streak formation

Stable plaque formation

Plaque rupture thrombosis

Atherosceloris   Normal

Figure 11.4

Aort/o > linking form for the largest artery of the body, the aorta. It begins immediately after the aortic valve opens from the left ventricle of the heart, to push oxygenated blood out to the body. It is named by its location along the way (Figure 11.5). These are the main arteries, and there are many arteries branching into the thoracic cage as well.

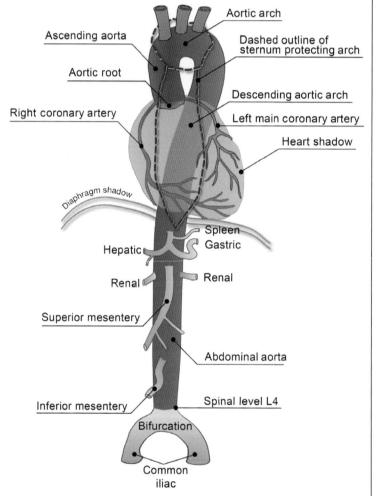

Figure 11.5

The average garden hose has a 5/8 inch diameter. The aorta is larger at about 1 inch. It is approximately 12–14 inches long. Its high pressure load and elastic component drive blood to the vital organs at a rate of about 280 liters an hour.

Bi/furc/ate > to split into two branches. Furc/o > Latin for fork, *furca*.

Artery locations

Tempor/o > temporal (near ear)

Mandibul/o > jaw line

Carotid > neck

Axill/o > under arm

Brachi/o > arm (antecubital region)

Radi/o > lateral wrist

Femor/o > groin

Tibi/o > tibial bone

Ped/o > foot (on top of)

- **Ascending aorta** (ay-**or**-tah) > upgoing behind the sternum, it turns at the manubrium. The left and right coronary arteries are the first branches supplying the heart itself.

- **Aortic arch** > the curve will send three branches to the neck, shoulders, and head where they will divide further.

- **Descending** aorta > dives deep into the thoracic cavity on the way to the abdomen. It is protected by the thoracic spine.

- **Abdominal** aorta > from the diaphragmatic 'aortic hiatus' until it bifurcates into the large iliac arteries. On the way branches go to the

  - Hepatic artery > the liver occupies the right upper quadrant, directly under the diaphragm.
  - Splenic artery > the spleen occupies the far left upper quadrant, directly under the diaphragm.
  - Gastric artery > the stomach shares the space of both the left and right medial areas (epigastric), directly under the diaphragm.
  - Renal arteries > short, branching laterally to the kidneys, keeping them high and medial in the retroperitoneal space.
  - **Superior** and **Inferior mesenteric** (**mes**-en-**tear**-ik) **arteries** > vast blood supply to the small and large intestines.

- **Aneurysm** (**an**-yur-izm) > localized weakening of an arterial wall enlarging over time. A rupture at any location can be life threatening, as seen in the brain (Figure 11.6). It can rupture into the cavity or it can rip between the layers of the artery itself.

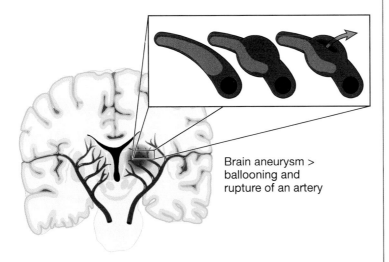

Brain aneurysm > ballooning and rupture of an artery

Figure 11.6

Kitchen lab

To take your pulse, you place a finger on an artery. It has the pressure to feel the impulse of each heartbeat. Look up and find on your body the following pulse points:

Temporal; Mandible: Carotid; Axillary; Brachial; Radial; Femoral; Posterior popliteal; and Dorsalis pedis. They should be equal side to side.

Discuss your findings with your instructor.

 Arteriectasis means _____

 Construct a medical term for 'cut into the vein'.

✓ Construct a medical term for 'pertaining to the vessels'.

11.4 artery dilation

11.5 Venotomy or phlebotomy
11.6 Vascular

Word building

Using the word roots with the linking vowel to build as many valid terms with the suffixes given. Please define each term.

Angi/o Arteri/o Phleb/o

-logy -tomy -itis -ectomy -stasis -pathy

11.7
The instructor has the list!

Large arteries have more elasticity to cope with the higher pressures; as the arteries become smaller (branching to organs) they are considered muscular or distributing. These smaller arteries and eventual arterioles (smallest arteries) branch into the tissues. They have greater vasoconstriction and vasodilation ability to adjust blood pressure locally. These finally give way to the capillaries (Figure 11.7).

- **Capill**/o > fine, hair-like vessel > single cell-thickness endothelial tube where oxygen and nutrients are exchanged at the cellular level of all the tissues. There are three types (Figure 11.8).
  - Continuous > tight cell junctions with minimal exchange, such as in the muscles.
  - Fenestrated > allows external diffusion, such as in the kidneys and brain via pores.
  - Discontinuous > loose cell junctions to maximize exchange of fluids and some solid cells, such as in the liver, spleen, and bone marrow.

11.8
Endo- > inside

Theli/o > cellular layer

The endothelial lining of the blood vessels is much like the lining tissues throughout the body. It is the single-cell layer where the exchange of gases, nutrients, hormones, and waste occurs.

CAPILLARY BLOOD FLOW

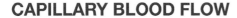

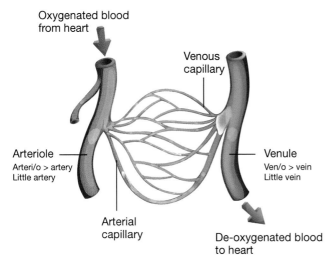

Figure 11.7

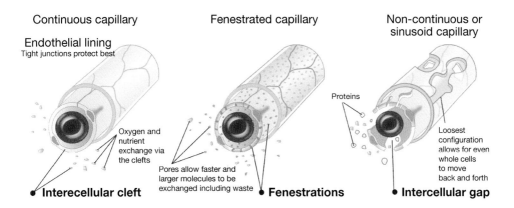

· **Continuous** > tight cell junction with minimal exhange such as in the muscles.

· **Fenestrated** > allows cell junctions with minimal exchange such as in the muscles.

· **Discontinuous** > loose cell junctions which maximize exchange of fluids and
                some solid cells such as in the liver, spleen, and bone marrow.

Figure 11.8

SURGERY AND ICD-10-PCS*

In the United States (USA), the Centers for Medicare and Medicaid Services (**CMS**) and the National Center for Health Statistics (**NCHS**) provide the coding method for procedures affecting repair on all systems of the body. The current version is called the ICD-10-PCS (Procedure Coding System). Like its counterpart, the ICD-10-CM, it standardizes guidelines for coding (in this example, an angioplasty). Atherosclerosis, as seen in Figure 11.9, slowly clogs a vessel thus blocking the flow of nutrient-rich blood. The placement of a stent restores flow to the vessel and its corresponding tissue. The coding of this procedure begins in the Index of Diseases and Injuries, *Angioplasty, dilation, heart and great vessels 027.*

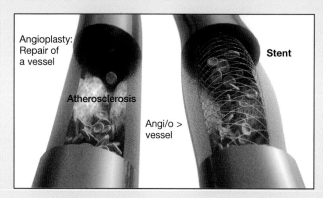

Figure 11.9

In the subsequent section, 027 reveals the information for the 6- or 7-digit alphanumeric. The evidence for the coding is found in the **surgical note** much as the SOAP note yields a diagnosis. Final code 02714D based on:

- 0 > the first digit will be a zero for 'medical and surgical' treatment
- 2 > is the next digit for the body system being repaired – in this case, the heart
- 7 > stands for dilation, opening a lumen of any tube (vessel, uterine tube, etc.)
- 1 > A choice of body part locations, in this example – two areas of the coronary arteries
- 4 > A choice of approach, one of three: open, percutaneous, and *percutaneous endoscopic*
- D > a device (or not) is used, in this example, intraluminal device – the stent.

For routine procedures, these codes will generate a 'bundle'. A bundle includes all the standard procedures and equipment needed for a specific surgery including the use of the operating arena, surgical tools, surgical devices (the stent), and more.
If a procedure deviates from the standard for some reason, it must be documented to account for additional billing codes. 'Unbundling' a code to maximize payment for billing is considered fraud.

* IMPORTANT NOTE: The reader is notified that these examples are from an online search done in 2016. Do **not** use these codes for patient care episodes; look up new ones!

VEINS AND DIAGNOSTICS

Veins > low-pressure return system like the plumbing taking waste back to the city water reclamation system. Blood is pushed up against gravity by the action of skeletal muscle, the diaphragm, and the one-way valves to prevent backflow. Venous blood is usually deoxygenated and the veins always carry blood back to the heart (Figure 11.10), with the exception of the four pulmonary veins bringing oxygenated blood back to the heart from the lungs. Unlike arteries, the discussion on veins begins with the venules (little veins) getting progressively larger on the way back to the heart.

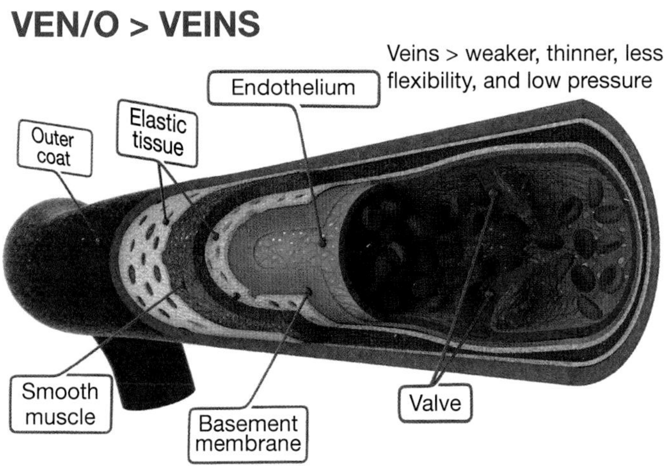

VEN/O > VEINS

Veins > weaker, thinner, less flexibility, and low pressure

Endothelium
Elastic tissue
Outer coat
Smooth muscle
Basement membrane
Valve

Figure 11.10

- **Ven/o** > veins > describe the anatomy. Ven/i and Ven/a are linking forms as well.
  - **Venipuncture** (**ven**-i-**punkt**-shur) > to puncture the vein to withdraw blood.
  - **Vena cava** > largest veins of the human body.
- **Phleb/o** > veins > Greek for procedures and disease conditions.
  - **Phlebotomy** (fleh-**bot**-oh-me) > to draw blood via a tiny needle.
  - **Phlebostasis** (fleh-**bos**-tay-sis) > abnormally slow motion of blood in the veins.

11.9
Phleb/o suffixes:

–ectasias > dilation

–ectomy > to cut out

–itis > inflammation

–clysis > to flush through

–meter > to measure

–stasis > to halt

Vena cava > cave-like vein. **Cavae** is the proper plural form.

When a surgeon uses a clamp or electrical system to stop bleeding, it is called hemostasis. The clamp is called a **hemostat**.

Vena cavae > Superior and inferior vena cavae are the culmination of the venous blood's return to the heart. Figure 11.11 illustrates how the superior vena cava (**SVC**) drains the arm, chest, neck, and head into the superior aspect of the right atrium. The return pathway is used to insert catheters to measure heart pressures or endoscopes to perform procedures.

Superior vena cava > SVC

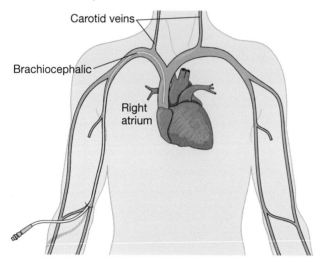

Figure 11.11

11.10

The hepatic portal system allows the liver to process venous blood for detoxification and use of the nutrients to build proteins, cholesterols, and hormone carriers, to name a few.

Veins do NOT pulse and tend to be noticed only if blocked. A phlebotomist uses the tourniquet to block flow when drawing blood.

The inferior vena (**IVC**) drains the legs, pelvis, and abdomen. It is unique in the portal vein enters the liver with the gathered venous blood from the entire digestive system (Figure 11.12). It carries the nutrients from food intake. The venous blood disburses throughout the hepatic tissue and recollects, exiting the superior liver essentially as the inferior vena cava, crossing the diaphragm to enter the inferior area of the right atrium of the heart, a distance of approximately 1/2 inch or 1.5 centimeters.

During the third trimester of pregnancy, the patient should always lie in the left recumbent position to avoid blocking the inferior vena cava.

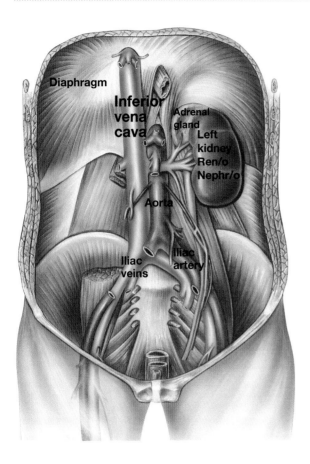

Figure 11.12

Deep arteries and veins tend to travel together along with the lymphatics. They are named by their locations in the body. Here are a few examples:

- The basilar (**bay**-si-lar) artery and occipital artery are branches of the internal carotid (ka-**rot**-id) artery. Their counterparts are the basilar and occipital veins. These are part of the brain's blood supply.

- The radial artery of the lateral wrist may be used to obtain 'arterial blood gases' (**ABGs**) to evaluate the level of oxygenation. There is a radial vein.

- The femoral vein is used during vascular procedures to inject dye, a catheter, or endoscope. The femoral artery is easily felt at the groin.

- The **superficial** veins seen and felt in the subcutaneous layers of the extremities may or may not have a corresponding artery of the same name.

11.11
The saphenous (sah-**fen**-us) vein is unique to the length of each posterior leg. There is no corresponding artery. The saphenous vein is harvested for use in coronary artery bypass surgery (**CABG**).

- **Deep vein thrombosis (DVT)** > large clot(s) (usually blood) forms in a limb (Figure 11.13). Frequently seen in the legs but can occur anywhere. The clot blocks the vein and if it breaks loose it is termed an embolus (em-**bow**-lus) or embolism. It tends to travel until it gets lodged in the wrong place. It can cause heart, lung, or brain failure depending on location.

A **thrombus** is a clot, usually associated with blood or a mixed atherosclerotic plaque.

An **embolus** is a clot in motion until it gets stuck. Air, fat, blood, or foreign bodies can all cause an embolus.

The terms tend to be used interchangeably.

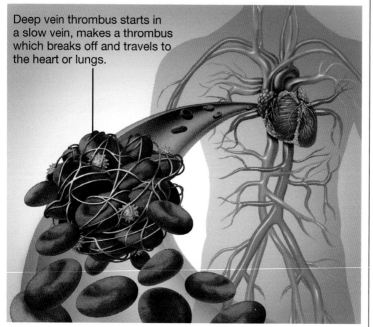

Deep vein thrombus starts in a slow vein, makes a thrombus which breaks off and travels to the heart or lungs.

Figure 11.13

✓ What would the medical term 'venoocclusive' disease mean?

11.12 The veins are blocked

✓ The head and neck venous blood drains into the _____ vena cava.

11.13 superior

✓ An X-ray procedure to trace the flow of a vessel is best called a/an _____ .

11.14 angiography

Diagnostic procedures evaluating the vessels of the cardiovascular system begin with a **simple pulse** count. In a report or SOAP note it is designated by a 'P': The pulse rate is a reflection of the speed and intensity of the heart's pumping action. The normal rate is a range of 60–100 per minute.

11.15 It is best to check a pulse with the pad of your index finger as it is the most sensitive.

- A **weak pulse** > indicates a cardiac change or a blockage of a particular pulse. Causes include dehydration, blood loss, injury, and heart failure.

- **Thready pulse** > weak pulse felt only intermittently.

- **Bounding pulse** > brisk in intensity due to stress, anxiety, being out of condition, or pregnancy.

Blood pressure (BP) > function of the pressure created by the pump (the heart) and the pressure of the vessels (the pipes) in a closed system.

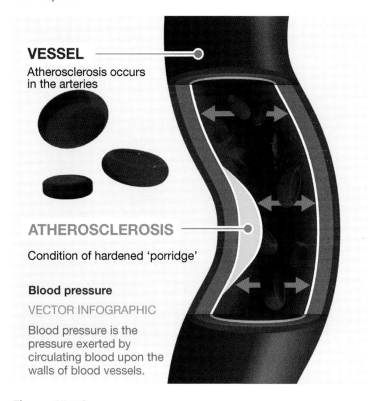

VESSEL
Atherosclerosis occurs in the arteries

ATHEROSCLEROSIS

Condition of hardened 'porridge'

Blood pressure
VECTOR INFOGRAPHIC

Blood pressure is the pressure exerted by circulating blood upon the walls of blood vessels.

Figure 11.14

- **Systolic** (sis-**tol**-ik) > contraction of the heart, the squeezing increases the pressure throughout the arterial system.

- **Diastolic** (**die**-ah-**stol**-ik) > ambient resting pressure *between* heartbeats. It should always be lower than the systolic because the system is at rest.

As Figure 11.14 demonstrates, things taking up space in the vessel increase the pressure readings, such as atherosclerosis, diabetes (glucose molecules take up space), or excess fluids to name a few.

Count over 60 seconds. Count yours at rest and then check it as you hold your breath. It should increase with the change in resistance.

11.16

LIKE ALERT!
BP > blood pressure

HBP > high blood pressure, a single elevated number set

HTN > hypertension, chronic elevated BP

Sphygmos > Latin for pulsation.

The **BP** is taken with a sphygmomanometer (**sfig**-mo-mah-**nom**-eh-tur) > comes in hand-held kits, wall-assemblies, and any number of computerized configurations. All close the artery off and slowly release blood to capture the first pump (systolic) and the last pump (diastolic) (Figure 11.15).

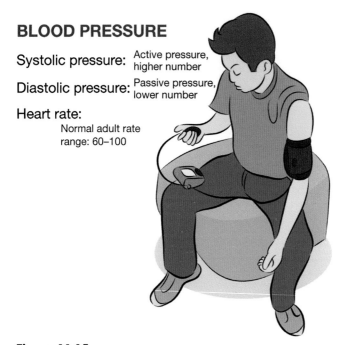

BLOOD PRESSURE

Systolic pressure: Active pressure, higher number

Diastolic pressure: Passive pressure, lower number

Heart rate:
Normal adult rate range: 60–100

Figure 11.15

Kitchen lab

Take your blood pressure twice a day for a week. Share with your instructor. Do you fit in the normal range for your age?

Flow studies > many types using X-ray imaging with contrast materials (dyes) and nuclear medicines. Most are done with the injection of the dye or nuclear tracer into a vein.

- **CTA, computerized tomogram** angi**ography** > can take hundreds of images of the vessel or heart per second (Figure 11.16).

- **DSA, digital subtraction angiography** > utilizes pre and post injection of the dye to define changes in the vessel's anatomy.

11.17
Angiogram is used for imaging any vessel.

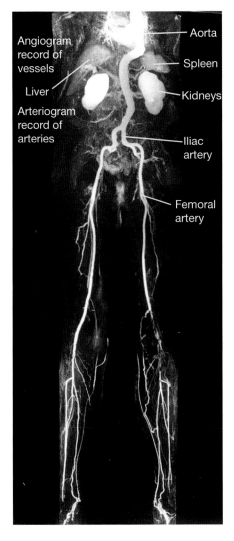

Angiogram
record of
vessels

Liver

Arteriogram
record of
arteries

Aorta

Spleen

Kidneys

Iliac
artery

Femoral
artery

Figure 11.16

- **EBCT, electron beam computed tomography** > excellent to define calcium deposits in vessels such as the carotid and abdominal aorta to evaluate arteriosclerosis.

- **Doppler** (dop-plur) **ultrasound** (**US**) > uses sound waves (not dye) to measure blood flow around the cardiac valves, chambers, and larger arteries. Useful for detecting peripheral vascular thrombosis.

- **ECHO, echocardiography** (**ek**-oh-kar-dee-oh-**graf**-ee) > uses high-intensity sound waves to review the heart valves and chambers. Today, the **TEE**, transesophageal (**tranz**-ee-so-**fah**-jeel) ultrasound can be quite definitive in detecting cardiac masses, aneurysms, and fluid in or around the pericardium.

Arteriogram is specific to arteries.

Venogram is specific to veins.

Nuclear scans are a method of tracking radioactive dye within the vascular system. Because the dye travels to the tissues via capillaries, it is used to evaluate injury to tissues.

PHARMACY CORNER*

Approximately 1 in 3 Americans will be treated for HTN, hypertension. The causes of HTN are many including simply aging. Aging makes the vessels a little stiffer, increasing the diastolic pressure. There are 11 groups of medications utilized to decrease HTN, with a variety of mechanisms.

- Diuretics (**die**-U-**ret**-iks) > decrease the water/fluid volume in the pipes. Less volume means decreased pressure.

- Beta-blockers > work at the pump, the heart, decreasing both workload and rate.

- **ACE** (angiotensin-converting enzyme) inhibitors > work at the arterial level, particularly in the kidneys, preventing constriction of the vessels.

- **ARBS** (angiotensin II receptor blockers) > work to block the 'key' which unlocks vasoconstriction of the arteries, keeping them open.

- Calcium channel blockers > reduce heart rate and force and also relax the arteries to a degree.

- Alpha-blockers > reduce the muscle tone of the arterial walls, decreasing constriction.

- Alpha-2 receptor agonists > help relax all the vessel muscles by blocking adrenaline, the fight-or-flight response of the nervous and hormone systems.

- Combined alpha-beta blockers > primarily used in intravenous (IV) administration to drop the BP in hypertensive crisis.

- Central agonists > work via the nervous system to keep blood vessels open.

- Peripheral adrenergic inhibitors > block neurotransmitters in the brain, thereby blocking the constricting message and keeping the vessels open.

- Vasodilators > working at the arteriole level, these dilate or widen the lumen allowing easier flow.

* IMPORTANT NOTE: All discussions of medications are for basic education. A medical provider should be consulted on any medication options. Do **not** use this information for patient care.

THE PUMP, THE HEART

The human heart > unique unto itself in the body. It is a one-of-a-kind, four-chambered pump pushing blood throughout the body from the 4th week as a fetus to death – a lifetime. It is intimately connected to the pulmonary system where the red blood cells go to pick up life-sustaining oxygen. The heart and great vessels sit in the mediastinal cavity, the center of the thoracic cavity.

- **Cardi**/o > heart > one of the most used linking forms with over 200 medical dictionary references (Figure 11.17).

  - **Myocardial infarction** (**my**-oh-**kar**-dee-al in-**fark**-shun) (**MI**) > death of heart muscle, a heart attack. A nuclear scan can define the area of injury.

  - **Endocarditis** (**en**-doe-kar-**die**-tis) > inflammation of the inner lining of the heart.

  - **Electrocardiogram** (ee-**lek**-tro-**kar**-dee-**oh**-gram) (**ECG** or **EKG**) > record of the electrical action of the heart. This is a diagnostic tool.

  - **Cardiogenic** (**kar**-dee-oh-**jen**-ik) > of heart origin; there are many sensations and symptoms which may be attributed to the heart.

11.18
Terms associated with the heart:
Atri/o > atrium
Ventricul/o > ventricle
Coron/o > crown, round
Valvul/o > valve
Ather/o > porridge
Steth/o > chest
Circul/o > circle

Suffixes
–pathy > disease
–rrhaphy > suture
–plasty > repair
–spasm > random contraction
–megaly > enlargement
–itis > inflammation
–genic > beginning
–vert > take back to normal

ANATOMY OF HUMAN HEART
Cari/o > heart

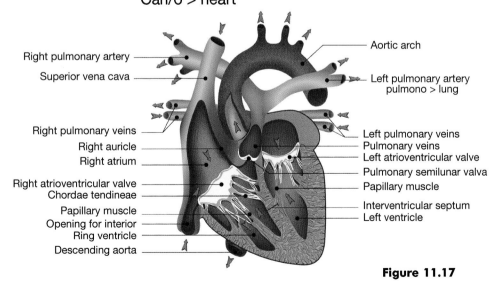

Right pulmonary artery
Superior vena cava
Right pulmonary veins
Right auricle
Right atrium
Right atrioventricular valve
Chordae tendineae
Papillary muscle
Opening for interior
Ring ventricle
Descending aorta

Aortic arch
Left pulmonary artery pulmono > lung
Left pulmonary veins
Pulmonary veins
Left atrioventricular valve
Pulmonary semilunar valva
Papillary muscle
Interventricular septum
Left ventricle

Figure 11.17

Atrium and ventricle both mean chamber or cavity. They are not unique to the heart but both are used to describe the four chambers of the heart.

Atri/o > small chamber > top set of chambers of the heart, right and left.

- **Right Atrium (RA)** receives deoxygenated blood from the superior and inferior vena cava. It is the location of the
  - **Sinoatrial (sigh-no-ay-tree-al) (SA)** node > self-starting electrical tissue is the normal trigger for the heartbeat (Figure 11.18).
  - **Atrioventricular (ay-tree-oh-ven-trik-u-lar) (AV)** node > way-station for the electrical impulse, it slows it just a bit to allow the ventricles to finish filling.

THE CARDIAC CONDUCTION SYSTEM

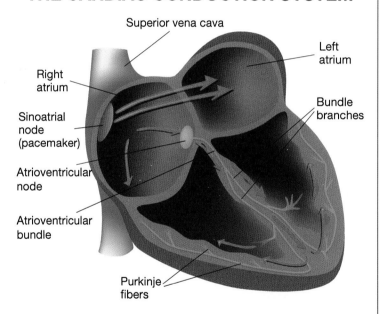

Figure 11.18

- The SA node is most involved with normal sinus rhythm (NSR).
  - **Bradycardia** (braid-ee-kar-dee-ah) > slow heart rate, less than 60 bpm.
  - **Tachycardia** (tak-ee-kar-dee-ah) > fast heart rate, greater than 100 bpm.
  - **Trigeminal rhythm** (try-jem-i-nal ri-thum) > cardiac arrhythmia where the QRS occurs in sets of three. It indicates a block between the atria (plural) and ventricles. Termed an **AV block**.

- **Atrial flutter** (**AF**) > the squeezing of the atria is NOT followed by a QRS complex (ventricular squeeze) in a rhythmic pattern: usually two to three unanswered to one QRS. Synonym: sawtooth pattern.
- **Atrial fibrillation** (**AFib**) (fib-ri-**lay**-shun) > atria are firing in a totally random manner with no relationship to ventricular contraction (Figure 11.19).

Arrhythmia (a-**rith**-me-ah) > abnormal heart rhythm versus NO heart rhythm.

Asystole (a-**sis**-toe-lee) > is used when there are NO heart contractions at all. If it persists, the person will die.

BBB > bundle branch block, a rhythm reflecting blocks in the ventricular septum.

Left atrium (**LA**) > receives oxygenated blood back from the lung via the four pulmonary veins.

A pacemaker replaces a dysfunctional SA node with a set rate of impulses via a wire placed in the RA.

NORMAL AND PATHOLOGICAL ELECTROCARDIOGRAMS

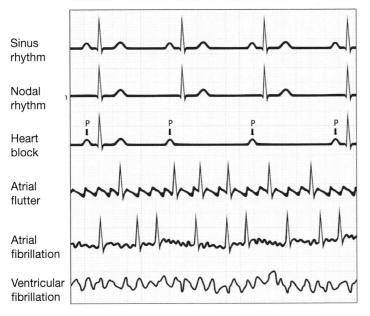

Sinus rhythm

Nodal rhythm

Heart block

Atrial flutter

Atrial fibrillation

Ventricular fibrillation

Figure 11.19

Word building

Using the word roots with the linking vowel to build as many valid terms with the suffixes given. Please define each term.

Cardi/o Vas/o Atri/o

-logy -ous -logist -oma -tomy -megaly

11.20
The instructor has the list!

Of the four chambers of the heart, which set is smallest receiving blood from the veins?

 Construct a medical term meaning 'of heart origin'.

11.21
Atria (plural)
Atrium (singular)

11.22 Cardiogenic

The ventricles are the larger heart chambers due to their increased muscle mass. All the chambers receive about 1/4th cup (45 ml) of blood during each cycle (Figure 11.20).

11.23
Other ventricular structures:

Interventricular septum > wall between the right and left ventricles. The electrical system travels here first after an **AV** node pause.

Did you know ligaments tear and tendons rupture? The chordae tendineae will leave part of the heart valve ineffective.

Defibrillation is 'undoing or breaking fibrillation'.

Defib is the abbreviation – when electrical stimulus is used to re-order the contractions of the heart.

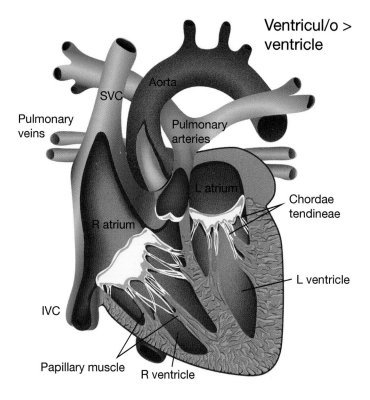

Figure 11.20

Ventricul/o > Latin for dark or dim room, this pertains to the heart and brain chambers.

- **Right ventricle (RV)** has thinner muscular walls as it pushes blood to the much closer and shorter pulmonary circulation to pick up oxygen.
  - **Chordae tendineae** (**kor**-day ten-**din**-ay) > tiny tendons supported by the papillary muscles and attached to the respective valve to prevent backflow.

- – **Papillary muscles** (**pap**-il-lar-ee) > sit on the floor of each ventricle; slight contractions pull on the chordae to keep valves closed under pressure, like an umbrella.

- **Left ventricle** (**LV**) has a 3×-thicker muscle mass to push oxygenated blood into the systemic circulation.

- **Ventricular fibrillation** (**VF** or **VFib**) > life-threatening arrhythmia where the normal impulses triggering an ordered contraction of the heart muscle become disorganized to the point where the heart is quivering. Quivering does not move blood or support life (Figure 11.21).

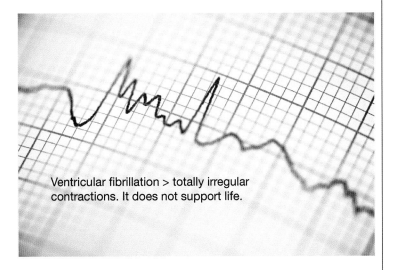

Ventricular fibrillation > totally irregular contractions. It does not support life.

Figure 11.21

The valves of the heart are designed like a one-way road, one direction keeping blood on its path to the lungs and into the systemic circulation. The valves are the source of the cardiac sounds, lubb-dubb (Figure 11.22).

- Tricuspid (try-kus-pid) > between the right atrium and ventricle; has three leaflets held by 4–6 chordae tendineae.

- Bicuspid or Mitral (my-tral) > between the left atrium and ventricle; has two leaflets held by 2–3 chordae tendineae.

- **Pulmonary** (**pul**-moe-nar-ee) > between the right ventricle and pulmonary arteries (2). When the ventricle contracts, this blood is sent to the pulmonary circulation to pick up oxygen and unload CO_2.

11.24
Cuspis > Latin for point.

Bi- > two

Tri- > three

Mitral is derived from the term for the shape of a Bishop's headgear > mitre. Mitral is an eponym.

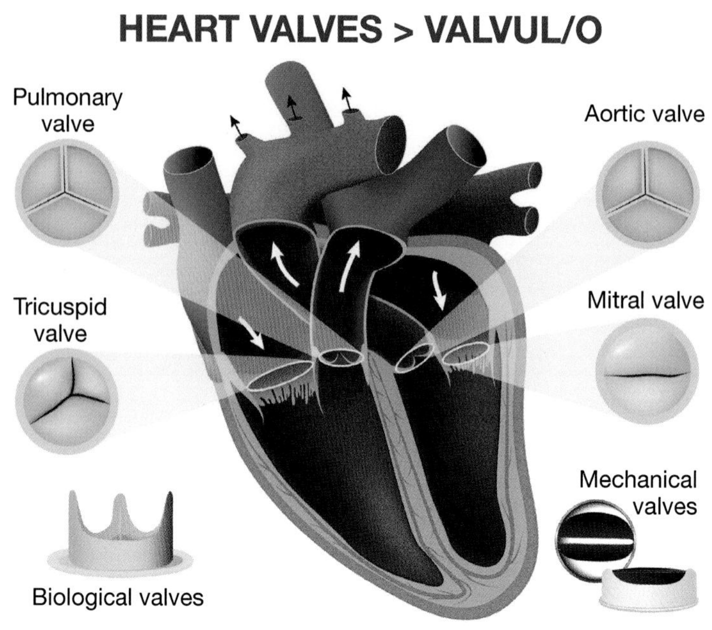

HEART VALVES > VALVUL/O

Pulmonary valve

Aortic valve

Tricuspid valve

Mitral valve

Mechanical valves

Biological valves

Figure 11.22

- **Aortic** > between the left ventricle and the ascending aortic artery. When the ventricle contracts this blood is sent out to the 75 billion cells of the body to deliver the oxygen and nutrients.

If a valve becomes stiff (**stenosis**) or **incompetent** (floppy) the result is similar: there is backflow across the valve, overfilling the corresponding chamber. Depending on the location and duration of the condition, heart failure occurs because the chambers get stretched out and do not contract as well, causing further congestion. This decreases the efficiency of the pump.

- **Congestive heart failure (CHF)** > inability of the heart to pump properly. It may be specific to systolic (contraction) or diastolic (at rest) mechanisms or both.

- **Mitral valve prolapse (MVP)** > murmur when the left ventricular blood backflows to the left atrium.

- **Pulmonary heart failure** > when the lungs are congested, the backflow affects the right heart and liver in particular. There is increased vascular resistance. The old term is 'cor pulmonale'.

The **Lubb** is the 1st heart sound (**S1**) and reflects the closure of the tricuspid and bicuspid valves.

The **Dubb** is the 2nd heart sound (**S2**) reflecting the closure of the pulmonary and aortic valves.

When the left ventricle is enlarged, a **LVAD**, left ventricular assist device, can help the severe CHF.

Other terms related to the valves concern the sounds or mechanisms of valve illness or injury. These are found with the physical exam of auscultation and palpation:

- **Murmur** (**mer**-mur) > sound created by the rush of blood over a valve or vessel. Incompetent valves or septal defects cause murmurs.

- **Gallop** (**gal**-up) > addition of a third and/or fourth heart sound (**S3**, **S4**) because valves are closing off the cycle; it sounds like a running horse.

- **Thrill** > vibration of a heart or vessel felt on palpation. Most associated with a blockage.

- **Bruit** (**brew**-ee) > an abnormal swishing or blowing sound associated with blocked blood vessels. It is the vessels' 'murmur'.

- **Regurgitation** (ree-**gur**-jeh-**tay**-shun) > the back-up of blood through an incompetent valve; it gurgles.

- **Palpitations** (**pal**-pee-**tay**-shuns) > sensation of the force of or irregular heartbeat. Patient may feel their heart in their chest. The provider may be able to palpate and/or auscultate the difference as well.

- **Vegetations** (**vej**-eh-ta-shuns) > growing on structures such as the leaflets of the cardiac valves. Bacteria and fungi are most frequent – these will cause murmurs.

11.25
Auscultation > the process of hearing sounds associated with the body.

Palpation > process of touching the body to feeling vibrations or discern pain.

Claudication (**klaw**-di-**kay**-shun) > limping seen due to pain in the legs caused by ischemia.

 The tricuspid on the right and bicuspid on the left are the valves creating this heart sound.

 A 'ventriculoatriostomy' creates what?

 What is the correct medical term for 'a slow heart rate'?

11.26
1st Lubb (S1)

11.27 A new opening between the ventricle and atrium

11.28 Bradycardia

Word building

 Using the word roots with the linking vowel to build as many valid terms with the suffixes given. Please define each term.

Aort/o Ven/o Capill/o

-logy -itis -ic -al -megaly -oma -tomy

11.29
The instructor has the list!

The coronary (**kor**-oh-nar-ee) arteries are no different from the other arteries: they supply the heart muscle with a supply of oxygen it cannot live without. They are also the first branching arteries as the aortic valve opens to fill the ascending aorta.

Coron/o > encircling, resembling a crown > refers to the left and right coronary arteries of the heart. Figure 11.23 shows a coronary arteriogram revealing the flow of the major arteries.

- 'Widow-maker' is a reference to a blockage of the left main coronary artery. A lesion here will block blood flow to the entire left heart often resulting in death.

- A **CABG** will use a vein linked in above the lesion and then below the lesion to divert blood supply to the arterial tree feeding the heart.

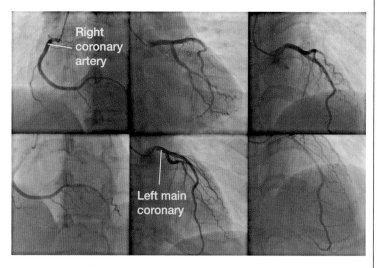

Figure 11.23

Besides the arteriogram, laboratory testing can help define damage to the heart muscle.

- **Troponin** (**trow**-poe-nin) (**Tn-I** or **Tn-L**) > muscle proteins of troponin I and troponin T increase with cardiac damage; this is a blood test.

- **Brain natriuretic** (**nay**-tree-you-**ret**-ik) **peptide** (**BNP**) > another protein unique to the heart and brain. It is a parahormone, helping relax blood vessels; it will be elevated post-injury in an effort to decrease the stress on the heart. It is a blood test.

11.30
The crown of the tooth is the corona.

CAD > coronary artery disease

CABG > coronary artery bypass graft

ASHD > Arteriosclerotic (hard arteries) heart disease

ACS > Acute coronary syndrome

Ischemia (is-**key**-me-ah) > local 'anemia', not enough blood due to obstruction of blood flow. It can be transient.

Lipid profile is a blood test assessing the level of circulating lipid proteins. Elevated LDL is predictive of heart or stroke events.

Angina pectoris (**an**-je-nah pek-**toe**-ris) > 'chest vessels' > severe pain in the chest secondary to ischemia of the heart muscle. It is called 'stable' when it occurs with exertion only. It is 'unstable' or 'ACS' > acute coronary syndrome when it occurs randomly.

Atherosclerosis (**ath**-ur-oh-sklar-**oh**-sis) > primary cause of cardiovascular disease (Figure 11.24). It begins with inflammation at the endothelial level of the vessel walls. It may be initiated as early as infancy. Risk factors include sedentary lifestyle, tobacco use, diabetes, elevated lipids, and hypertension (HTN).

- **Ather**/o > porridge or gruel > Greek for sticky, pasty foods.

- **Scler**/o > hard, hardening > thus atherosclerosis is an abnormal condition of hard porridge stuck in the arteries.

11.31
Cholesterol is made by the liver; it is vital for cell repair and the building of hormones and other proteins. Some is good.

LDL > low-density lipoprotein (bad guys)

HDL > high-density lipoproteins (good guys)

VLDL > very low-density lipoproteins

UNSTABLE ATHEROSCLEROSIS

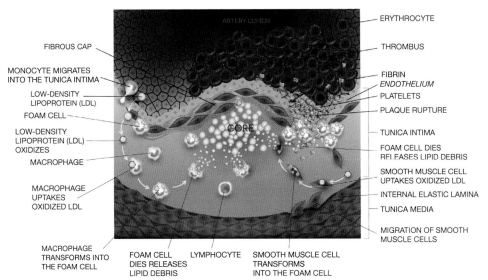

Figure 11.24

✓ Construct a medical term meaning 'porridge tumor'.

✓ 'Dysrhythmia' means _____ .

✓ An abbreviation of the process of recording the electrical activity of the heart.

11.32 Atheroma

11.33 bad or poor rhythm

11.34 ECG or EKG

DOCUMENTING HEART PAIN

It is a wonder people are able to communicate their perception of pain. Our language carries so many definitions. An example is, 'Don't be hyper', which could mean manic or wired, or excitable – 3 of 28 different possibilities. Even in medicine, the prefix 'hyper-' can mean increased, elevated, more, higher than, or above normal. Documentation is all about providing the most accurate information on the patient's story as possible.

Cardiac pain has many possible physiologic expressions and the descriptives typically involve related systems such as the lungs and gastrointestinal tract. Terms include: dull, sharp, squeezing, lancinating, piercing, burning, heavy, pushing, penetrating, stabbing, drilling, cutting, or slicing pain. The pain may be linked to dyspnea, shortness of breath 'SOB', heartburn, tightness, and smothering, a punched sensation, out of breath or can't breathe, indigestion, food-stuck sensation, and colic.

In defining the symptoms, the provider needs to use the patient's words and ensure the meaning is as close as possible to the patient's intent. This does involve expanding on how the pain starts, where it starts and its radiation pattern, length of time, and the things effecting the pain for better or worse. The words used in documentation impact care of the patient diagnosis because there is a significant difference in treating an acute myocardial infarction (AMI) versus gastroesophageal reflux disease (GERD).

PERICARDIUM

The support of the heart, great vessels, and lungs comes from a double-layered connective tissue sac. The **pericardium** is specific to the heart as the **pleura** is to the lungs. They are, in fact, intimately connected to allow the heart, lungs, and diaphragm to work in unison during each breath and heartbeat, as illustrated by Figure 11.25.

- **Pericardium** (**pear**-ee-**kar**-dee-um) > pertaining to around the heart.
  - **Visceral** (**vis**-sur-al) pericardium is the layer enveloping the heart itself.
  - **Parietal** (pah-**rye**-eh-tal) pericardium folds back on the visceral layer to become the second layer communicating with the connective tissues of the diaphragm and lungs.
  - **Potential space** > there is a minute amount of fluid between the two layers to lubricate the motion. It is a potential space for excess fluids or bleeding.

11.35
The abdominal contents, lungs, and heart all have this double-layer sac permitting movement without friction. Given the number of heartbeats, respirations, and abdominal movements over a lifetime, it is vital.

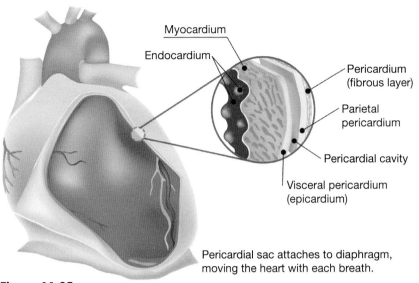

Myocardium

Endocardium

Pericardium (fibrous layer)

Parietal pericardium

Pericardial cavity

Visceral pericardium (epicardium)

Pericardial sac attaches to diaphragm, moving the heart with each breath.

Figure 11.25

- **Pericarditis** > inflammation of the pericardial sac due to infection or injury. Bacterial, viral, parasitic, and fungal infections can cause production of fluid between the visceral and parietal layers surrounding the heart. Sharp chest pain and dyspnea are typical symptoms.

- **Pericardial tamponade** (**tam**-poe-nad) > compression of the heart due to fluid and/or blood in the pericardial sac (Figure 11.26). This is a medical emergency. A pericardial centesis is performed to relieve the fluid compression or the action of the heart will not have room to function.

11.36

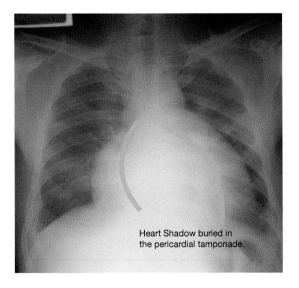

Heart Shadow buried in the pericardial tamponade.

Figure 11.26

Kitchen lab

Take two plastic bags, one inside the other. Place a rubber ball inside the inner sac. This is a 'pericardial' sac. Place a little drop of oil between the sacs to smooth movement. Now, carefully fill the outside bag with water. What happens to the ball?

Ischemia and hemorrhage can cause the same damage to tissues but the mechanisms and treatment for each are different. This is especially important in the brain as bleeding takes up space, crushing tissues (Figure 11.27).

ISCHEMIC AND HEMORRHAGIC STROKE

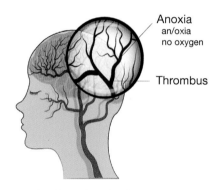

Anoxia
an/oxia
no oxygen

Thrombus

Ischemic stroke
Loss of oxygen, a blockage or similar

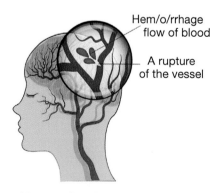

Hem/o/rrhage
flow of blood

A rupture
of the vessel

Hemorrhagic stroke
Rupture (-rrhexis) > blood loss

Figure 11.27

11.37
A stroke is any vascular impairment of the cerebral circulation. Thus, no matter the mechanism, a blood flow anomaly can cause temporary or permanent damage.

A transient ischemic attack (**TIA**) is usually due to a blockage. Anticoagulants are used to break up the clot.

A **hemorrhage** requires an intervention to stop the bleeding (**hemostasis**) and to remove the hematoma.

- **Ischemia** > localized loss of blood due to a mechanical blockage. The vessel remains intact but constriction or a clot (thrombus) or crushing (injury) prevents blood flow beyond that point.

  - Tissues below the blockage get little or no blood and tissue death (**necrosis**) is likely.

- **Hemorrhage** (**hem**-or-ahj) > flowing blood > the vessel has ruptured (like a pipe) or been cut or torn (injury) and blood is escaping into the surrounding tissues. In a closed space such as the skull this can be catastrophic to the brain. In the abdomen or chest, there is more space but the loss of blood decreases overall oxygenation to vital organs. Neither is good.

Construct a medical term meaning 'hardening of the arteries'.	**11.38** Arteriosclerosis
In which part of a SOAP note would this be found? 'John reports severe lancinating chest pain near his sternum. He has SOB and is sweating profusely.'	**11.39** Subjective. It is John's story
Circle the correct answer: Instead of 2 heart sounds there are 3 or even 4. Murmur Gallop Bruit Thrill	**11.40** Gallop

---

UNIT SUMMARY

1 The cardiovascular system is a closed system of blood flow via the heart (the pump) and vessels (pipes) to deliver life-giving oxygen, nutrients, hormones, and more to the human body.

2 The arteries (arteri/o) are the larger of the two pathways. They move blood away from the heart and are stronger, having more smooth muscle to maintain a safe blood pressure via vasoconstriction and vasodilation.

3 The veins (phleb/o or ven/o) are thinner, with little muscle action. They are unique, with one-way valves acting as an escalator moving blood back to the heart.

4 The heart (cardi/o) is a four-chambered muscle weighing about 11 ounces. It is found in the mediastinum of the thorax and it is intimately connected to the pulmonary system. The two top chambers are atria (small chambers) and the two stronger lower chambers are the ventricles.

5   There are two major disease processes affecting the arteries: arteriosclerosis (hardened arteries) and atherosclerosis (hardened fatty plaques). These can occur alone or in unison to slow the pump or change the peripheral resistance of the vessels.

6   The thousands of miles of capillaries are where the minute arterioles and venules meet. One cell thickness allows for the vital exchange of oxygen, wastes, and nutrition at the tissue/cellular level.

7   The connective tissues of the pericardial sac protect the heart, lungs, and diaphragm from friction injury resulting from constant motion.

8   The ICD-10-PCS provides standard codes for all procedures including therapy type, body system, actions performed, specific body anatomy involved, surgical approach, and any devices used in repair.

9   Hypertension (HTN) affects 1 in 3 adults in the USA. There are 11 medication groups representing approximately 100 medications designed to improve the efficiency of the pump (heart) or relax the pipes (vessels).

UNIT WORD PARTS

Word roots with linking vowel		
Angi/o; Vas/o; Vascul/o > vessel	Aort/o > aorta	Arteri/o > artery
Ather/o > fatty deposits, porridge	Atri/o > chamber, atrium	Brachi/o > arm
Capill/o > capillary	Cardi/o > heart	Coron/o > crown, surrounding like a crown
My/o; Muscul/o > muscle	Phleb/o; Ven/o > vein	Sphygm/o > pressure
Steth/o > chest	Theli/o > layers, tissue	Thromb/o > clot

Prefixes: attached to the front of the word root to change meaning		
A-, An- > no, not, absent	Anti- > against	Bi- > two; Tri- > three
Brady- > slow	Dys- > bad, poor, difficult	Endo- > within
Eu- > good, normal	Hyper- > more, elevated	Hypo- > less, decreased
Peri- > around, near	Tachy- > fast	Trans- > across

Suffixes change the meaning of the word, linking vowel is usually 'o' with consonants		
-ase > to break apart	-centesis > puncture, to draw out	-clysis > to flush
-ectasias > to dilate	-gram or graph > record	-ism > pertaining to a collection
-itis > inflammation	-lysis > to break, to destroy	-megaly > enlargement
-osis > abnormal condition	-pathy > disease	-plasty > to repair
-rrhaphy > to suture	-rrhexis > rupture	-sclerosis > condition of hardening

Acronyms, abbreviations, and initial sets*		
AAA > abdominal aortic aneurysm	ABG > arterial blood gases	ACE > angiotensin converting enzymes
ACS > acute coronary syndrome	AF or AFib > atrial fibrillation	ARBS > angiotensin II receptor blockers
ASHD > arteriosclerotic heart disease	BNP > brain natriuretic peptide	BP > blood pressure; HBP > high blood pressure
CABG > coronary artery bypass graft	CAD > coronary artery disease	CHF > congestive heart failure
DVT > deep vein thrombosis	ECG or EKG > electrocardiogram	ECHO or echo > echocardiogram
HTN > hypertension	MI or AMI > myocardial infarction (acute)	MVP > mitral valve prolapse
NSR > normal sinus rhythm	TEE > transesophageal echo	TIA > transient ischemic attack
VF or VFib > ventricular fibrillation	Heart chambers: RA, LA: right and left atria RV, LV: right and left ventricle	Cholesterol lab: HDL > high-density lipoprotein LDL > low-density lipoprotein

* The use of any acronyms, abbreviations, or initial sets depends on the context of the note. BBB, AAA, CVA, etc., all have different meanings in other settings. When in doubt, spell it out.

UNIT WORKSHEETS

Building terms: Use the proper prefix/word root/linking vowel/suffix as appropriate.

Example: to cut into the stomach > gastr/o/tomy

a) Inflammation of the heart > _____

b) Repair of an artery > _____

c) The study of the heart > _____

d) To break up fibrillation > _____

e) To cut into a vein > _____

f) To remove fluid from the heart sac > _____

g) Pertaining to the inner lining of the tissue > _____

h) A moving thrombus > _____

Know your initial sets/acronyms! For the initial set or acronym given, spell it out correctly.

a) AMI   _____

b) CABG   _____

c) NSR   _____

d) LV   _____

e) VF   _____

f) BBB   _____

g) AAA   _____

h) ECHO   _____

Best choice: Pick the most appropriate answer.

1 The term 'cardiovascular' contains _____ word roots.

   a) One

   b) Two

   c) Three

   d) None

2 A vasopressor is likely to
   a) Stop muscle action
   b) Crush the vein
   c) Increase the vascular resistance
   d) Slow the heart rate

3 If the tricuspid valve is incompetent, this condition may occur
   a) CHF
   b) ADA
   c) CVA
   d) PVS

4 An arteriogram is specific to
   a) Lymph vessels
   b) Veins
   c) Arteries
   d) All vessels

5 The descending aorta is found in the
   a) Anterior chest
   b) Abdomen
   c) Under the manubrium
   d) Deep, posterior chest

Name the condition or term! Based on the description and/or function.

a) This artery goes to the large organ in the right upper quadrant _____

b) This term means to 'split into two branches' _____

c) To flush out the vein _____

d) The enlargement of the ventricle _____

e) Receives returning blood from the head, neck, and arms _____

f) The device measuring blood pressure _____

g) To suture the heart _____

h) To open or dilate the vessels _____

Multiple correct: Select ALL the correct answers to the question or statement given.

1 Mark all structures associated with the heart?

   a) Chordae tendineae   d) Aortic valve

   b) Femoral vein   e) Left ventricle

   c) Atrium   f) Aortic arch

2 Which of these characteristics is consistent with the veins?

   a) Strong smooth muscle   d) Takes blood away from heart

   b) Thinner   e) Carries oxygenated blood

   c) One-way valves   f) Low pressure system

3 Which of the following are hypertensive medication groups?

   a) Diuretics   d) Calcium channel blocker

   b) Aminoglycosides   e) Tricyclics

   c) ARBS   f) ACE

Spelling challenge! Circle the correct spelling based on the definition given.

1 'Abnormal condition of hard fatty plaque'

   Aterisklerosis   Atherocytosis   Arteriosclerosis   Atherosclerosis

2 'Pertaining to vascular origin'

   Angegenesis   Vascogenesis   Angiogenic   Venogenial

3 'To breakdown a clot'

   Thombolytik   Throbostenosis   Thromace   Thrombolysis

Define the term: Spelling *does* count in your definition too!

1 Regurgitation > _____

2 Claudication > _____

3 Myocardiopathy > _____

4 Cerebrovascular> _____

5 Phlebectasis > _____

6 Ventriculoscopy > _____

7 Angioplasty _____

8 Thrombophlebitis > _____

Find it! Using the words in the table – match the definition given or answer the statement. Some may not be used. It is recommended you know all the choices.

vasoneuropathy	ventriculectomy	parietal	prothrombin
arteriography	asplenic	atrioseptoplasty	vascularization
aortorrhaphy	phlebotomy	endovascular	thrombosis
myocarditis	cardiomalacia	capillaropathy	

1 _____ Suturing the aorta

2 _____ Disease of the hair-like tubes

3 _____ Disease involving both the nerves and vessels

4 _____ Softening of the heart

5 _____ The process of recording the arteries

6 _____ Inflammation of the heart muscle

7 _____ Pertaining to within the vessels

8 _____ Abnormal condition of clotting

Matching: Some will not be used.

	Letter	Defined as
Bruit		a) specific circulation into the liver
Visceral		b) bacteria, viruses, fungus can form these in the heart
Auscultation		c) weakening of the vessel wall
Ischemia		d) the process of listening
Arteriorrhexis		e) connective tissue enveloping the organ
Vegetations		f) flushing the vein
Thrill		g) rupture of an artery
Portal		h) the sensation of vibration
		i) sound made by the rushing of blood in a vessel
		j) localized 'anemia', not enough blood

An essay: Explain the process of asking a patient about chest pain. What are the important elements in your own words?

Note challenge: Define the underlined terms. You may need to look up a few terms. Answer the questions which follow. Student is reminded this is an incomplete SOAP note used for the learning experience. Do not use this for patient encounters.

S. Philamon is a 56 <u>yo</u> man with a history of a mitral <u>systolic</u> murmur. He is complaining of fatigue, <u>dyspnea</u>, and <u>palpitations</u>. He reports one episode of severe, stabbing, <u>substernal</u> pain lasted about a minute when he was jogging. <u>PMH</u>: <u>HTN</u> × 10 years. No <u>DM</u>, thyroid issues, or past <u>MI</u>s. Medications: <u>ACE</u> for HTN.

O. 56 yo man NAD. BP: 146/86 P: 84 R: 16 Pulse Ox: 94%

Heart: irregular rhythm with a <u>gallop</u>. 4/6 systolic murmur 5th ICS, MCL. Palpable thrill in same area. No evidence of <u>cardiomegaly</u>.

A. Mitral insufficiency
<u>Angina pectoris</u>
HTN

P. Schedule <u>TEE</u> this week and <u>ECG</u> with Exercise Stress Test.

Questions:

1 Translate all the acronyms and give meaning to the words which are underlined in the note.

2 Where is the mitral valve located (which chambers does it serve)?

3 Why does the insufficiency cause a murmur?

4 The TEE is a procedure. Which book would be used to code the procedure?

Unit 12

Respiratory system

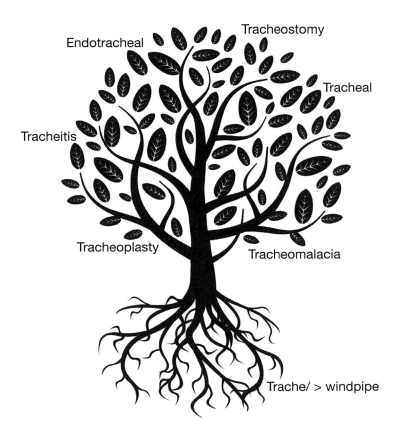

Tracheostomy

Endotracheal

Tracheal

Tracheitis

Tracheoplasty

Tracheomalacia

Trache/ > windpipe

TARGETED LEARNING

1 Recognize word parts and assemble medical terms related to the respiratory system.

2 Correctly construct, define, pronounce, and spell medical terms.

3 Explore disease tracking via respiratory illnesses post September 9, 2001.

4 Link respiratory illness and injury with appropriate pharmacotherapeutics and other therapeutic options.

KEY WORD PARTS

Word roots with linking vowel	Prefixes	Suffixes
Alveol/o > air sacs, alveoli	A-, An-	-centesis
Bronchi/o or Bronch/o > airway tube	Bi-	-desis
Capn/o > carbon dioxide	Brady-	-ectomy
Epiglott/o > above an opening	Dys-	-itis
Laryng/o > voice box, larynx	Endo-, In-	-osis
Nas/o or Rhin/o > nose	Epi-	-ostomy
Pharyng/o > throat, pharynx	Hyper-	-pnea
Pneum/o; Pneumon/o; Pulmon/o > lung or air	Hypo-	-ptysis
Spir/o > breathing	Ortho-	-rrhea
Tonsill/o > tonsils	Para-	-scope, -scopy
Trache/o > windpipe, trachea	Tachy-	-tomy

BREATHING EASY

Like the heart, the lungs' function of moving air in and out is a matter of both physiology and philosophy. A familiar saying after danger has passed is, 'We can breathe easy now'. Unfortunately, breathing easy is increasingly difficult because of the health impact of fine particulate pollution. The human hair is about 70 micrometers (μm) wide versus the fine particulates we are breathing in everyday at a tiny 2.5 μm (Figure 12.2). These minuscule particles are made of dust, smoke, dirt, soot, rust, and the off-gassing of materials effected by the sun's rays, to name a few. The protective mechanisms built into the respiratory system are little help in keeping these particles out of the deep tissues of the lungs, the alveoli.

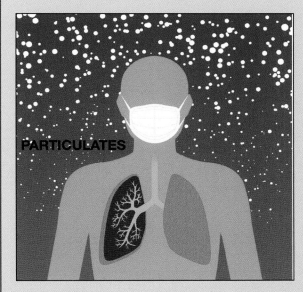

Figure 12.2

The consequences of inhaling pollution on a regular basis include the development of asthma, severe allergies, coronary artery disease (it starts the inflammation process), pneumonias, and pulmonary cancers. In highly industrial areas, the annual number of deaths due to pollution runs at about 400. We can't afford to truly breathe easy until the world addresses methods to decrease the dangers.

UPPER RESPIRATORY TRACT

When 'breathing' is discussed, the lungs are the anatomy considered first. In fact, they are last in the process of inhaling oxygen. The environmental gas called 'air' contains about 21% oxygen and the respiratory tract will utilize approximately 5% with each breath. It begins with our nose and mouth (Figure 12.3).

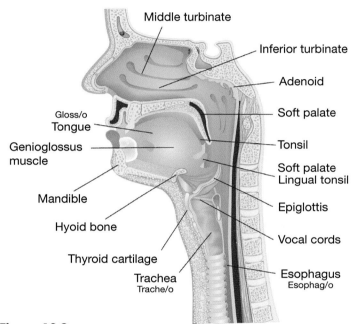

UPPER RESPIRATORY

- Middle turbinate
- Inferior turbinate
- Adenoid
- Soft palate
- Gloss/o
- Tongue
- Tonsil
- Genioglossus muscle
- Soft palate
- Lingual tonsil
- Mandible
- Epiglottis
- Hyoid bone
- Vocal cords
- Thyroid cartilage
- Trachea
- Trache/o
- Esophagus
- Esophag/o

Figure 12.3

12.1

Did You Know?

Air is composed of only about 0.4% of carbon dioxide (CO_2) but the human body exhales about 4.2% as a waste gas. The CO_2 is used by plants and they produce the O_2 we need.

Suffixes

–pathy > disease

–plasty > repair

–algia > pain

–dynia > pain

–rrhea > discharge, flow

–scope > instrument to look at . . .

–scopy > process of using an instrument to look at . . .

- **Or/o or Os** > mouth, opening > draws environmental air in when needed. The nose does most of the work. Mouth-breathing can dry the mouth out. Second word root: stomat/o or stom/o.
  - **Orolingual** (**or**-oh-**ling**-gwal) > pertaining to the tongue and mouth. Or/o is used to denote the anatomy.
  - **Stomatitis** (**stoy**-mah-**tie**-tis) > inflammation of the mouth.
  - **Stomatodynia** (**stoy**-mat-oh-**die**-knee-ah) > pain of the mouth. Stomat/o is used for medical conditions.
- **Nas/o** > nose > the primary function of the nose is to pull air into the respiratory tract. The sense of smell includes a nose constructed to moisten and warm the air on its way to the lungs.

It also provides some cleanup duty with sticky mucus and nose hair to capture particles. Second word root: rhin/o

- **Nasopharyngeal** (**nay**-zo-fa-**rin**-jee-al) > pertaining to the nose and throat. Nas/o is used to designate anatomy.
- **Rhinitis** (rye-**nigh**-tis) > inflammation of the nose.
- **Rhinolith** (rye-**no**-lith) > a nose stone.
- **Rhinorrhea** (**rye**-no-**ree**-ah) > runny nose. Rhin/o is used for conditions and procedures.
- **Epistaxis** (**ep**-ee-**stay**-xis) > Greek for nose bleed, for 'dropping'.

The defense mechanisms of the respiratory system begin with the nose with the

- **Muc/o** or **Muc/i** > sticky, viscous fluid produced by the goblet cells. This is the material blown out of the nose and sinuses during a cold or infection.
- **Vibrissae** (vie-**bris**-ay) (plural) > nose hairs which are visible; these are designed to capture larger particles of dust, sawdust, and dirt. Vibrissa > singular
- **Microvilli** (**my**-krow-**vil**-lie) (plural) > minute finger-like projections of the mucosal lining of the nose and sinuses. Microvilli or micro**cilia** (**see**-lee-ah) line most of the respiratory surface. They increase the surface area to capture debris (Figure 12.4).
- A forceful exhalation can blow fluids and debris from the nose.

12.2

Mucus (**mew**-kus) is the substance, the noun of sticky fluid

Mucoid (**mew**-koyd) > like mucous

Mucous > (**mew**-kus) > pertaining to sticky (the descriptive)

Microvillus > singular

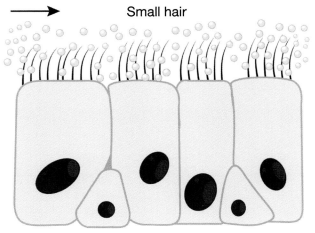

MICRO CILIA

Small hair

Nasal mucosa cells

Figure 12.4

Paranasal (**pear**-ah-**nay**-zal) **sinuses** are bony cavities surrounding the nose. They add a soundboard to our voice and they provide the increased surface to warm and moisten air (Figure 12.5). When the mucosal tissues of the sinuses are swollen, facial congestion follows.

- **Antr/o** > antrum, a small room > the maxillary sinuses (under the maxillary facial bone) are termed 'antral'. They are the first and largest 'rooms' the air passes through.
  - **Antroscope** (an-**trow**-skop) > instrument to look at the maxillary sinuses.
  - **Antrostomy** (an-**tros**-toe-me) > to create a new opening in the maxillary sinus. This would be done to evacuate a closed, painful sinus.

12.3
Paranasal sinuses include the

Maxillary

Sphenoid

Ethmoid

Frontal

All named for the facial bone overlaying the cavities. The maxillary and frontal sinuses are associated with **sinusitis**.

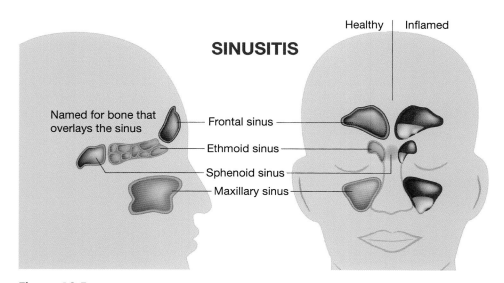

Figure 12.5

✓ Nasopharyngolaryngitis has _____ word roots.

✓ What is the meaning of the medical term antritis?

✓ Construct a medical term for 'mouth pain'.

12.4
three: nose, throat, and voice box

12.5
Inflammation of maxillary sinuses

12.6
Stomatodynia or stomatalgia

Word building

*Using the word roots **with the linking vowel to build as many valid terms with the suffixes given.** Please define each term.*

Rhin/o Stomat/o Antr/o

–logy –tomy –itis –ectomy –al –pathy

12.7
The instructor has the list!

The **throat** and **voice box** regions have several structures affecting the air flow on the way to the lungs including uvula, tonsils, adenoids, three areas of the pharynx, and the larynx.

- **Pharyng/o** > pharynx (**fair**-inks) > throat has air and food pass by it day in and day out. There are three specific areas:

  – **Nasopharynx** (**nay**-zo-**fair**-inks) > nose and posterior throat area (Figure 12.6); this allows the flow of air into the pharynx. When giggling with fluid in the mouth, this is the path it takes to the nose! ☺

  – **Oropharynx** (**or**-oh-**fair**-inks) > mouth and posterior throat area; this is the area a provider can see when the patient says 'ah'. The tonsils and adenoids are located in this area.

    o **Tonsill/o** > tonsils (**tohn**-sils) > tonsillitis, inflammation of the tonsils may be caused by *Streptococcus* Group B (**GBS**) or viruses.

    o **Aden/o** > glands > adenoid is 'to be like glands'. Both tonsils (a set) and adenoids (a set) are lymphatic tissues

12.8
Suffixes

–itis > inflammation

–ectomy > remove or cut out

–cele > hernia, diverticulum

–al > pertaining to

–pexy > fix in place

–tomy > to cut into

–osis > abnormal condition

–plegia > paralysis, weakness

–stenosis > narrowing

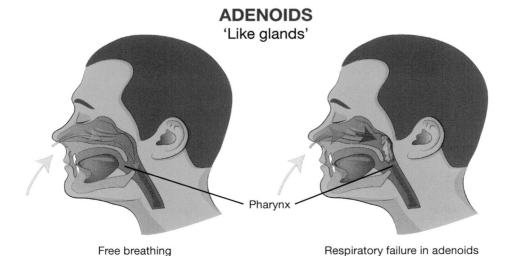

ADENOIDS
'Like glands'

Pharynx

Free breathing   Respiratory failure in adenoids

Figure 12.6

intended to capture bacteria, fungi, viruses, and other foreign bodies.

o **Uvul/o** > small grape > this is the fleshy mass of tissue hanging from the soft palate. During swallowing it rises to shield the nasopharynx from regurgitation. Uvulitis is caused by the same infections of the pharynx or allergies.

— **Hypopharynx** (**high**-poe-**fair**-inks) > below or under the throat is a very short link to the larynx (voice box). Laryngopharynx (**lair**-ink-go-**fair**-inks) is an alternate term.

A **T&A** procedure is the removal of the tonsils and adenoids: tonsillectomy and adenoidectomy.

An uvulectomy may be done to decrease snoring or sleep apnea.

Tonsillomegaly > enlarged tonsils can block air flow. This is a medical emergency.

Diseases of the **pharynx** are caused by either infections or cancers.

• **Pharyngitis** (**fair**-in-**jie**-tis) > inflammation of the pharynx can occur from shouting at the game too much, but more often there is swelling due to infection (Figure 12.7).

— **Viruses** predictably cause a pharyngodynia, abundant drainage and mucosal erythema. **PND** > post-nasal drip is part of the drainage felt on the pharynx.

— **Bacteria** such as *Streptococcus* Group B or diphtheria. Diphtheria (dif-**thear**-ee-ah) is a particularly bad infection creating a leathery membrane over the oropharynx endangering breathing. In centuries past, it killed thousands. The **DTP** vaccination prevents this in most countries.

— **Fungal** conditions such as 'thrush', properly called pharyngomycosis (fair-**ing**-oh-my-**ko**-sis), can occur in the immunosuppressed.

12.9
Vir/o > virus
Bacteri/o > bacterium
Fung/o > fungus
Eryth/ > red
Erythr/o > is also red.

DISEASES OF THE MOUTH AND THROAT

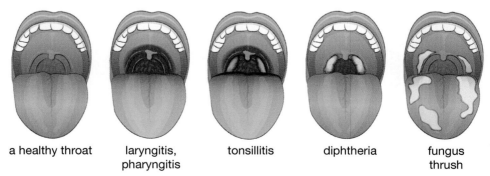

a healthy throat | laryngitis, pharyngitis | tonsillitis | diphtheria | fungus thrush

Figure 12.7

- **Pharyngeal cancer** occurs in patients who abuse chewing tobacco or snuff. The chemicals create a chronic inflammation in and around the tongue and pharynx.

LIKE ALERT!

Erythema is the color of the tissues. Erythrocytes are the red blood cells

---

- **Laryng/o** > larynx (**lair**-inks) > voice box; this is the transition space from the upper and lower respiratory tracts (Figure 12.8) — about one inch of specialized cartilage and several muscles with one bone (the hyoid). The vocal folds vibrate the exhaled air, allowing speech, coughing, and sneezing.

  - **Laryngitis** (**lair**-in-**jie**-tis) > inflammation of the voice box creates **dysphasia** (diss-**fay**-zee-ah) > poor or difficult speech. A familiar cause is a viral infection but cancer, polyps, and neurological damage can also cause the loss of speech. Dysphonia (diss-**foe**-knee-ah) > difficult speech (phonation) is another valid term.

DTP > diphtheria, tetanus, and pertussis vaccination given first in early infancy.

12.10

Pharynx and larynx are two words which change in pronunciation from a hard 'g' or a soft 'g'. If a suffix begins with an 'e' or 'i' it will be soft. Laryngeal > lair-in-**jeel**

LIKE ALERT!

Dysphagia > difficult swallowing

Dysphasia > difficult speech. Only ONE letter difference and they sound alike.

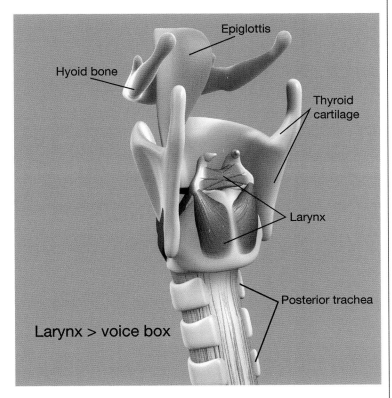

Epiglottis

Hyoid bone

Thyroid cartilage

Larynx

Posterior trachea

Larynx > voice box

Figure 12.8

- **Laryngismus** (**lair**-in-**jiz**-mus) > spasm of the vocal cords.
- **Croup** (crewp) > a childhood illness associated with a barking cough and stridor caused by the respiratory syncytial (sin-**sish**-al) virus (**RSV**). The sound is created by the swollen larynx.

The larynx has two unique structures vital to speech and protection of the airway.

- **Epiglottis** > glott/o > Greek for opening; epi- > near, above > making this flap of flexible cartilage 'above the opening', acting similarly to a door with a hinge. It closes over the larynx when food and drink passes into the esophagus (Figure 12.9). This is why eating, speaking, and breathing should not be done together. ☺

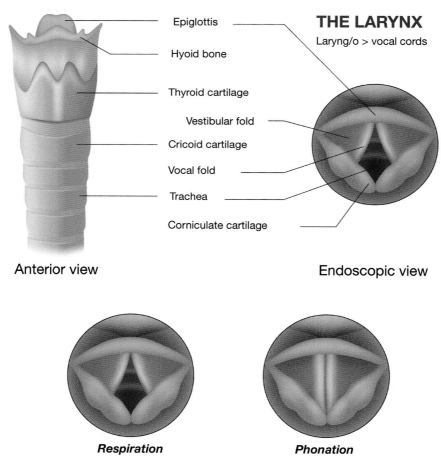

Epiglottis

Hyoid bone

Thyroid cartilage

Vestibular fold

Cricoid cartilage

Vocal fold

Trachea

Corniculate cartilage

THE LARYNX

Laryng/o > vocal cords

Anterior view

Endoscopic view

Respiration

Phonation

Figure 12.9

- – Epiglottitis (**ep**-ee-**glot**-tie-tis) > medical emergency when the inflammation creates swelling of the 'swinging door'. If stimulated it can close over the glottis and prevent all air flow.

- Chordae vocalis > vocal cords or folds > pair of ligamentous, yellowish tissues pulled tautly over the thyroid cartilage. When an endotracheal tube (ET) is placed to help a patient breathe, it passes through these cords or, more properly, 'folds'. The folds are the last defense to keep food and drink out of the trachea.

- Vocal cord polyps tend to develop in singers, an overuse syndrome.

- **Hyoid** (**hi**-oyd) **bone** > only bone in the body without a bone-to-bone interaction. It is suspended in the neck, supporting attachments for many swallowing and speech muscles. Strangling trauma of any sort breaks the hyoid and collapses the support structures for breathing. This is one of the reasons hanging kills a person.

 What is the correct definition of 'laryngeal stenosis?'

 Kia is a 5 y/o girl with recurrent tonsillitis. She is scheduled to have them removed. What is the proper medical term for this procedure?

Adenomalacia means?

12.11

Did You
Know?

To speak, exhalation must vibrate the vocal folds, the average length of time being about 15 seconds between breaths.

Whispering actually makes the vocal folds work harder. This is why silence is the fix for laryngitis.

The muscles moving the vocal folds also aid in swallowing.

Any food or fluid getting past the epiglottis stimulates forceful coughing to clear the airway.

12.12
Narrowing of the voice box

12.13
Tonsillectomy

12.14
Softening of the gland

UPPER RESPIRATORY DOCUMENTATION

'Kellie can't come out to play, she has a cold'. A 'cold' is the everyday word for an upper respiratory infection, **URI**. The terminology began with the false thinking that 'colds' occur only during cold weather. This never explained the 'summer cold'. In fact, a 'cold' can properly be called by a variety of medical terms: pharyngitis, laryngitis, sinusitis, rhinitis, tonsillitis, adenoiditis, or any combination of those names. Perhaps, it is easier just to say a 'cold'. Whatever we call it, it is a viral infection irritating the entire upper respiratory system from nose to larynx and all structures on the way. The irritation generates a defense mechanism: the massive production of mucus to flush the virus out. This is accompanied by sneezing (also to propel the virus out the door) and a low-grade fever. It runs a characteristically viral course, bad one day, better the next, and back to miserable the next. It tends to last 7–14 days (Figure 12.10).

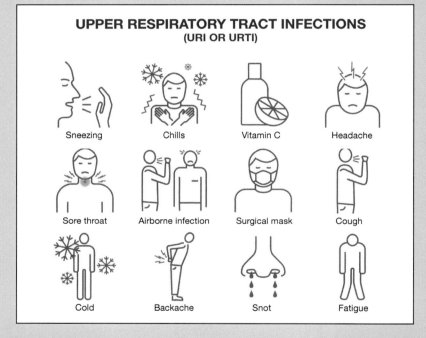

UPPER RESPIRATORY TRACT INFECTIONS
(URI OR URTI)

Sneezing	Chills	Vitamin C	Headache
Sore throat	Airborne infection	Surgical mask	Cough
Cold	Backache	Snot	Fatigue

Figure 12.10

Medical terms associated with a 'cold' include: rhinorrhea, nasal exudates, congestion, mucosal edema and erythema, pharyngodynia, otodynia, anorexia, and fatigue. There are also some non-scientific descriptions such as 'my face feels like it's falling off' or 'my ears and nose are plugged' or 'a scratchy throat'. Capturing the language is important to the diagnosis and treatment. What appears to be a viral 'cold' can be a bacterial or fungal infection of the sinuses, throat, ears, nose, or tonsils. The treatments are quite different. Another differentiation with the term 'cold' is it is NOT the 'flu'. The 'flu' is influenza, a severe lower respiratory infection.

LOWER RESPIRATORY TRACT

The trachea (tray-**key**-ah) begins immediately after the larynx; it is built of a series of 15–20 C-shaped cartilages, this is the windpipe. The trachea extends from the palpable anterior neck down into the thoracic cage to T–5 (nipple level). It terminates at the **bifurcation** (two branches) becoming the two main bronchi. The bifurcation is also called the carina (**kar**-eye-nah).

Trache/**o** > air tube > transportation of air in and waste gases out. It has a mucosal layer to moisturize the air, cilia to grab foreign bodies – moving these up and out like an escalator, and smooth muscle (Figure 12.11).

- **Trache**o**bronch**itis (tray-key-oh-brong-**keye**-tis) > inflammation of the trachea and bronchi is seen with the childhood disease **pertussis** (purr-**tus**-is), also called **whooping cough**.

- **Trache**ostomy (tray-key-**os**-toe-me) > creation of a new opening of the windpipe > done when air flow is blocked above the new opening due to trauma, unconsciousness, or inflammation (Figure 12.12).

- **Trache**oscopy (tray-key-**os**-kop-ee) > process of looking into the windpipe. This procedure allows a tube for breathing to be inserted, or a camera to investigate disease or foreign bodies, in the windpipe and into the bronchi.

  - Children accidentally inhale small objects all too readily. This causes a **stridor** or odd-sounding cough. Coins, small objects, or food (grapes, raisins) can be quite dangerous.

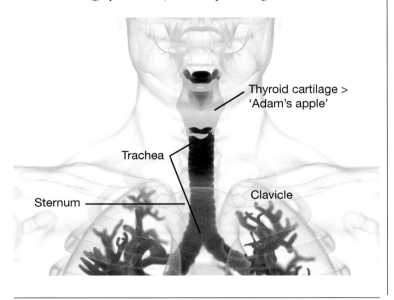

Thyroid cartilage > 'Adam's apple'

Trachea

Sternum

Clavicle

12.15

Trachea > Greek for a 'rough artery'. An artery is a conduit.

The term, '**bronch**i**al tree**' is often used. The trachea is the tree trunk part and the bronchi and bronchioles are the roots.

A procedure prior to surgery is the placement of an endotracheal tube (**ET**) > pertaining to inside the trachea > protects the patient's airway while they are sedated.

Suffixes

–scope > instrument to look

–plasty > repair

–rrhagia > hemorrhage

–stenosis > narrowing

–tomy > cut into

Figure 12.11

TRACHEOSTOMY

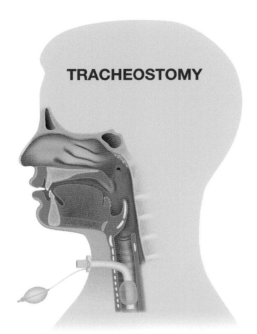

Creating a new opening in the trachea **Figure 12.12**

The **bronchi** (plural) are the right and left branches from the bifurcation of the trachea. Bronchus (**brong**-kus) is the singular.

ASTHMA – INFLAMED BRONCHIAL TUBE

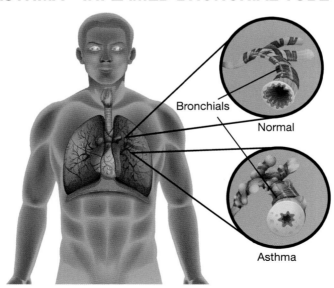

Bronchials

Normal

Asthma

12.16

Did You Know?

The right bronchus is longer and straighter than the left. Providers take care NOT to put the endotracheal tube into the right side only.

The bronchial tree consists of approximately 30,000 branches covering 1,500 miles.

Figure 12.13

These are mucus-lined airway tubes, transporting the gases deeper into the tissues of the lungs.

Bronch/o or **bronchi/o** > air pipes > short, cartilage-supported tubes quickly give way to multiple segmented bronchi or branches.

- **Bronchitis** (bronk-**eye**-tis) > inflammation of the bronchial tubes is a general term including the segmental bronchi (Figure 12.13). Besides an active mucosal surface, the bronchials have abundant smooth muscles to move air. **Asthma** (**az**-mah) causes loss of air passage.

The bronchioles (**brong**-key-oh-les) are six levels of progressively smaller and thinner air tubes ending at the alveolar sac – the tissues of the lungs (Figure 12.14). They maintain the mucus and smooth muscle effect all the way to the terminal bronchioles just above the 30–50 million alveoli.

Bronchiol/o > tiny air tubes > like the arterioles of the circulatory system, the bronchioles are extensive air flow tubes approximately 1 mm across.

- Bronchiolitis (**brong**-key-oh-**lie**-tis) > inflammation of the bronchioles associated with RSV and influenza viruses. Cough, fever, and body aches (malaise) are hallmark symptoms.

Pulmonary Function Tests (**PFT**s) check airway functions, lung volumes, and capacity.

12.17
Bronchospirometry > studies the volume of air flow into each lung. It is useful to determine the severity of asthma or bronchiolitis.

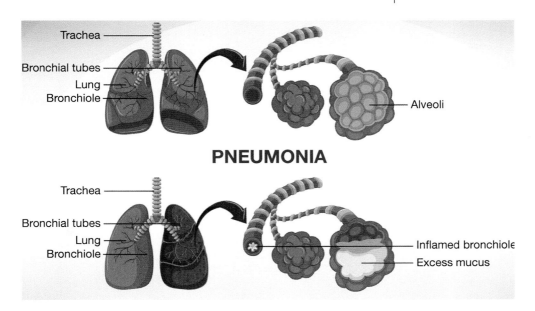

Figure 12.14

The **alveoli** (al-**vi**-oh-lie) (plural) are the gas exchange area of the lungs; these are air sacs, between 30–50 million in the two lungs (Figure 12.15). These are like linked balloons with very thin walls (1 cell thick) and elastic recoil. The heart sends the deoxygenated blood via the pulmonary arteries to the millions of capillary beds, gases are exchanged, and the oxygenated blood returns via the pulmonary veins.

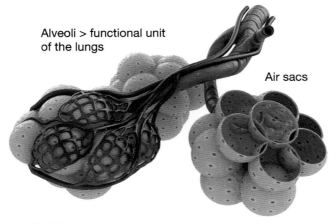

Alveoli > functional unit of the lungs

Air sacs

Figure 12.15

12.18

LIKE ALERT!

The alveolus (singular) also refers to the socket (basin) of each tooth socket. Most of the anatomical terms such as alveolar duct or alveolar ridge are concerning the teeth.

Causes of ARDS

Sepsis

Burns

Pneumonia

Chemical inhalation

Lung contusions

Alveol/**o** > a tiny basin > the functional units of the respiratory system. This is where oxygen and CO_2 are exchanged by passing 11,000 liters of air through each day.

- **Alveolar macrophage** (**mak**-row-fahj) > a protective foreign body (particulate) eater on the epithelial lining of the air sacs.

- **Surfactant** (sir-**fak**-tant) > a lipoprotein acting as a wetting agent to the internal alveoli. This helps prevent collapse of the tiny balloons. Premature infants do not produce enough surfactant, thus they need respiratory support. In adults, loss of surfactant leads to **ARDS** (Adult Respiratory Distress Syndrome) – fluids leak and the lungs stiffen.

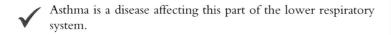 Asthma is a disease affecting this part of the lower respiratory system.

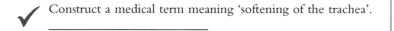 Construct a medical term meaning 'softening of the trachea'.
_____

✓ Herman is having a bronchogram to investigate a possible cancer. What is a bronchogram?

12.19
Bronchi and bronchioles

12.20
Tracheomalacia

12.21
A record of the bronchi (air tubes)

Word building

Using the word roots with the linking vowel to build as many valid terms with the suffixes given. Please define each term.

Trache/o Bronch/o

–logy –tomy –itis –ectomy –al –pathy –cele

12.22
The instructor has the list!

RESPIRATORY MEDICATIONS*

Medications of the respiratory tract are aimed at keeping the airway clear for the passage of oxygen. The disease process of asthma offers medications designed to keep the bronchials open by decreasing bronchial constriction and decreased mucus production. These are used for other respiratory conditions such as severe allergies, pneumonia, and chronic obstructive pulmonary disease (**COPD**). Most of these dampen the body's response to inflammation triggers such as dust, pollens, smoke, chemicals, and more.

- Long-acting beta-agonist (**LABA**) > are strong bronchodilators, opening up the bronchi and bronchioles.
- Leukotriene (**lew**-ko-**try**-enz) modifiers > are thought to block chemicals such as histamine and prostaglandin causing inflammation.
- Mast cell stabilizers > decrease the activity of specific white blood cells arising during inflammation. Like the leukotriene modifiers, decreasing inflammation lowers swelling allowing more air to pass.
- Theophylline (thee-**off**-i-lyn) > an older medication utilized as a bronchodilator. Levels must be followed to avoid adverse reactions.
- Immunomodulators (**im**-mew-no-**mod**-U-**lay**-tors) > these target specific immunologic protective mechanisms. By targeting eosinophils and IgE levels associated with severe allergies, the triggers will not start an asthma-type reaction.
- Corticosteroids (**kor**-ti-ko-**ster**-oyd) may be used as a spray, pill, or injection to decrease the body's response to allergic triggers.
- Antihistamines (**an**-tea-**his**-tah-meanz) > dry the secretions of the bronchial mucus opening up the airway a bit. This is true in the upper respiratory tract as well.
- Mucolytics (**mew**-ko-**lit**-iks) > break up or help liquify the thick mucus making it easier to cough and move air.

Antibiotics are the other medication set employed extensively in both the upper and lower respiratory tract to fight infections. Antibiotics are best used to limit or cure bacterial infections of the sinuses, ears, tonsils, adenoids, pharynx, larynx, tracheal, bronchials, and lung tissues (alveoli).

---

* **IMPORTANT NOTE: All discussions of medications are for basic education. A medical provider should be consulted on any medication options. Do <u>not</u> use this information for patient care.**

THE LUNGS

The **pulmonary** (**pul**-moe-nar-ee) **system** has many parts but the functional part moving oxygen into the bloodstream is the lungs – a pink, slightly spongy collection of millions of tiny balloons and air passages.

- **Pulmon/o** > lung > word root is used almost exclusively to indicate anatomy. The lungs fill the thorax minus other structures from apex at rib 1 to the base (when inhaling) of rib 10 (Figure 12.16).
  - Pulmonary edema > collection of interstitial fluid between tissues and alveoli.

- **Pneum/o** or **Pneumon/o** > air, breathing, or lungs > utilized extensively to describe disease of the lung or of breathing. Aer/o > air, gas is alternate term used primarily in the laboratory.
  - Pneumonia (new-**mow**-knee-ah) > inflammation of the lung tissues (alveoli), tending to consolidate in a specific lobe.
  - Pneumatocardia (**new**-mat-toe-**kar**-dee-a) > presence of air or gas in the blood of the heart.

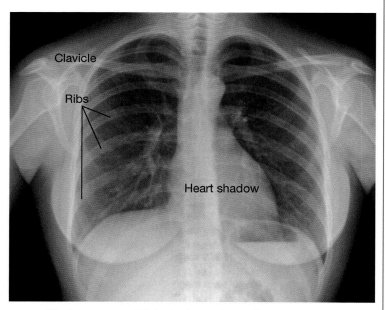

Black is pure air. White is dense tissue like bone. Grays are air in lung tissues.

Figure 12.16

12.23
Pn > Greek is normally a silent 'P'

Dyspnea (diss-**knee**-ah) > difficult breathing, an example of the silent 'p' with a consonant in front or the beginning of a word.

Orthopnea (or-**thop**-knee-ah) > having to sit up to breathe is an example of a hard 'p' because of the vowel (e, i, y).

Apnea (**ap**-knee-ah) > no breath

-pnea > breathing

Tachypnea > fast breathing

Bradypnea > slow breathing

Pneumococcus is a bacterium associated with respiratory infections.

- **Spir/o** > breathing > respiration is repetitive breathing. The average adult has 12–17 cycles of respiration every 60 seconds.
  - Inspiration > to breathe in.
  - Expiration > to breathe out.

LIKE ALERT!

Spir/o also means to coil or coil-shaped. It is used to describe bacteria of the genus *Spirillum*. A spirochete (**spy**-row-keet) is a flexible, spiralling bacterium. Syphilis and Lyme's disease are caused by spirochetes.

 What is the word root found in 'respiratory' therapist?

 The pulmonary pleura is irritated causing subcostal pain. What does the term 'pulmonary' mean?

 Jose had a partal pneumograph. What did the machine measure?

12.24
Spir- > to breathe

12.25
Pertaining to the lungs
12.26
Lungs or air flow

Word building

 Using the word roots with the linking vowel to build as many valid terms with the suffixes given. Please define each term.

Pneum/o or Pneumat/o Laryng/o

-logy –ous –logist –oma –tomy –it is –osis

12.27
The instructor has the list!

The lungs are partitioned by lobes. The right side has three lobes: superior, middle, and inferior. The right lung is slightly higher because the large, solid liver is pushing up on it. The left lung has two lobes: superior and inferior, with the cardiac notch (room for the heart).

Lob/o > a division > the lung lobes provide divisions used to identify location of conditions such as pneumonia, lung masses, or foreign bodies.

- **Lobectomy** (low-**bek**-toe-me) > surgical removal of a lobe.

Atelectasis (**at**-eh-**lek**-tah-sis) > 'incomplete extension'; it is essentially a complete or partial collapse of a lobe (Figure 12.17). It is like crumbled plastic wrap that can no longer be separated. It is also called a 'lung scar'. The effect is loss of air motion in this part of the lobe.

12.28
Lobes are not unique to the lungs. The brain has five distinct divisions. There are ear lobes and lobes of the liver.

LLL > left lower lobe; **LUL** > left upper lobe; **RLL** > right lower lobe; **RML** > right middle lobe; **RUL** > right upper lobe

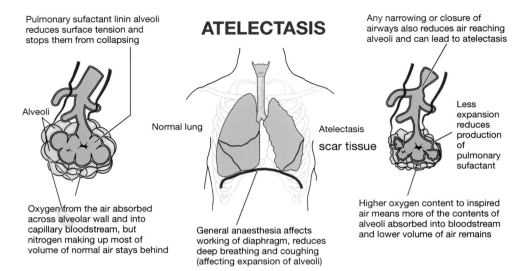

Pulmonary sufactant linin alveoli reduces surface tension and stops them from collapsing

ATELECTASIS

Any narrowing or closure of airways also reduces air reaching alveoli and can lead to atelectasis

Alveoli

Normal lung

Atelectasis

scar tissue

Less expansion reduces production of pulmonary sufactant

Oxygen from the air absorbed across alveolar wall and into capillary bloodstream, but nitrogen making up most of volume of normal air stays behind

General anaesthesia affects working of diaphragm, reduces deep breathing and coughing (affecting expansion of alveoli)

Higher oxygen content to inspired air means more of the contents of alveoli absorbed into bloodstream and lower volume of air remains

Figure 12.17

The lung's primary responsibility is to exchange life-giving gases at the alveolar level. The vital gases are oxygen and carbon dioxide (Figure 12.18).

- **Ox/o** > oxygen, **O** is the chemical designation. Each of the four hemoglobin protein structures of a red blood cell will hold one million oxygen molecules.
  - **Hypoxia** (hi-**pok**-see-ah) > abnormally low levels of oxygen in arterial blood. Synonym: hypoxemia.
  - **Anoxia** (an-**ock**-see-ah) > absence of oxygen. Synonym: anoxemia. Both persistent hypoxia and anoxia can be life threatening.

A '**pulse ox**' is the estimated oxygen saturation (**O$_2$ sat**) measured by looking at the red blood cells flowing at the finger or toe tips or an ear lobe. A pulse ox of 92% or less is concerning.

- **Capn/o** > carbon dioxide or smoke, **CO$_2$** is the chemical designation. This is a waste gas, blown out with each expiration.
  - **Hypercapnia** (hi-purr-**kap**-knee-ah) > abnormal elevation of CO$_2$ in the arterial blood indicating either respiratory and/or renal disorders. COPD patients have chronic hypercapnia because they cannot exhale completely.
  - **Hypocapnia** (hi-poe-**kap**-knee-ah) > abnormal decrease in arterial CO$_2$ associated with hyperventilation. Anxiety and illness induce the patient to breathe too fast, blowing off too much CO$_2$. The fix is slowing the breathing and rebreathing the air (using a paper bag).

12.29
Note the exception of adding a prefix directly to the word root:

Hypo- > under, less than and Ox/o > oxygen. Only one 'o' is used hypoxia.

O$_2$ and CO$_2$ are properly written as O$_2$ and CO$_2$ (subscript) but are seen regularly in both configurations.

Arterial blood gases (**ABG**) provide partial pressure levels of O$_2$ (**PaO$_2$**) and **PaCO$_2$**. It also provides a HCO$_3$ (bicarbonate) level to buffer the acidity of the blood. The pH is a measure of hydrogen ions, a healthy pH is between 7.35–7.45

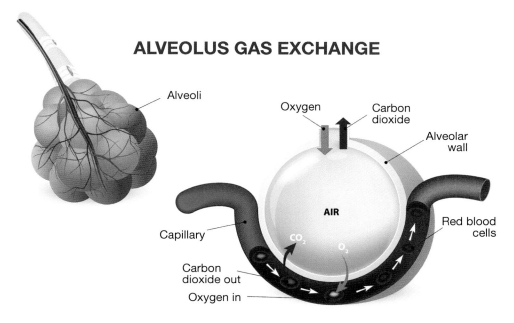

ALVEOLUS GAS EXCHANGE

Alveoli

Oxygen

Carbon dioxide

Alveolar wall

Capillary

AIR

CO_2

O_2

Red blood cells

Carbon dioxide out

Oxygen in

Figure 12.18

The **diaphragm** (**die**-ah-fram) > large muscle providing the negative pressure motion to pull air into the tubes and alveoli (Figure 12.19). Inspiration is the contraction of the muscle. Exhalation is generally by gravity and elastic recoil. Inhalation can be increased by use of the accessory muscles:

12.30

- Sternocleidomastoid (**ster**-no-**klie**-eh-doe-**mas**-toyd) muscles > neck muscles.

- External intercostal muscles > rib muscles.

To push more air out (exhale), to shout, or sing, or cough, these muscles help empty the lungs.

- Internal intercostal muscles > rib muscles.

- Abdominal muscles.

The function of the diaphragm and accessory muscle is obviously essential for breathing, but their activity during illness gives providers' clinical clues. An asthmatic patient will pull air in deeply, activating all the inspiratory muscles. The COPD and emphysema (**em**-fi-**see**-mah) patient will drape themselves over a table to expand the chest as much as possible to force gases out. Emphysema stretches out the alveoli, becoming like a flabby balloon – no elasticity to empty the lungs.

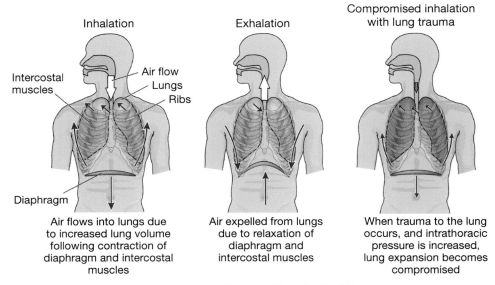

Inhalation

Exhalation

Compromised inhalation with lung trauma

Intercostal muscles

Air flow
Lungs
Ribs

Diaphragm

Air flows into lungs due to increased lung volume following contraction of diaphragm and intercostal muscles

Air expelled from lungs due to relaxation of diaphragm and intercostal muscles

When trauma to the lung occurs, and intrathoracic pressure is increased, lung expansion becomes compromised

DIAPHRAGM > PHREN/O

Figure 12.19

- **Phren/o** > diaphragm > used exclusively to describe the phrenic nerve innervating the muscle. Trauma to the right or left phrenic nerve or the spinal cord injury at C2 or C3 can paralyze breathing.

LIKE ALERT!
Phren/o also means 'mind' as it is the 'seat of emotions' (the heart sits on the diaphragm), from the Greek.

Kitchen lab

The intercostal muscles (between the ribs) are at 90-degree angles from each other. They keep the rib cage from flaring out during inhalation or collapsing during exhalation. Place your hands on your rib cage and take some slow, deep breaths. Can you feel the contractions?

The pulmonary pleura (**plur**-ah) is the double-layer membrane surrounding the lung in conjunction with the heart pleura (pericardium) and the diaphragm. This allows them to work in unison and decrease the friction of non-stop motion.

- **Pleur/o** > side of rib > the two pleural layers slide over each with respiration.
  - Visceral pleura touches the organ, in this case the surface of the lungs.
  - Parietal pleura touches the inside wall of the thoracic cage, the ribs.
  - The potential space is between the two layers.
- **Pleurisy** (**plur**-i-see) or **pleuritis** (**plur**-eye-tis) > inflammation of the pleura, instead of moving easily it is more like Velcro pulling.
- **Pneumothorax** (**new**-moe-**thor**-aks) > when the potential space fills with air between the layers, it crushes the tissue as it enlarges (Figure 12.20). Dyspnea results.
  - Hemothorax (**he**-moe-**thor**-aks) > when the potential space fills with blood. This patient may exhibit hemoptysis (he-**mop**-tea-sis) > spitting or coughing up blood.

PNEUMOTHORAX > AIR IN THE CHEST

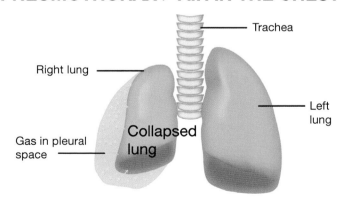

Figure 12.20

- **Pleurodesis** (plur-ow-**dee**-sis) > artificial production of scar tissue of the pleura to seal a reoccurring pneumothorax or hemothorax.

12.31

A pleural effusion is when fluid fills the potential space. It may create a pleural friction rub easily heard by stethoscope or felt as a vibration, pleural fremitus.

Pneum/o > air, lung

Thorac/o > chest

Cost/o > ribs

Hem/o > blood

-cele > hernia

-clysis > wash out

-centesis > to draw out by puncture

-desis > binding together

-lysis > destruction

-genic > beginning, formation

-ptysis > spitting

✓ Kevin has a stitch in his right lateral chest. It hurts when he takes in a deep breath, like Velcro pulling. This is _____ .

12.32
pleurisy or pleuritis

✓ A phrenectomy will remove the nerve to the _____ .

12.33
diaphragm

✓ What is the proper medical term for 'low level of oxygen' in the arterial blood?

12.34
Hypoxia or hypoxemia

Word building

Using the word roots with the linking vowel to build as many valid terms with the suffixes given. Please define each term.

Lob/o Pleur/o Hem/o or Hemat/o

–ectomy –cele –clysis –ptysis –itis –al

12.35
The instructor has the list!

9/11/2001 SURVEILLANCE*

On 9/11/2001 mankind experienced another tragedy of violence on a mass scale, with the attack on the World Trade Center in New York City (NYC). There were thousands of deaths and injuries and the effects are and will be felt well into the future. Tons of debris caused by the collapse of the towers generated enormous levels of concrete dust, and an estimated 2,500 contaminants which were inhaled by responders and citizens alike. The Centers of Disease Control and Prevention (**CDC**) is tracking the effects of the widespread contamination illustrated by the plume caught on radar (Figure 12.21).

From the first responders to the survivors in the NYC area, over 75,000 people are being tracked for 15 primary disease processes and dozens of other conditions. By far, lung fibrosis, scarring of the lung tissue due to silicosis, is a typical finding. The method used to track all the possible ramifications of this incident is via the ICD coding of the conditions. Like those exposed to Ebola or Zika due to travel, the question is asked of all NYC patients if they were exposed in or around the date of 9/11/2001. This flags their diagnoses to the CDC. Examples would include:

Reactive airways dysfunction syndrome (RADS) > J68.3

Silicosis > chronic, massive peribronchial > J62.8

Lymphoid leukemia > C91.92

Multiple myeloma > C90.0

Tracheobronchitis, chronic > J42

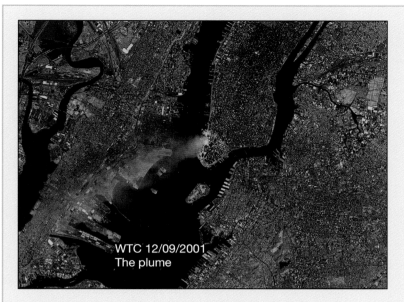

WTC 12/09/2001
The plume

Figure 12.21

When these codes and many others are entered during an office visit, they are also tagged with the code for 'Terrorism, secondary effects' > Y38.9. Documentation and the ICD system allows researchers and clinicians to track and treat the diseases associated with the event no matter where in the world the patient may travel.

★ **IMPORTANT NOTE: The reader is notified that these examples are from an on-line search done in 2016. Do <u>not</u> use these codes for patient care episodes, coding, or billing; look up the new ones!**

LUNG CONDITIONS

Pneumon**ia** is the term used to describe an infection of the lungs, its tissue, the alveoli, and bronchioles. There are 30+ causes with four classification sets:

- **Bacterial** infections may be triggered by a weakened immune system: age, poor nutrition, and other illnesses. These are treated with oral or intravenous antibiotics. Cure for each episode is the usual.
  - *Streptococcus* (**strep**-toe-**kock**-us) *pneumoniae* is seen most frequently.
  - *Staphylococcus aureus* (**staf**-ee-loe-**kock**-us **aw**-ree-us).
  - *Haemophilus influenzae* (he-**mof**-ee-lus in-**flew**-en-za).

12.36
Strept/o > curve, twisted
Staphyl/o > grapes, as in bunches of
Cocc/i > round
Vir/o > virus
Bacteri/o > bacteria
Myc/o > fungus

- **Viral** infections occur frequently. There are no curative antiviral medications but they can diminish the viral load and decrease the severity.
  - Influenza (**in**-flew-**en**-zah).
  - Adenovirus (**ad**-eh-no-**vie**-rus).
  - Coronavirus (kor-**row**-no-**vie**-rus).

- **Fungal** infections are not as common and they tend to be harder to treat. Fungal infections begin by inhaling spores found in the dirt. The treatment is with Amphotericin B (am-foe-**ter**-i-**sin** B).
  - Histoplasmosis (**his**-toe-plaz-**mow**-sis)
  - *Cryptococcus* (krip-tow-**kock**-us)
  - Coccidioidomycosis (kok-**sid**-ee-**oy**-doe-my-**ko**-sis)

- **Atypical** pneumonias range from what is termed 'walking pneumonia' to deadly epidemics due to a perfect storm in the environment.
  - Legionnaires' (**lee**-jo-**narz**) disease.
  - *Mycoplasma* (**mi**-ko-**plaz**-ma) *pneumoniae* > 'walking pneumonia' or 'community acquired pneumonia' are alternate names.
  - *Chlamydophila* (kla-**mid**-oh-**fil**-a) pneumonia.
  - *Pneumocystis* (**new**-mow-**cis**-tis) *pneumonia* (**PCP**) > seen in immunocompromised patients.
  - Mycobacterium tuberculosis (tu-**ber**-Q-**low**-sis) > **TB** can affect any tissues of the body and is seen in the lungs (Figure 12.22). It creates cavities by destroying entire areas

Most pneumonias no matter the cause are associated with:

Cough

Fatigue/Weakness

Fever

Shaking chills

Night sweats

Shortness of breath (**SOB**) or dyspnea especially dyspnea on exertion (**DOE**)

Anorexia

Sputum (**spew**-tum) production. Sputum is the debris (pus) of the pneumonia being moved up and out by bronchial cilia and the cough.

Hemoptysis > blood in the sputum

Chest X-rays (CXR), CT scans, MRI can all be used to help define the location and severity of the infection. Cultures (**C&S**) or biopsy is definitive.

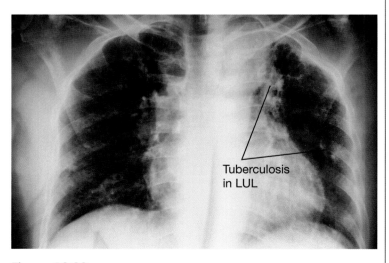

Tuberculosis in LUL

Figure 12.22

of alveoli. It is seen in immunocompromised patients and is becoming drug resistant. An **acid-fast bacterium** (**AFB**) test can help identify TB; a culture is definitive. A skin test, **PPD** (purified protein derivative) screens for exposure to TB.

- Other causes of pneumonia are irritants weakening the pulmonary system such as dust, inhaled food, liquids, chemicals, or smoke.

- **Sarcoidosis** (**sahr**-koy-**doe**-sis) > a chronic inflammatory disease of unknown origin; it is associated with granular nodules in the lungs and lymph nodes. Many patients are asymptomatic.

Lung cancer continues to be a major killer worldwide due to tobacco use and exposures to toxic dusts and chemicals (Figure 12.23). In fact, most lung cancers or carcinomas (**kar**-sin-**oh**-mas) are **bronchogenic**, beginning in the bronchi or bronchioles. Carcin/o > cancer, generally a malignant tumor.

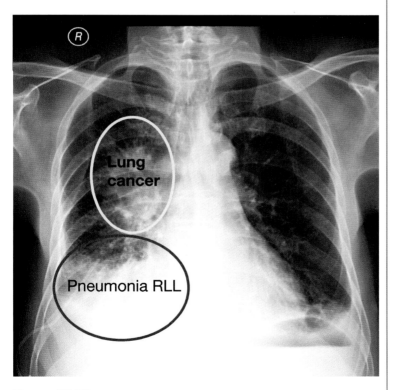

Figure 12.23

12.37

Did You Know?

There is no redeeming value in the use of tobacco products. Each cigarette has a complex mix of over 4,000 chemicals and toxins. Repeated attacks on the protective mechanisms of the respiratory system lead to chronic inflammation. Recurrent inflammation and the genetic damage to cell replication incite cancer production.

- **Non-small cell lung cancer** (**NSCLC**) accounts for approximately 85%, and there are three types.:
  - – Adenocarcinoma (**ad**-eh-no-kar-**sin**-oh-ma) tends to begin on the periphery of the lungs and is more likely to spread via the lymph nodes > aden/o.
  - – **Squamous cell** carcinoma occurs toward the center of the chest in the epithelial layers of the bronchi, which fight inflammation and damage from tobacco in particular.
  - – **Large cell** carcinoma or undifferentiated, fortunately, is rare because it tends to be aggressive, with distant metastasis.
- **Small cell lung carcinoma** (**SCLC**) is considered the most aggressive and is strongly related to tobacco smoking. It metastasizes rapidly to liver, bone, and brain.
- **Mesothelioma** (**mez**-oh-**thee**-lee-oh-ma) is associated with exposure to asbestos (as-**bes**-toes). It arises in the pleura and it is malignant.

Inhaling dust, fumes, or chemicals can set up a chronic inflammation in the respiratory system. These are due to occupational exposures even in weekend do-it-yourself folks. This is a short list.

- Pneumoconiosis (**new**-mow-ko-knee-**oh**-sis) or Black Lung is from coal dust. The term may be used for other dusts as well.
- Silicosis (**seal**-ee-**ko**-sis) > inhalation of sand dust of any type.
- Organic dust such as farm dust, sugar, or cotton or flour dust.
  - – Byssinosis (**bis**-ee-**no**-sis) > inhalation of cotton dust.
  - – Bagassosis (**bag**-ah-**sew**-sis) > sugar cane dust.
  - – Farmer's lung > plant matter with dust.
  - – Bird handler's lung > droppings and feathers.
- Burning organic materials: wood, leaves, dung, or trash.
- Gases can include ammonia and bleach, but also inhaled gases from burning plastics and oils, such as:
  - – Carbon dioxide > foundry work.
  - – Ozone > aircraft workers, arc welding.

12.38
All inhalation disease tends to present the same way with inflammation, cough, and eventually dyspnea as the COPD progresses.

Prevention, especially in occupational exposures, is part of the mandate from OSHA, Occupational Safety and Health Administration.

Circle the viral cause for a pneumonia.

Streptococcus Asbestos Influenza Tuberculosis

 Myc/o/bacteri/um > what is the meaning of each of the word roots.

✓ Mesothelioma is most commonly caused by _____
.

12.39
Influenza

12.40
Myc/o > fungus and
bacteri/o > bacteria

12.41
asbestos

The respiratory systems can create a myriad of **sounds**. These are terms used for these sounds and some other diagnostic terms.

- **Wheezing** (**we**-zing) is usually described as musical and tends to be a higher pitch. Occurs with obstruction such as asthma. Occurs with both inspiration and expiration.

- **Rhonchi** (**rong**-ki) are similar to a wheeze but deeper in tone and can be continuous or intermittent. Heard with pneumonias.

- **Rales** (rahls) are intermittent bubbling sounds or rattles with inspiration.

- **Crackles** (**krak**-els) are the sound of rice crisps in milk, popping sounds which tend to be a deeper tone. Linked with pneumonia and TB.

- **Stridor** (**stri**-dur) is a deep, discordant whistle because the air is struggling to squeak by. Epiglottitis, croup, and a foreign body tend to present with stridor.

- **Friction rub** or crepitus sounds like Velcro being pulled apart; associated with pleurisy, pulmonary embolisms, edema, or lung masses.

12.42
Prior to the invention of X-rays, watching the chest rise (observation), percussion (tapping), and auscultation (listening) with or without a stethoscope was the only way to define pulmonary illness. Crepitus can also describe a sensation of crackling under the skin which can occur with a pneumothorax.

Auscultation (**aws**-kul-**tay**-shun) methods utilize the stethoscope > chest scope to listen to the air flow or sounds.

- **Pectoriloquy** (**pek**-toe-**real**-oh-kwee) > a whisper is generally not heard until it passes through a consolidation, a more solid area of the lung indicating pneumonia or mass-effect. Pect/o > chest and −loquy > Latin, to speak.

- **Egophony** (ee-**gof**-oh-knee) > the patient says an 'E' but is heard as an 'A' with consolidation of fluid, pneumonia, or mass.

- **Bronchophony** (bronk-**off**-oh-knee) > increased clarity and intensity when the spoken word passes through an area of consolidation.

12.43
Auscultation and percussion is done over several areas of the lungs to evaluate each lobe, base, and apices.

Percussion (purr-**kus**-shun) methods utilize tapping on the chest wall (anterior and posteriorly) to discern hollow (air-filled) versus dull (solid consolidation) (Figure 12.24). It is similar to finding the wood stud in a wall.

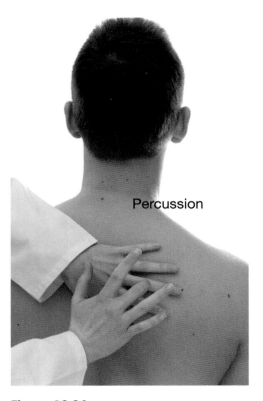

Percussion

Figure 12.24

The level of the diaphragm can be discerned using percussion by having the patient inhale and hold their breath. It creates approximately 2 inches of increased air-filled area. On expiration, it rises back into place. A mass or paralysis can change this side to side.

An apex is a point. **Apex** is the singular and **apices** is the plural. In the lungs, the apices are high at the clavicles. The apex of the heart is the tip found in the 5th intercostal space, mid-clavicular line (**5th ICS MCL**).

Diagnostics and abbreviations

- **Imaging** studies include:
  - **CXR** > chest X-ray, AP and Lateral.
  - **MRI** > magnetic resonance imaging.
  - **CT** > computerized tomography.
  - **PET** > positron emission tomography.

12.44
Imaging studies are not unique to the respiratory system, except the V/Q scan is used to

– **V/Q scan** > ventilation-perfusion scan is done with a nuclear medicine tracer following the blood volume and rate as it is exchanging its gases.

• **Abbreviations**

– **CF** > cystic fibrosis (**cis**-tik fi-**bro**-sis), congenital metabolic disorder associated with abnormally high secretions causing pulmonary congestion and edema.

– **CPAP** > continuous positive airway pressure is used to treat obstructive sleep apnea (**OSA**) and respiratory support.

– **CPR** > cardiopulmonary resuscitation.

– **C&S** > culture and sensitivity of sputum, nasal smear, throat culture (**TC**), or products of a bronchoscope lavage.

– **MDI** > metered-dose inhaler used by asthma, COPD, and emphysema patients.

evaluate pulmonary embolism (**PE**) > a blood clot in a pulmonary artery or arteriole that is blocking the function of a section of the lobe.

UNIT SUMMARY

1 The respiratory system begins at the nose and mouth in a repeating cycle of moving air deep to the lung tissues, 15 times a minute for life. The primary function of the system is exchange of oxygen and carbon dioxide with the bloodstream.

2 The upper respiratory structures are the nose (rhin/o or nas/o), mouth (or/o or stomat/o), throat (pharyng/o), voice box (laryng/o), tonsils (tonsill/o), and adenoids (aden/o). The function is to moisturize, warm, and filter the air on its way to the lungs.

3 The lower respiratory structures are the windpipe (trache/o), large airway tube (bronchi/o), the smaller airway tubes (bronchiol/o), and the tiny air-basins (alveol/o). From the trachea to the tiny bronchioles the function continues to be to filter and moisturize the air into the alveoli where the gas exchange takes place.

4 Supporting structures enable the air to move in and out (respirations). These include the diaphragm (phren/o), ribs (cost/o), and the pleural (pleur/o) membranes. When the diaphragm contracts the lungs are pulled down pulling air in, requiring muscle action. Expiration is done primarily by the elastic recoil though expiratory muscle can increase the push-out to give a louder voice.

5 The respiratory system is susceptible to two major condition sets: pneumonias and inhalation damage from dust, smoke, chemicals, and other toxins. Pneumonia triggers include bacterial, viral, fungal, and the

atypical presentations such as tuberculosis (TB) and sarcoidosis. The cardiorespiratory illnesses include pulmonary edema and pulmonary embolism.

6   Respiratory carcinoma from throat cancer to mesothelioma arises due to repeated injury from agents diminishing the protective mechanism of the system. Tobacco, occupational exposures, and immunodeficiencies lead to cancers.

7   Respiratory medications are designed to keep the airway open and gas exchange happening. Antibiotics are used to treat bacterial infections. Bronchodilators and mucolytics are used to keep the airways open and clear.

8   Documentation of symptoms, their timing, and severity helps make a diagnosis. Laboratory and diagnostic imaging can confirm illness or injury. The CDC and other agencies track those codes when respiratory illnesses are caused by natural disasters or terrorism acts such as those of 9/11/2001 in New York City, the Pentagon, and a field in Pennsylvania.

UNIT WORD PARTS

Word roots with linking vowel		
Aden/o > node, lymph node	Alveol/o > tiny basin	Antr/o > small room, entry
Arteri/o > artery	Bronchi/o or Bronchiol/o > airway tubes	Capill/o > capillary
Capn/o > carbon dioxide (CO_2)	Glott/o > opening	Laryng/o > voice box, larynx
Lob/o > lobe	Muc/o > sticky liquid	Nas/o or Rhin/o > nose
Phren/o > diaphragm	Pleur/o > side of rib	Pneum/o, Pneumon/o > lung, air
Pulmon/o > lung	Or/o or Stomat/o > mouth	Spir/o > breathe
Tonsill/o > tonsil	Trache/o > windpipe	Uvul/o > small grape

Prefixes: attached to the front of the word root to change meaning		
A-, An- > no, not, absent	Bi- > two	Brady- > slow
Dys- > bad, poor, difficult	Endo-, In- > inside	Epi- > on top of
Hyper- > increased, more	Hypo- > under, less than	Inter- > between
Ortho- > straight	Para- > surround, near	Tachy- > fast

Suffixes change the meaning of the word, linking vowel is usually 'o' with consonants		
-algia or –dynia > pain	-cele > hernia	-centesis > puncture, remove fluid
-desis > bind together	-ectomy > surgical removal, to cut out	-lysis > destruction, break down
-osis > abnormal condition	-ostomy > new opening	-ous > condition of
-pathy > disease	-pexy > fix in place	-phasia > speech
-plasty > repair	-ptysis > spitting	-rrhagia > hemorrhage
-rrhea > discharge, runny	-scope, -scopy > instrument to look, process of	-stenosis > narrowing

Acronyms, abbreviations, and initial sets		
ABG > arterial blood gases	AFB > acid fast bacilli	C&S > culture and sensitivity
CF > cystic fibrosis	COPD > chronic obstructive pulmonary disease	CPAP > continuous positive airway pressure
CPR > cardiopulmonary resuscitation	CXR > chest X-ray	DOE > dyspnea on exertion
DPT > diphtheria, pertussis, and tetanus vaccination	ET > endotracheal tube	LLL > left lower lobe
LUL > left upper lobe	MDI > meter-dosed inhaler	PCP > pneumocystis pneumoniae
PE > pulmonary embolism	PFT > pulmonary function tests (PFS (studies))	PND > post nasal drip or paroxysmal nocturnal dyspnea
PPD > purified protein derivative (TB skin test)	RLL > right lower lobe	RML > right middle lobe
RSV > respiratory syncytial virus	RUL > right upper lobe	SOB > short of breath (dyspnea)
T&A > tonsillectomy and adenoidectomy	TB > tuberculosis bacillus	T/C or TC > throat culture

UNIT WORKSHEETS

Building terms: Use the proper prefix/word root/linking vowel/suffix as appropriate.

Example: to cut into the stomach > gastr/o/tomy

a) To bind together the pleura >   _____

b) Repair of a bronchus >   _____

c) Pertaining to tiny air sacs >   _____

d) To break up mucus >   _____

e) To cut into the trachea >   _____

f) Inflammation of the tonsils >   _____

g) On top of the opening (of the voice box) >   _____

h) Inflammation of the smallest air tubes >   _____

Know your initial sets/acronyms! For the initial set or acronym given, spell it out correctly.

a) SOB   _____

b) DOE   _____

c) ET   _____

d) PFT   _____

e) MDI   _____

f) RLL   _____

g) COPD   _____

h) RSV   _____

Best choice: Pick the most appropriate answer.

1   The term 'emphysema'

   a) refers to the maxillary sinuses

   b) associated with loss of elasticity of lungs

   c) mass effect of the pleura of the lungs

   d) creates rales under the skin

2   Wheezing

   a) Popping sounds

   b) Motion of the diaphragm

   c) Musical sounds

   d) Long E's to A

3   This atypical lung disease causes cavities in the lung tissues

   a) CF

   b) RSV

   c) COPD

   d) TB

4   A bronchogram will record the

   a) Lymph vessels

   b) Veins

   c) Arteries

   d) Airway tubes

5   Hemoptysis

   a) blood in the nose

   b) spitting blood

   c) blood in the voice box

   d) throat bleeding

Name the condition or term! Based on the description and/or function.

a) The pollution is extraordinarily tiny (2.5 μm) _____

b) This term means to 'split into two branches' _____

c) A painful mouth _____

d) John put a stone up his nose _____

e) A tube placed inside the windpipe to help a person breathe (two words)

   _____ _____

f) These larger nose hairs capture dust and debris _____

g) Difficult or poor breathing _____

Multiple correct: Select ALL the correct answers to the question or statement given.

1 Mark all structures associated with upper respiratory system?

a) Trachea

b) Ethmoid sinuses

c) Adenoids

d) Alveoli

e) Hypopharynx

f) Surfactant cells

2 Which of gases are exchanged at the alveolar level?

a) K^+

b) Cl^-

c) O_2

d) HCO_3

e) CO_2

3 Which of the following are medication groups is designed to open the bronchial tubes?

a) Beta-agonists

b) Mucolytics

c) Antibiotics

d) Theophyllines

e) Antihistamines

Spelling challenge! Circle the correct spelling based on the definition given.

1 'Inflammation of the windpipe and airway tubes'

Traceobrongitis   Bronchitracheoitis   Tracheobronchiti   Laryngobroncitis

2 Most common cause of bacterial pneumonia

Steptococcus   Stafococcus   Septococcus   Streptococcus

3 'Abnormal condition of fungus in the throat'

Farynomykosis   Pharyngomycosis   Pharynxomycosis   Mykopharyngosis

---

Define the term: Spelling *does* count in your definition too!

1 Atelectasis > _____

2 Cilia > _____

3 Rhonchi > _____

4 Pneumonitis > _____

5 Epistaxis > _____

6 Anoxia > _____

7 Bronchiostenosis > _____

8 Dysphasia > _____

Find it! Using the words in the table – match the definition given or answer the statement. Some may not be used. It is recommended you know all the choices.

apnea	leukotriene	orthopnea	laryngitis
spirometer	lobectomy	pleurisy	influenza
bronchoscopy	bradypnea	croup	corticosteroid
diaphragmatic	aerobic	silicosis	dyspneic

1 _____ The process of using an instrument to look at the airways

2 _____ An instrument to measure breathing

3 _____ To surgically remove a lobe of the lung

4 _____ A viral infection of the lungs

5 _____ Pertaining to the diaphragm

6 _____ No air

7 _____ Associated with a barking cough

8 _____ Having to sit up straight to breathe

Matching: Some will not be used.

	Letter	Defined as
Tonsillectomy		a) congenital disorder associated with excessive secretions
Mycoplasma pneumoniae		b) undifferentiated lung cancer, very aggressive
Adenocarcinoma		c) saying an E to see if it changes to an A when listening to the chest
Byssinosis		d) also called 'walking pneumonia'
Stridor		e) inflammation of the mouth
Egophony		f) condition caused by cotton dust
Cystic fibrosis		g) inhalation of asbestos fibers
Stomatitis		h) surgical removal of the tonsils
		i) cancer occurs on the periphery of the lungs
		j) deep discordant whistle of airway obstruction

An essay: Research what medical supplies might be needed for another large act of terrorism. What will we need and in what quantities?

Note challenge: Define the underlined terms. You may need to look up a few terms. Answer the questions which follow. The student is reminded this is an incomplete SOAP note used for the learning experience. Do not use this for patient encounters.

S. Daizha is a 47 yo woman with a deep, wet cough for the last 7 days. It is progressively worse with sputum production, <u>dyspnea</u> and 2 days of <u>orthopnea</u>. She is having night sweats, fever, and <u>anorexia</u>. She does smoke 1 pack of cigarettes a day for 20+ years. History of <u>asthma</u> in the past.

O. 47 yo female is in obvious distress. BP: 158/96 P: 102 R: 28 <u>Pulse Ox</u>: 89%

Heart: mild <u>tachycardia</u>, regular with no murmurs or gallops. Lungs: some use of accessory muscle for <u>inspiration</u> and <u>expiration</u>. <u>Percussion</u> changes in the RLL. There is <u>pectoriloquy</u> changes in the <u>RLL</u> and <u>rales</u> noted as well. <u>CXR</u>: <u>infiltration</u> in the RLL.

A. <u>Pneumonia</u>, RLL <u>etiology</u> unknown
Tobacco abuse
HTN

P. <u>PPD</u> ordered
Sputum <u>C&S</u> ordered
Begin <u>O</u>$_2$ by <u>NC</u> at 2 l/min

Questions:

1 Translate all the acronyms and give meaning to the words which are underlined in the note.

2 What are the different types of pneumonia possible in this patient?

3 Should you code the diagnosis of 'tobacco abuse'? Why or why not?

4 What is the anatomy associated with the diagnosis of 'pneumonia'?

Gastrointestinal system

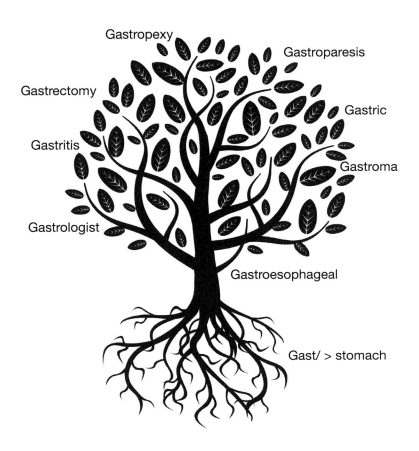

Gastropexy

Gastroparesis

Gastrectomy

Gastric

Gastritis

Gastroma

Gastrologist

Gastroesophageal

Gast/ > stomach

TARGETED LEARNING

1 Recognize word parts and assemble medical terms related to the gastrointestinal system.

2 Correctly construct, define, pronounce, and spell medical terms.

3 Link gastrointestinal illness and injury with appropriate pharmacotherapeutics and other therapeutic options.

4 Explore the unique terms associated with dental care.

5 Use the online resources to perform basic coding from ICD Index of Illness and Injury.

KEY WORD PARTS

Word roots with linking vowel	Prefixes	Suffixes
Chole/o > gall, bile	A-, An-	-algia
Col/o > colon	Brady-	-cele
Duoden/o > duodenum, C-loop	Dys-	-ectomy
Enter/o > small intestines (as a whole)	Endo-, In-	-itis
Esophag/o > esophagus	Epi-	-malacia
Gastr/o > stomach	Exo-	-ostomy
Hepat/o > liver	Hyper-	-paresis
Ile/o > ileum	Hypo-	-pathy
Intestin/o > intestines	Mal-	-plasty
Jejun/o > jejunum	Mega-	-rrhage
Pancreat/o > pancreas	Micro-	-rrhea
Stom/o or Stomat/o or Or/o > mouth, opening	Sub-	-tomy

FOOD

The alimentary canal is about 45 feet of mucus-lined tube; it sounds simple, a place where humans eat and process food. For humanity, food is actually multifaceted. Food and water intake is vital for living and an essential part of society. Unlike oxygen and the function of the heart and lungs, food intake is full of many choices. In some countries, the choices and abundance are so high many people suffer from obesity. Yet, in places in those same countries and others, people are starving to death with protein deficiency and clean water scarcity. This is one of the many areas when ethics intersects medicine, the inequality of food availability across all of society.

Documentation of food intake and its effect on the body is part of most visits. In pediatrics, if the child is 'eating, drinking, peeing, and pooing' a provider and parent can be less worried. The extremes of weight have a whole set of negative effects on a patient. Children, in particular, are susceptible to growth changes and learning disability when food is inadequate. Noting the appropriate diagnoses helps agencies such as the World Health Organization (WHO) determine where and when to recommend support of entire populations. The challenge is to spread the food and clean water to every population to maintain the health of all peoples.

THE ORAL CAVITY

Our **mouth** has several functions and structures. The digestive process of food is one of them. The teeth, salivary glands, tongue, lips, and cheeks contribute to making food into a bolus (**bow**-lus) to be swallowed (Figure 13.2).

- **Stom/o** or **Stomat/o** > mouth, opening or **Or**/o > mouth
  - **Stomatitis** (**stow**-mah-**tie**-tis) > inflammation of the mouth.
  - **Stoma** (**stow**-mah) > an opening, this may refer to the artificial opening of the colon to the skin level to bypass a portion of the colon as an example.
  - **Oral** (or-al) > pertaining to the mouth, the oral cavity. Or/o denotes anatomy or the oral language.

- **Gloss/o** or **Lingu/o** > tongue
  - **Glossitis** (glos-sigh-tis) > inflammation of the tongue.
  - **Glossotrichia** (glos-oh-**trik**-ee-ah) > hairy tongue occurs due to habit of chewing tobacco.
  - **Lingual** (**ling**-gwal) > pertaining to the tongue. Lingu/o denotes anatomy.

13.1
Suffixes:

-itis > inflammation

-pathy > disease

-plasty > repair

-algia > pain

-dynia > pain

-malacia > softening

-rrhea > discharge, flow

-rrhagia > bleeding

-al > pertaining to

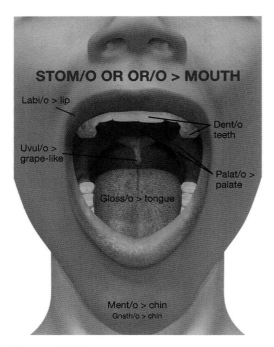

Figure 13.2

- **Sublingual** (sub-**ling**-gwal) > under the tongue > used typically for medication delivery.
- **Bucc/o** > cheeks > an important element for the act of chewing (mastication); these are essentially the lateral walls of the oral cavity.
  - Buccal (**buc**-kal) > pertaining to the cheeks.
- **Cheil/o** or **Labi/o** > lips > help with eating and speech.
  - **Cheiloschisis** (key-**low**-ski-sis) > cleft lip.
  - **Labiogingival** (**lay**-be-oh-**jin**-ji-val) > pertaining to the lips and gums.

Mastication (**mas**-ti-**kay**-shun) > the act of grinding and chewing food

Digestion (die-**jest**-shun) > to force apart, to break up

Absorption (ab-**sorp**-shun) > to take in, incorporate, to add to

The teeth sit in the alveoli (sockets) of the upper jaw (maxilla) and lower jaw (mandible) and provide the hard surfaces for grinding and tearing food. The gums (gingiva) are like suction cup material, helping the teeth to stay in place and protecting the roots.

- **Dent/o** or **Odont/o** > teeth > dentin is the ivory forming the major portion of the tooth (Figure 13.3).
  - Dental > pertaining to the teeth, used primarily to denote anatomy.

13.2

- Odontiasis (**o**-don-**tea**-ah-sis) > teething > multiple eruptions of baby teeth.
- Orthodontist (**or**-tho-**don**-tist) > specialist who straightens teeth.

TOOTH

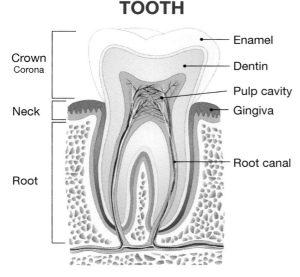

Crown
Corona

Neck

Root

Enamel

Dentin

Pulp cavity

Gingiva

Root canal

Figure 13.3

- **Gingiv/o** > gums of the teeth > used for both anatomy and disease.
  - Gingivitis (**jin**-ji-**vie**-tis) > inflammation of the gums can occur with vitamin deficiency or medication side effects.
- **Palat/o** > plate, palate > hard and soft palate form the upper area of the mouth cavity.
  - Palatoplasty (**pal**-ah-toe-plaz-tee) > repair of the palate is a surgery to effect snoring.
  - Palatoschisis (**pal**-ah-toe-**ski**-sis) > cleft palate.

There are three sets of **salivary** (**sal**-i-**ver**-ee) glands deep in the mucosa of the oral cavity. They produce a liter of saliva a day to moisten our mouth and help liquify food. Saliva contains alpha-amylase, which starts carbohydrate digestion. It also contains special bacteria destroying lysosomes (Figure 13.4).

13.3

-iasis > infestation, many of . . .

-ase > breaking up

Lith/o > stone

Doch/o > duct, passageway

SALIVARY > SIAL/O

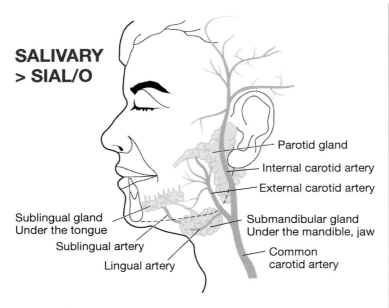

- Parotid gland
- Internal carotid artery
- External carotid artery
- Submandibular gland
  Under the mandible, jaw
- Common carotid artery

Sublingual gland
Under the tongue
Sublingual artery
Lingual artery

Figure 13.4

- **Sial/o** > saliva, salivary glands > three major sets
  - Sialolithiasis (**sigh**-ah-low-lee-**thigh**-ah-sis) > infestation of salivary gland stones.
  - Sialodochoplasty (**sigh**-ah-low-**do**-ko-**plaz**-tee) > repair of salivary ducts.

Lys/o > to break up (lysis)

Amyl/o > starch

Muc/o > mucus, sticky liquid

✓ Dilantin is a medication known to cause gingival hyperplasia. What does the term 'gingival' mean?

✓ Construct a medical term for 'tongue pain'.

✓ 'Odontopathy' means _____

13.4
Gums

13.5
Glossalgia or glossodynia
13.6
disease of the teeth

Word building

*Using the word roots **with the linking vowel to build as many valid terms with the suffixes given. Please define each term.***

Odont/o Sial/o Gloss/o

–logy –tomy –itis –ectomy –al –lysis

13.7
The instructor has the list!

DENTAL DOCUMENTATION

A dental examination has a very different look from the average SOAP note. Since teeth sit in round sockets and have a top or 'occlusive' surface, there are many directional notations required to describe their health. The universal system counts permanent teeth in numbers 1 to 32. The primary (baby) teeth are counted by the alphabet, A–T and the oral cavity with all of its surfaces is noted in double digits such as '10 upper right quadrant' or '40 lower right quadrant' (Figure 13.5).

Directions such as mesial (middle), distal, and apex (tip) of the tooth root are utilized extensively. Here are some terms unique to dental care.

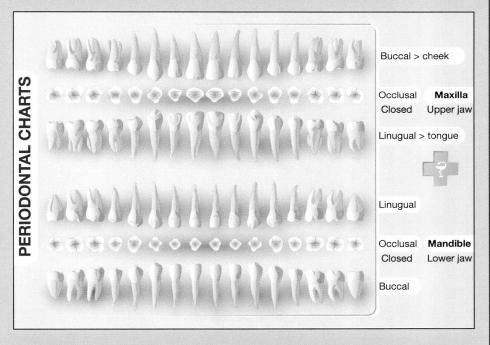

PERIODONTAL CHARTS

Buccal > cheek

Occlusal **Maxilla**
Closed Upper jaw

Lingual > tongue

Lingual

Occlusal **Mandible**
Closed Lower jaw

Buccal

Figure 13.5

- Incisal (in-**sigh**-zal) > pertaining to the biting edges of the incisor teeth.

- Malocclusion (**mal**-oh-**klue**-shun) > poor alignment of the bite or chewing.

- Interproximal > between neighboring surfaces of adjacent teeth.

- Cementum (seh-**men**-tum) > tough connective tissue surrounding the root of the tooth.

- Diastema (**die**-ah-**steh**-mah) > space between adjacent teeth.

- Orthognathic (**or**-thog-**nath**-ik) > pertaining to the 'straightness' between the maxilla and mandible (chin > gnath/o).

An X-ray of the teeth is called a bitewing radiograph; it is designed to reveal the coronal halves of both the upper and lower jaw. Like all bone X-rays, these can demonstrate bone erosion, cracks, fractures, chips, and malunions. The panoramic X-ray can locate oral masses and sialoliths (salivary stones).

As with all documentation, precision is required to ensure the next reader will understand the odontopathy. Continuity of care from provider to provider with proper coding and billing helps offer each patient quality care.

UPPER GASTROINTESTINAL (UGI)

The **alimentary** (**al**-i-**men**-tar-ee) canal begins at the esophagus and ends at the anus (Figure 13.6). It has several unique names and functions. The **esophagus** (eh-**sof**-ah-gus) carries the food bolus from the pharynx to the stomach, passing through the diaphragm.

- **Esophag/o** > gullet for food intake.
  - Esophagitis (eh-**sof**-ah-**jie**-tis) > inflammation of the esophagus.
  - Esophagogastroanastomosis (eh-**sof**-ah-go-**gas**-tro-ah-nas-toe-**mow**-sis) > surgical formation of a connection between the esophagus and stomach.
- **EGD**, Esophagogastroduodenoscopy (eh-**sof**-a-go-**gas**-tro-**due**-oh-deh-**nos**-ko-pee) > diagnostic procedure to evaluate the inner mucosal surface for masses, ulcers, bleeding, and other conditions.
- **Peristalsis** (**pear**-ee-**stal**-sis) > rhythmic squeezing moving food (the bolus) down the alimentary canal. Esophagospasm is the term used when the rhythm is broken.
- **Achalasia** (ak-ah-**lay**-zee-ah) > when a sphincter fails to relax, in the case of the lower esophageal sphincter (**LES**), this allows food to collect in the esophagus causing an esophagomegaly.
- **Regurgitation** (ree-**gur**-jeh-**tay**-shun) > to bring food up or burp gas (eructation).
- **Nausea** (**naw**-zee-ah) > sensation of a queasy stomach, the sensation of needing to vomit.
- **Vomiting** > emesis (**em**-e-sis) > violent expulsion of the chyme from the stomach. Emesis is both the product and the process.

13.8
The esophagus traverses the thorax behind the heart. The **TEE**, transesophageal echocardiogram allows the heart structures to be evaluated easily.

The esophagus can also generate pain with spasm and **GERD** can mimic heart disease.

An **anastomosis** is a connection procedure occurring in the GI system, but coronary artery bypass surgery utilizes it as well.

It may also be termed an –ostomy, creating a new opening.

UGI > upper gastrointestinal section (esophagus, stomach, and small intestine).

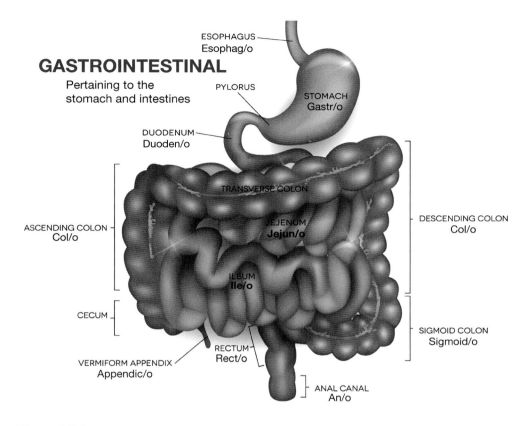

GASTROINTESTINAL

Pertaining to the stomach and intestines

ESOPHAGUS
Esophag/o

PYLORUS

STOMACH
Gastr/o

DUODENUM
Duoden/o

TRANSVERSE COLON

ASCENDING COLON
Col/o

JEJENUM
Jejun/o

DESCENDING COLON
Col/o

ILEUM
Ile/o

CECUM

SIGMOID COLON
Sigmoid/o

VERMIFORM APPENDIX
Appendic/o

RECTUM
Rect/o

ANAL CANAL
An/o

Figure 13.6

- **Hematemesis** (**he**-mah-**tem**-ee-sis) > bloody vomit associated with **UGI** bleeding. It can be bright red or coffee-ground appearance (older blood).

LGI > lower gastrointestinal section, the colon.

The **stomach** functions like a washing machine with both mechanical mixing and chemicals with enzymes. It actively churns from the **LES** to the pyloric sphincter. It is well protected – tucked under the left anterior ribs.

- **Gastr/o** > stomach or the belly.
  - Gastroenteritis (**gas**-tro-en-tur-**eye**-tis) > inflammation of the stomach and small intestines. **AGE** > Acute gastroenteritis, associated with diarrhea and vomiting.
  - Gastromegaly (**gas**-tro-**meg**-ah-lee) > overeating may cause enlargement of the stomach.

13.9

Suffixes

–itis > inflammation

–cele > hernia

–algia > pain

–dynia > pain

–tomy > to cut into

–ectomy > to cut out, remove

GASTROESOPHAGEAL REFLUX DISEASE
GERD

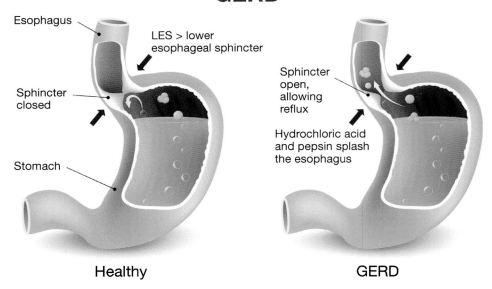

Figure 13.7

- Gastroparesis (**gas**-tro-**par**-ee-sis) > when the gut stops due to inflammation, injury, medication, or neurologic changes. Churning stops as does peristalsis.
- **GERD**, gastroesophageal reflux disease > when gastric acid is able to splash up into the esophagus (Figure 13.7).

• **Gastric ulcer** > peptic ulcers rarely occur in the stomach because the mucosa is designed for acid, BUT a *Helicobacter pylori* infection can make it happen.

• **Pyloric stenosis** (pie-**lor**-ik **sten**-oh-sis) > narrowing of the sphincter between the stomach and duodenum. It may be congenital or occur due to peptic ulcer disease (**PUD**).

The upper gastrointestinal area is investigated by:

- **UGI** > X-ray procedure; the patient swallows barium, which traces the alimentary canal from an esophageal swallow to a small bowel followup.
- **CT scan** or **MRI** > reveals masses or significant changes.
- **Nasogastric lavage** (**nay**-zo-**gas**-trik la-**vahj**) > irrigation of the stomach via a tube (**NG tube**) placed via the nasopharyngeal route.

–ic or –al > pertaining to

–oma > tumor

–logy > study of

–pathy > disease of

–paresis > paralysis

Peptic > pertaining to the stomach. Pept/o is digestion, from the Greek

Chyme (kime) > partially digested food, enzymes, and fluid mix of the stomach. A bolus becomes chyme.

Chyme nutrients are absorbed and the waste is called feces.

The **small intestine** is approximately 26 feet of the tube; it will finish digestion and absorb nutrients and water along its entire length. It has a name for the entire distance and three specific names as well:

- **Enter/o** > small intestines > beginning at the pyloric sphincter and ending at the ileal sphincter. The term is used for anatomic locations. Synonym: intestines. While there is an enteritis, there is no '*intestinitis*'. The word 'intestines' is used for anatomy only.

- **Duoden/o** > '12 finger-breadths (duo > two; den > ten)', this first and shortest piece of the small intestines is also called the **C-loop** (Figure 13.8) as it curves around the head of the pancreas. It will also communicate with the liver via the bile duct. It is a major area of digestion and absorption of nutrients into the bloodstream.
  - Duodenitis (**dew**-oh-**den**-eye-tis) > inflammation of the C-loop of the small intestines. This can be caused by **PUD**, infections, and autoimmune diseases.

13.10

Gest/o > to bear

Enter/o > intestines

Duoden/o > C-loop

Jejun/o > 2nd section of intestines

Ile/o > 3rd section of intestines

Hepat/o > liver

Pancreat/o > pancreas

Pylor/o > gate keeper, between stomach and duodenum

LIKE ALERT!

Ile/o > Ileum, is the 3rd portion of the small intestines.

Ili/o > top section of the pelvic bone. They are pronounced the same and look very similar.

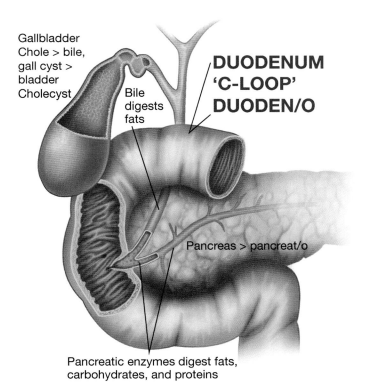

Gallbladder
Chole > bile,
gall cyst >
bladder
Cholecyst

Bile digests fats

DUODENUM 'C-LOOP' DUODEN/O

Pancreas > pancreat/o

Pancreatic enzymes digest fats, carbohydrates, and proteins

Figure 13.8

- **Jejun/o** > Latin for 'empty', is the second section of the small intestines. It is not empty but its job is to continue absorption of nutrients and water, thus becoming increasingly empty.

  − Jejunoplasty (jeh-**jun**-oh-plaz-tee) > repair of the jejunum.

- **Ile/o** > near the groin, the ileum > third and last section of the small intestines. It is found in the **RLQ**. The ileocecal sphincter carries the leftover chyme into the cecum where it is properly called **feces** (**fee**-seez).

- **Sphincter** (**sfink**-tur) > a band, like a purse string > the GI tract has several rate limiters which open and close depending on hormonal, mechanical, and some voluntary controls.

- **Microvilli** (**my**-krow-**vil**-lie) > tiny finger-like structures on the surface of the small intestines, which increase the surface area for absorption. They are most dense in the duodenum and almost absent in the ileum (Figure 13.9).

- **Lacteal** (**lak**-teels) > specialized lymph tissue residing in the center of each microvilli. It absorbs **chyle** (kile) (emulsified fat) from the duodenum (Figure 13.9).

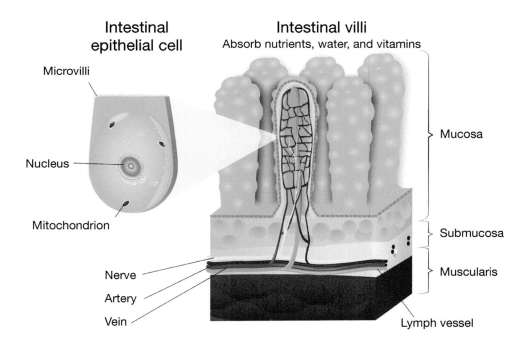

Figure 13.9

Kitchen lab

Look around the house and find things functioning like the GI tract.

Example: When a toothpaste tube is squeezed > peristalsis. Are there structures which increase surface area? Discuss with your instructor.

 On an X-ray exam Amelia's small intestine is enlarged with air and fluid lines. The proper term of an 'enlarged intestine' is?

13.11
Enteromegaly

 Construct a medical term meaning 'a new opening of the jejunum'.

13.12
Jejunostomy

Tang's stomach has stopped its mechanical action; this would be properly called?

13.13
Gastroparesis

Word building

Using the word roots ***with the linking vowel to build as many valid terms with the*** suffixes ***given. Please define each term.***

Esophag/o Gastr/o Duoden/o

–itis –ostomy –malacia –dynia –tomy –oma

13.14
The instructor has the list!

CODING PRACTICE

The gastrointestinal tract comes with many conditions, infections, and injuries. Use the internet to look up the ICD codes from the list given below. Use the *Index of Illness and Injury* exclusively. As stated, this text will not make the student a coder but the exercise will illustrate the importance of proper documentation and spelling. Look under the finding (caries, ulcer) first. Check your work with your instructor.

- Sialolithiasis
- Leukoplakia (buccal)
- Acute gastric ulcer with both hemorrhage and perforation
- Adult hypertrophic pyloric stenosis
- Dental caries on smooth surface limited to enamel
- Achalasia (esophagus), congenital
- Hematemesis, newborn, neonatal
- Diverticulum of the esophagus, acquired

LOWER GASTROINTESTINAL

The **colon** or **large intestine** is approximately 15 feet of the tube. It is larger and functions to move feces out and reabsorb water and other elements on the path. There are five distinct areas.

- **Col/o** > colon (**ko**-lon), large intestines > colon/o is an alternative.

COLON > COL/O
5 DISTINCT AREAS

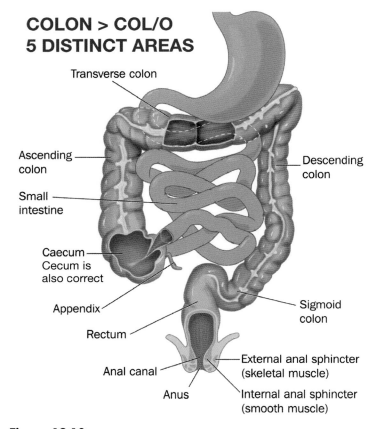

Transverse colon

Ascending colon

Descending colon

Small intestine

Caecum
Cecum is also correct

Appendix

Sigmoid colon

Rectum

Anal canal

External anal sphincter (skeletal muscle)

Anus

Internal anal sphincter (smooth muscle)

Figure 13.10

13.15

RUQ > right upper quadrant > liver, gallbladder, ascending colon.

RLQ > right lower quadrant > ascending colon, appendix, ovary, kidney, and ureter.

LUQ > left upper quadrant > stomach, spleen, pancreas, descending colon.

LLQ > descending and sigmoid colon, kidney, ureter, ovary.

Epigastrium > stomach, pancreatic head, major vessels

Pubic region > bladder, uterus or prostate, ureters, rectum, and anus.

Umbilical region > small intestines (jejunum), abdominal aorta, and vena cava.

- **Ascending colon** > the first section begins in the **RLQ** and ascends to the hepatic (liver) flexure. A flexure is a turn.
  - Cec/o > cecum > blind corner, Figure 13.10 demonstrates that the cecum is closed at the base with the appendix hanging from it.
  - Appendic/o > to hang down > appendix is lymph tissue designed to capture and process pathogens via the lymphatics.

- **Transverse colon** > second section begins at the hepatic flexure to the splenic flexure. It hangs like a volleyball net between the two poles.

- **Descending colon** > third section begins at the splenic flexure to the slight medial turn of the sigmoid colon.

- **Sigmoid/o** > 'like an S', sigmoid colon > S-shaped section takes the colon from the far and deep lateral wall toward the midline.

- **Rect/o** > straight > rectal colon or rectum > short, fifth section serves to store feces until evacuation.

col/o or colon/o terms:

- Colonoscopy (ko-lon-os-ko-pee) > instrument to look into the colon.

- Colectomy (ko-lek-toe-me) > surgical removal of the colon, usually partial.

- Colostomy (ko-**los**-toe-me) > surgically create a new opening, typically bringing the colon up to skin level for evacuation into a colostomy bag.

- Colopexy (**ko**-low-pek-zee) > surgically fix the colon in place.

- Colorectal (**ko**-low-**rek**-tal) > pertaining to the descending colon and rectal area.

The **anus** (**a**-nus) > last part of the tube, only one to two inches long. It has two sets of muscles, involuntary and voluntary.

- **An/o** > exit orifice for the digestive tract > the anus (ani is plural) has both internal smooth muscles under control of the nervous system and external skeletal muscles permitting voluntary control of defecation (Figure 13.11).

- **Hemorrhoids** (**hem**-or-oydz) > the varicose (**var**-i-kos) veins of the anus. Compression of the veins from constipation or sitting too long causes enlargement and stasis.

- **Constipation** (**kon**-sti-**pay**-shun) > infrequent bowel movements tend to be small and hard.

- **Defecation** (**def**-eh-**kay**-shun) > discharge of feces, a bowel movement or 'stooling'.

- **Diarrhea** (**die**-ah-**ree**-ah) > 'flow through', the passage of watery stool on a regular basis. A defense mechanism to wash irritants out of the system.

13.16
A digital rectal exam (**DRE**) allows the provider to feel the sphincter tone (neurological) and check for internal hemorrhoids and other masses. In men, the posterior prostate is palpated through the rectal wall.

An anoscope is a short scope to look at the anal mucosa.

A rectoscope is similar, just a bit longer.

ANUS > AN/O

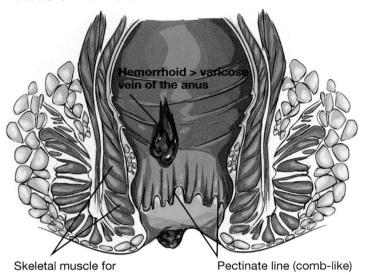

Hemorrhoid > varicose vein of the anus

Skeletal muscle for voluntary release of waste

Pectinate line (comb-like)

A **hemoccult** is a method to check stools for blood. Stools can be investigated for worms and other foreign invaders.

Figure 13.11

- **Hematochezia** (**hem**-ah-toe-**key**-zi-ah) > passage of bloody stool, bright red from local mass or hemorrhoids.

- **Melena** (meh-**leh**-nah) > passage of tarry (black) stool indicating bleeding higher up the GI tract.

Other terms associated with the GI tract include:

- **Haustra** (**haw**s-trah) > pouches > the colon has a series of these pouches pushing the feces up and around and enabling water reabsorption. Haustrum is singular.

- **Diverticula** (**die**-ver-**tik**-U-lah) > hernias of the mucosa and submucosal layers of the colon. These occur due to repeated stress against the walls (constipation). Diverticulum is singular.
  - Diverticulosis > abnormal condition of 'turning away' (Figure 13.12).

- **Volvulus** (**vol**-vyu-lus) > twisting of the intestines causing an obstruction.

- **Intussusception** (**in**-tu-sue-**sep**-shun) > telescoping of the intestine on itself, causing an obstruction. Currant-like stool (blood + mucus).

- **Obstruction** (ob-**struk**-shun) > blockage of any sort from masses, stool impaction, volvulus, or intussusception.

13.17
With the exception of haustra, all these terms can occur anywhere along the alimentary canal.

Obstipation (**ob**-sti-**pay**-shun) > an obstruction due to severe constipation. It can cause a **megacolon** (**meh**-ga-**ko**-lon) > enlarged colon.

Adynamic > no motion

DIVERTICULOSIS AND DIVERTICULITIS

To divert > to turn away

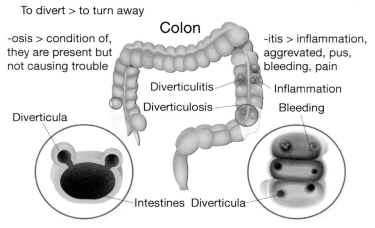

-osis > condition of, they are present but not causing trouble

Colon

-itis > inflammation, aggrevated, pus, bleeding, pain

Diverticulitis

Diverticulosis

Inflammation

Bleeding

Diverticula

Intestines Diverticula

Figure 13.12

- **Ileus** (**il**-ee-us) > mechanical or adynamic obstruction of the intestines. Associated with cramping pain, distention, and vomiting. **Do not confuse ileus** with ileum (3rd section of small intestines) or ilium, the top bony portion of the pelvis.

Cancers of the gastrointestinal tract account for a high number of deaths worldwide yearly. Caught early, cure is possible but most are not found early and they tend to metastasize.

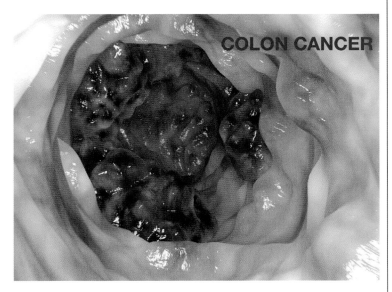

COLON CANCER

Figure 13.13

13.18
A **colonoscopy** is the study most recommended to evaluate the entire colon for polyps and cancers. Diverticula may be seen as well. This allows visualization of changes and enables biopsy and polypectomy.

A **BAE**, barium enema is an X-ray study. It is often done first, prior to a CT or MRI.

- **Esophageal cancer** occurs more frequently in Asia, but in the USA the incidence is rising due to tobacco abuse.
  - Squamous cell carcinoma (**SCC**) affects the upper two-thirds of the esophagus.
  - Adenocarcinoma tends to affect the lower one-third and is seen in industrialized countries.
- **Gastric cancer** (adenocarcinoma) is the 2nd most common cause of death worldwide.
- **Colon cancer** tends to increase due to aging. Adenocarcinoma generally begins in the descending colon or the rectum. The mass effect begins to affect stool passage and is associated with occult bleeding (Figure 13.13).

The **GI polyp** (pol-ip) > mass of tissue protruding outward from the inner mucosal surface anywhere along the alimentary canal. It may have a broad base, appearing flat (sessile) or slightly mobile on a stalk as noted in Figure 13.14.

- **Benign polyps** (non-cancerous) in limited numbers is a normal finding.
- **Polyposis** (**pol**-ee-**poe**-sis) > abnormal condition of multiple polyps; these are more likely to be converted to a cancer.

13.19
A colonoscopy is recommended every five years after age 50.

Polyps may occur anywhere in the body including on the skin.

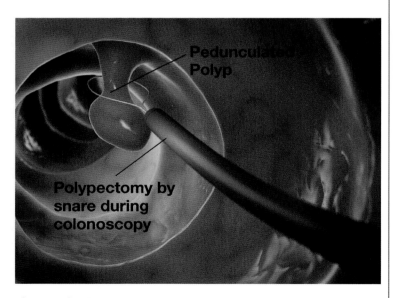

Figure 13.14

✓ Following a partial colectomy, the surgeon created a new opening for the colon, moving it out to the skin level. This is properly called a _____ .

✓ The proper medical term for 'black tarry stools'.

✓ Which section of the colon would have a rectal polyp?

13.20
colostomy

13.21
Melena

13.22
5th section

Word building

Using the word roots *with the linking vowel to build as many valid terms with the suffixes given. Please define each term.*

Col/o An/o Rect/o

–itis –ostomy –centesis –pexy –plasty
–tomy –ectomy

13.23
The instructor has the list!

Crohn's (kronz) **disease** > inflammatory bowel disease (**IBD**), a specific type as described by Dr. Crohn in the 1930s. It is thought to be an autoimmune disease with some environmental and bacterial triggers (Figure 13.15). Synonyms: **Regional enteritis** because it is

13.24
A stool evaluation can help define the two IBD types. Crohn's stools tend to be like oatmeal with fatty stools (steatorrhea). **UC** tends to produce bloody stools with mucus.

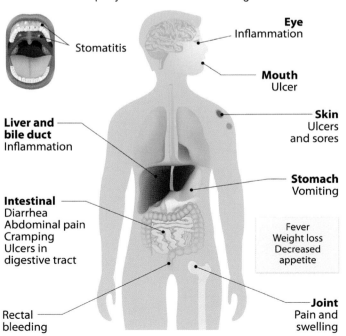

CROHN'S DISEASE
Crohn's is an eponym. It is also known as regional enteritis

Stomatitis

Eye
Inflammation

Mouth
Ulcer

Skin
Ulcers and sores

Liver and bile duct
Inflammation

Stomach
Vomiting

Intestinal
Diarrhea
Abdominal pain
Cramping
Ulcers in digestive tract

Fever
Weight loss
Decreased appetite

Rectal bleeding

Joint
Pain and swelling

Figure 13.15

seen in the ileum, characterized by thickening intestinal walls, longitudinal ulcers, bleeding, and weight loss.

Ulcerative Colitis (ul-sir-ah-tiv ko-**lie**-tis) (**UC**) > inflammatory bowel disease (**IBD**), a specific type related to the colon more than the small intestines. The symptoms are similar to Crohn's disease. The distinction is between the location and microscopic changes noted from biopsy.

Irritable bowel syndrome (IBS) > specific to the motility of the colon. In the past it was called a 'nervous stomach' or 'stress gut'. Unlike the two **IBD** disorders it is NOT associated with major inflammation or bleeding. All of the patterns are characterized by cramping, bloating, and gas (flatulence). Pain seems to be associated with a heightened perception of colonic motion.

- Alternating diarrhea/constipation pattern.

- Diarrhea pattern.

- Constipation pattern.

13.25
Triggers for IBS may include foods, stress, and hormone changes. Almost all teens or adults will have an IBS episode at some time.

Mesenteric (mes-en-ter–ik) **Artery Ischemia** (is-**key**-me-ah) > loss of blood supply to either the superior or inferior mesenteric artery. These supply the small intestines and colon. It is characterized by severe abdominal pain after eating and diarrhea (Figure 13.16).

13.26
Mesentery > middle area of the peritoneum, the double-layer sac holding much of the intestines. Similar to the pulmonary pleura and the pericardial sac.

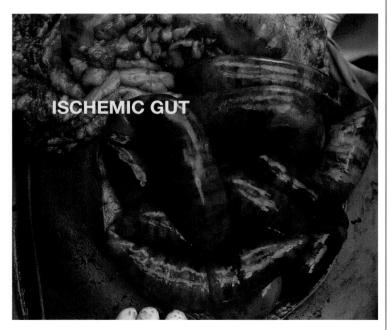

ISCHEMIC GUT

Figure 13.16
Blood loss turns intestines deep purple, it is necrotic.

MEDICATIONS AND THE GI TRACT*

As often as people eat and drink on a daily basis, so to is medication ingested in tablets, capsules, liquids, and sublingually. With rare exceptions, the process by which medication works to control pain or hypertension or diabetes or allergies is dependent on the GI tract. Illness can slow absorption making a medication less likely to work. Medications can also change the flora of the gut, killing the good bacteria along with the bad and causing diarrhea. Some foods with medications don't mix. Here are some specific effects of medications and the GI tract:

- Antihistamines dry fluids (mucus) – utilized for allergies and sneezing but they can cause the gut to slow, drying out the mouth (xerostomia) and promoting constipation.

- Narcotics work well to control pain in a variety of areas but they do slow the gut and severe constipation is a serious side effect. It needs to be considered during their use.

- Anti-ulcer and GERD medications work by turning off the chemistry of the stomach, decreasing the work of pepsin and hydrochloric acid. This does decrease the likelihood of GERD or ulcer but it also affects the absorption of B_{12} from our foods.

- Statins, HMG-CoA reductase inhibitors are a type of lipid-lowering medication. The liver makes cholesterol (HDL, LDL, and VLDL) on purpose as the foundation of many hormones and proteins. When adjusting the liver's function to decrease the bad guys' LDLs, liver damage may occur. They can also cause muscle soreness and damage.

This is just a small survey on the importance of understanding the pros and cons of any medication use. While it may accomplish the goal, it is impacting the gastrointestinal tract and other areas of the body as well. Documentation of allergies, food choices, and other medications is vital to the safe delivery of care.

★ IMPORTANT NOTE: All discussions of medications are for basic education. A medical provider should be consulted on any medication options. Do <u>not</u> use this information for patient care.

ACCESSORY GLANDS TO DIGESTION

The accessory organs of digestion are the **liver** and the **pancreas**. These are involved in both the digestion of food and the use of the absorbed nutrients.

- **Hepat/o** > liver > largest solid organ of the body. It is responsible for detoxification of absorbed products, processing most medications and alcohol, and producing a variety of proteins. The proteins will build hormones and cholesterols (Figure 13.17).

Liver, Gallbladder, Pancreas, and Bile Passage

HEPAT/O > LIVER

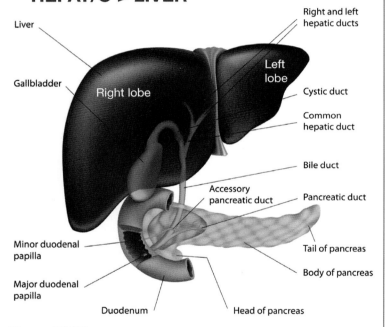

Figure 13.17

- **Hepatitis** (**hep**-ah-**tie**-tis) > inflammation of the liver. This can include any disease process and also reflect specific viral infections:
  - o Hepatitis A > mild, food-borne, and person to person.
  - o Hepatitis B > serious, blood-borne.
  - o Hepatitis C > potentially serious, converts to liver cancer, blood-borne.
  - o There is Hepatitis D, E, F, G, and perhaps an H.

- Hepat**oma** (**hep**-ah-**toe**-mah) > tumor of the liver. While the liver can be the primary site of a carcinoma, especially in patients with Hepatitis C, it is frequently a secondary cancer with metastasis from lung, breast, or colon cancers.

- Hepat**omegaly** (**hep**-at-oh-**meg**-ah-lee) > enlargement of the liver > quite painful due to the tough connective tissue capsule surrounding it.

- **Ascites** (ah-**sigh**-teez) > accumulation of fluids in the peritoneal sac secondary to liver failure. It is essentially a backup of fluids.

- **Anasarca** (**an**-ah-**sahr**-ka) > systemic infiltration of fluids into all the subcutaneous tissues (body-wide edema) associated with heart and/or liver failure.

- **Cirrhosis** (**sear**-oh-sis) > Abnormal condition of the liver (cirrh = yellow in Latin). This term is used for a chronically ill liver due to conditions such as alcohol, medication overdoses, or viral illnesses.

- **Jaundice** (**jahn**-dis) > collection of bile pigments in the dermis and eye sclera indicating liver malfunction.

The liver's many functions can be evaluated by various serum laboratory studies (Figure 13.18).

- **Albumin** (al-**bu**-min) > most abundant protein produced by the liver. Hypoalbuminemia (**hi**-poe-al-**bu**-mi-**knee**-me-ah) will cause ascites and anasarca as albumin is vital to fluid balance in the body. Hyperalbuminemia may indicate dehydration or a high-protein diet.

- **Alkaline phosphatase** (**al**-ka-lin **fos**-fa-taz) (liver ALP) may be elevated with cholecystitis, fatty liver, and drug intoxication.

- **ALT** > alanine transaminase > elevation indicates inflammation or damage to hepatic cells. This is often temporary. Statin medications may cause mild elevations.

- **AST** > aspartate transaminase > elevation indicates inflammation or damage to hepatic cells.

- **Bilirubin**, Total > found in bile, this is the breakdown of old RBCs, a function of the liver. Hyperbilirubinemia (**hi**-purr-**bil**-ee-rue-bi-**knee**-me-ah) indicates inflammation (hepatitis) or cirrhosis.

- **Protein**, Total > combination measure of the albumin and globulin proteins. Lower levels can indicate injury such as bleeding or burns. High levels indicate chronic inflammation such as Hepatitis C or multiple myeloma.

13.28
Transaminases (tranz-**am**-ee-naz) > These are catalytic enzymes. They are important in the synthesis of 20 amino acids – the building blocks for proteins utilized throughout the body for all cell functions.

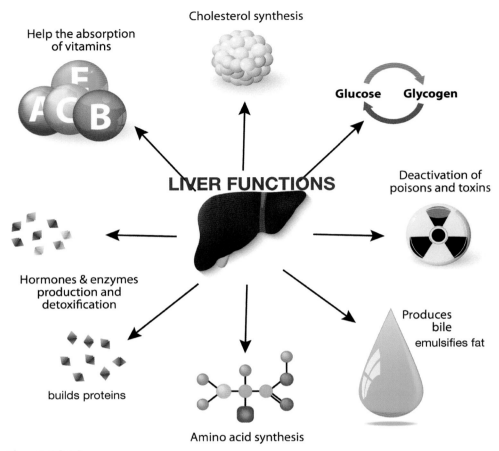

Help the absorption of vitamins

Cholesterol synthesis

Glucose   Glycogen

LIVER FUNCTIONS

Deactivation of poisons and toxins

Hormones & enzymes production and detoxification

Produces bile emulsifies fat

builds proteins

Amino acid synthesis

Figure 13.18

Cholesterol (ko-**les**-tur-ol) > lipoprotein (fat + protein) and the most abundant steroid of the human body. It combines with other proteins to create sexual and stress-related hormones (Figure 13.19).

- **HDL-C** > high-density lipoprotein > the good cholesterol. It begins the transportation of fats for cell replication and repair. It also cleans up LDLs.

- **LDL-C** > low-density lipoprotein > the so-called sticky bad cholesterol, this is essentially the leftover fatty part of the molecule. It is part of the negative process of atherosclerosis of blood vessels.

Triglyceride (tri-**glis**-ur-ide) > most abundant fat of the body made up of a glycerol and three fatty acids; this is 'stored' fat. Because of their composition they may be converted by the liver into glucose (glyconeogenesis) when food is scarce for energy.

13.29

Lip/o > fat

Prote/o > protein

Ather/o > porridge

Steroids and hormones are complex proteins affecting body tissues.

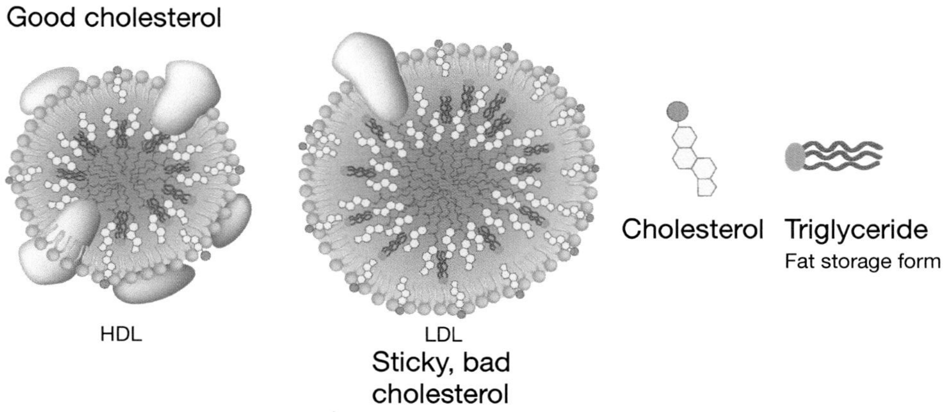

Good cholesterol

HDL

LDL

Sticky, bad cholesterol

Cholesterol   Triglyceride
Fat storage form

Figure 13.19

The Gallbladder (**GB**) > storage sac for the bile the liver produces. There are three linking forms (Figure 13.20):

- **Chole/o** or **Chol/o** > bile or gall > formed by the liver, bile may go directly to the duodenum via the common bile duct or be stored by the gallbladder. Bile is an emulsifier; it breaks down fats like soap breaks up grease on dishes.

- **Cyst/o** > bladder, sac > bile sac is stimulated by the presence of fat in the chyme. The sac contracts to push bile into the common bile duct. Cyst- is NOT unique to the gallbladder – the urinary bladder also uses this word root.
    - Cholecystitis (**ko**-leh-sis-**tie**-tis) > inflammation of the bile sac (gallbladder).
    - Cholecystokinin (**ko**-leh-**sis**-toe-**ki**-nin) (**CCK**) > GI hormone released by the duodenum in the presence of a fatty meal. It stimulates the gallbladder to release bile.

- **Doch/o** > duct, passageway > refers to any small passageway.
    - Choledocholith (**ko**-leh-**doe**-ko-lith) > stone in the bile duct.
    - Choledocholithotripsy (**ko**-leh-doe-ko-**lith**-oh-trip-see) > to break up (fragment) the stone in the bile duct, -tripsy > to break up, done chemically or by ultrasound vibration.

- **Chol**angiogram (ko-lan-gee-oh-gram) > record of the study of the bile duct. Angi/o > vessel.

- A **GB ultrasound** (**US**) > uses sound waves to reveal echoes of choleliths (gall stones).

13.30
The compound linking form 'cholecyst/o' has many possible suffixes:

–tomy > to cut into

–ectomy > to remove

–ostomy > to create a new opening

–centesis > to puncture, remove fluid

–tripsy > to break up

–ectasia > dilation

–pexy > to fix in place

–gram > the record

–graphy > process of recording

–plasty > to repair

GALLBLADDER > CHOLECYST

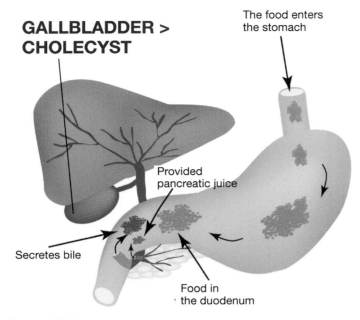

The food enters the stomach

Provided pancreatic juice

Secretes bile

Food in the duodenum

Figure 13.20

PANCREAS > PANCREAT/O

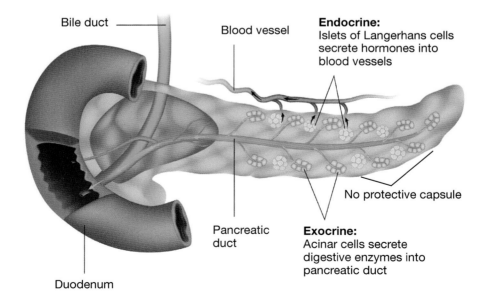

Bile duct

Blood vessel

Endocrine:
Islets of Langerhans cells secrete hormones into blood vessels

No protective capsule

Pancreatic duct

Exocrine:
Acinar cells secrete digestive enzymes into pancreatic duct

Duodenum

Figure 13.21

The **pancreas** > smallish, friable, un-encapsulated organ; its primary function is producing a variety of digestive enzymes and hormones which impact protein, carbohydrate, and fats (Figure 13.21).

- Pancreat/**o** > pancreas, sweetbread > elongated and deep in the retroperitoneum stretching from the duodenum to the spleen.

  - Pancreat**itis** (**pan**-kree-ah-**tie**-tis) > inflammation of the pancreas. It is associated with some medications, alcoholism, tobacco use, and the presence of gallbladder disease.

  - Pancreat**ic** (**pan**-kree-at-ik) **cancer** > arises in the exocrine glands of the pancreas. Because there is no capsule to distend and cause pain, cancer here tends to be silent. In fact, it is found because of symptoms caused by metastasis to other areas such as the bone, liver, brain, and lungs.

  - Pancreat**ectomy** (**pan**-kree-ah-**tek**-toe-me) > excision or removal of a part of the pancreas.

The pancreas may be investigated by an **ERCP** > endoscopic retrograde cholangiopancreatography. A CT scan and/or MRI can evaluate the entire area as well including the liver, duodenum, and pancreas with all related ducts.

The **peritoneum** (**pear**-i-toe-**knee**-um) > to stretch over > double-layer serous membrane lining the abdomen and covers most of its organs (Figure 13.22). It is similar in function to the pleura of the lung and pericardial sac of the heart. The linking form is **periton/o**:

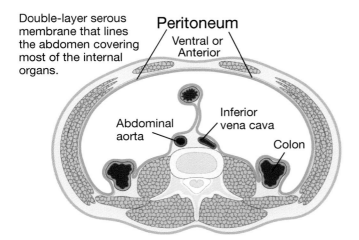

Double-layer serous membrane that lines the abdomen covering most of the internal organs.

Peritoneum
Ventral or Anterior

Abdominal aorta

Inferior vena cava

Colon

Retroperitoneal
Behind the peritoneum
Dorsum or Posterior

13.31

The pancreas is both an endocrine organ and exocrine organ.

Endo- > inside

Crin/o > to secrete

These are the hormones regulating glucose levels: insulin and Glucagon.

13.32

Did You Know?

In the presence of renal (kidney) failure, **periton**eal **dialysis (PD)** is used to remove waste toxins. A dialysis solution is introduced, left to absorb toxins and then removed.

Figure 13.22

- **Peritonitis** (**pear**-i-toe-**nigh**-tis) > inflammation of the peritoneal sac or space due to inflammation of another organ such as the appendix, or to enteritis.

- **Peritoneal lavage** or **peritoneoclysis** (**pear**-i-toe-knee-oh-**klie**-sis) > to flush out or rinse the peritoneum to remove pus and debris.

- **Retroperitoneal** (**ret**-row-**pear**-i-toe-kneel) > behind the peritoneum > the ascending colon, descending colon, pancreas, and the kidneys with the adrenal glands are protected and steadied by this deep position in the trunk.

✓ Construct a medical term meaning 'tumor of the bile vessel'.

✓ A 'hepatocyte' is a _____?

✓ '-clysis' means _____ .

13.33
Cholangioma

13.34 liver cell

13.35 to irrigate or rinse out

Word building

 *Using the word roots **with the linking vowel to build as many valid terms with the suffixes given.** Please define each term.*

Cholecyst/o Hepat/o Pancreat/o

-logy –centesis –lith –ostomy –clysis
–ectomy –itis

13.36
The instructor has the list!

The chemistry of digestion is seen in laboratory reports for a variety of reasons. These three complex molecules make up the macronutrients required to live and two of the hormones balance the use of those nutrients.

- **Carbohydrates** (**kahr**-bow-**hi**-draytz) > sugars and starches in our foods > contain carbon, hydrogen, and oxygen. The body runs on two major elements: glucose and oxygen.
  - **Amylase** (**am**-il-ace) > enzyme breaks down carbohydrates. Two types: salivary and pancreatic.
  - **Glucose** (**glue**-kose) > functional carbohydrate used by all cells for energy production in the mitochondria making ATP. It requires insulin to move into the cells.

- **Protein** (**pro**-teen) > combination of amino acids, nitrogen, carbon, hydrogen, and carboxyl group. Vital to all cell activities including repair and replication.

13.37
Gluc/o, Glyc/o > sugar, glucose

Prote/o > protein

Adip/o or Lip/o > fat

Steat/o > oil

–ase > to break down

Macro- > large

Micro- > small

- Proteins are denatured (broken apart) by the **pepsin** in the stomach; this initiates digestion.
- Proteases (pro-**tee**-ayses) > two enzymes to break down proteins are secreted by the exocrine functions of the pancreas.
    - o **Trypsin** (**trip**-sin) > enzyme to break down proteins to esters, amides, and peptides.
    - o **Chymotrypsin** (**ki**-mow-**trip**-sin) > enzyme to break down proteins.

- **Fats** are required for a number of vital life functions such as building and repairing all cell walls.
    - **Bile** > acts as a detergent to break up fats, like dish soap. It is produced by the liver.
    - **Lipase** (**lie**-pace) > enzyme breaks fats into monoglyceride (**mon**-oh-**glis**-er-ides) and two fatty acids. This is produced by the pancreas as well, allowing the lacteals to absorb fats into the circulation.

Insulin (in-**sue**-lin) > endocrine hormone secreted by the pancreas. It reduces the level of glucose in the blood by enabling glucose to cross into the cells.

Glucagon (**glue**-ka-gon) > endocrine hormone secreted by the pancreas. It increases the level of glucose in the blood from stored energy when food is not available, such as during sleep or fasting.

Laboratory tests:

Serum amylase

Serum lipase

Serum glucose

Serum insulin levels and **HgbA1C**

Serum glucagon level

 How many word roots are used in the term 'cholangiopancreatogram'?

 Wayne has been diagnosed with a hepatomegaly. What is the meaning of the medical term?

✓ An accumulation of fluid in the abdomen (peritoneum) is called _____ .

13.38 Three: Chol/o, Angi/o, and Pancreat/o

13.39 Enlarged liver

13.40 ascites

UNIT SUMMARY

1   The gastrointestinal system begins at the mouth and ends as the anus.
     The long and varied tube is also called the alimentary canal. Each section
     has a specific anatomy and function permitting humans to ingest, digest,
     and absorb food nutrients vital for living. There are a multitude of linking
     forms.

2   The upper gastrointestinal (**UGI**) area includes the mouth, salivary glands,
     teeth, tongue, lips, and cheeks of the oral cavity. Working together, a
     food bolus is formed and swallowed. The esophagus carries the bolus to
     the gastrum, the stomach, for mechanical and chemical digestion. The
     small intestine will continue digestion with the aid of enzymes from the
     pancreas and liver and absorption of nutrients will take place.

3   The lower gastrointestinal tract is made up of the five sections of the colon
     and the end point for waste, the anus. Its primary duty is to move waste
     along the path while reabsorbing water and other elements.

4   The liver has a variety of functions, from building new proteins and
     cholesterol from the nutrients to detoxifying ingested elements and
     medications. A healthy liver is required for living. Disease of the liver is
     described as hepatitis (acute) or cirrhosis (chronic). Bile is produced by the
     liver to break up fats in the duodenum.

5   The pancreas is also a major accessory digestive organ vital to nutrition.
     The powerful exocrine enzymes digest all of the major nutrients: fats,
     proteins, and carbohydrates. The endocrine hormones are vital to glucose
     metabolism in every cell: insulin and glucagon.

6   Diseases of the GI tract are many including cancers, infections,
     infestations, with acute and chronic inflammation. Medications can help
     but they do affect many other systems as well and most will be processed
     through the busy liver.

7   Documentation of anatomy, functions, and distress is vital from dental
     to anal care. Precision in noting diet, medications, and allergies is vital to
     proper continuity of care.

UNIT WORD PARTS

Word roots with linking vowel		
Adip/o; Lip/o > fat	Amyl/o > starch	An/o > anus
Bucc/o > cheek	Cheil/o; Labi/o > lips	Chole/o or Chol/o> bile or gall
Col/o or Colon/o > colon	Cyst/o > bladder, sack	Dent/o; Odont/o > teeth
Doch/o > passage, tunnel	Duoden/o > C-loop	Enter/o > small intestines
Esophag/o > gullet, food tube	Gastr/o > stomach	Gingiv/o > gums
Gloss/o; Lingu/o > tongue	Gluc/o; Glyc/o > glucose, sugar	Gnath/o or Ment/o > chin
Hepat/o > liver	Ile/o > 3rd section of small intestines	Jejun/o > empty, 2nd section of small intestines
Muc/o > sticky liquid	Or/o; Stomat/o > mouth, opening	Palat/o > palate (hard and soft)
Pancreat/o > pancreas, sweetbread	Prote/o > protein	Pylor/o > gatekeeper
Rect/o > rectum	Sial/o > salivary	Steat/o > oily

Prefixes: attached to the front of the word root to change meaning		
A-, An- > no, not, absent	Brady- > slow	Dys- > difficult, poor, painful
Endo-, In- > inside	Epi- > on top, upon	Exo- > outside, outer
Hyper- > more, increased	Hypo- > less, under, decreased	Mal- > bad, poor
Mega- > large	Micro- > small, smallest	Para- > surrounding, near
Peri- > around, near	Sub- > under, below	Tachy- > fast

Suffixes change the meaning of the word, linking vowel is usually 'o' with consonants		
-cele > hernia	-ectomy > to cut out, remove	-iasis > infestation, many
-itis > inflammation	-logy > knowledge of	-lytic or lysis > to break down
-malacia > softening	-megaly > enlargement	-osis > abnormal condition of
-ostomy > to create a new opening	-paresis > paralysis, stopping	-pathy > disease
-plasty > to repair	-rrhagia > bleeding	-rrhea > discharge, runny
-schsis > split, cleft	-stasis > to stop	-tomy > to cut into

Acronyms, abbreviations, and initial sets		
ALT and AST > liver function test	ANA > Antinuclear antibody	BAE > barium enema, X-ray procedure
CT > computerized tomogram	DRE > digital rectal exam	EGD > esophagogastro-duodenoscopy
ERCP > endoscopic retrograde cholangio-pancreatogram	GERD > gastroesophageal reflux disease	HDL > high-density lipoproteins
Hep A, B, C . . . > hepatitis A, B, C > viral illness of the liver	HgbA1C > hemoglobin A1C	IBD > inflammatory bowel disease
IBS > irritable bowel syndrome	LDL > low-density lipoproteins	MRI > magnetic resonance imaging
NG Tube > nasogastric tube	PD > peritoneal dialysis	PUD > peptic ulcer disease
SCC > squamous cell carcinoma	UC > ulcerative colitis	UGI > upper gastro-intestinal (X-ray procedure)

UNIT WORKSHEETS

Building terms: Use the proper prefix/word root/linking vowel/suffix as appropriate.

    Example: to cut into the heart > cardi/o/tomy

a) Teething, multiple eruptions of the teeth >   _____

b) Sialolithiasis >   _____

c) The study of the stomach >   _____

d) To break up fat >   _____

e) To cut a new opening in the jejunum >   _____

f) Tumor of the liver >   _____

g) To stop bile >   _____

h) To break down proteins >   _____

Know your initial sets/acronyms! For the initial set or acronym given, spell it out correctly.

a) ERCP   _____

b) DRE   _____

c) BAE   _____

d) UC   _____

e) RUQ   _____

f) IBD   _____

g) SCC   _____

h) LDL   _____

Best choice: Pick the most appropriate answer.

1 The term 'hematochezia'

    a) refers to vomiting blood   c) urination of blood

    b) passage of bloody stool   d) stopping bleeding

2 Cirrhosis

    a) Abnormal stomach lining   c) Chronic liver damage

    b) Autoimmune condition of colon   d) Fungal infection of duodenum

3 Ileus
   a) obstruction of intestines
   b) top portion of pelvis
   c) outpouching of colon
   d) pouches which enable peristalsis

4 A cholecystogram will investigate the
   a) Pancreas
   b) Gallbladder
   c) Jejunum
   d) Liver

5 'Dyspepsia'
   a) blood in the nose
   b) poor digestion
   c) vomiting
   d) runny stool

Multiple correct: Select ALL the correct answers to the question or statement given.

1 Mark all structures associated with colon.
   a) Esophagus
   b) Sigmoid
   c) Rectum
   d) Duodenum
   e) Haustra
   f) Pylorus

2 Which of following are macronutrients?
   a) B_{12}
   b) Fats
   c) Vitamin K
   d) Carbohydrates
   e) Proteins

3 Which of the following linking forms are associated with mouth structures?
   a) Odont/o
   b) Sial/o
   c) Ile/o
   d) Gloss/o
   e) Chole/o
   f) Cheil/o

Spelling challenge! Circle the correct spelling based on the definition given.

1 'Pertaining to under the tongue'
              Hyperglossal   Subbuccal   Sublinqual   Sublingual

2 'Create a new opening between stomach and 2nd section of small intestines'
         Gastrojejunostomy   Jejenogastrotomy   Gastojejunectomy   Gastojejunoschisis

3 'When the esophagus sphincter fails to relax'
              Acalsisia   Achalasia   Anhalasia   Ahchalasia

Define the term: Spelling *does* count in your definition too!

1 Orthognathic >   _____

2 Anastomosis >   _____

3 Gastroparesis >   _____

4 Microvilli >   _____

5 Hyperbilirubinemia > _____

6 Appendectomy > _____

7 Uvulectomy > _____

8 Pylorostenosis> _____

Find it! Using the words in the table – match the definition given or answer the statement. Some may not be used. It is recommended you know all the choices.

polyposis	palatoschisis	stomatitis	hepatomalacia	rectotomy
pancreatitis	orthodontist	gingivosis	peritoneoclysis	cholecystectomy
ascites	coleocele	megacolon	rectorrhagia	sialoadenitis

1 _____ Inflammation of the mouth

2 _____ Fluid accumulation in the abdominal cavity

3 _____ Abnormal condition of the gums

4 _____ Split palate

5 _____ Surgical removal of the gallbladder

6 _____ Inflammation of the salivary glands

7 _____ Flushing out the peritoneum

8 _____ Someone who straightens teeth

Matching: Some will not be used.

	Letter	Defined as
Alimentary		a) salivary stone
Labiogingival		b) create a new opening in the sigmoid colon
Sialolith		c) absorbs chyle from duodenum, specialized lymph
Regurgitation		d) partially mobile mass of tissue
Lacteal		e) long tube where food is eaten, digested, and absorbed
Sigmoidostomy		f) most common cause of colon cancer
Flexure		g) loss of blood supply
Adenocarcinoma		h) pertaining to the lips and gums
		i) to bring food up
		j) a turn or turning

An essay: Investigate the extremes of food: starvation and obesity. What can you do to make a change to bring people to a healthy normal?

Note challenge: Define the underlined terms. You may need to look up a few terms. Answer the questions which follow. The student is reminded this is an incomplete SOAP note used for the learning experience. Do not use this for patient encounters.

S. Timeka is a 42 yo woman with severe <u>epigastric</u> pain radiating to the back for the last 24 hours. She is also complaining of left chest and arm pain. She is <u>nauseated</u> and vomiting. No diarrhea. No <u>hematochezia</u> or <u>hematemesis</u>. Fever began about 12 hours ago. No previous history of <u>PUD</u>, <u>GERD</u>, or <u>colitis</u>. No tobacco use. No allergies.

O. 42 yo female is in obvious distress. BP: 162/98 P: 118 R: 20 Pulse Ox: 96%

Heart: mild <u>tachycardia</u>, regular with no murmurs or gallops. Lungs are clear. Abdomen: slow bowel sounds, tender in the epigastric region with rebound. No <u>ascites</u>, no <u>jaundice</u>. Tender over the left CVA. No <u>hepatomegaly</u>. Pelvic exam with in normal limits.

<u>GB US</u>: <u>cholecystolithiasis</u> CT scan: edema and possible mass effect over <u>duodenal</u>/pancreatic region.

A. <u>Pancreatitis</u>
   Cholecystolithiasis
   HTN
   <u>Tachycardia</u>

P. <u>NG</u> Tube ordered to be inserted to rest gut
   Morphine 4 mg, <u>sublingually</u> q 4 hours for pain
   Admit to 2A.

Questions:

1 Translate all the acronyms and give meaning to the words which are underlined in the note.

2 What are some of the causes for pancreatitis?

3 What endocrine hormones are made by the pancreas?

4 Where would you look up the diagnoses to code them?

Renal system

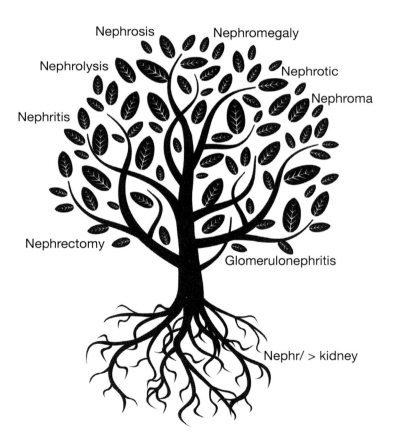

Nephrosis
Nephromegaly
Nephrolysis
Nephrotic
Nephroma
Nephritis
Nephrectomy
Glomerulonephritis
Nephr/ > kidney

TARGETED LEARNING

1 Recognize word parts and assemble medical terms related to the renal and urinary system.

2 Correctly construct, define, pronounce, and spell medical terms.

3 Link renal and urinary system illness and injury with appropriate pharmacotherapeutics and other therapeutic options.

4 Use the online resources to perform basic coding from *ICD Index of Illness and Injury*.

5 Explore medical documents as related to law.

KEY WORD PARTS

Word roots with linking vowel	Prefixes	Suffixes
Cort/o > outer surface	A-, An-	-al, -ary
Cyst/o > bladder, sac	Dia-	-cele
Glomerul/o > capillary loops	Dys-	-ectasia
Kal/o > potassium	Endo-, En-	-ectopia
Ket/o > ketones	Hyper-	-iasis
Lith/o > stones	Hypo-	-osis
Pyel/o > trough, vat	Nocto-	-paresis
Ren/o or Nephr/o > kidneys	Oligo-	-poiesis
Ur/o or Urin/o > urine	Peri-	-ptosis
Ureter/o > ureters	Poly-	-tripsy
Urethr/o > urethra	Retro-	-uria

END-STAGE RENAL DISEASE (ESRD)

The kidneys, like the brain and liver, have impressive longevity. In healthy conditions these organs are likely to work error-free for over 100 years. However, disease or injury can damage the reserves and result in renal failure or end-stage renal disease (**ESRD**). The most common cause of ESRD remains poorly treated diabetes mellitus (**DM**). Diabetes and hypertension rupture the many miles of tiny capillary beds filtering waste out of the body. ESRD patients often need regular dialysis to live. This is at a tremendous cost in quality of life, money, and resources.

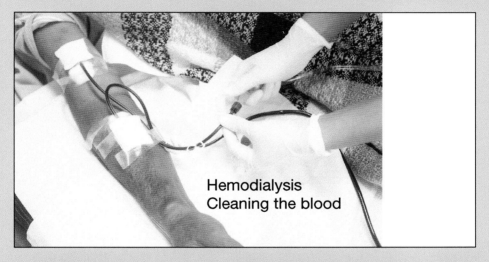

Hemodialysis
Cleaning the blood

Figure 14.2

Hemodialysis (**hem**-oh-die-**al**-lee-sis) utilizes an inserted port process to clean the blood. This is done at least three times a week for five to six hours each time for every patient. It requires specific machinery and skilled medical care. The cost, on average, is over $1000 for each treatment. The loss of quality of life is even larger as many of these patients will be on dialysis > 'breaking through' for years. The hemodialysis does remove toxins but it cannot perform the other functions of the kidneys. The alternatives are a kidney transplant or death. The challenge to society is to prevent this level of chronic care by preventing diabetes and hypertension with healthy lifestyles.

THE RENAL SYSTEM

The renal or urinary system could easily be grouped with the circulatory system because its main function is filtering waste from the bloodstream. It is like a strainer in the sink capturing and holding the debris while letting the water continue down the pipes. The system utilizes the fenestrated capillaries (Figure 14.3) to force waste into the sink (Bowman's capsule) and then it reabsorbs water and electrolytes into the circulation.

FENESTRATED CAPILLARY

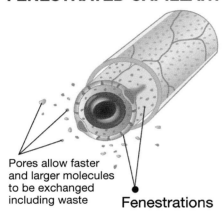

Pores allow faster
and larger molecules
to be exchanged
including waste   **Fenestrations**

Figure 14.3

The linking forms for this system include:

- Ren/o > Latin for kidney.

- Nephr/o > Greek for kidney.

- Ur/o or Urin/o > urine, the waste byproduct of renal function.

The term renal describes the anatomy of the kidney. Nephr/o is used for disease of the kidneys though there are several exceptions to both. Ur/o and Urin/o are used most often for the lower tract including the ureters, bladder, and urethra.

The kidneys are the physiologic functioning part of the urinary system. They are doing the work of filtering the bloodstream and isolating the waste to be washed out and into the urinary bladder, the storage sac.

There are two kidneys located in the retroperitoneal, high and deep for protection. They are more midline as the renal arteries come

---

14.1

Did You Know?

Each kidney contains about 1.2 million nephrons, the functional units of the kidneys.

Each day approximately a half gallon of urine is produced by filtering 50 gallons of blood across about 140 miles of tubules.

14.2

Suffixes with ren/o:

–al > pertaining to

–genic > originating

–graphy > to record

ANATOMY OF THE KIDNEY
Ren/o or Nephr/o

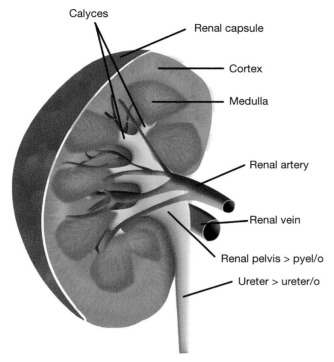

Calyces

Renal capsule

Cortex

Medulla

Renal artery

Renal vein

Renal pelvis > pyel/o

Ureter > ureter/o

Figure 14.4

directly off the abdominal aorta. The following cover the large or macro-anatomy terms (Figure 14.4):

- **Ren/o** > renal (**ree**-nal) > pertaining to the kidney such as the renal capsule, the tough connective tissue cover binding and protecting the kidney. When the kidney enlarges (renomegaly), the stretching of the capsule creates substantial pain.

- **Cort/o** > cortex (**kor**-teks) > outer zone of the kidney, the location of glomerular sections of the nephrons and capillary loops. Cortices (**kor**-tea-sez) is plural.

- **Medulla** (meh-**due**-lah) > center part of the kidney tissues is the location of the rest of the nephron's convoluted tubules, dumping the waste in the calyces. Medullae (meh-**due**-lay) is plural.

- **Calyx** (**ka**-liks) > Greek for 'cup of a flower' > funnel-shaped connective tissue captures the liquid waste and dumps it into the renal pelvis (pyel/o). Calyces (**kay**-lee-sez) is plural.

–megaly > enlargement

Cortex and medulla are used for other organs as well, such as the adrenal glands, bone, and brain.

- **Pyel/o** > trough, vat, or pelvis > collects all the urine in the center of the kidney and transitions to the ureters, the urine tubes to the bladder.
  - Pyelogram (**pi**-el-oh-gram) > X-ray exam of the ureter and renal pelvis done to check for stones, inflammation, or kinks.
  - **IVP** > intravenous pyelogram, X-ray dye (iodine derivative) is injected into the vein, highlighting the renal system.
  - **RGP** or **RP** > retrograde pyelogram, the dye is sent up the system from the urethra.
  - **Pyelonephritis** (**pi**-eh-low-neh-**fry**-tis) > inflammation of the renal pelvis and kidneys. This is a serious condition and if left untreated it can lead to renal failure.

✓ The function of the calyces is to collect _____ .

✓ Deconstruct the medical term for 'study of the kidneys'.
   _____/__/_____

Word building

*Using the word roots **with the linking vowel to build as many valid terms with the suffixes given. Please define each term.***

   Ren/o Pyel/o

   –logist –tomy –itis –ectomy –al –megaly

The microscopic anatomy of the kidneys is where the exchange of fluids, electrolytes, and waste occurs. Like the alveoli of the lungs, the nephron is a unit with several parts linked together to sift out the waste.

- **Nephr/o** > nephron (**neh**-fron) > functional unit of the kidneys. Each kidney has 1.5 million units (Figure 14.5).

- **Glomerul/o** > glomeruli (glo-**mar**-U-lie) > Latin for 'ball of yarn'. The arteriole (little artery) becomes a capillary cluster within the 'sink' of Bowman's capsule. This is the sink and beginning of the tubules (pipes) processing the waste. The fluid is pushed out of the fenestrated capillaries by a localized increase in the blood pressure. Glomerulus (glo-**mar**-U-lus) is singular.
  - **Glomerulopathy** (glo-**mar**-U-**lop**-ah-thee) > disease of the glomeruli may be induced by medications, congenital, or autoimmune diseases.

Suffixes with **pyel/o**:

–itis > inflammation

–gram > record

–tomy > cut into

–plasty > repair of

–ostomy > new opening

–ectasis > dilate

–scope > instrument to look

14.3
urine
14.4
Nephr/o/logy or ren/o/logy

14.5
The instructor has the list!

14.6

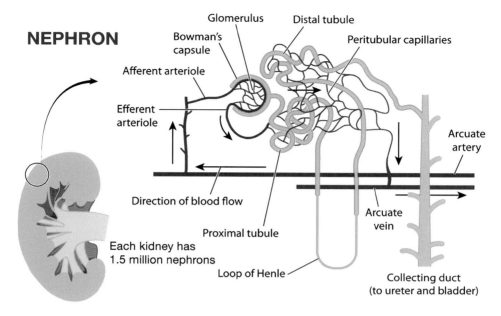

NEPHRON

Glomerulus

Distal tubule

Bowman's capsule

Peritubular capillaries

Afferent arteriole

Efferent arteriole

Arcuate artery

Direction of blood flow

Arcuate vein

Proximal tubule

Each kidney has 1.5 million nephrons

Loop of Henle

Collecting duct (to ureter and bladder)

Figure 14.5

- **Convoluted** (**kon**-voh-**loo**-ted) **tubules** > coiled segments of renal tubules (pipes). There are four distinct areas: proximal, loop of Henle (**hen**-leh), distal, and collecting. They convey and exchange by virtue of the one-cell thickness of the tubules and capillary beds:

  - **Water** > H_2O, most will be reabsorbed.

  - **Glucose** (Gl), Sodium (Na^{++}), Potassium (K^+), Chloride (Cl), Calcium (Ca^{++}), Magnesium (Mg^{++}), Bicarbonate (HCO_3), and Phosphate (P). Most of these will be immediately reabsorbed for recycling and use in the body.

  - **Amino acids** (building blocks for proteins) and protons > approximately 65% will be reabsorbed.

- The waste being pushed out with the excess water (urine) includes urea, nitrogen, uric acid, and ammonia – all wastes of liver, muscle, and cell activity.

Kitchen lab

To get an idea of how the kidneys work, take a sponge and soak up 20 ml of water. This represents the blood circulating. Now squeeze the sponge as hard as you can. This is increasing pressure and

pushing water OUT of the sponge and into a bowl, just as the glomeruli do. You will notice the sponge is still damp. You cannot squeeze it to become absolute dry. Then reabsorb the water with the sponge. Most of it is absorbed but not all. The leftover water would be the urine.

The linking form, nephr/o is used to describe any number of disease conditions of the kidney. Most are associated with slow or inappropriate functions of the nephrons of one or both kidneys. Here are a few terms:

- **Nephrolithiasis** (**nef**-row-li-thigh-ah-sis) > infestation of kidney stones. Renolith is also correct for kidney stones. Usually associated with abnormalities in calcium reabsorption (Figure 14.6).

- **Nephrotic** (neh-**fro**-tik) **syndrome** > pertaining to a set of symptoms including edema, proteinuria, and fatty urine casts indicating the glomeruli are leaking larger elements – renal disease. Synonym: Nephrosis

- **Nephroblastoma** (**nef**-row-blast-**oh**-ma) > tumor of the cells which build the nephrons. Eponym: Wilms' tumor.

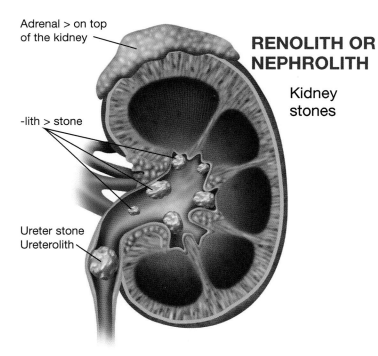

Adrenal > on top of the kidney

RENOLITH OR NEPHROLITH

Kidney stones

-lith > stone

Ureter stone
Ureterolith

Figure 14.6

14.7

Proteinuria > protein in the urine

Glycosuria > glucose in the urine

Pyuria > pus in the urine

Phenylketonuria (**PKU**) > phenylalanine, an amino acid in the urine

Hematuria > RBCs in urine

Ketonuria > ketones in urine

Suffixes

-logy > study of

-gram > record or

-osis > abnormal condition

-cele > hernia

-tomy > cut into

-ectomy > cut out

-ostomy > create new opening

-uria > in urine

LIKE ALERT!

Hydr/o > water

Hidr/o > sweat

POLYCYSTIC KIDNEY DISEASE

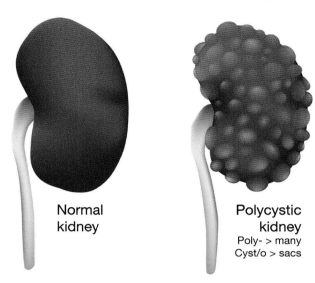

Normal
kidney

Polycystic
kidney
Poly- > many
Cyst/o > sacs

Figure 14.7

- **Nephritis** (neh-**fry**-tis) > inflammation of the kidneys due to infection, injury, congenital abnormalities, or autoimmune disease.

- **Polycystic Kidney Disease** (**PKD**) > hereditary disease characterized by multiple cysts on both kidneys. Worse in the presence of **DM** and likely to cause **ESRD** (Figure 14.7).

- **Hydronephrosis** (**hi**-drow-**nef**-row-sis) > abnormal condition of 'water on the kidney'. Urine is retained in the kidney due to obstruction from stones, masses, or inflammation. This is quite painful as the capsule does not like being stretched into a fat water balloon.

Renal function and disease conditions may be evaluated by a variety of laboratory tests:

- **UA** > urinalysis (**yur**-in-**al**-i-sis) > set of tests done on the urine, usually collected by clean catch. It should be clear of all cells with a **pH** of around 6.0.

  - **Catheterization** (**kath**-eh-tur-i-**za**-shun) > sterile tube (catheter) inserted in the urethra to the bladder to retrieve sterile urine for analysis.

- **BUN** > blood urea nitrogen > serum test gives an indication of kidney, circulatory, and/or heart disease.

14.8
Urea (yur-**ee**-ah) > nitrogen waste of cell metabolism, processed first by the liver.

Ketones (**key**-tones) > fatty acid waste producing a variety of 'alcohol' esters.

- **Creatinine** > waste of muscle activity indicates urinary blockage, dehydration, myolysis, pre-eclampsia, or malnutrition.

- **Creatinine clearance** > 24-hour urine collection; low results indicate kidney disease or failure, or marked dehydration.

- **GFR** > glomerular filtration rate > a ratio based on age, sex, and race, and creatinine indicates the function of the nephrons.

- **Urine Casts** > due to slow flow and solid cells leaking from the glomeruli, indicating the kidneys are not functioning well; the cells get molded or 'cast' in the shape of the ureters. There are RBC casts (Figure 14.8), WBC casts, bacterial casts, fat and protein casts seen on a UA.

Excess blood ketones cause a dangerous acidosis. Elevated with high-protein diets because fat is broken down to create energy.

Ammonia (NH$_3$) is a nitrogen waste; it is quite toxic to the brain.

CVA > costovertebral angle > tapping over the kidneys to elicit pain.

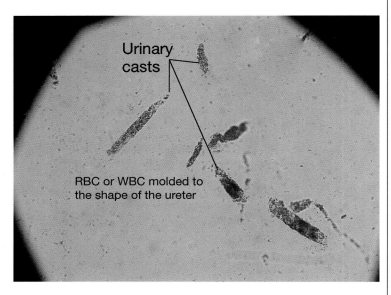

Urinary casts

RBC or WBC molded to the shape of the ureter

Figure 14.8

✓ Recovering from a Strep B pharyngitis, Jasmine developed 'glomerulonephritis'. How many linking forms are seen with this diagnosis?

✓ Howard is asked to provide a urine sample. What is the abbreviation for a urinalysis?

✓ Olivia's report reveals a proteinuria. This indicates she has _____ in her urine.

14.9
Two, glomerul/o and nephr/o

14.10
UA

14.11
protein

MEDICAL RECORDS AS LEGAL DOCUMENTS

Signs and symptoms, laboratory results, standard of care, surgery, and rehabilitation – all of this is called the practice of medicine. It is often pointed out that 'practice' is the correct word for delivery of medical care; it is not perfect! No matter the technology or research, we will never understand all the functions of this machine, the body. Intentional and unintentional errors do occur in medicine. Some errors are avoidable. Other errors are the nature of life and death. The legal system is part of the process to determine which is which.

- **Malpractice** > patient is harmed when a provider fails to competently perform their medical duties. An extreme example of this is doing a nephrectomy on the wrong kidney. All providers must know their craft and their own limitations. It is important to ask for help when needed.

- **Misadventure** > patient is harmed due to inadvertent outcome of an intended action. This is typically termed an unforeseen 'complication'. It can be as simple as an unexpected side effect from a medication.

- **Neglect** > failure to provide adequate care resulting in physical illness or injury. This is a failure to treat, a sin of omission such as not noting a high blood pressure or an elevated glucose and leaving it untreated. It can also be a family member withholding care to an individual.

Medical documentation is vital to discern how an injury or illness occurred. With rare exceptions, the errors are NOT intentional. It is usually a confluence of errors leading to injury, i.e., when noting an injury is to the right toe instead of the left toe or a medication is 10% instead of 1%. Every misspelling, error in direction, the placement of a decimal point, or the hours between therapies can lead to a significant injury or death. Charting errors do occur. Legally, they may be corrected. The written word may be struck out once with initials, date and time of the change. On an electronic health record (EHR) an addendum is placed at the end of the note with the date and time as well. Additionally, the safety and privacy of the records are vital to patient care and are protected by the Health Insurance Portability and Accountability Act of 1996 (**HIPAA**). Use of the language of medicine comes with an admonition to utilize it correctly to deliver the highest level of quality care to all people.

CHEMISTRY AND THE KIDNEYS

Since the functions of the kidneys include filtering out waste and managing electrolytes, it is important to know how these linked forms relate to the chemistry of the body.

- **Natr/o** > sodium, **Na** > primary extracellular electrolyte for all cell functions. The control of circulating sodium is a combination of renal function and two hormones managed by the pituitary gland in the brain. Too high or too low can be life-threatening.
  - Hyponatremia (**hi**-poe-nah-**tree**-me-ah) > low blood (serum) sodium.
  - Hypernatremia (**hi**-purr-nah-**tree**-me-ah) > high blood sodium.
- **Kal/o** > potassium, **K⁺** > primary intracellular electrolyte for all cell functions. Like sodium, potassium levels have a narrow range before significant illness or death is likely.
  - Hypokalemia (**hi**-poe-kay-**lee**-me-ah) > low blood potassium.
  - Hyperkalemia (**hi**-purr-kay-**lee**-me-ah) > high blood potassium.

14.12

Did You Know?

Salt, sodium in particular, is vital to our existence. A familiar saying, 'Where salt goes water follows' is true in human physiology. A high-sodium diet typically causes swelling (edema). A person who is dehydrated will crave salt as well. This is why salt was and still is a valuable commodity worldwide.

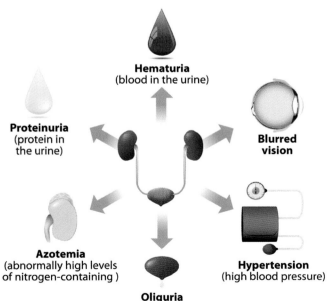

NEPHRITIC SYNDROME
Severe renal inflammation

Hematuria
(blood in the urine)

Proteinuria
(protein in the urine)

Blurred vision

Azotemia
(abnormally high levels of nitrogen-containing)

Hypertension
(high blood pressure)

Oliguria
(low output of urine)

Figure 14.9

- **Calci/o** or **Calce/o** > calcium, **Ca⁺⁺** > major electrolyte functioning in all neurologic, bone, and muscular activities.
  - Hypocalcemia (**hi**-poe-kal-**see**-me-ah) > low blood calcium.
  - Hypercalcemia (**hi**-purr-kal-**see**-me-ah) > high blood calcium.
- **Azot/o** > nitrogen, **N** > waste product of all cellular activity, specifically proteolysis.
  - Azotemia (**a**-zoe-**tea**-me-ah) > excess levels of nitrogen in the blood. Synonym: uremia
- **Ket/o** or **Keton/o** > waste product of adipolysis (fat breakdown).
  - Ketoacidosis (**key**-toe-ass-ee-**doe**-sis) > high level of acid in the bloodstream associated with starvation or uncontrolled diabetes mellitus (**DM**).
  - Ketonemia (**key**-toe-**knee**-me-ah) > ketone bodies in the blood.

- **PKU**, Phenylketonuria (**fen**-il-**key**-toe-**nyur**-ee-ah) > an inherited disorder interrupting the breakdown (-lysis) of phenylalanine, an amino acid. Normally, the liver produces an enzyme to do this but it is missing in these individuals. The accumulation in the bloodstream is toxic to the brain.
- **Albumin/o** > albumin (al-**bue**-min) > most abundant circulating protein, vital to water balance.
  - Albuminuria (al-**bue**-me-**nyur**-ee-ah) > protein in the urine indicating malfunction of the kidneys.
- **Bilirubinemia** (**bil**-i-rue-bi-**knee**-me-ah) > yellow pigment > result of hemolysis of recycled RBCs by the liver. If the liver is not processing well there is an elevation of bilirubin in the blood and it is seen in the urine as well, urobilinogen (**yur**-oh-bi-**lin**-oh-jen).

14.13
PKU is a condition of childhood. There is a simple blood stick done on infants at birth to check for the condition. Low protein diet and no artificial sweeteners are required to avoid damage to the central nervous system (CNS).

 The term 'uremia' can also be stated as _____ .

 Hypercalcemia pertains to which chemical?

Kevin has liver cirrhosis. He is likely to have 'elevated blood level of yellow pigment'. What is the correct medical term?

14.14
azotemia

14.15
Calcium

14.16
Hyperbilirubinemia

Word building

What word root is noted in the terms below? What do the prefixes mean?

Hyponatremia

Anuria

Hypermagnesemia

Hypoglycemia

Hematuria

Dysuria

14.17
The instructor has the answers!

The kidneys are influenced by **hormones** from the distant brain, heart, liver, and lungs; they produce some hormones as well.

- **ADH** > antidiuretic hormone > produced by the posterior pituitary (brain). It encourages retention of sodium and where salt goes water follows. It is important to balance water when intake is low.

- **ACTH** > adrenocorticotropic hormone > produced by the anterior pituitary. It stimulates the adrenal gland to release the following.

- **Aldosterone** (al-**doss**-tur-ohn) > from the adrenal gland; it stimulates sodium reabsorption at the distal convoluted and collecting tubules. Water follows the sodium so it retains water. It affects potassium reabsorption as well.

14.18
As noted earlier, hemodialysis is useful to eliminate toxic waste from the system in the absence of renal function. However, the process does not replace any of the hormones and their interactions so vital to water and electrolyte balance.

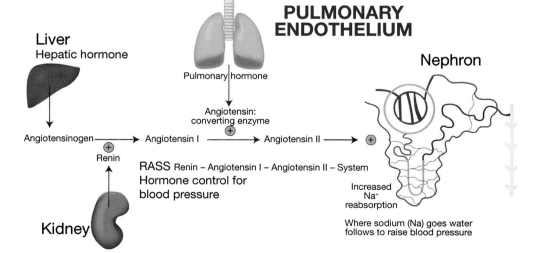

Figure 14.10

- **Renin** (**rey**-nin) > specific to the kidneys, it raises the blood pressure (**BP**) in the glomeruli by causing vasoconstriction to force fluid into the tubules. It acts as an enzyme for

- **Angiotensin I** (**an**-jee-oh-**ten**-sin) > protein peptide, localized hormone > 'vessel tension', it promotes vasoconstriction as well.

- **Angiotensin II** > produced by the liver and works with renin and angiotensin I system, termed RAAS, managing BP.

- **Erythropoietin** (eh-**rith**-row-**poe**-eh-tin) > 'to produce RBCs', a protein hormone produced by the kidneys to stimulate RBC production in the bone marrow.

- **Calcitriol** (**kal**-see-**tri**-ol) > physiologically active form of vitamin D. Calcitriol circulates as a hormone in the blood, regulating the levels of both calcium and phosphorus.

✓ Where sodium goes _____ follows.

✓ Erythropoietin, a renal hormone will stimulate the _____ to make more red blood cells.

Without the erythropoietin and calcitriol these patients are frequently anemic and have osteoporosis. The solution is to avoid renal failure with healthy choices.

Linking forms

Erythr/o > red

Angi/o > vessels

Adren/o > on top of the kidney

Physi/o > function

14.19
water

14.20
bone marrow

MEDICATIONS AND THE KIDNEYS*

Like its counterpart the liver, the kidneys process toxins and medications out of the body. There are several medications associated with acute and/or chronic nephritis and the loss of tubular function leading to edema. Chronic nephritis and nephrotoxicity results in reduced kidney size and GFR.

- Antibiotics > methicillin, penicillin, some cephalosporins, tetracycline, rifampin, erythromycin, and sulfonamides. Basically, any class of antibiotic can cause nephritis, indicating the indiscriminate use of these antibiotics should be avoided.

- NSAIDs > any non-steroidal antiinflammatory drug can trigger a nephritis. Like antibiotics, these are used regularly for a number of conditions. It is crucial to remember all medications carry risks.

- Other medications include those affecting the reabsorption of water and electrolytes in the tubules > diuretics, allopurinol (uric acid), cimetidine, and phenytoin.

- Antiviral medications can cause tubular cell toxicity > Adefovir, Cidofovir, Indinavir.

- Cardiovascular medications may modify intraglomerular blood flow > ACE inhibitors, Plavix, Ticlid, and the cholesterol medication class of 'statins'.

Antibiotic medications are used to treat the kidneys or the lower urinary tract for infections. Infections can cause glomerulonephritis, cystitis, urethritis, and pyelonephritis.

- Bacteria: *Streptococcus* Group B and *Escherichia coli* are treated with sulfonamides and cephalosporins.

- While not as frequent, viruses can cause infection: HIV, Epstein–Barr, and CMV.

- Other unique infections include TB, toxoplasmosis, and Rocky Mountain Spotted-fever.

★ IMPORTANT NOTE: All discussions of medications are for basic education. A medical provider should be consulted on any medication options. Do <u>not</u> use this information for patient care.

THE URINARY SYSTEM

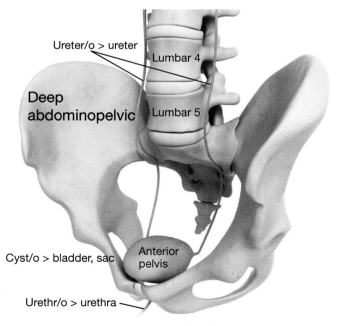

URINARY SYSTEM

14.21
The urinary system is sometimes referred to as the lower renal tract. Similar to the differentiation of the upper and lower respiratory tract. The kidneys are the upper tract.

Figure 14.11

Upon leaving the renal pelvis, the urine travels down via the ureters, dropping into the bladder for storage. Figure 14.11 demonstrates how deep the kidneys and ureters are in the abdominopelvic cavity. The ureters progress down and forward to meet the bladder in the midline and ventral, sitting right behind the pubic bone.

Ureter/o > ureter (**yur**-eh-tur) > urinary canal with its thick connective tissue, muscular layer, and transitional epithelium (same as the bladder) transports urine to the bladder. The transitional tissue is like elastic, it can stretch and rebound.

The horseshoe kidney depicted in Figure 14.12 is an anomaly of the kidneys. These are two functional kidneys fused at an isthmus. Each ureter will still be about 10–12 inches long, flowing into the urinary bladder posteriorly. This aids in preventing reflux.

- **Ureterectasia** (yur-**ee**-tur-ek-**tay**-zee-ah) > dilating the ureter > done when disease or injury narrows the tube (stenosis).

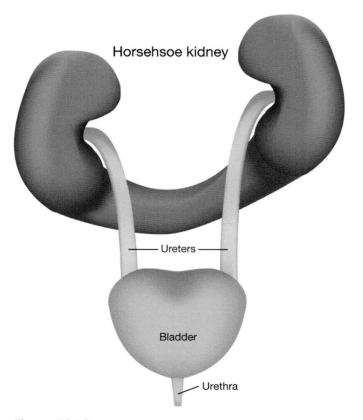

Horsehsoe kidney

Ureters

Bladder

Urethra

Figure 14.12

14.22

LIKE ALERT!

Ureter and Urethra are quite similar and part of the same system. Take care to use each properly.

Suffixes

–al > pertain to

–cele > hernia

–ectopia > out of place

–algia > pain

–ectomy > surgical removal

–itis > inflammation

–rrhaphy > suturing

–graphy > process of recording

–ostomy > create a new opening

Corp/o > body

Py/o > pus

LITHOTRIPSY
'Stone breaking'

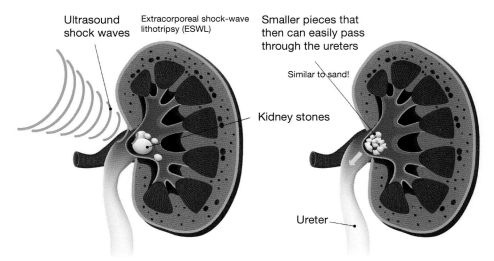

Ultrasound shock waves

Extracorporeal shock-wave lithotripsy (ESWL)

Smaller pieces that then can easily pass through the ureters

Similar to sand!

Kidney stones

Ureter

Figure 14.13

- **Ureterolith** (yur-**ee**-tur-**oh**-lith) > stone in the ureter > painful contractions by the ureter tries to clear the stone. A lithotripsy can be performed to split it into pieces; **ESWL** is the abbreviation for extracorporeal shock-wave lithotripsy.

- **Ureteropyeloplasty** (yur-**ee**-tur-oh-**pie**-eh-low-**plaz**-tee) > surgical repair or reconstruction of a ureter from the renal pelvis.

- **Ureteropyosis** (yur-**ee**-tur-oh-**pie**-oh-sis) > accumulation of pus in the ureter. Urinary casts are formed here.

Cyst/o or **Vesic/o** > bladder, sac > the urinary bladder lays flat as it fills with urine on the floor of the pelvis. It resembles a hot-air balloon as it fills. It is a storage unit for urine; as the bladder fills the transitional epithelium and the detrusor (deh-**tru**-sur) muscle expands. There is an internal smooth muscle sphincter to prevent urinary leaks. It also signals the bladder is ready to empty. The levator ani (leh-**vay**-tor a-**nigh**) muscles provide the voluntary skeletal muscle sphincter to allow micturition.

- **Vesic/o** > bladder > term is most associated with the urinary bladder.
  - **Vesicoclysis** (**ves**-i-**kok**-lie-sis) > washing out the bladder or irrigation.

14.23
Did You Know?

The urinary bladder generally holds 2 cups or one liter of urine.

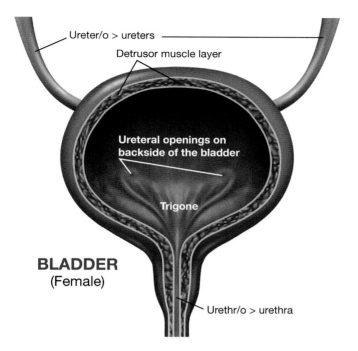

Ureter/o > ureters

Detrusor muscle layer

Ureteral openings on backside of the bladder

Trigone

BLADDER
(Female)

Urethr/o > urethra

Figure 14.14

Cystoscope > instrument to look into the bladder

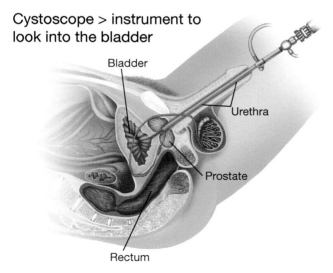

Bladder

Urethra

Prostate

Rectum

Figure 14.15

The detrusor muscle contracts to push urine out.

The openings allowing the ureters to carry urine to the bladder are located very low and posterior on the bladder. This helps prevent reflux of the urine back to the kidneys.

Women are more likely to have bladder infections (UTI) than men.

Suffixes

–ptosis > fallen, falling out

–paresis > paralyzed

–ectomy > to cut out, remove

–clysis > to rinse or irrigate

–rrhea > discharge, flow from

–rrhage > excessive bleeding

- – **Vesic**ou**ter**ine (**ves**-i-ko-**U**-tur-ine) fistula > abnormal opening between the bladder and uterus.
  - – **Vesic**otomy (**ves**-i-**kot**-oh-me) > to cut into the bladder.
- **Cyst/o** > bladder, sac, hollow organ > term may be applied for any sac or bladder in the body. It is best to document the urinary bladder to be specific.
  - – **Cyst**oscopy (sis-**toss**-ko-pee) > instrument to look into the urinary bladder (Figure 14.15).
  - – **Cyst**ocele (**sis**-toe-seal) > herniation of the urinary bladder.
  - – **Cyst**itis (sis-**eye**-tis) > inflammation of the urinary bladder. **UTI**, is a urinary tract infection, associated with the urethra and the urinary bladder. It is an imprecise term.
  - – **Cyst**oplegia (**sis**-toe-**pleh**-jee-ah) > paralysis of the urinary bladder. Injury of S1 (sacral spinal nerve), S2, or S3 may cause this.
  - – **Cyst**ostomy (**sis**-tos-**toe**-me) > creating a new opening to allow urine escape.

- **Urethr/o** > urethra > urogenital canal, a short 4 cm in women and the length of the penis in men. It is the exit tube. The opening is called the meatus (**me**-ah-tus).

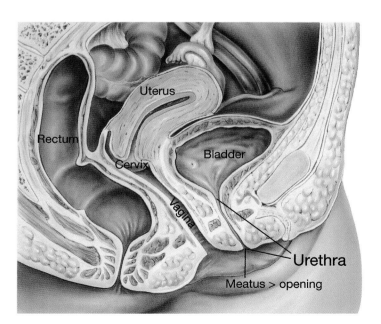

Figure 14.16

14.24
X-ray dye is properly termed radiocontrast agent.

Iodinated dye is used intravascularly (**IV**). It can be used by other routes as well such as for the voiding cystourethrogram (VCUG).

Barium and air is used in the GI tract.

A **KUB** is a plain X-ray of the kidneys, ureters, and bladder. It is basically an X-ray of the abdominopelvic area.

- **Urethritis** (**yur**-ee-**thri**-tis) > inflammation of the urethra. Commonplace in women because of the short length and proximity to the vaginal and rectal flora.
- **Urethrocystometry** (**yur**-ee-throw-sis-**toe**-meh-tree) > procedure measuring the pressure required for release of urine at the urethral and urinary bladder levels.

• **Voiding cystourethrogram** (**VCUG**) (**voy**-ding **sis**-toe-yur-ee-**throw**-gram) > X-ray image made as a patient voids (urinates) a bladder full of X-ray dye. It illustrates stenosis, neurological weakness, stones, or masses. Figure 14.17 is a cystogram of a 51-year-old woman with a pelvic fracture and multiple myeloma. She has anuria or urinary retention.

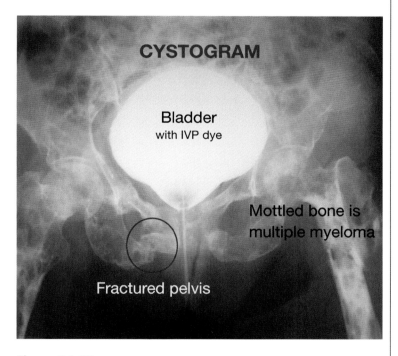

CYSTOGRAM

Bladder
with IVP dye

Mottled bone is
multiple myeloma

Fractured pelvis

Figure 14.17

✓ Which anatomical structure(s) carries urine from the renal pelvis to the bladder?

✓ Ida has been diagnosed with a bladder stone. What is the best medical term for this diagnosis?

✓ A cystorectostomy refers to an opening between _____ and the _____ .

14.25
Ureters

14.26
Cystolith

14.27
urinary bladder; rectum

Word building

Using the word roots with the linking vowel to build as many valid terms with the suffixes given. Please define each term.

Cyst/o Ureter/o Urethr/o

–lith –ostomy –clysis –ectomy –itis

14.28
The instructor has the list!

Urinary terms abound for descriptions of what is going on with the urine on its way out.

- **Micturition** (mik-thur-**ish**-on) > pertains to the neurologic feedback loops triggering the internal sphincter to empty the bladder. This also activates the detrusor muscle to contract several times (Figure 14.18).

- **Voiding** or **Urination** (**yur**-i-**nay**-shun) > evacuating urine.

- **Nocturia** (nok-**tyur**-ee-ah) > night urination, specifically having to rise too often to empty the bladder.

14.29
Diabetes mellitus is associated with polyuria, nocturia, and polydipsia > excessive thirst

polyphagia > excessive eating with

glycosuria > glucose in the urine

Prefixes

Poly- > many

Dys- > bad, poor, difficult

Oligo- > scant

An- > no, not, absent

Nocto- > night

En- > in

Extra- > outside

Urgency > sensation of needing to urinate despite an empty bladder.

Incontinence > unable to control urine flow.

NEURAL CONTROL OF MICTURITION

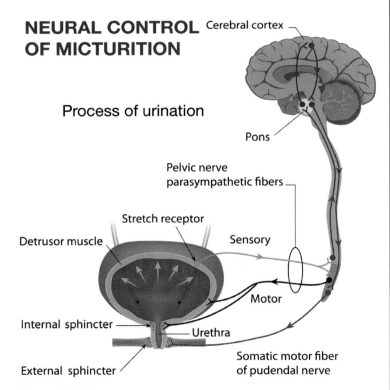

Figure 14.18

- **Oliguria** (**ol**-ee-**gyur**-ee-ah) > scant flow of urine with obstructions, BPH, and UTIs.

- **Enuresis** (en-yur-**ee**-sis) > urinary incontinence, particularly at night. This is also called 'bed wetting'. Seen in young children whose neurologic signals have not kicked in completely yet.

- **Dysuria** (dis-**yur**-ee-ah) > difficult or painful urination associated with UTIs and sexually transmitted diseases (STDs) such as gonorrhea (**gon**-ah-**rhee**-ah) in men.

- **Diuresis** (die-yur-**ee**-sis) > 'through (dia) urine' > recurrent urination with large volumes. A diuretic medication is designed to produce water loss to decrease edema.

- **Polyuria** (**pol**-ee-**yur**-ee-ah) > many urinations, may be due to medications but it can also be hormone driven by diabetes insipidus affecting the pituitary with blockage of ADH.

- **Anuria** (**an**-yur-**ee**-ah) > no urination due to blockage, renal failure, or neurologic damage.

The **prostate** (**pros**-tat) is unique to men and is part of the urinary system. The urethra runs right through the middle of the prostate, like a car through a tunnel. During urination, the fluids associated with sexual ejaculation are blocked and during sex the internal bladder sphincter is locked down tight. The prostate is about the

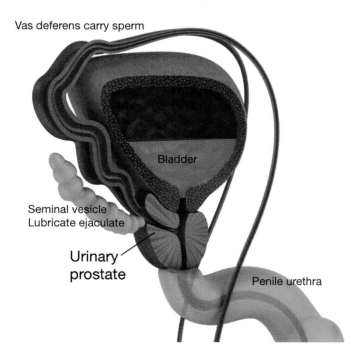

Vas deferens carry sperm

Bladder

Seminal vesicle
Lubricate ejaculate

Urinary
prostate

Penile urethra

14.30

LIKE ALERT!

Prostate > unique to men, it is part of the urinary and reproductive systems.

Add an 'r'

Prostrate > lying extended on the ground facedown, being prone.

Figure 14.19

size of a walnut, weighs about one ounce, and sits just below the urinary bladder.

- **Prostat/o** > from the Latin, one who stands before, protector.
  - **Prostatitis (pros**-tah-tie-tis) > inflammation of the prostate.
  - **Benign prostatic hypertrophy (hi**-purr-**trow**-fee) (**BPH**) > enlargement of the prostate.
    - o A transurethral resection of the prostate (**TURP**) is done to open the passageway, like cleaning out a drain.

 As we age, the bladder's sphincters are not as receptive to neurologic stimulus, and this can cause urine leakage. What is the best medical term for this?

 Ian is on Lasix, a diuretic. How will this effect urination?

 A prostatectomy would mean Jonathan had his _____ removed.

14.31 Incontinence

14.32 More frequent urination and larger volume

14.33 prostate

CODING PRACTICE

The renal system comes with many conditions, infections, and injuries. Use the internet to look up the ICD codes from the list given below. Use the *Index of Illness and Injury* exclusively. As stated, this text will not make the student a coder but the exercise will illustrate the importance of proper documentation and spelling. Check your work with your instructor.

- Incontinence, post-dribbling
- Renal calculus
- Prostatitis, hypertrophic
- Nephrogenic diabetes insipidus
- Urethritis, gonococcal, acute
- Proteinuria, membranous (diffuse)
- Ureterocele
- Nephropathy, potassium depletion
- Dysuria
- Tuberculosis, renal
- Anuria, following molar pregnancy

CANCER AND AUTOIMMUNE DISEASE

Cancers can occur anywhere within the renal system, but the kidneys and bladder are the most frequent locations. Hematuria is a shared symptom with all renal systems cancers and masses.

Renal cell carcinoma > an estimated 90% will involve the renal tubules with their epithelial cells. Risk factors include tobacco use, long-term dialysis for ESRD, obesity, and uncontrolled hypertension. A nephrectomy is the best option for care currently. Neither chemotherapy nor radiation therapy has much impact on the progression of the disease.

Transitional cell carcinoma of the bladder > rapid uncontrolled group of the transitional epithelial cells: tobacco, aging, men, petroleum chemicals, and some diabetic medications. Early cancer may be treated with fulguration (**ful**-gue-**ray**-shun) > destruction of the innermost transitional epithelium by high-frequency electric current. Surgery, radiation, chemotherapy, biological therapies are possible as well.

Tests for cancer and other renal diseases include:

- Ultrasound of the kidneys or bladder.
- Abdominal CT scan
- Renal arteriogram
- Liver function tests
- IVP
- Basic laboratory: CBC, UA

14.34

Did You Know?

Epithelial cells are the most abundant in the body. They reproduce by the millions as a method of cleaning debris from the skin, GI tract, respiratory and urinary tract.

Tobacco increases the risk factor for all cancers because it disrupts blood flow to these continuously producing tissues.

Diminished blood flow and oxygen weakens cell production and contributes to errors in the DNA.

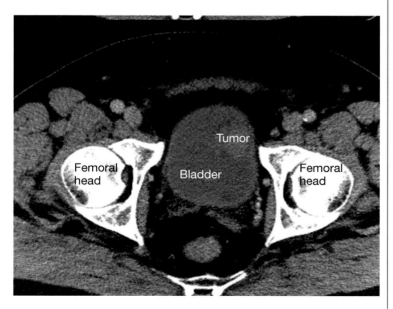

Figure 14.20

Autoimmune disease occurs in the renal system both specifically and by virtue of peripheral effects.

- **SLE,** Systemic Lupus Erythematosus (**lew**-pus er-**ith**-ee-mah-**toe**-sus) > connective tissue disorder that disrupts glomerular function in the renal system. It is also affects skin, eyes, and joints, resulting in pericarditis and anemia.

- **Goodpasture's syndrome** > loss of reproduction of the epithelial cells rapidly causing destruction leading to renal failure and death. It effects the lungs in the same way.

- **IgA nephropathy** (neh-**frop**-ah-thee) > the abnormal deposit of the IgA protein in the glomeruli. This plugs them up and proteinuria and hematuria occur. It takes 10–20 years to reach **ren**al failure on average.

- **Infectious disease:** HIV, CMV, EPV, and TB have a high incidence of renal failure.

✓ What is a 'vesical calculus'?

✓ The most common renal cancer occurs in the _____

ureters   glomeruli   tubules   afferent arterioles

14.35
HIV > human immunodeficiency virus
TB > tuberculosis
CMV > cytomegalovirus
EBV > Epstein–Barr virus

14.36
Another term for bladder stone

14.37
tubules

UNIT SUMMARY

1   The renal or urinary system is intimately associated with blood circulation and the control of blood pressure, electrolytes, and water balance. There are three linking forms: ren/o, nephr/o, and ur/o or urin/o. The major function of the system is to detoxify the blood and evacuate the waste via the ureters, bladder, and urethra.

2   The macro-anatomy includes several linking forms including: ren/o > the kidney; cort/o > the outer zone of the kidney; medulla > inner or middle zone of the kidney; the funnels of urine are called calyx, and the renal pelvis > pyel/o.

3   The micro-anatomy includes the complex nephrons, the function units of the kidneys. The beginning of the nephron unit is the glomeruli where a slight increase in BP forces fluids into Bowman's capsule and tubules. Here the water, electrolytes, amino acids, and waste will be processed by single-cell layer exchanges.

4   Several chemistry linking forms are seen due to the primary function of the kidneys. Natr/o > sodium (salt); Kal/o > potassium; Calci/o > calcium; Azot/o > nitrogen, and Ket/o > ketones. The feedback loop for controlling the flow or reabsorption of these electrolytes, amino acids, hormones, and water is controlled by the brain, adrenal glands, and the kidneys themselves.

5   Disease occurs with a disruption of the filtering process. Nephrotic syndrome, End-Stage Renal Disease (**ESRD**) due to diabetes and hypertension, cancers, and some of the autoimmune diseases can lead to renal failure and death. Hemodialysis and peritoneal dialysis can slow the progression of these conditions.

6   The lower urinary tract is occupied with moving the urine (waste) from the kidneys via the ureters > ureter/o to the urinary bladder (the storage sac > cyst/o) and out via the urethra > urethr/o. Disease and injury can obstruct flow including infections, stones, swelling of the prostate (in men), and stenosis.

7   There are several diagnostic tools to evaluate the function of the kidneys and urinary bladder including urinalysis (UA), electrolyte levels in both the blood and urine, and an IVP, intravenous pyelogram. Procedures include lithotripsy to crack the stones into sand and cystoscopes to look at and take samples from the urethra and bladder.

8   We are reminded the kidneys should function well for approximately 100 years. Prevention of diabetes and hypertension would decrease the number of people who lose quality of life and years of living to renal failure. Also, documentation is utilized to evaluate quality of care. Errors do occur. The task is to be aware of the possibilities of failure to recognize an issue and ensure all steps are taken to avoid mistakes.

UNIT WORD PARTS

Word roots with linking vowel		
Albumin/o > albumin, protein	Angi/o > vessel	Azot/o > nitrogen
Bacteri/o > bacteria	Calc/o or Calci/o > calcium, Ca++	Capill/o > capillary
Cort/o or Cortic/o > outer zone	Cyst/o > bladder, sac	Electr/o > charge, electrical
Glomerul/o > ball of yarn	Gluc/o or Glycos/o > glucose, sugar	Hem/o or Hemat/o > blood
Hydr/o > water	Kal/o > potassium, K+	Ket/o > ketones
Lith/o > stone	Meat/o > opening	Natr/o > sodium, Na++
Nephr/o or Ren/o > kidney	Prote/o > protein	Py/o > pus
Pyel/o > renal pelvis	Sten/o > narrowing	Ur/o or Urin/o > urine
Ureter/o > tubule, ureter	Urethr/o > tube, end point	Vesic/o > bladder, sac

Prefixes: attached to the front of the word root to change meaning		
A-, An- > no, not, absent	Anti- > against	Dia- > through
Dys- > difficult, painful, bad	Endo-, En- > inner, inside	Hyper- > increased, more
Hypo- > less, decreased	Nocto- > night	Oligo- > scant
Peri- > around, near	Poly- > many, frequent	Retro- > behind

Suffixes change the meaning of the word, linking vowel is usually 'o' with consonants		
-al, -ary > pertaining to	-cele > herniation	-dynia or -algia > pain
-ectasis or -ectasia > dilate	-ectomy > to remove, cut out	-gram > record of
-iasis > infestation	-itis > inflammation	-logy > knowledge of
-megaly > enlargement	-osis > abnormal condition	-ostomy > create a new opening
-paresis > paralysis	-poiesis > to make, produce	-ptosis > falling, fallen
-rrhaphy > suturing	-rrhea > discharge, flow	-scope > instrument to look
-stenosis > narrowing	-tripsy > break up	-uria > urine, in urine

Acronyms, abbreviations, and initial sets		
ADH > antidiuretic hormone	BPH > benign prostatic hypertrophy	BUN > blood urea nitrogen
CBC > complete blood count	CVA > costovertebral angle, physical exam	DM > diabetes mellitus
Epo > erythropoietin (medication)	ESRD > end-stage renal disease	ESWL > extracorporeal shock-wave lithotripsy
GFR > glomerular filtration rate	IVP > intravenous pyelogram	KUB > X-ray kidney, ureter, bladder
PD > peritoneal dialysis	pH > acid level, hydrogen	PKD > polycystic kidney disease
PKU > phenylketonuria	RP or RGP > retrograde pyelogram	Sp gr > urine test, specific gravity
TURP > transurethral resection of the prostate	UA > urinalysis	UTI > urinary tract infection
VCUG > voiding cystourethrogram	HCO_3 > bicarbonate	Na^{++} > sodium
K^+ > potassium	Ca^{++} > calcium	N > nitrogen
NH_3 > ammonia	Mg^{++} > magnesium	

UNIT WORKSHEETS

Building terms: Use the proper prefix/word root/linking vowel/suffix as appropriate.

   Example: to cut into the heart > cardi/o/tomy

a) Inflammation of the glomeruli and nephrons > _____

b) Stone infestation of the ureter > _____

c) The study of kidneys > _____

d) Process of using an instrument to look into the urinary bladder > _____

e) To cut a new opening in ureter > _____

f) Low blood sodium > _____

g) Glucose in the urine > _____

h) Tumor of the kidney > _____

Know your initial sets/acronyms! For the initial set or acronym given, spell it out correctly.

a) VCUG _____

b) IVP _____

c) TURP _____

d) BUN _____

e) GFR _____

f) UTI _____

g) BPH _____

h) PKD _____

Best choice: Pick the most appropriate answer.

1 The term 'hemodialysis'

   a) refers to vomiting blood   c) urination of blood

   b) cleaning of the blood   d) RBCs in the casts

2 Aldosterone

   a) Stimulates calcium   c) Stimulates sodium reabsorption

   b) Produces RBCs   d) Releases potassium

3 Enuresis

   a) no urine flow   c) nerve supply for urination

   b) scant urination   d) urinary incontinence

4 'Ureteropyosis' refers to _____ in the ureter

   a) Blood   c) Pus

   b) WBC   d) Glucose

5 A renal arteriogram will demonstrate the

   a) blood supply of the kidneys   c) stones in the ureter

   b) expansion of the bladder   d) urethral inflammation

Multiple correct: Select ALL the correct answers to the question or statement given.

1 Mark all conditions associated with autoimmune renal disease?

   a) SLE   d) Cystocele

   b) Hepatitis C   e) Goodpasture's syndrome

   c) IgA nephropathy   f) Nephromegaly

2 Which of the following structures of the kidney are considered as macro-anatomy?

a) Calyx

b) Cortex

c) Tubules

d) Medulla

e) Renal pelvis

3 Which of the following hormones are associated with renal function?

a) ACTH

b) Renin

c) Epinephrine

d) Erythropoietin

e) Prolactin

Spelling challenge! Circle the correct spelling based on the definition given.

1 'Abnormal condition of water on the kidney'

Hidronephosis   Hydronephrosis   Hytronefrosis   Hypernephrosis

2 PKU

Fenolketonuria   Phenokeytonuria   Phenylketonuria   Finolykeatonuria

3 Production of red blood cells (the hormone)

Erythemopoyetin   Eyrthropoyetin   Erthromoetin   Erythropoietin

Define the term: Spelling *does* count in your definition too!

1   Bilirubinemia > _____

2   Ureteropyeloplasty > _____

3   Micturition > _____

4   Urgency > _____

5   Cystourethrogram > _____

6   Ketoacidosis > _____

7   Prostatectomy > _____

8   Vesicorectostomy > _____

9   Nephrocalcinosis > _____

10 Cystolithotomy > _____

Find it! Using the words in the table – match the definition given or answer the statement. Some may not be used. It is recommended you know all the choices.

cystometry	hematuria	glomerular	cystodynia	prostatitis
nephroma	urethrostenosis	ureterectasia	oliguria	nephroblastoma
pyelogram	nephritis	lithotripsy	ureterostomy	pyelonephritis
cauterization	Staphylococcus	nephrolith	polyuria	pyuria

1 _____ Inflammation of the kidney

2 _____ Measurement of bladder pressure

3 _____ Scant urination

4 _____ Tumor of the developing cells of the kidney

5 _____ Pertaining to the glomeruli

6 _____ Blood in the urine

7 _____ Bladder pain

8 _____ Breaking stones

Matching: Some will not be used.

	Letter	Defined as	
Pyelolithotomy		a)	disease of the glomeruli
Meatal		b)	elevation of blood sodium
Ketonuria		c)	absorbs sodium from the loop of Henle
Glomerulopathy		d)	suturing the ureter
Creatinine		e)	to cut stone in the renal pelvis
Hypernatremia		f)	ketones in the urine
Ureterorrhaphy		g)	paralysis of the bladder
Cystoplegia		h)	pertaining to an opening
		i)	reflux of urine
		j)	waste of muscle activity

An essay: In your own words what is the difference between malpractice and misadventure? Why is documentation important to the law of medicine?

Note challenge: Define the underlined terms. You may need to look up a few terms. Answer the questions which follow. Student is reminded this is an incomplete SOAP note used for the learning experience. Do not use this for patient encounters.

S. Kevin is a 74-year-old man in the office today due to progressive <u>dysuria</u>, <u>urgency</u>, and <u>nocturia</u>. He has a diagnosis of <u>BPH</u> but this seems much worse in the last 4 weeks. Yesterday his urine was darker and he is worried it is bleeding, <u>hematuria</u>. He reports a 15# weight loss with a mild nausea. No specific pain just a sense of unwellness. No fever, chills, vomiting or change in bowel habits. He has a 50 year/pack history of tobacco smoking.

O. 74-year-old man in no acute distress. BP 163/94; R 16; T 98.6; P 96; Pulse Ox 94%.

Heart: RRR without murmurs. Lungs: shallow air flow, no rales or rhonchi. Abdomen: soft, nontender with a mass effect just above the pubic bone on the left. <u>CVA</u>'s nontender. No <u>edema</u>, no <u>jaundice</u>, no <u>cyanosis</u>. Left <u>inguinal</u> area with enlarged lymph node.

UA:

Color:	Red
Clarity:	Turbid
pH	6.1
Protein UA	>410**
Glucose UA	Negative
Ketones UA	Trace
Blood UA	Abundant
Nitrite UA	Positive
Bacteria	few
WBC	+80
Epithelials	Many
CBC:	<u>microcytic</u>, <u>hypochromic</u> anemia
<u>IVP</u>:	Mass within the bladder, left superior aspect

A. Bladder carcinoma, presumed diagnosis

Microcytic anemia
Hypertension
Tobacco Abuse

P. Schedule for *Cystoscope* for *biopsy* and lavage

Order <u>CXR</u>, <u>ECG</u>, <u>Cardiopulmonary</u> consult

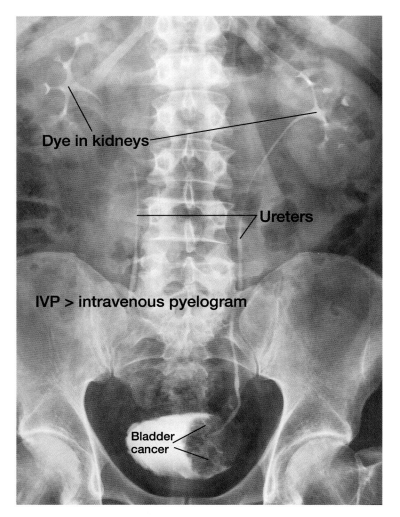

Figure 14.21

Questions:

1 Translate all the acronyms and give meaning to the words which are underlined in the note.

2 What is the most common tissue type associated with bladder carcinoma?

3 There is protein and blood in the urine. What are the proper terms for these findings?

4 What is the significance of noting the tobacco use? Is it a risk factor for this cancer?

5 Which ICD table would include the diagnosis of bladder carcinoma?

Unit 15

Reproductive system

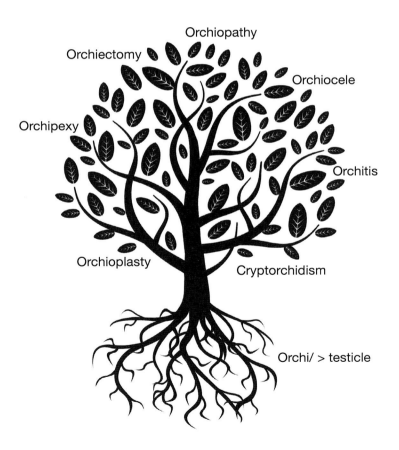

Orchiopathy

Orchiectomy

Orchiocele

Orchipexy

Orchitis

Orchioplasty

Cryptorchidism

Orchi/ > testicle

TARGETED LEARNING

1 Recognize word parts and assemble medical terms related to the reproductive system.

2 Correctly construct, define, pronounce, and spell medical terms.

3 Link reproductive illness and injury with appropriate pharmacotherapeutics and other therapeutic options.

4 Explore ethical terms considerations as part of proper documentation.

KEY WORD PARTS

Word roots with linking vowel	Prefixes	Suffixes
Balan/o > glans penis	Ante-	-algia
Cervic/o > neck	Crypto-	-arche
Colp/o or Vagin/o > vagina	Dys-	-cyesis
Epididym/o > epididymis	Endo-	-ectomy
Gonad/o > seed, sexual organ	Hydro-	-parous
Hyster/o or Uter/o> uterus, womb	Multi-	-pexy
O/o > egg	Neo-	-plasty
Oophor/o or Ovari/o > ovary	Nulli-	-ptosis
Orchid/o or Test/i > testicles	Peri-	-rrhagia
Prostat/o > prostate	Post-	-rrhaphy
Salping/o > tube, trumpet	Primi-	-tocia
Scrot/o > sac, scrotum	Secundi-	-trophy

MEDICAL ETHICS AND REPRODUCTION

The reproductive system is not required for life. It does not move blood or filter toxins or take in food or air. It *does* populate the species – building societies, communities, and cultures over thousands of years. The mystic of the anatomy of sexual reproduction continues even today, with each culture having specific terms and slang to describe the act of procreation.

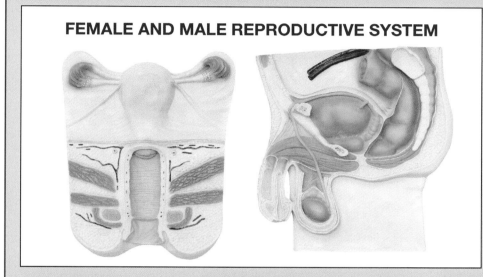

FEMALE AND MALE REPRODUCTIVE SYSTEM

Figure 15.2

Reproductive health has always had many ethical questions swirling nearby. Here are a few:

- *Religion*: sex should only take place for the act of procreation, not for enjoyment.
- *Responsibility*: since the woman bears the child she should be responsible for birth control.
- *Timing*: when is the product of conception alive? Does the fetus have rights?
- *Language*: should advertisers use words such as 'erectile dysfunction' during family viewing time? How and who educates young people on sexual matters?
- *Health*: sexually transmitted diseases should be private, not an issue for Public Health?
- *Genetics*: if we can fix the gene for Down syndrome or other genetic diseases, should we? What do we do with the errors in genetic manipulation?

Medical care and documentation provides the starting place and perhaps the ending place for some of these questions. These are real and sometime volatile topics merging with politics, private beliefs, and public health on a regular basis. As providers and patients, it is important to listen and provide quality education and care to all people equally to avoid the angst of the ethics.

THE MALE REPRODUCTIVE SYSTEM

The male reproductive system is designed to produce, transport, and discharge the male gamete, the sperm in the process of reproduction (Figure 15.3). There are three hormones effecting this process directly and a number of word roots to describe the anatomy.

15.1
Gamete (gam-eat)
> germ cell, a haploid cell when joined with its counterpart (ovum) produces an embryo or offspring.

Suffixes
-algia > pain
-ectomy > to cut out
-tomy > to cut into

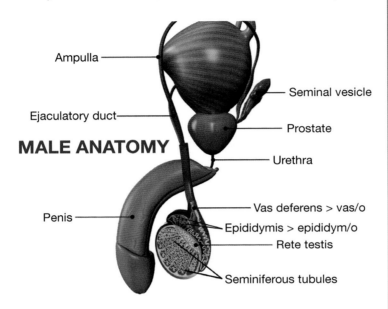

MALE ANATOMY

Ampulla
Ejaculatory duct
Penis
Seminal vesicle
Prostate
Urethra
Vas deferens > vas/o
Epididymis > epididym/o
Rete testis
Seminiferous tubules

Figure 15.3

The external genitalia of men is more noticeable and there is a dictionary's worth of slang terms for the anatomy and activity of these body parts.

• **Phall/o** > the penis > copulation (**kop**-U-**lay**-shun) organ for men, it changes in size when stimulated to allow the ejaculation of the semen. The base of the penis is at the abdominopelvic wall. The shaft is the length of the penis with loose skin, and the glans penis is the head.

  – Phallodynia (**fal**-oh-**din**-ee-ah) > pain in the penis.
  – Phalloplasty (**fal**-oh-**plaz**-tea) > repair of the penis.

The head of the penis has three structures including the meatus of the urethra.

• **Balan/o** > the glans penis is the expansion of the corpus spongiosum forming the head of the penis (Figure 15.4). It is most sensitive during sexual activities.

15.2
Meat/o > opening
Meatorrhea > discharge from the opening

GENITAL HERPES
Glans penis > balan/o

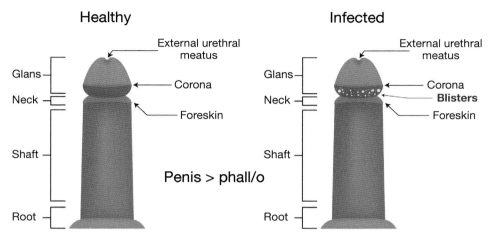

Healthy   **Infected**

Glans — External urethral meatus — Corona — Foreskin — Neck — Shaft — Root

Glans — External urethral meatus — Corona — **Blisters** — Foreskin — Neck — Shaft — Root

Penis > phall/o

Figure 15.4

- – Balanitis (**bal**-ah-**nigh**-tis) > inflammation of the glans penis. More common in uncircumcised men but sexually transmitted diseases (**STDs**) are seen in circumcised men as well: syphilis, trichomonas, herpes, and gonorrhea.

- **Prepuce** (**pre**-pyus) > foreskin > loose, folded skin covering the glans penis.
  - – **Smegma** (**smeg**-mah) > cheese-like substance forms under the foreskin if the glans covered by the foreskin is not cleaned properly.

Meatoplasty > repair of the opening is done to repair a hypospadia; when the meatus is located on the underside of the glans penis versus in the center.

The **corpus cavernosum** and **spongiosum** are two parallel columns of highly vascular tissue. The filling of these tissues allows the erection of the penis; this is required for copulation and ejaculation (Figure 15.5). Systemic diseases which diminish blood supply such as diabetes and hypertension can cause **erectile dysfunction, ED**.

- **Corpus cavernosum** (**kor**-pus ka-vur-**no**-sum) > 'body cavern'; this tissue is where the majority of blood floods the penis to enable erection.

- **Corpus spongiosum** (**kor**-pus spon-je-**oh**-sum) > 'body sponge'; this tissue is more central and ends in the glans penis. Its main function is to protect the urethra from collapsing with the filling of the corpus cavernosum.

15.3
The **pudendal nerve** provides both movement and sensing function to the external genitalia in both men and women. It controls the muscles of urination. During sex, the sphincter is tightened to prevent mixing of urine and semen.

MEDICAL ANATOMY OF PENIS

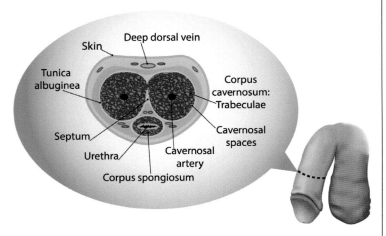

Figure 15.5

 Jorge slipped on the ice and he sustained a laceration of his penis. What is the medical term for 'repair of the penis'?

 The urethra moves through the center of the penis, what is the urethra?

The **scrotum** is the other obviously exterior element of the male anatomy (Figure 15.6). It is a cutaneous (skin) and muscular sac containing the male gonad, the testicle, on each side. The **cremasteric muscle** contracts to pull the scrotum close to the body.

- **Scrot/o** > scrotum (singular), scrota (plural)
  - **Scrotal raphe** (**skro**-tal **ray**-fee) > tendinous connective cord running the length of the scrotum to the **an**us.
  - **Scrotal septum** > incomplete wall between the right and left scrotum.
  - **Scrotal hydrocele** (hi-**drow**-seal) > trauma or inflammation can cause fluid to fill the scrotum.
  - **Scrotal varicocele** (**var**-ee-**ko**-seal) > varicose veins of the scrotum. It may cause decreased sperm production.

15.4
Phalloplasty

15.5
Urinary tube

15.6

Did You Know?

The left testicle tends to hang lower than the right. There is no clinical significance either way.

The scrotum protects the testicles from extremes of temperature, keeping them about two degrees cooler than body temperature.

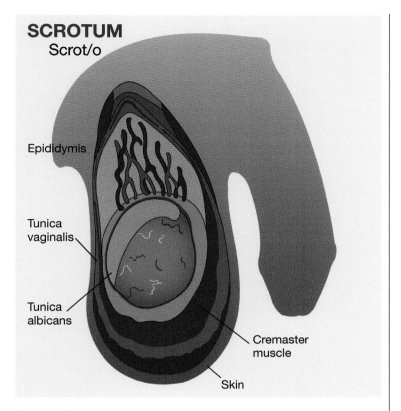

SCROTUM
Scrot/o

Epididymis

Tunica vaginalis

Tunica albicans

Cremaster muscle

Skin

Figure 15.6

The testis (plural) or testicles are the gonads of the male. The male testis produces sperm from puberty until death. Total numbers do decrease with age. In a single ejaculation between 40 million and 1 billion sperm will be released to fertilize a single ovum.

- **Gonad/o** > seed, the organ of producing sex cells.
  - **Gonadotropin** (go-**nad**-oh-**trow**-pin) > hormone promotes growth and function of the gonads (testicles and ovaries). Synonym: Follicle-Stimulating Hormone (**FSH**).
- **Test/i or Testicul/o** > testicles, used most for the anatomy (Figure 15.7).
  - **Testicular cancer** (tes-**tik**-U-lar) > typically found in young men, 15–35 years old. It creates a painless mass. Self-exams are useful during this age-range to catch it early.
  - **Torsion testicle** (**tor**-shun **tes**-tea-kel) > when the testicle rotates around the spermatic cord, blocking blood supply. It is a medical emergency.

15.7
The sperm of the testicle matures under the influence of **testosterone** (tes-**tos**-tur-own) it produces. The sperm mature in the epididymis.

The almond-shaped testicle will have approximately 350 seminiferous tubules; the sperm ascends to the epididymis sitting atop the testi.

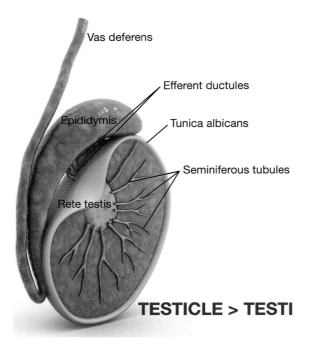

Vas deferens

Efferent ductules

Epididymis

Tunica albicans

Seminiferous tubules

Rete testis

TESTICLE > TESTI

At puberty, **FSH** and **luteinizing hormone (LH)** from the pituitary gland will trigger the production of testosterone. The hormone will activate the development of secondary male characteristics.

Sperm requires the sweetened fluids of the prostate and seminal vesicles to provide energy for about 36 hours of motility. The sugar is specifically fructose.

Figure 15.7

Orchi/o or Orch/o or Orchid/o > testicles, used for disease and injury:

– **Orchialgia** (or-**key**-al-**jee**-ah) > pain in the testicle. Orchalgia and testalgia are also correct.

– **Cryptorchidism** (krip-**toe**-key-dizm) > hidden testicle, when the testicle does not descend at birth from the pelvis into the scrotum.

– **Orchidopexy** (or-**key**-doe-**pek**-see) > fixing the testicle in place so it does not sneak back up into the pelvis, where it is too warm for sperm survival.

• Sperm/o or Spermat/o > sperm, male reproductive cells (gametes) (Figure 15.8).

– **Spermatogenesis** (**spur**-mat-oh-**jen**-eh-sis) > process of producing sperm.

– **Spermatocide** (**spur**-mat-oh-side) > process of killing sperm. Heat, radiation, and some medication can destroy sperm.

– **Semen** (**sea**-men) > penile ejaculate, a thick, slightly sweet, sticky fluid combining the sperm and other fluids to push the sperm into the cervix of the woman.

SPERMATOGENESIS > SPERM BEGINNINGS

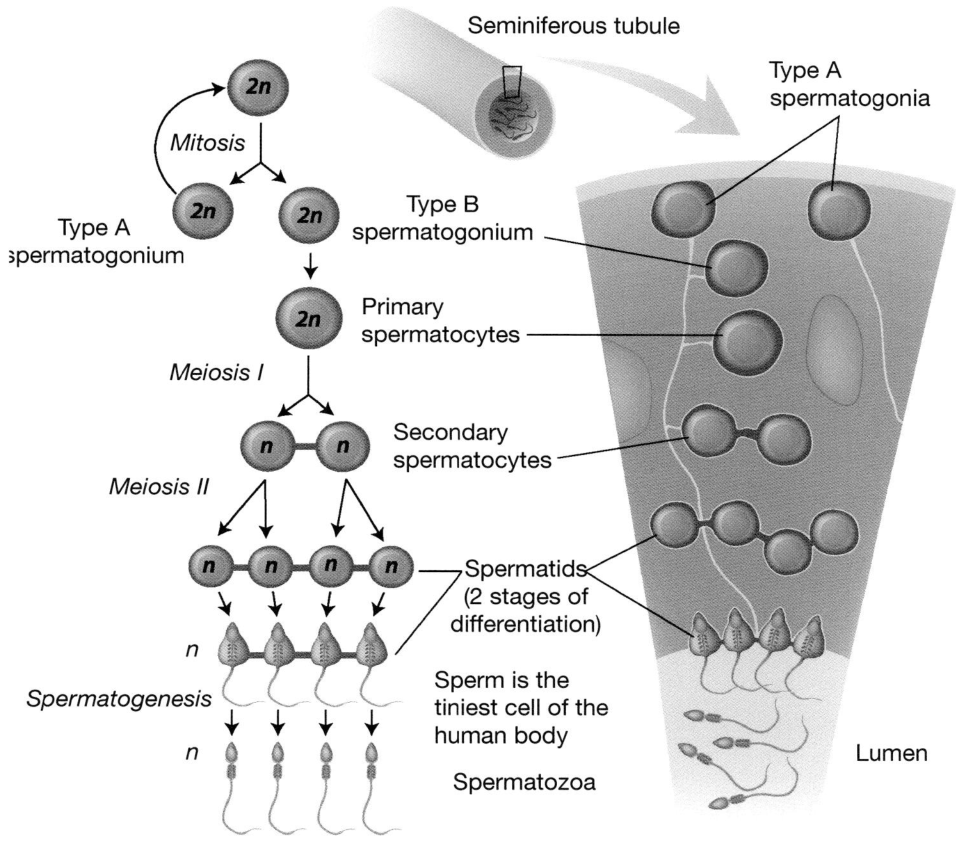

Figure 15.8

The **epididymis** (ep-ee-**did**-ee-mis) > described as a 'comma' atop the testi, a convoluted tubule; it is the storage place for sperm (Figure 15.9). Sperm will mature here and the tail of the epididymis becomes the **vas deferens** transporting sperm up and around to the posteriolateral prostate.

Epididym/o > from the French 'on top of twins' (two testes).

- **Epididymitis** (**ep**-ee-**did**-ee-**my**-tis) > inflammation of the epididymis (Figure 15.9). This condition causes a great deal of pain and may be due to trauma, urinary or prostate infections, or rarely, tuberculosis. It is seen with STDs such as gonorrhea and chlamydia (kla-**mid**-ee-ah).

- **Epididymoorchitis** (ep-ee-**did**-ee-moe-or-**keye**-tis) > inflammation of both the testi and epididymis.

15.8
Chlamydia > *Chlamydia trachomatis* is a bacterial **STD**. It is typically silent, presenting with no symptoms. With symptoms, dysuria is likely in both men and women. In women it can cause PID, pelvic inflammatory disease. Treatment: antibiotics.

Healthy epididymis

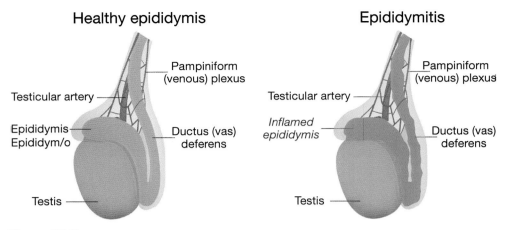

Pampiniform (venous) plexus

Testicular artery

Epididymis
Epididym/o

Ductus (vas) deferens

Testis

Epididymitis

Pampiniform (venous) plexus

Testicular artery

Inflamed epididymis

Ductus (vas) deferens

Testis

Figure 15.9

✓ An epididymotomy means?

✓ Some condoms and cervical diaphrams contain a spermatolytic. What does the medical term mean?

Word building

Using the word roots with the linking vowel to build as many valid terms with the suffixes given. Please define each term.

Orchid/o Epididym/o Balan/o

-itis -pexy -plasty -ectomy -algia -cele

The **vas deferens** (vas **def**-ur-enz) > 'to carry away up the tube'. This tube begins at the tail of the epididymis and travels via the inguinal canal to the prostate where it joins with the seminal vesicles. Synonym: ductus deferens.

- **Vasectomy** (vas-**ek**-toe-me) > to cut out or remove the vas deferens. A section is removed and the ends are tied off to prevent sperm progression.

- **Vasovasostomy** (vah-so-vah-**sos**-toe-me) > the repair of a vasectomy, a new opening is created by joining the two cut ends together. This is also called an **anastomosis** (Figure 15.10).

15.9
To cut into the epididymis

15.10
To destroy sperm

15.11
The instructor has the list.

15.12

Did You Know?

About 6% of men will have a vasectomy compared to 16% of women having a tubal ligation.

Vas/o > vessel, tube

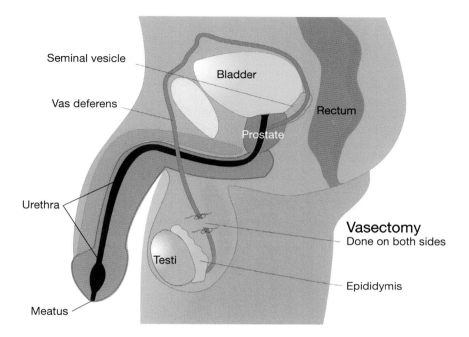

Seminal vesicle

Bladder

Vas deferens

Rectum

Prostate

Urethra

Vasectomy
Done on both sides

Testi

Epididymis

Meatus

Figure 15.10

The **prosta**te is at once an organ of the urinary tract and the reproductive system. The fluid of the vas deferens (sperm), seminal vesicles, and the prostate converge to become the ejaculate from both sides of the prostate during sexual intercourse. The remainder of the time, it is part of the male urethra.

Prostat/o > gland, sits below the urinary bladder in men; it receives fluid from the vas deferens and seminal vesicles. It also produces a sweet fluid to support the energy needs of the sperm.

• Prosta**titis** (**pros**-tah-**tie**-tis) > inflammation of the prostate.

• **Benign** prosta**tic hypertrophy** (**BPH**) > slow enlargement of the prostate is part of aging in men. It affects urine flow in many men: polyuria and nocturia. It is like crimping a straw. There are medications and procedures available to help with these symptoms.

• Prosta**tic cancer** > adenocarcinoma of the prostate occur when the prostate gland tissue grows uncontrollably (Figure 15.11). Treatment includes surgery, radiation, cryosurgery, hormone, and chemotherapy.

15.13
PSA > prosta**te specific antigen** is a blood test utilized to follow post-therapy care in patients.

DRE > **digital rectal exam** allows the provider the ability to feel the posterior prostate from the rectal wall. It should be firm and smooth.

STAGES OF PROSTATE CANCER
Prostat/o

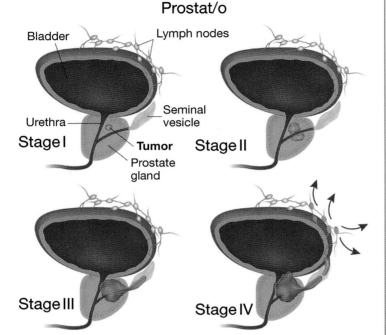

Bladder
Lymph nodes

Urethra

Seminal vesicle

Stage I

Tumor

Prostate gland

Stage II

Stage III

Stage IV

Figure 15.11

Suffixes:

–centesis > to remove fluid with needle

–ectomy > to cut out

–tomy > to cut into

–algia > pain

–dynia > pain

–rrhea > discharge

✓ Kenneth has a prostatocystitis. This means he has inflammation of the _____ .

✓ A gentleman with BPH needs a TURP to deal with the polyuria and urinary retention. What is a TURP?

Word building

Using the word roots with the linking vowel to build as many valid terms with the suffixes given. Please define each term.

Prostat/o Test/i Scrot /o

–itis –pexy –plasty –ectomy –dynia –cele

15.14 prostate and urinary bladder

15.15 Transurethral resection of prostate

15.16 The instructor has the list!

TREATING SEXUALLY TRANSMITTED DISEASE (STD)*

In 2015, over 100,000 cases of STD were reported. There has been a steady increase of STDs in the last 10 years in the United States; in fact, it is estimated one-half of all sexually active 25-year-olds have had one or more STDs. **HPV**, Human papilloma virus (genital warts) is #1, followed by herpes (**HSV**), chlamydia, gonorrhea, and syphilis. Some of these have striking symptoms bringing a patient in for care; others are almost silent until chronic conditions present such as HPV and cervical cancer.

The accurate diagnosis and documentation of STD enables public health offices to impact the spread of the disease and ensures treatment when available. The CDC provides STD treatment guidelines including proper culture and sensitivities prior to treatment and after to confirm the cure.

- **Gonorrhea** (**gon**-or-**rhee**-ah) > bacterial infection causing severe dysuria in men and generally asymptomatic in women. Like many bacterial infections, resistance to fluoroquinolones has been noted. This leaves cephalosporins as the only class of antibiotics likely to cure gonorrhea. The good news is a single injection of Ceftriaxone is sufficient for cure. An alternate is Azithromycin 1 gram orally.

- **Chlamydia** > bacterial infection can cause PID in women and tends to be asymptomatic in men. Both may be treated with any of the following: Azithromycin, Doxycycline, Erythromycin, Levofloxacin, or Ofloxacin.

- **Syphilis** (**sif**-i-lus) > systemic disease caused by *Treponema pallidum*. It has three stages and it can evaluated with a blood test, **RPR**, Rapid Plasma Reagin or other immunoassays. Penicillin G given by intramuscular injection remains the best

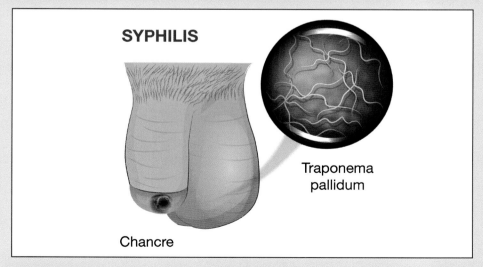

SYPHILIS

Traponema pallidum

Chancre

Figure 15.12

treatment no matter the stage of the disease, though longer therapy may be required in stage 3.

- Viral infections such as HPV, Herpes (HSV), and HIV have no cures – only medication to slow the replication of the virus. This limits the amount of virus in the area and the bloodstream keeping the infections at a relative neutral.

- There is a vaccination to prevent HPV. It is recommended for all teens.

The CDC tracks numbers and results for the USA; the World Health Organization (WHO) tracks STDs and more conditions worldwide. Anyone can access these reports by checking their web sites online. The goal of the WHO and CDC is to continue education and prevention methods for these diseases as they have real and potentially deadly consequences.

★ **IMPORTANT NOTE: All discussions of medications are for basic education. A medical provider should be consulted on any medication options. Do not use this information for patient care.**

THE FEMALE REPRODUCTIVE SYSTEM

Like the male counterpart, the female reproductive system is designed to generate a gamete, the egg or ovum, and deliver it via a tube to the uterus. It is also designed to carry the product of the union, an embryo. The female system is more internal versus external and involves four hormones. The external area has several structures sharing the same muscles, tissues, and sensations of the male, but in a different configuration (Figure 15.13).

- **Perineum** (**pear**-ee-**knee**-um) > the area between the anus and vagina in women and the penis in men.
  - Episiotomy (ee-**piz**-ee-**ot**-oh-me) > to cut into the vulva and proximal perineum to expand space for birthing. Episi/o > perineal area.

- **Vulva** (**vul**-vah) > general term describing the area including the clitoris, labia, hymen, and vaginal opening.
  - **Vulvitis** (**vul**-vie-tis) > inflammation of the vulva, associated with yeast infections or similar.

- **Labia** (lay-**bee**-ah) > lips, in this case, the outer (majora) and inner (minora) set protecting the vaginal opening.
  - **Labioplasty** (lay-**bee**-oh-**plaz**-tea) > repair of the lips. This is used primarily for dental repair. **Vulvoplasty** is used for perineum.

15.17
LIKE ALERT!
Peritoneum > the double-layer sac encasing some of the abdominal contents.

Perineum > genital area.

Labia > lips, check the documentation to ensure discussion concerns female anatomy versus the lips of the mouth (dental notes).

Word parts:
Labi/o > lips
Vulv/o > roll (of skin)
–megaly > enlargement
–ectomy > to cut out, remove
–itis > inflammation

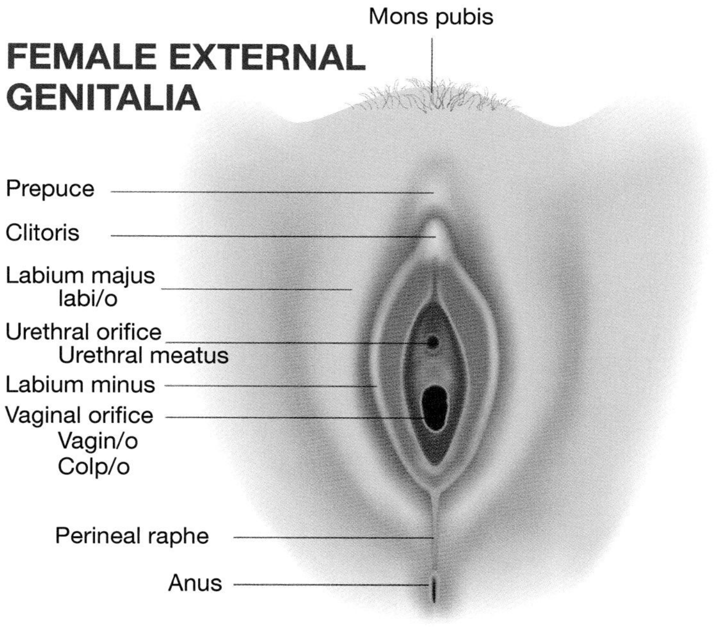

FEMALE EXTERNAL GENITALIA

Mons pubis

Prepuce

Clitoris

Labium majus
    labi/o

Urethral orifice
    Urethral meatus

Labium minus

Vaginal orifice
    Vagin/o
    Colp/o

Perineal raphe

Anus

Figure 15.13

- **Clitoris** (**klit**-or–is) > erectile body, superior aspect of vulva. It is analogous to the male penis with the same sensitivity. It is protected by a small prepuce as well.
  - In some cultures the clitoris of young women is damaged or removed (clitorectomy).

- **Hymen** (**high**-men) > thin membrane covering the vaginal opening prior to use of tampons or sexual activity. It may be complete or incomplete.

The **vagina** is the copulation organ of the female. It is muscular with a thick mucosa layer producing mucus for protection and lubrication. Like the average penile length, the vagina is approximately 6 inches (15 cm) long.

- **Vagin/o** > 'sheath', associated with anatomy and clinical conditions.
  - **Vaginitis** (**vaj**-ee-**nigh**-tis) > inflammation of the vagina. A typical cause is a yeast infection (Figure 15.14).
  - **Vaginosis** (**vaj**-ee-**no**-oh-sis) > abnormal condition of the vagina frequently used to describe vaginal discharge until culture return of bacterial, viral, or fungal infection.

15.18

Suffixes

–scopy > process of using an instrument to look

–pexy > to fix in place

–plasty > to repair

–dynia > pain

–cele > hernia

–pathy > disease of

–rrhaphy > suturing

VAGINITIS

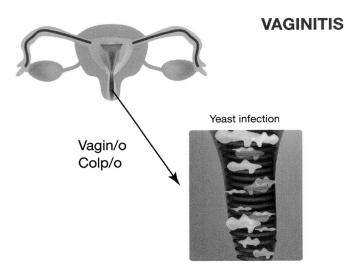

Vagin/o
Colp/o

Yeast infection

Inflammation in the vagina due to candidiasis

Figure 15.14

- **Colp/o** > Greek for 'hollow fold' > vagina.
  - **Colposcopy** (kol-**pos**-ko-pee) > instrument to look at the vagina.
  - **Colporrhexis** (**kol**-por-**rek**-sis) > tear or rupture of the vagina.
  - **Colpocleisis** (**kol**-po-**kleye**-sis) > surgical closure of the vagina.
- **Cul-de-sac** (kul-deh-**sahk**) > deep vaginal blind pouch merges with the cervix. This is a convenient space to access the distal uterus with a needle for an amniocentesis.
  - **Amniocentesis** (am-**knee**-oh-**sen**-tea-sis) > needle inserted into the amniotic sac supporting the fetus. Fluid is tested for a variety of genetic and laboratory values.

–cleisis > closure

–centesis > puncture

–ptosis > falling, prolapse

–rrhexis > tear, rupture

Amni/o > fluid within the sac floating the fetus in the uterus.

Vaginitis occurs due to trauma or infection. These are frequently seen especially in women with multiple partners. Many of these are considered STDs and all of them can be cycled between the man and woman.

- **Monilia candidiasis** (moe-**nil**-ee-ah **can**-dee-**die**-ah-sis) > yeast or fungal infestation presents with thick, white discharge (cottage-cheese look) and pruritus (prue-**ree**-tus) > itchy.

- **Trichomoniasis** (**trik**-oh-moe-**nigh**-ah-sis) > infestation of malodorous, green–yellow, thin discharge with colpodynia. It is a **protozoan** (pro-toe-**zoh**-ahn) as seen in Figure 15.15. Abbreviated: Trich (trik). Treated with antibiotics.

15.19

Did You Know?

The fungus 'candida' is also associated with oral thrush, diaper rash, athlete's foot, and respiratory infections. These are worse with immune-deficient

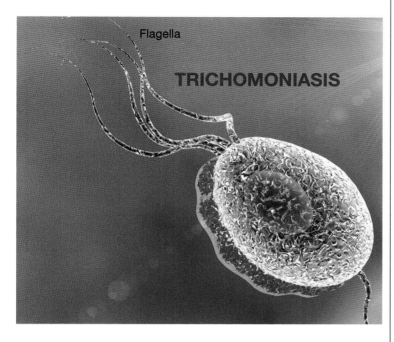

Flagella

TRICHOMONIASIS

Figure 15.15

diseases such as HIV. Treatment includes fluconazole, amphotericin, and topical nystatin or clotrimazole.

–iasis > infestation

–osis > abnormal condition

–trophy > growth

- **Bacterial vaginosis** > grayish-white, fish-smelling discharge.

- **Vaginal atrophy** (at-row-fee) > loss of hydration and hormone stimulation causes the mucosal layer to be dry and friable.

- **STDs** > chlamydia, gonorrhea, herpes (HSV), and genital warts (HPV).

 What is the suffix meaning 'infestation'?

 A vaginoperineorrhaphy was performed on Bianca. What is the meaning of the term?

Which vaginitis presents with a cottage-cheese discharge?

15.20
–iasis
15.21
Suturing the vagina and perineum
15.22
Yeast or candidiasis

Word building

 Using the word roots with the linking vowel to build as many valid terms with the suffixes given. Please define each term.

Colp/o Vulv/o Labi /o

–itis –pexy –plasty –ectomy –dynia –cele

15.23
The instructor has the list!

The **cervix** of the uterus is the last point of external exposure for the female reproductive organs. It is the neck of the uterus or the womb.

- **Cervic/o** > neck > approximately 3 cm long, it presents at the most superior aspect of the **vagina**. There is an external **os** (opening) and internal os which opens to the internal uterus. Between the two openings is the endocervical canal.

  - **Cervicitis** (**ser**-vee-**sigh**-tis) > inflammation of the cervix. The infections of the vagina bathe the cervix in the same process. Excess inflammation over time can lead to cervical cancer, particularly from HPV (Figure 15.16).

  - **Cervical cultures** > pertaining to the cervix > cultures done during a PAP test or independently help define infections.

  - **PAP test**, **Papanicolaou test**, can detect abnormal cells in the cervical mucosa. Cervical cancer diagnoses are found in the ICD Table of Neoplasms.

  - **Cervical cancer** > HPV infections are the most common cause of this cancer. Approximately 12,000 women will be diagnosed each year and over 1/4 will die with the disease.

  - **Biopsy of the cervix** can be done by punch biopsy, an endocervical curettage, or a cone biopsy.

15.24

LIKE ALERT!

Cervic/o > neck is the neck of the uterus AND the neck holding up the head.

Cervix (singular)

Cervices (plural)

Punch > 1 to 5 mm core biopsy.

Curettage (kyur-eh-**tahz**) > shave biopsy with curved loop.

Conization (ko-nigh-**zay**-shun) > deep, cone-shaped removal of tissue (Figure 15.17). This can also achieve cure in some cases.

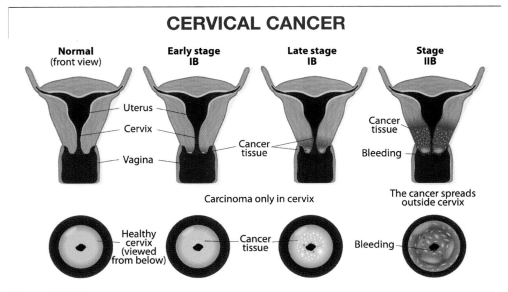

CERVICAL CANCER

Normal (front view) **Early stage IB** **Late stage IB** **Stage IIB**

Uterus
Cervix
Vagina
Cancer tissue
Cancer tissue
Bleeding

Carcinoma only in cervix

The cancer spreads outside cervix

Healthy cervix (viewed from below)
Cancer tissue
Bleeding

Figure 15.16

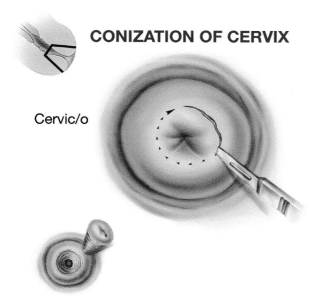

CONIZATION OF CERVIX

Cervic/o

Figure 15.17

The **womb** over the eons, in most cultures, is a revered place because life is born of the womb. The uterus is the anatomical term for this muscular, pear-shaped pouch. It is about 8 cm long at rest (Figure 15.18). There are four combining forms:

- **Men/o** > Greek for month or Latin for honor > used to describe the cycle of the reproductive system occurring on a monthly basis in the absence of pregnancy.
  - Menstruation (**men**-stru-**ay**-shun) > cyclic shedding and discharge of vascular fluids and tissues from the uterus.

- **Hyster/o** > Greek for womb > used primarily for conditions and procedures.
  - **Hyster**ectomy (**his**-tur-**ek**-toe-me) > removal of the uterus.
  - **Hyster**ocleisis (**his**-tur-oh-**kleye**-sis) > surgery to close the uterus.
  - **Hyster**omy**oma** (**his**-tur-oh-**my**-oh-mah) > a muscle tumor of the uterus. The majority of the uterus is muscular.

- **Uter/o** > Latin for uterus > most associated with anatomic descriptions but there are some terms for procedures.
  - **Uter**ine atony (**U**-tur-ine **at**-oh-knee) > failure of the myometrium (muscle layers of the uterus) to contract.

15.25

Did You Know?

The word root, hyster/o is also the root for the term hysterical > extreme emotion with screaming, crying, and/or laughter. During childbirth this is an apt description of a woman in labor.

FEMALE REPRODUCTIVE SYSTEM
Uter/o or Hyster/o or Metri/o

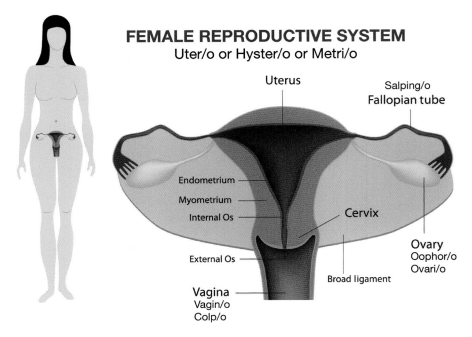

Uterus

Salping/o
Fallopian tube

Endometrium

Myometrium

Internal Os

Cervix

External Os

Ovary
Oophor/o
Ovari/o

Broad ligament

Vagina
Vagin/o
Colp/o

Figure 15.18

THE OCCURRENCE OF ENDOMETRIOSIS
Endo- > inside   Metri/o > lining of uterus

Pieces of the endometrium take root.
These are the locations of endometriosis.

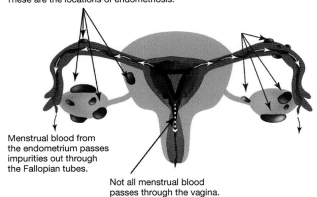

Menstrual blood from
the endometrium passes
impurities out through
the Fallopian tubes.

Not all menstrual blood
passes through the vagina.

Figure 15.19

Suffixes

–itis > inflammation

–atresia > closed

–tomy > cut into

–cele > hernia

–rrhexis > rupture

–lysis > destruction
of

–gram > record of

–algia or –dynia >
pain

–spasm > cramps

–plasty > repair

–rrhea > discharge

–rragia > excessive
bleeding

–scopy > instrument
to look

–osis > abnormal
condition

- Uterosalpingography (**U**–tur–oh–**sal**–ping–**goh**–graf–ee) > process of recording the uterine tube and uterus for open passageway.

- Metri/o > Greek for uterus > generally used to describe the internal layer of the uterus, the vascular bed shed monthly or that hosts the embryo in pregnancy.
  - **Endometritis** (**en**–doe–me–**try**–tis) > inflammation of the inner lining of the uterus. Causes include recent miscarriage, abortive procedures, chlamydia, gonorrhea, tuberculosis, and a mix of normal vaginal bacteria.
  - **Endometriosis** (**en**–doe–me–tree–**oh**–sis) > abnormal condition of the inner lining of the uterus being 'out of place' (Figure 15.19).
  - **Metrorrhagia** (**me**–trow–**ra**–jee–ah) > off-cycle bleeding from the uterus. It is also used for excessive bleeding.
  - **Endometrial** carcin**oma** is seen in postmenopausal women. Since it is associated with a return of menses, it tends to be found early and treated successfully.

 A uterine fibroid is causing dysmenorrhea for Gloria. What is the meaning of 'dysmenorrhea'?

 A Papanicolaou test will evaluate the cervix for abnormal cells. The abbreviation for this test is _____ .

15.26
Painful menses

15.27
PAP test

The **ovary** is the female gonad, producing the eggs to the male sperm. While the paired ovaries will produce approximately 1 million ova over a lifetime, only about 500 will be viable for fertilization. Unlike men, the female gonad will stop producing in the late 50s for most women.

- O/o or Ov/o > egg > like the sperm, each egg or ovum develops in stages under the influence of **FSH (Gonadotropin)**, **LH**, Estrogen, and Progesterone.
  - **O**ocyte (**oh**–ou–site) > female sex cell.
  - **O**ogenesis (**oh**–ou–**jen**–ee–sis) > process of developing eggs.
- Oophor/o > Greek for 'egg bearing', ovary > used to discussed conditions or procedures concerning the ovaries.
  - **Oophorectomy** (**oh**–ou–for–**ek**–toe–me) > removal of an ovary.
  - **Oophoropexy** (**oh**–ou–for–oh–**pek**–see) > to fix the ovary in place.

15.28
The pronunciation of o/o is also heard as '**oh**-oh-site' or '**oh**-oh-for-**ek**-toe-me'

Specific menses terms:

Amen**orrhea** (a–**men**–or–**ree**–ah) > no flow

Oligomen**orrhea** (**ol**–ee–go–**men**–oh–ree–ah) > scant flow

Dysmen**orrhea** (dis–**men**–oh–**ree**–ah) > painful or difficult flow

- **Ovari/o** or **Ovar/o** > Latin for ovary > seen for the anatomy and some conditions such as
  - **Polycystic ovarian (PCO) disease** > ovarian cysts form, fill with fluid, and change hormone levels. This causes dysmenorrhea, prolonged menses, acne, and facial hair in most women with this condition (Figure 15.20).
  - **Ovarian follicle** (oh-**ver**-ee-an **fol**-i-kel) > one of the stages of development, a spherical cell accretion in the ovary containing an oocyte.

Menarche > first menses

Menopause > last menses

The timing of puberty in women is dependent on both hormones and adequate food intake. Starvation or extreme athleticism can cause amenorrhea.

FEMALE REPRODUCTIVE SYSTEM DISEASES:
polycystic ovarian syndrome

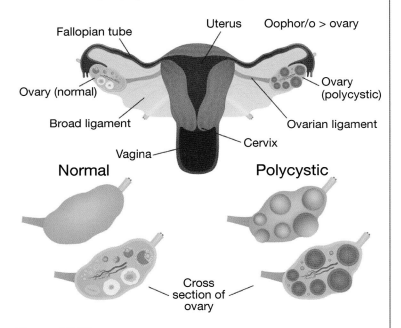

Figure 15.20

✓ The neck of the uterus is properly called the _____ .

✓ A 'hysteromyotomy' means _____ _____ .

✓ Jeanine is having a hysteroscope today to investigate a polyp. What is a 'hysteroscope'?

15.29
cervix

15.30
to cut into the uterine muscle

15.31
An instrument to look in the uterus

The **uterine tubes** or **Fallopian tubes** (an eponym) are essentially similar to the vas deferens in men: they carry the ovum to the uterus. Each tube is approximately 10 cm (4 inches) long and 1 cm wide (Figure 15.21). They are uniquely populated by specialized cilia to move the ovum or zygote along the tube until it enters the uterus. They also produce special glycoproteins to nourish the cells in transit.

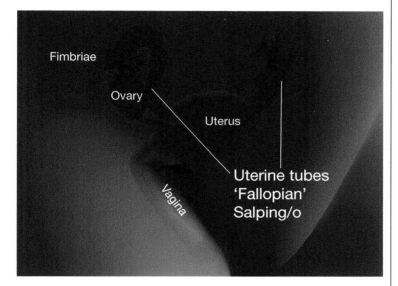

Fimbriae

Ovary

Uterus

Vagina

Uterine tubes
'Fallopian'
Salping/o

Figure 15.21

- **Salping/o** > Greek for trumpet > the shape of the tube lends itself to the name as the fimbriae (**fim**-breh) > fingers or fringe forming a funnel over each ovary to capture the released ovum.
  - **Salping**oscope (sal-**ping**-go-skop) > instrument to look at the uterine tube; done when a patient has difficulty getting pregnant to see if there is a blockage.
  - **Salping**ectomy (**sal**-pin-**jek**-toe-me) > removal of uterine tube usually secondary to an ectopic pregnancy.
  - **Salping**opexy (sal-**ping**-go-pek-see) > fixing the uterine tube in place.

Pelvic inflammatory disease (PID) > complication usually involving the cervix, uterus, salpinges, and ovaries on one or both sides (Figure 15.22). It is typically caused by **STDs**, such as gonorrhea and chlamydia. PID patients have infertility issues due to scar tissue and swelling of the salpinx or swelling of the ovaries and cervix.

15.32

Salpinx > singular

Salpinges > plural

Fimbria > singular

Fimbriae > plural

Suffixes

–itis > inflammation

–tomy > to cut into

–ostomy > to create a new opening

–plasty > repair of

–lysis > destruction of

–cele > herniation

–graphy > process of recording

–rrhaphy > suturing

15.33

Pelvic inflammatory disease
PID

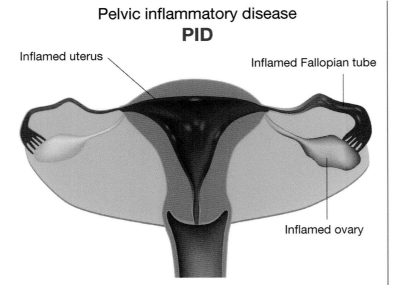

Inflamed uterus

Inflamed Fallopian tube

Inflamed ovary

Figure 15.22

The uterine tube has segment names associated with these two conditions:

Ampulla (am-**pew**-lah) > dilated end of a tube.

Isthmus (**is**-mus) > constriction or narrowing of a tube or structure.

- **Ectopic** (ek-**top**-ik) pregnancy > 'out of place' > zygote implants outside of the uterus (Figure 15.23). It can occur from the fimbria, anywhere along the uterine tube, the uterine interstitial tissue, in the cervical canal or even in the abdominal or pelvic cavities. An ectopic rupture can be a medical emergency.

TYPES OF ECTOPIC PREGNANCY

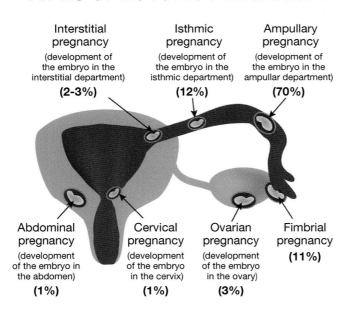

Interstitial pregnancy
(development of the embryo in the interstitial department)
(2-3%)

Isthmic pregnancy
(development of the embryo in the isthmic department)
(12%)

Ampullary pregnancy
(development of the embryo in the ampullar department)
(70%)

Abdominal pregnancy
(development of the embryo in the abdomen)
(1%)

Cervical pregnancy
(development of the embryo in the cervix)
(1%)

Ovarian pregnancy
(development of the embryo in the ovary)
(3%)

Fimbrial pregnancy
(11%)

Figure 15.23

Word building

Using the word roots with the linking vowel to build as many valid terms with the suffixes given. Please define each term.

Hyster/o Salpingo/o Cervic/o

–plasty –rrhaphy –otomy –gram –ectomy –itis

15.34
The instructor has the list!

MEDICAL ETHICS TERMS

Documentation is used for many things from tracking the progress of the patient to keeping statistics on spontaneous abortions. It is also used to evaluate the ethics of a situation. There are four key medical ethical terms which are mirrored in documentation in a variety of ways.

1 **Autonomy** (aw-**ton**-oh-me) > patient's right to make their own decisions. This right is protected specifically by the 1996 law, Patient Rights Act in the United States, and it is upheld in any number of worldwide documents as well. In day-to-day documentation the most evident function of autonomy is the signed consent form. By law and several guidelines, patients must understand why they need a procedure, how it will be done, by whom, and all the benefits and risks involved. Additionally, it must be in language the average person will understand. Patients should feel confident that their team is working responsibly to manage their health. If consent forms are absent or incomplete they never happened, just like all documentation.

2 **Beneficence** (be-**neh**-fee-sens) > practice of doing what is good and correct for the patient. It is incumbent on every person working in healthcare to do their very best to deliver the finest healthcare to all patients. Providers are to do what is right for the patient – perhaps it is recommending a surgery or a specific medication. It is found in the language of documentation as 'chart reviews' for standard of care or the practice of clinical guidelines. If a provider chooses to deviate from the norm, the rationale for such action must be evident in the documentation of patient care. There are times when autonomy and beneficence conflict, such as when a provider thinks it is in the best interest of the mother to abort a doomed fetus but Mom wants to carry the child to term; it is her right.

3 **Nonmaleficence** (**non**-mah-**leh**-fee-sens) > if a provider cannot do 'good' – at least do no harm. This occurs more frequently than one might anticipate. An example is the presence of terminal breast cancer which medicine and the providers cannot cure but providers should do nothing to make it worse AND protect the patient's quality of life. This ethical premise is tested in documentation in the chart reviews and in malpractice courts. Make sure the language, the intent, and the expectations of any treatment are clear in documentation with the correct terms and spelling.

4 **Justice** (**jus**-tis) > giving equal treatment to all patients. Every patient with pelvic inflammatory disease deserves the same investigation and options for treatment no matter their location or ability to pay. It is not just to withhold proper medical care for one patient and then deliver it for another. All patients should be treated with compassion and dignity. This precept is upheld by a number of laws including **HIPAA**, Patient Right Act, and **EMTALA** (Emergency Medical Treatment and Labor Act). It is also addressed in the Fraud laws – not taking advantage of loopholes or un-bundling coding to make an undue profit from the illness or injury of others.

BIRTHING A NEW PERSON

Copulation is the sexual act between a man and woman (Figure 15.24). There are many terms for the act of reproduction (e.g., sexual intercourse).

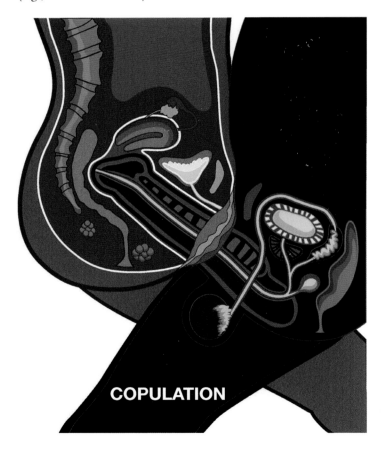

COPULATION

15.35
Sexual intercourse can be painful for one or both partners for a variety of reasons. The medical term is **dyspareunia** (dis-pahr-ou-knee-ah).

Honeymoon cystitis describes the dysuria encountered after first-time sexual activity. The skin and mucosal surfaces suffer from abrasion and the urethra tends to be populated with more contaminants than usual.

Figure 15.24

- **Sex** (seks) > features distinguishing male from female. It is based on gonads, internal and external physical findings, chromosome pattern, and hormones.

  - **Sexuality** (**sek**-shu-**al**-i-tee) > sum of a person's preferred sexual behaviors and tendencies.

  - **Andr/o** > male human being. Symbol is ♂

    o Androgen (an-**drow**-jen) > hormone agent stimulates male characteristics.

  - **Gyn/o** or **Gynec/o** > female human being. Symbol is ♀

    o Gynecology (**gi**-neh-**kol**-oh-gee) > study of women.

- **Copulation** > joining, the merging of two independent cells (or people) which then separate.

- **Coitus** (**ko**-i-tus) > sexual union or **pareunia** (pa-**rue**-knee-ah) > French for lying beside.

There are three hormones produced by the **pituitary gland** in the brain. These stimulate sexual characteristics and play a role in post-pregnancy activities. It creates a feedback loop.

- **Follicle-stimulating hormone** or **Gonadotropin-releasing hormone (FSH** or **GnRH)** > at puberty, this activates the gonads to produce their own specific hormones.

HORMONAL CONTROL OF OVULATION

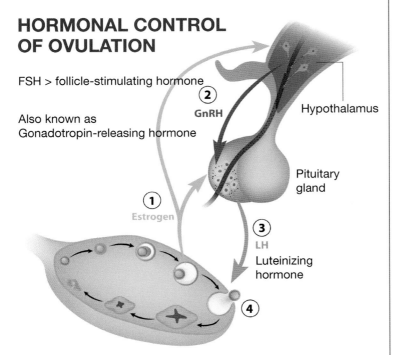

FSH > follicle-stimulating hormone

Also known as Gonadotropin-releasing hormone

② GnRH

Hypothalamus

① Estrogen

Pituitary gland

③ LH Luteinizing hormone

④

15.36

Did You Know?

Despite millions of sperm being released at the cervical os, only a small fraction will make it into the uterus and move up into the uterine tube to fertilize an ovum. The acidity of the vagina, mucus plug at the os, and relative lack of fructose to generate motion limit the viable sperm to dozens.

Figure 15.25

- **Luteinizing hormone (LH)** > supports both gonads on maintaining gonadal health and in the case of the woman, the menstrual cycle (Figure 15.25).

- **Oxytocin** (**ock**-see-**toe**-sin) > one of only two produced by the posterior pituitary, this will
  - Stimulate the uterus to contract during labor.
  - 'Let down' milk from the breast as the baby is born.

The gonads will produce their own hormones to develop and deliver the sex-cells – gametes. They also trigger and maintain the secondary sexual characteristics. Both testosterone and estrogen are present in the opposite sexes, at much lower levels.

- **Testosterone** (tes-**tos**-tur-ohn) > male, stimulates sperm formation, the smallest cell by volume of the body, at about 5 micrometers.

- **Estrogen** (**es**-trow-jen) > female, triggers ovum formation, the largest cell type by volume of the body, at about 1,000 micrometers.

- **Progesterone** (pro-**jes**-tur-ohn) > female, provides the balance of the menstrual cycle or preparation for the zygote implantation. The spent follicular cyst produces it.

 Hugo is using androgenic hormones to bulk up his muscles. What does 'androgenic' mean?

Rebecca has a small vaginal vault, which is adding to her dyspareunia. What does 'dyspareunia' mean?

There are specific terms associated with the joining of the sperm and ova, including conception (kon-**sep**-shun). They bring their distinctive 23 chromosomes to create a new life with a complete set of 46 chromosomes. This is reproduction of life – **meiosis** (me-**oh**-sis). The cycle is seen in Figure 15.26.

LIKE ALERT!
Mitosis (my-**toe**-sis) > reproduction of cells to replace old or damaged cells.

- **Zygote** (**zeye**-goat) > fertilization of an oocyte by a sperm, joining chromosomes.

- **Embry/o** > fullness, swelling > early stages of development, the embryo (**em**-bree-oh) will implant in the uterine wall. This stage

The sperm has approximately 72 hours to make it to its destination.

A **retroverted** (positioned backward) uterus can slow the sperm.

15.37
Pertaining to male beginnings
15.38
Pain with intercourse

15.39
Meiosis > joining of chromosomes to create a new life.

Abortion (ab-**or**-shun) (**Ab**) > Latin for 'fail at onset' or away from normal.

Spontaneous is due to natural causes or a **miscarriage**. Induced is elective or therapeutic.

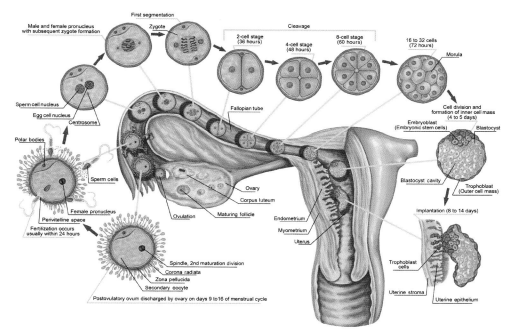

Figure 15.26

is 8 weeks long. It is the most vulnerable time to the child as many toxins can disrupt the neurologic development. Between 8–12 weeks is associated with spontaneous abortion secondary to genetic malformation.

- **Fetus** (**fee**-tus) > Latin for off-spring; used from the end of week 8 until the moment of birth. The pregnancy is evaluated in terms of trimesters, each 3 months long.

- **Infant** > live-birth, from the moment of delivery.

Pregnancy (**preg**-nan-see) > female condition of carrying the product of conception until termination of the product. It seems a cold definition for a new life but it is the purely scientific perspective. Related terms and word parts:

- **Gestation** (jes-**tay**-shun) > to bear, the act of bearing (a child).

- **Gravida** (**grav**-ee-dah) (**G**) > pregnant, to be heavy with (a child).
  - **Nulligravida** (**nul**-lee-**grav**-ee-dah) > no pregnancies.
  - **Primigravida** (**pre**-me-**grav**-ee-dah) > first pregnancy.
  - **Secundigravida** (seh-**kun**-di-**grav**-ee-dah) > second pregnancy.

15.40

Gest/o > to bear or carry

Estr/o > Greek for being in 'heat', able to produce offspring.

- **Parous** (pahr-us) (**P**) > Latin for to bear, to carry.
  - Antepartum (an-tee-pahr-tum) > before birth.
  - Post**partum** > after birth.

- **G4P3Ab1** > abbreviation set to indicate the number of pregnancies, live births, and abortions. The noted set means the woman has had 4 pregnancies, 3 live births, and 1 abortion. It is not specific regarding the type of abortion.
  - G3P4Ab0 would indicate 3 pregnancies, 4 live births (1 set of twins), and 0 abortions.

- **-cyesis** > pregnancy. **Pseudocyesis** (**sue**-doe-sigh-**ee**-sis) > false pregnancy. A **hydatiform** (**hi**-da-**tid**-oh-form) mole is a polycystic mass which mimics pregnancy with elevated HCG numbers.

- **-tocia** > childbirth, dystocia (dis-**toe**-see-ah) > difficult childbirth.

- Nat/**i** > birth, neonatal (knee-oh-**nay**-tal) > newborn.
  - Perinatal care > 'around birth' care.

 These abbreviations of '**G**' for gravida and '**P**' for parous do NOT stand alone. They are part of the set G P Ab. Define these sets for your instructor:

G1P3Ab1   G6P5Ab1   G2P5Ab0

The **placenta** (pla-**sen**-tah) > organ of pregnancy; part of the implantation of the embryo is the formation of the chorionic villi into the fetomaternal connection (Figure 15.27). This permits the mother's physiology to do the work for the developing fetus by circulating blood, providing nourishment, and removing toxins. It is highly vascular. It will detach after delivery of the child. The placenta produces the **HCG**: *human chorionic gonadotropin* (**kor**-ee-**on**-ik go-**nad**-oh-**trow**-pin) hormone is checked to determine pregnancy, making it an endocrine organ too.

- **Abruptio** (ah-**brupt**-she-oh) **placenta** > premature separation of the placenta; this can interrupt and end the pregnancy.

- **Placenta previa** (pre-**vee**-ah) > placenta is located in the wrong place in the distal uterus, often covering the cervical canal.

15.41
Qualitative HCG by urine denotes pregnancy but does not define a length of time estimate.

Quantitative HCG from blood gives a specific number; it is associated with gestation time such as – at 13–16 weeks it is likely to be 13,300–250,000 units. It is a wide range. A decreasing **HCG** tends to indicate a miscarriage.

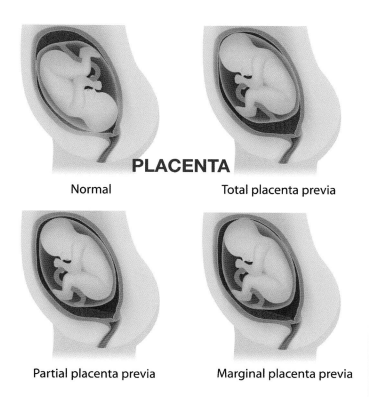

PLACENTA

Normal   Total placenta previa

Partial placenta previa   Marginal placenta previa

Figure 15.27

The **breast** is not part of the procreation process of pregnancy but it is essential to the postpartum infant (Figure 15.28).

- Mamm/o > breast > primarily used for anatomy such as mammary glands, but there are some procedure terms as well.
  - **Mammogram** (**mam**-oh-gram) > a record of the breast (tissue).
- Mast/o > breast > seen with conditions and procedure.
  - **Mastectomy** (mas-**tek**-toe-me) > to remove the breast.
  - **Mastodynia** (**mas**-toe-**die**-knee-ah) > pain in the breast.
- **Mastitis** (mas-**tie**-tis) > inflammation of the breast, common with early breast feeding.

Breast cancer remains one of the top cancers to inflict women worldwide. It is most associated with aging but weight, body composition, estrogen levels, and genetics all play a role in the disease. As noted in Figure 15.29, not all things lumpy in the breast indicate cancer BUT these should always be investigated.

15.42

Suffixes

–itis > inflammation

–algia > pain

–oid > resembling

–oma > tumor

–rrhea > discharge

–plasia > development

–pexy > fix in place

–ptosis > sagging or drooping

–rrhagia > hemorrhage, bleeding

–pathy > disease of

MEDICAL STRUCTURE OF THE FEMALE BREAST

Mast/o or Mamm/o > breast

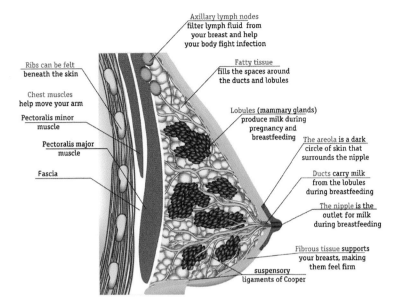

Figure 15.28

BREAST DISEASE

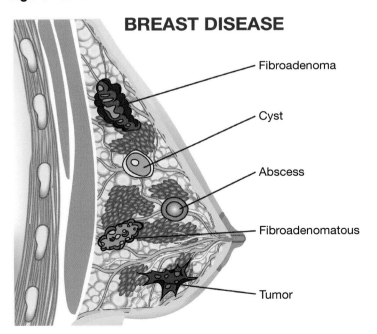

Figure 15.29

- **Fibrocystic breast disease** > fibrous tissue and cysts tend to enlarge and become tender during menses.

- **Cystic breast disease** > cyst (tiny bladders) fills and empties via hormone changes. Since the breast is designed to fill with milk, the sacs and ducts are susceptible to these changes.

- **Fibroadenoma** > fibrous, glandular tumor, benign.

- **Ductal carcinoma** > metastatic breast cancer; the number of lymphatics in the breast, axilla, and thoracic cavity make metastasis likely.

The gene markers of **BRCA1** and **BRCA2** can be useful to guide women at risk for breast carcinoma.

Breast disease can be checked via ultrasound (US), mammogram, CT, or MRI. Biopsy is most definitive.

 Anita is a 43-yo woman who is G5P7Ab1. What does this notation mean?

 Spelling for the organ of pregnancy:

        Playsenta Phlacenta Placenta Plehcenta

15.43
Pregnancy 5, live births 7, and abortion 1
15.44
Placenta

Word building

 Using the word roots with the linking vowel to build as many valid terms with the suffixes given. Please define each term.

    Mast/o Testicul/o Embry/o

    –logy –plasty –rrhaphy –otomy –gram
    –ectomy –itis

15.45
The instructor has the list!

Birthing is a complex process relying on a variety of hormones and some mechanical requirements. The placenta will slowly increase both estrogen and progesterone during the pregnancy to help the uterus expand without becoming irritable.

- **Human placental lactogen** (**lak**-toe-jen) (HPL) > stimulates maternal fat and protein actions to provide adequate nutrition to the growing fetus. It also activates the milk-producing glands of the breasts.

- Oxytocin from Mom and adrenocortical stress hormones from the fetus start labor. The cervix dilates and flattens as the baby progresses down the cervical canal. This is called **effacement** (ef-**fas**-ment).

Presentations > position of the fetus as they progress through the cervical canal (Figure 15.30).

15.46
C-section > abbreviation for an eponym, **Cesarean**.

Procedure to remove the fetus via transverse abdominal incision. The reasons for a C-section include fetal distress, mechanical difficulty in traversing the birthing canal, maternal eclampsia, or other metabolic

PRESENTATION

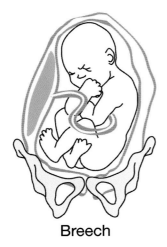
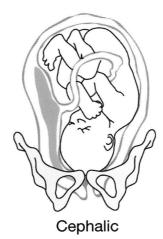

Breech   Cephalic

Figure 15.30

- **Cephalic** (ceh-**fal**-ik) > head first into the cervical canal, this is the preferred or normal position. It allows the infant's mouth to clear the compression of delivery first so a breath may be taken.

- **Breech** > buttock first or a combination. A foot may present or a hip. Mechanically, this is not a good position and it leaves the respiratory tract susceptible to inhaling inside the fluid-filled uterus.

- **Shoulder** and **Compound** positions are as similarly difficult as the breech. These presentations may end in a C-section to protect the newborn.

- **Meconium** (me-**ko**-knee-um) > green-yellowish stool may be expelled prior to birth by the fetus. This is called meconium staining. The danger comes if the fetus/infant inhales the meconium causing a hypoxic event for the infant.

issues, and the presence of cervical or vaginal infections in Mom.

A drop in fetal heart rate (less than 150 per minute) indicates distress. Slowing heart rate suggests hypoxia (hi-**pok**-ee-ah) > low oxygen.

Genetic disorders exceed 1200 types to date. These occur because of the diversity of the human genome. These are a few of the common hereditary DNA mutations, the test, and the **cpt**® code from an online search.

- **Cystic fibrosis** > Cystic Fibrosis Transmembrane Regulator (**CFTR**) gene, cpt® code 81220–81224.

- **Huntington's disease** > **HD** gene on chromosome 4, cpt®81401.

15.47

cpt > current procedural terminology is the coding manual for testing, procedures, and some materials.

- **Down syndrome** or Trisomy 21> Fetal chromosomal aneuploidy (e.g., trisomy 21, monosomy X) genomic sequence analysis panel, cpt® 81420.

- **Duchenne muscular dystrophy** > *DMD* gene specifies instructions for making of the protein called dystrophin, cpt® 81161, 81408.

- **Sickle cell anemia** > Mutations in the *HBB* gene cause sickle cell disease, cpt® 81401, 81403, 81404.

- **Celiac disease** > variants of the *HLA-DQA1* and *HLA-DQB1* genes, cpt® 81382, 81376.

Since the human genome was mapped (1990s), the number of genetic tests available is up to about 1200. A commercial oral swab can give anyone an estimate of genetic propensities. Besides the value in pre-pregnancy planning for a couple, the genetic knowledge may in time allow changes to be made **en-utero** (in the uterus) to the developing embryo or fetus. This would negate disabilities and chronic disease if successful.

★ **IMPORTANT NOTE: The student is reminded these cpt® codes are likely to be different in the current edition of the cpt®. Do <u>not</u> use these for patient encounters.**

 Because Jasmine's baby is breech and her pelvis is small, which of the following is a reasonable method to deliver the child? Hysterectomy C-section Oophorostomy Salpingotomy

 A benign fibroadenoma is defined as _____ .

Between day 0 and 56, the product of conception is called the _____ .

Aneuploidy (**an**-yu-**ploy**-dee) > state of having abnormal number of chromosomes with incomplete sets versus duplication of sets.

15.48 C-section

15.49 tumor of fiber and glands

15.50 embryo

UNIT SUMMARY

1   The reproductive system is the only system of the body NOT required for survival of the individual. It is required for the survival of the species. It requires the two sex gametes, an ovum and sperm to meet and the support of the maternal womb to produce a child.

2   The male genitalia are more external, including the testicles suspended in the scrotum. The testicles produce testosterone and the sperm. The sperm travels to the epididymis to mature. Millions of sperm will travel up into the pelvis via the vas deferens. Joining with the seminal vesicle and prostate fluids, it becomes the semen, the ejaculate. The penis is the copulation organ for males and part of the urinary system as well.

3   The external anatomy of the female as a whole is called the vulva and includes the labia majora and minora, vagina opening, clitoris, and urethra. The vaginal vault is the copulation organ of women and gives way to the cul-de-sac and cervical os. The cervix is the neck of the internal uterus where a fetus will mature during pregnancy. The uterine tube conveys the ovum (the egg) from the ovary to the uterus approximately every 28 days.

4   Hormones involved with the reproductive system include three from the pituitary gland: follicle-stimulating hormone (**FSH**), luteinizing hormone (**LH**), and oxytocin. The male testis will produce testosterone guiding the production of sperm. The female ovary and the placenta will produce estrogen and progesterone in a balance to maintain the health of the uterus.

5   Both sexes are susceptible to a variety of sexually transmitted diseases (**STDs**) which are easily swapped back and forth when one partner remains untreated. Infections include **HIV, HPV, HSV** – all viruses and uncurable. There is a vaccination for HPV. Bacterial infections include gonorrhea, chlamydia, and syphilis. Fungal infections are not considered STDs but they can persist in the absence of treatment.

6   When the millions of sperm are released at climax, only a few will make it to the destination, the ovum. Once joined, the conception is called a zygote until it implants on the uterine wall. During the first 56 days, the growing cells are called the **embryo** and after 56 days, the **fetus** until delivery. A vaginal delivery is the preferred method but it does depend on the health of the mother, fetus, and presentation at the time of labor. A **HCG**, human choriogonadotropin level can give an indication of and progress of the pregnancy.

7   There are many possibilities of genetic flaws particularly in the first trimester. The embryo is susceptible to toxins and injury and DNA errors. A spontaneous abortion (miscarriage) is often the result of the body being unable to maintain growth due to the errors. Elective or induced abortions are done as related to maternal decisions or specific therapeutic needs.

UNIT WORD PARTS

Word roots with linking vowel		
Amni/o > fluid of uterus	Balan/o > glans penis	Cervic/o > neck
Colp/o or Vagin/o > vagina	Corp/o > body	Embry/o > full, swelling
Epididym/o > epididymis	Episi/o > perineal area	Estr/o > able to bear children
Gest/o > to bear, to carry	Gonad/o > seed, sexual organ	Hyster/o or Uter/o > uterus, womb
Labi/o > lips	Mamm/o or Mast/o > breast	Meat/o > opening
Men/o > month, honor	Metri/o > inside lining of uterus	O/o > egg
Oopor/o or Ovari/o > ovary	Orchid/o or Test/i or Testicul/o > testicles	Phall/o > penis
Prostat/o > prostate	Salping/o > trumpet, tube	Scrot/o > sac, scrotum
Spermat/o > sperm	Urethr/o > urethra	Vas/o > vessel, tube

Prefixes: attached to the front of the word root to change meaning		
Ante- > before, forward	Crypto- > hidden	Dys- > bad, poor, difficult
Ec- > outside	Endo- > inner, inside	Hydro- > water
Intra- > between	Multi- or Poly- > many	Neo- > new
Nulli- > none, zero	Peri- > around	Post- > before, behind
Pre- > before	Primi- > first, one	Secundi- > second, two

Suffixes change the meaning of the word, linking vowel is usually 'o' with consonants		
-algia or -dynia > pain	-arche > beginning	-cele > hernia
-centesis > puncture	-cyesis > pregnant	-ectomy > to remove, cut out
-gram or -graphy > record, process of recording	-iasis > infestation	-ism > pertaining to a collection of
-itis > inflammation	-lysis > destroy	-megaly > enlargement
-oma > tumor	-osis > abnormal condition	-ostomy > create a new opening
-parous > to bear, to carry	-pathy > disease of	-pexy > to fix in place
-plasty > repair	-ptosis > sagging, falling	-rrhagia > hemorrhage
-rrhaphy > suture	-rrhea > discharge	-rrhexis > rupture
-scope or –scopy > instrument to look and the process	-spasm > contractions	-tocia > labor
-tomy > to cut into	-trophy > growth, development	

Acronyms, abbreviations, and initial sets		
BPH > benign prostatic hypertrophy	BRCA 1 and 2 > breast cancer gene marker	CDC > Centers of Disease Control and Prevention
Colpo > slang for colposcope	DMD > Duchenne's muscular dystrophy	DRE > digital rectal exam
ED > erectile dysfunction	EMTALA > Emergency Medical Treatment and Labor Act	FSH > follicle-stimulating hormones or GnRH (Gonadotropin-releasing hormone)
GPAb > gravida, parous, abortion	HCG or hCG > human chorionic gonadotropin	HD > Huntington's disease
HIPAA > Health Information Portability and Accountability Act	HIV > human immunodeficient virus	HPL > human placental lactogen
HPV > human papilloma virus	HSV > human simplex virus	LH > luteinizing hormone
PAP > Papanicolaou test	PID > pelvic inflammatory disease	PSA > prostate specific antigen
RPR > rapid plasma reagin	STD or STI > sexually transmitted disease or infection	WHO > World Health Organization

UNIT WORKSHEETS

Building terms: Use the proper prefix/word root/linking vowel/suffix as appropriate.

Example: to cut into the heart > cardi/o/tomy

a) Inflammation of the glans penis > _____

b) Infestation of yeast > _____

c) The study of women > _____

d) Surgical removal of the uterus > _____

e) Many pregnancies > _____

f) Inflammation of the uterine tube > _____

g) Tumor of the testicle > _____

h) An instrument to look at the vagina > _____

Know your initial sets/acronyms! For the initial set or acronym given, spell it out correctly.

a) HPV _____

b) DRE _____

c) GPAb _____

d) BRCA1 _____

e) PAP _____

f) ED _____

g) PSA _____

h) GnRH _____

Best choice: Pick the most appropriate answer.

1 The term 'Phallorrhea'

   a) Refers to vomiting blood   c) Urination of blood

   b) Flow from the penis   d) Stopping bleeding

2 Beneficence

   a) To do no harm   c) Patient decision

   b) To do what is good   d) Equal care for all

3 Product of conception is called
   a) Fetus
   b) Gamete
   c) Zygote
   d) Smegma

4 A collection of fluid around the testicle
   a) Seminal varices
   b) Scrotal raphe
   c) Cryptorchidism
   d) Hydrocele

5 Semen combines all of the following **EXCEPT**
   a) sperm
   b) urine
   c) prostate fluids
   d) seminal fluids

Multiple correct: Select ALL the correct answers to the question or statement given.

1 Mark all bacterial STDs.
   a) HPV
   b) Chlamydia
   d) Candida
   c) Syphilis
   e) Gonorrhea
   f) HSV

2 Which of the following linking forms is associated with the internal structures of the female reproductive system?
   a) Labi/o
   b) Salping/o
   c) Oophor/o
   d) Clitor/o
   e) Metri/o

3 Which of the following hormones originate from the pituitary gland?
   a) FSH
   b) Testosterone
   c) HPL
   d) LH
   e) Oxytocin

Spelling challenge! Circle the correct spelling based on the definition given.

1 'Removal of the uterus and ovary'
   Ophorohisterectomy   Colpohysterostomy
   Oophorohysterectom   Salpingohysterostomy

2 'Reproduction of a new life'
   Mieosis   Miteosis   Mioesis   Meiosis

3 'Product to kill sperm'
   Spermoside   Spermatocide   Spurmatoside   Spermosidal

Define the term: Spelling *does* count in your definition too!

1 Epididymosis > _____

2 Trichomoniasis > _____

3 Endometritis > _____

4 Embryology > _____

5 Aneuploidy > _____

6 Conization > _____

7 Colporrhexis > _____

8 Multiparous > _____

Find it! Using the words in the table – match the definition given or answer the statement. Some may not be used. It is recommended you know all the choices.

oocyte	vasovasostomy	menarche	balanitis	hematocele
cervicitis	oophoropexy	clitorectomy	fibroadenoma	orchidomegaly
mastectomy	neonatal	prostatectomy	nulligravida	dystocia

1 _____ Fixing the ovary in place

2 _____ Enlargement of the testicle

3 _____ Difficult labor

4 _____ Egg cell

5 _____ Beginning of monthly periods

6 _____ Tumor of fibers and glands

7 _____ Removal of the prostate

8 _____ Inflammation of the glans penis

Matching: Some will not be used.

	Letter	Defined as	
Gonadotropin		a)	pointed backward
Isthmus		b)	to cut into the perineum
Hysteromyoma		c)	constriction or narrowing of a tube
Amniocentesis		d)	sex organ development
Anteverted		e)	repair of the opening
Breech		f)	abrasion of the glans penis
Meatoplasty		g)	puncture to remove fluid from sac
Episiotomy		h)	tumor of the uterine muscle
		i)	buttocks presentation
		j)	pointed forward

An essay: Write a short paper on your opinion on whether we should use genetic manipulation to prevent birth-defects, Yes or No? Use the four concepts of medical ethics to explain why.

Note challenge: Define the underlined terms. You may need to look up a few terms. Answer the questions which follow. Student is reminded this is an incomplete SOAP note used for the learning experience. Do not use this for patient encounters.

S. Julia is a 32-year-old woman: <u>nulligravida</u> with <u>metrorrhagia</u>, <u>dyspareunia</u>, and <u>dysmenorrhea</u>. Symptoms have increased steadily for the last 6 months. <u>PAP</u> test and <u>C&S</u> reveals no evidence of cervical cancer or infections.

O. Bimanual exam reveals an <u>anteverted</u> uterus, enlarged, and non-tender. <u>hCG</u> is negative. US is done revealing a <u>leiomyoma</u>.

A. Leiomyoma

P. Three options presented to the patient:

a) Hormone trial to shrink tumor
b) Limited <u>leiomyectomy</u>
c) Hysterectomy

Questions:

1 Translate all the acronyms/initial sets and give meaning to the words which are underlined in the note.

2 What hormones would be lost with a bilateral oophorectomy?

3 Are there any ethical questions in recommending a hysterectomy for a nulliparous woman? Why?

Glossary and pronunciation

Unit

Amblyopia > **am**-blee-**oh**-pee-ah > condition of dim vision, visual impairment.   8

Amenorrhea > a-**men**-or-**ree**-ah > absence of the discharge of menses (monthly period in women).   1, 15

Amitotic > **a**-my-**tot**-ik > cells cannot replicate or duplicate.   3, 7

Amnesia > am-**knee**-ze-a > temporary or permanent loss of memory.   7

Amniocentesis > am-**knee**-oh-**sen**-tea-sis > needle inserted into the amniotic sac supporting the fetus.   15

Amphiarthrosis > **am**-fee-are-**throw**-sis > joints slightly mobile in two directions (planes).   5

Amygdala > a-**mig**-da-la > resembling an 'almond', concentration of nuclei is most associated with our emotions and motivation when interacting with others.   7

Amylase > **am**-il-ace > enzyme, breaks down carbohydrates.   13

Amyloidosis > **am**-ee-loy-**doe**-sis > disease typified by an accumulation of the protein, amyloid in tissues of the body including the skin. The lesions appear pink or pale red.   4

Amyotrophic lateralizing sclerosis (ALS) > a-**my**-oh-**trow**-fik > progressive muscle disease.   6, 7

Anabolic steroid > an-ah-bal-ik > medication: increases growth/metabolism of muscle cells.   6

Anabolism > a-**nah**-bowl-ism > building up or creating a new product from smaller pieces or elements.   3

Anaerobic > **an**-a-**roe**-bik > pertaining to an organism that can live without air.   1, 3, 5, 6

Anaphylaxis > **an**-ah-**fee**-lax-is > immediate immune reaction to foreign body or antigen.   9

Anasarca > **an**-ah-**sahr**-ka > systemic infiltration of fluids into all the subcutaneous tissues (body-wide edema).   13

Anastomosis > an-**as**-toe-**moe**-sis > surgical joining of tubes such as colon, vessel, or vas deferens.   1, 11, 13, 15

Anatomical > an-a-**tom**-mi-kal > relating to anatomy: the physical structures making up the human body in this case. A car has an anatomy too. It is all the pieces and parts.   2

Anatomy > a-**nah**-toe-me > all the pieces and part of a structure such as the human body. It is the form or shape or make-up of a structure. Literally: to cut into the body (dissection).   1

Androgen > an-**drow**-jen > hormone agent, stimulates male characteristics.   9, 15

Anemia > a-**knee**-me-a > relative lack of blood due to injury, diet, or illness. Literally, without (an) blood (emia).   1, 10

Aneuploidy > **an**-yu-**ploy**-dee > state of having abnormal number of chromosomes with incomplete sets versus duplication of sets.   15

Aneurysm > **an**-yur-izm > localized weakening of an arterial wall, enlarges over time.   11

Angina pectoris > **an**-je-nah pek-**toe**-ris > 'chest vessels': severe pain in the chest secondary to ischemia of the heart muscle.   11

Unit

Angioedema > **an**-gee-oh-eh-**dee**-ma > swelling of a large area of capillaries and tissues.   11

Angiosarcoma > **an**-gee-oh-sahr-**ko**-ma > rare soft tissue carcinoma arising from the fibroblastic cells of the blood vessels. The lesions appear as purple to purple-red.   4

Angioscotoma > **an**-gee-sko-**toe**-ma > visual field defect caused by damage to retinal vessels.   11

Angiotensin I > **an**-jee-oh-**ten**-sin > protein peptide, localized hormone > 'vessel tension', it promotes vasoconstriction as well.   14

Angiotensin II > produced by liver and works with renin and angiotensin I system, termed RAAS, managing BP.   14

Anion > **an**-eye-on > ion or electrolyte has a negative charge, attracted to cations, e.g., Chloride (Cl) or Phosphorus (P).   3

Anisocoria > an-**ee**-so-**kor**-ee-ah > condition of unequal pupils (side to side).   8

Ankylosing > **ang** key-los-ing > bent or crooked.   5

Annular > **an**-yule-ar > pertaining to ring-shaped skin lesions. Tinea corporis, ringworm is an example.   4

Anorexia > **an**-oh-**rek**-see-ah > condition of a steep decline in appetite. It can occur with acute or chronic illness or injury.   3, 12

Anorexia nervosa > **an**-oh-**rek**-see-a nur-**voe**-sah > eating disorder due to a self-perception of obesity.   7

Anosmia > an-**oz**-me-ah > condition of the inability to smell.   8

Anoxia > an-**ok**-see-ah > absence of oxygen. *Synonym*: anoxemia.   12

Antagonist > an-**tag**-oh-nist > muscle, provides resistance to the primary mover.   6

Antepartum > **an**-tee-**pahr**-tum > before birth.   15

Anterior > an-**tier**-ee-or > direction: term denoting the front of the human body. *Synonym*: ventral, near the front (opposite of posterior).   2

Antibiotic > **an**-tea-buy-**ot**-ik > general term for the medication group which fights against bacterial infections.   1, 9

Antibody > **an**-tea-bod-ee > immunoglobulin (protein) designed to react to specific foreign bodies or antigens.   9

Antidote > **an**-tea-dote > substance (medication), neutralizes or counteracts poisons.   1

Antigen > **an**-tea-jen > 'against beginning', a foreign body or invader of the human body.   9

Antihistamines > **an**-tea-**his**-tah-meanz > dry the secretions of the bronchial mucus which opens up the airway a bit.   12

Antipyretic > **an**-tea-pie-**ret**-ik > medication, lowers or reduces fever.   1, 9

Antronasal > **an**-trow-**na**-zal > pertaining to the maxillary sinus and nose.   8

Antroscope > an-**trow**-skop > instrument to look at the maxillary sinuses.   12

Antrostomy > an-**tros**-toe-me > to create a new opening in the maxillary sinus. This would be done to evacuate a closed, painful sinus.   12

Anuria > **an**-yur-**ee**-ah > no urination.   14

Unit

Anxiety > ang-**zi**-eh-tea > feeling of worry, uneasiness, dread.   7

Aortic > **ay**-or-tik > valve between the left ventricle and the ascending aortic artery.   11

Aphasia > a-**fay**-zee-a > condition of no speech.   7

Aplasia > a-**play**-ze-ah > absence of development of an organ or cell type.   1, 9

Aplastic > a-**plaz**-tik anemia > severe decreased production of all cells from the bone marrow.   10

Apnea > **ap**-knee-ah > no breath, absence of breathing.   12

Apocrine > **ap**-oh-krin > specialized sweat glands known from their odor.   4

Aponeurosis > **ap**-oh-**nur**-oh-sis > derived from sinew, the thick connective sheet binding muscle to muscle.   6, 13

Apoptosis > ap-**op**-toe-sis > programmed cell death, the cells are designed to die and be recycled.   3

Appendicitis > a-**pen**-di-**sigh**-tis > inflammation of the appendix at the end of the cecal area of the ascending colon.   10, 13

Arachnoid mater > ah-**rak**-noyd **ma**-tur > spider web matter. It is the fine but tough web, middle layer of the meninges.   7

Areolar > a-**re**-oh-lar > small place or delicate, refers to the cotton ball-like connective tissue, loose, providing padding and protection to many body areas.   3

Arrector pili > ah-**rek**-tor **pee**-lie > tiny muscle, pulls the hairs up; goosebumps.   4

Arrhythmia > a-**rid**-thee-me-ah > 'no rhythm' – in the heart a markedly irregular rhythm.   11

Arteriogram > ahr-**tier**-ee-oh-gram > imaging: a radiologic study of the arteries of the human body looking for blockage, tears, or enlargements.   1, 7, 11

Arterioles > ahr-**tier**-i-ohls > small arteries, progressively smaller to become capillaries.   11

Arteriorrhexis > ahr-**tier**-ee-or-**rek**-is > rupture of an artery such as an abdominal aortic aneurysm (**AAA**).   11

Arteriosclerosis > ahr-**tier**-ee-oh-**sklar**-oh-sis > hardening of the arteries.   11

Arteritis > **ahr**-tur-eye-tis > inflammation of the arteries.   1, 10, 11

Artery > **ahr**-tur-ee > largest blood vessels, stronger, thicker, more muscle, high pressure, carry oxygen.   10, 11

Arthritis > are-**thri**-tis > inflammation of the joints.   1, 5

Ascending aorta > a-**or**-tah > upgoing behind the sternum, it turns at the manubrium.   11

Ascites > ah-**sigh**-teez > accumulation of fluids in the peritoneal sac secondary to liver failure.   13

Asplenia > a-**sple**-knee-ah > without a spleen, increases risk of infections.   10

Assessment > a-**ses**-ment > area of the SOAP note where the diagnosis is listed and/or a problem list created to be investigated further.   2

Asterixis > as-tur-**ik**-is > involuntary jerking motion, no fixed position.   6, 7

Astigmatism > ah-**stig**-mah-tizm > lens of one eye has a slightly different refractivity (curvature) than the other.   8

Unit

Astrocytes > **as**–tro–sites > 'star' cells. These are the most abundant neuroglial
cells, blood–brain barrier. 3, 7

Asystole > a–**sis**–toe–lee > no pressure, the heart is no longer beating, a flat line. 11

Ataxia > aa–**tak**–see–ah > 'no order', the inability to coordinate muscle motion. 6, 7

Atelectasis > at–eh–**lek**–tah–sis > 'incomplete extension'; it is essentially a complete
or partial collapse of a lobe. 12

Atherosclerosis > **ath**–ur–oh–sklar–**oh**–sis > main cause of cardiovascular disease.
Condition of hardened porridge 11

Atom > **at**–om > functional unit of an element. There are sub (under)–atomic
particles: protons, electrons, and neutrons with even smaller pieces: quarks,
leptons, and hadrons. 3

Atony > **at**–oh–knee > no tone or tension, it is also seen as atonia or atonic. 6, 7

Atopic dermatitis > ay–**top**–ik **dur**–mah–**tie**–tis > genetic condition of
hypersensitivity of the skin associated with asthma and eczema. 4

Atopy > a–**top**–ee > Greek for 'strangeness (of) place'. 4

Atrial fibrillation (AFib) > **fib**–ri–**lay**–zhun > atria are firing in a totally random
manner with no relationship to ventricular contraction. 11

Atrial flutter (AF) > the squeezing of the atria is NOT followed by a QRS
complex (ventricular squeeze) in a rhythmic pattern. 11

Atrioventricular > **ay**–tree–oh–ven–**trik**–u–lar > (**AV**) node, way-station for the
electrical impulse, it slows it just a bit to allow the ventricles to finish filling. 11

Atrium > **a**–tree–um > chamber or cavity, used most commonly for the (2) atria
of the heart. Unit 11 (in second 11

Atrophy > **at**–row–fee > loss of thickness or matrix, skin looks flatter, more
depressed, paler. 4, 6

Auricle > **awr**–i–kel > the outer ear. 8

Auscultation > **aws**–kul–**tay**–shun > methods utilize the stethoscope, chest scope
to listen to the air flow or sounds. 11, 12

Autism > **ah**–tizm > difficulties in social interaction, verbal and nonverbal
communication, and repetitive behaviors. 7

Autograft > **awe**–toe–graft > replacement tissue from oneself. 4

Autoimmune > **aw**–toe–im–**mewn** > self-protection, in this case it is against
self, self-attacking healthy tissue. 9

Autonomy > aw–**ton**–oh–me > patient's right to make their own decisions. 15

Auto–rhythmicity > **aw**–toe ridh–**mis**–i-tea > local nervous system makes GI
and cardiac cells 'self-starters'. 6

Axial > **ak**–see–al > core, center skeleton on which the appendicular skeleton hangs. 5

Axolemma > **ak**–so–**lem**–ma > cytoplasm of the nerve axon. 3

Axon > **aks**–on > nerve fiber, takes off from the neuron's body carrying the signals
to its action destination. 3, 7

Azotemia > a–zoe–**tea**–me–ah > excess levels of nitrogen in the blood. *Synonym*:
uremia. 14

Bacteria (plural), **Bacterium** (singular) > bak–**tier**–ee–ah or bak–**tier**–ee–um >
one-celled organism found in and on the human body. Some are helpful,
others are pathogens, and others are opportunistic. 1, 7, 9

Balanitis > **bal**-ah-**nigh**-tis > inflammation of the glans penis.

Basophil > **bay**-sew-fil > laboratory: another WBC type which will stain deep blue or purple with basic stain.

Beneficence > be-**nef**-ee-sens > practice of doing what is good or correct for the patient.

Benign Prostatic Hypertrophy > **hi**-purr-**trow**-fee (**BPH**) > enlargement of the prostate.

Bicipital > **buy**-sip-**it**-al > having two heads.

Bicuspid or **mitral** > **my**-tral > valve between the left atrium and ventricle; has two leaflets held by 2–3 chordae tendineae.

Bifurcate > **buy**-fur-kate > to split into two branches. The trachea into bronchi or the abdominal aorta into iliac arteries.

Bile > acts as a detergent to break up fats like dish soap. It is produced by the liver.

Bilirubinemia > **bil**-i-rue-bi-**knee**-me-ah > yellow pigment, result of hemolysis of recycled RBCs by the liver.

Biopsy > buy-**op**-see > procedures: removal of cells, tissues, or fluids for inspection for changes of illness or injury.

Blepharitis > **blef**-ah-**rye**-tis > inflammation of the eyelids.

Botulism > **boch**-U-lizm > toxins block the release of the ACh at the synapse (NMJ).

Bradycardia > **braid**-ee-**kar**-dee-ah > slow heart rate, less than 60 bpm.

Bradykinesia > **braid**-ee-ki-knee-**see**-ah > slow to motion, halting movement.

Bradypnea > **braid**–ee-pee-**knee**-ah > slow breathing.

Brain natriuretic > **nay**-tree-you-**ret**-ik peptide (**BNP**) > another protein unique to the heart and brain.

Breech > buttock first or a combination. A foot may present or a hip.

Bronchial asthma > **brong**-key-al **az**-mah > condition of the airway tubes of the lungs associated with wheezing, tight air flow, increased mucus production.

Bronchioles > **brong**-key-oh-les > six levels of progressively smaller and thinner air tubes ending at the alveolar sac which are the tissues of the lungs.

Bronchiolitis > **brong**-key-oh-**lie**-tis > inflammation of the bronchioles associated with RSV and influenza viruses.

Bronchitis > brong-**eye**-tis > inflammation of the bronchial tubes is a general term which includes the segmental bronchi.

Bronchophony > brong-k**off**-oh-knee > increased clarity and intensity when the spoken word passes through an area of consolidation.

Bruise > brews > diffuse extravasation of the blood under the skin, usually a flat lesion, purple/red.

Bruit > **brew**-ee > abnormal swishing or blowing sound associated with blocked blood vessels. It is the vessels' 'murmur'.

Buccal > **buc**-kal > pertaining to the cheeks.

Bulla (singular) > **bull**-ah; **Bullae** (plural) > **bul**-lee > larger vesicle (greater than 0.5 cm), fluid-filled and generally translucent too.

Unit

BUN > blood urea nitrogen > serum test, can give an indication of kidney, circulatory, and/or heart disease. 14

Burrows > **bur**-rows > skin lesion looks like a subway pathway in the skin; usually associated with scabies. 4

Bursa, **bursae** > **burr**-sah, **burr**-say > tough connective tissue sac filled with gel-like center; cushions bone-to-bone actions. 5

Byssinosis > **bis**-ee-**no**-sis > condition of inhaled cotton dust. 12

Cachexia > ka-**kek**-see-ah > progressive loss muscle and body weight, wasting associated with severe illness. 9

Cacosmia > kah-**koz**-me-ah > condition of 'bad odors'. This is a subjective perception of a noxious odor. 8

Calcitonin > **kal**-see-**toe**-nin > secreted by PTH, it stimulates the osteoblasts to increase bone building, lowering blood calcium levels. 5, 9

Calcitriol > **kal**-see-**tri**-ol > physiologically active form of vitamin D. 14

Callus > **kal**-us > in response to injury or constant pressure, the skin or bone will form tissue to protect the area and/or heal a fracture. 5

Calyx > **ka**-liks > 'cup of a flower' (Greek), funnel-shaped connective tissue which captures the liquid waste and dumps it into the renal pelvis. 14

Capillary > ka-**pil**-la-ree > tiniest vessels, beds reach most cells for oxygen and nutrient exchange. 10, 11

Carbohydrates > **kahr**-bow-**hi**-draytz > sugars and starches in our foods, contain carbon, hydrogen, and oxygen. 13

Carbuncle > kar-**bun**-kel > enlarged, or confluence of, infected hair follicles. 4

Carcinoma (singular); **carcinomata** (plural) > **kar**-sin-**oh**-ma, kar-sin-**oh**-ma-tah > any of the many types of malignant neoplasms most commonly derived from the epithelial tissues. 3, 9, 12

Cardiac > **kar**-dee-ak > pertaining (-ac) to the heart. 1, 6, 11

Cardiocentesis > **kar**-dee-oh-sen-**tea**-sis > procedure: removal of fluid from the heart. 1, 11

Cardiodynia > **kar**-dee-oh-**dine**-ee-ah > pain in the heart. 6

Cardiogenic > **kar**-dee-oh-**jen**-ik > of heart origin, there are many sensations and symptoms presenting due to heart health. 11

Cardiologist > **kar**-dee-**ol**-oh-jist > specialist who studies and treats heart disease. 1, 11

Cardiomegaly > **kar**-dee-oh-**meg**-a-lee > enlargement (hypertrophy) of the heart. 1, 6, 11

Cardiomyopathy > **kar**-dee-oh-my-**op**-ath-ee > disease of the heart muscle. 1, 6, 11

Carina > **kar**-eye-nah > bifurcation of the trachea into the right and left bronchi. 12

Carotene > **kare**-oh-tin > yellow-orange, lipochromes are derived from food. 4

Catabolism > ka-**tab**-oh-lizm > breakdown to complex compounds into smaller pieces or elements. 3

Catecholamines > kat-ee-**kol**-ah-menz > class of neurotransmitters, which are a part of our fight-or-flight response. 7, 9

Unit

Catheterization > **kath**-eh-tur-i-**za**-shun > sterile tube (catheter) inserted into the urethra.   14

Cation > **cat**-eye-on > ion or electrolyte, a positive charge, attracted to anions, e.g., sodium (Na) or potassium (K).   3

Caudal > **kaw**-dal > direction: pertaining to the tail or downward motion.   2

Cavity > **cav**-it-ee > hollow place in the human body; we have air-filled cavities in the sinuses of the face or the organ-filled cavities of the thorax (chest) and abdomen, to name a few.   2, 13

Cellular > **sell**-U-lar > pertaining to the cells.   3

Cellulitis > **sell**-U-**lie**-tis > inflammation, infection of the skin cells.   1, 3, 4, 8

Cementum > seh-**men**-tum > tough connective tissue surrounding the root of the tooth.   13

Centigrade > **sen**-teh-grade > range, measures temperature; zero (0°C) (32 degrees Fahrenheit) is freezing.   2

Centimeters > **sen**-teh-**me**-ters > 1/100 of a meter (10^{-2}): a length measure, metric system.   2

Cephalad > **sef**-ah-lad > direction: toward the head, movement toward the head.   2

Cephaledema > **sef**-al-eh-**dee**-ma > swelling of the brain.   7

Cephalic > seh-**fal**-ik > direction: pertaining to the head or upward motion.   2

Cerebellar > ser-eh-**bel**-lar speech > pertaining to explosive utterance with slurring (loss of the fine tuning).   7

Cerebrospinal > **ser**-eh-bro-**spy**-nal > pertaining to the brain and spine.   7

Cerebrovascular > **ser**-eh-bro-**vas**-Q-lar > pertaining to the brain's blood vessels.   1

Cerebrum > **ser**-eh-brum > cortex of the brain, outer convoluted mass of the brain.   7

Cerumen > seh-**rue**-men > earwax.   4, 8

Ceruminous > se-**rue**-min-us > specialized apocrine glands found in the ear; moisturizes and protects the ear canals.   4

Cervicitis > **ser**-vee-**sigh**-tis > inflammation of the cervix.   15

Chalazion > kah-**lay**-zee-on > deeper, chronic, inflammatory granuloma of the eyelid. It is also called a tarsal cyst.   8

Cheiloschisis > key-**low**-ski-sis > cleft lip, split lip.   13

Chemoreceptors > **key**-moe-reh-**sep**-tours > activated with the detection of a chemical – taste and smell.   8

Chemotactic > **key**-mo-**tac**-tik > one or more biochemical elements attracting leukocytes to inflammation area.   9

Chiropractor > **ki**-roe-**prak**-tor > chir/o > hand, this practitioner works with their hands to manipulate bone and muscles.   5

Chlamydia > kla-**mid**-ee-ah > bacterial infection which can cause PID in women and tends to be asymptomatic in men.   15

Chloroma > **klor**-oh-ma > distinguished by bony tumors, have a green hue.   4

Unit

Chlorophyll > **klor**-oh–fil > light energy absorber of green plants; converts light energy to food nutrients.   4

Cholangiogram > ko-**lan**-gee-oh-gram > record of the study of the bile duct.   13

Cholecystitis > **ko**-leh-sis-**tie**-tis > inflammation of the bile sac (gallbladder).   13

Cholecystokinin > **ko**-leh-**sis**-toe-**ki**-nin (**CCK**) > GI hormone released by the duodenum in the presence of a fatty meal. It stimulates the gallbladder to release bile.   13

Choledocholith > ko-leh-**doe**-ko-lith > stone in the bile duct.   13

Choledocholithotripsy > **ko**-leh-doe-ko-**lith**-oh-trip-see > to break up (fragment) a stone in the bile duct.   13

Cholesteatoma > **ko**-leh-steh-ah-**toe**-ma > fatty mass occurring in the middle ear.   8

Cholesterol > ko-**les**-tur-ol > a lipid-protein vital to creation of steroids, hormones, and cell repair.   13

Chondroblasts > **kon**-dro-blasts > immature cells producing (or becoming) cartilage cells.   3, 4

Chondrodysplasia > **kon**-dro-dis-**play**-zee-ah > abnormal growth or development of cartilage.   5

Chondromalacia > **kon**-dro-ma-**lay**-shah > cartilage softening.   3, 5

Chondromyalgia > **kon**-dro-**my**-al-gee-ah > pain of the cartilage and muscle.   1

Chondropathy > kon-**drop**-ah-thee > disease of the cartilage.   5

Chorda vocalis > **kor**-da **voh**-ka-lis > vocal cords or folds, pair of ligamentous, yellowish tissues pulled tautly over the thyroid cartilage.   12

Chordae tendineae > **kor**-day ten-**din**-ay > tiny tendons supported by the papillary muscles and attached to the respective valve to prevent backflow.   11

Chyme > kime > product of the churning of the stomach; it is called chyme in the small intestine.   13

Cilia > see-**lee**-ah > hair-like structures that move fluids, increasing absorption found in many cells/tissue types.   3, 8, 12

Circular > sir-**Q**-lar > forms a circle, these muscles help form orifices such as the mouth.   6

Circulation > **sir**-Q-**lay**-shun > any movement or flow in a circle, as in the closed system of the arteries and veins in the human body.   2, 11

Circumduction > **sir**-kom-**duk**-shun > ability to turn the joint in a circle.   5

Circumscribed > **sir**-kum-scrybd > bound by a border, defined, or confined area. Used to describe skin lesions.   4

Cirrhosis > **sear**-oh-sis > abnormal condition of the liver (cirrh = yellow in Latin).   4, 13

Claudication > **klaw**-di-**kay**-shun > limping seen due to pain in the legs caused by ischemia.   11

Clitoris > **klit**-or-is > erectile body, superior aspect of vulva. It is analogous to the male penis with the same sensitivity.   15

Clonus > **cloy**-nus > tumult, rapid contractions and relaxation of the muscles.   6, 7

Cochlea > **kok**-lee-ah (singular)/**Cochleae** (plural) > snail shell; the mechanical sound wave will end deep in the shell at the Organ of Corti, the cochlear nerve.   8

Unit

Coitus > **ko**-ee-tus > sexual union or pareunia (pa-**rue**-knee-ah) > French for lying beside. 15

Colectomy > ko-**lek**-toe-me > surgical removal of the colon. 13

Collagen > **kol**-lah-jen > protein of white fibers building many connective tissues such as the meniscus and cartilage. 3, 4, 5

Colonoscopy > ko-lon-**os**-ko-pee > instrument to look into the colon. 13

Colopexy > **ko**-low-pek-zee > to surgically fix the colon in place. 13

Colorectal > **ko**-low-**rek**-tal > pertaining to the descending colon and rectal area. 13

Colostomy > ko-**los**-toe-me > surgical: surgery to create a new opening in the colon. 1, 13

Colpocleisis > **kol**-po-**kleye**-sis > surgical closure of the vagina. 15

Colporrhexis > **kol**-por-**rek**-sis > tear or rupture of the vagina. 15

Colposcopy > kol-**pos**-ko-pee > instrument to look at the vagina. 15

Coma > **ko**-mah > profound loss of unconsciousness even with noxious or painful stimuli. 7

Compact bone > com-**pakt** > tough, outer shell of the bone. 5

Compartment syndrome > intense pressure building up inside an enclosed space in the body. 6

Complement > **kom**-play-ment > set of 20 proteins sensitive to body temperature. Cascade activates phagocytosis. 9

Concussion > kon-**kush**-un > damage to the brain tissue with edema, usually secondary to trauma. 7

Conductive > kon-**duk**-tive > hearing loss is caused by something blocking the sound wave. 8

Conization > ko-nigh-**zay**-shun > deep, cone-shaped removal of tissue. 15

Conjunctivitis > kon-**junk**-tea-**vigh**-tis > inflammation of the inner lid area. 8

Consciousness > **kon**-shus-nes > state of awareness of self and the external environment. 7

Constipation > **kon**-sti-**pay**-shun > infrequent bowel movements, tend to be small and hard. 13

Contracture > kon-**trak**-shur > scar tissue or tight fascia locks tissue in place stopping complete motion. 4, 5

Contralateral > kon-tra-**lat**-er-al > structures on the other side or opposite side of concern. 2, 7

Contusion > kon-**two**-zun > tissue injury of the skin/soft tissue with trapped blood; may be elevated, nodular. 4, 10

Convergent > kon-**vur**-jent > muscle, strong, broad origin point inserts to a common point. 6

Convoluted > **kon**-voh-**lut**-ed tubules > coiled segments of renal tubules (pipes). 14

Convulsions > **kon**-vul-shuns > abnormal, uncoordinated muscle contractions. 6, 7

Coprolalia > kop-row-**lah**-lee-a > compulsive use of obscene words. 7

Copulation > kop-U-**lay**-shun > joining, the merging of two independent cells (or people) then separation. 15

Unit

Corectopia > **kor**-ek-**toe**-pee-ah > condition of the pupil not being in the center of the iris.   8

Corneal > **kor**-knee-al > pertaining to the cornea of the eye.   8

Coronal > **kor**-row-nal > direction: it refers to the crown, the head. An older term, it is the same as the frontal plane, cutting the head in sections – dividing front (anterior) and back (posterior).   2

Coronary > **kor**-oh-**nar**-ee > 'around the crown', refers to the arteries which surround the heart muscle.   11

Corpus cavernosum > **kor**-pus ka-vur-**no**-sum > 'body cavern'; this tissue is where the majority of blood floods the penis to enable erection.   15

Corpus spongiosum > **kor**-pus spon-je-**oh**-sum > 'body sponge'; this tissue is more central and ends in the glans penis.   15

Cortex > **kor**-teks > outer portion of an organ. The cortex of the brain is composed of 6 layers, each with millions of neurons and their axon terminals linking to millions of dendrites. The kidneys, adrenal glands, and bones all have a cortex.   7, 11, 14

Cortisol > **kor**-ti-sol > glucocorticoid produced by the adrenal cortex.   9

Costochondritis > **kos**-toe-kon-**dry**-tis > inflammation of the rib cartilage, anterior chest.   5

Cough > kawf > sudden, forceful expulsion of air from the trachea past the glottis and out the mouth.   3, 9

Coxal > **koks**-al > pertaining to the pelvis: fusion of the ilium, ischium, and pubis.   5

Crackles > **krak**-els > sound of rice crisps in milk, popping sounds, tend to be a deeper tone. Linked with pneumonia and TB.   12

Cranial > **kray**-knee-al > pertaining to the skull.   2, 5, 7

Craniectomy > **kray**-knee-**ek**-toe-me > to surgically remove part of the skull bone.   5, 7

Craniostomy > **kray**-knee-os-**toe**-me > surgical: to cut a new opening in the skull (cranium).   1, 7

Craniotomy > **kray**-knee-**ot**-oh-me > surgical: to cut into the skull.   1, 7

Creatinine > kree-**ah**-ti-nin > laboratory: final waste product (via kidneys) of liver and muscle functions. Analyzed via blood or urine.   3, 14

Creatinine clearance > laboratory: 24-hour urine collection; low results indicate kidney disease or failure, or marked dehydration.   14

Crepitus > **krep**-ee-tus > palpation technique of placing a hand over the joint during motion and *feeling* the crackling of an inflamed joint.   5

Crohn's > kronz **disease** > autoimmune disease, inflammatory bowel disease (**IBD**).   13

Croup > crewp > childhood illness associated with a barking cough and stridor caused by the respiratory syncytial (sin-**sish**-al) virus (**RSV**).   12

Cruciate > **krew**-she-ate > to cross; ligament crossing front to back of knee joint.   5

Crust > honey-colored dried serous fluid or exudate from opening vesicles or pustules.   4

Cryptorchidism > krip-**toe**-key-dizm > hidden testicle, when the testicle does not descend at birth from the pelvis into the scrotum.   15

Unit

Curettage > kyur-eh-**tahz** > shave biopsy with curved loop.   4, 15

Cutaneous > Q-**tay**-knee-us > pertaining to the skin.   4

Cutaneous candidiasis > Q-**tay**-knee-us **can**-did-**eye**-ah-sis > diaper rash, this is
a yeast infection (a type of fungus).   4

Cutaneous leishmaniasis > Q-**tay**-knee-us **lesh**-ma-**nigh**-ah-sis > skin infection
with leptomonads from the bite of a sand fly.   4

Cuticle > Q-tea-cal > growth plate of the nail, epithelial tissue.   4

Cyanosis > **sigh**-an-**oh**-sis > condition of being blue, a skin color description or
blue color associated with cyanide.   4

Cycloplegia > **sigh**-klo-**pleh**-jee-ah > condition of paralysis of the ciliary muscle.   8

Cyst > sist > soft, raised, and encapsulated lesion; it is usually deep to the dermis
or even in the subcutaneous layer in the soft tissue. Cyst is also any bladder
conditon.   4, 12, 14

Cystitis > sis-**eye**-tis > inflammation of the urinary bladder.   14

Cystocele > **sis**-toe-seal > herniation of the urinary bladder.   14

Cystoplegia > **sis**-toe-**pleh**-jee-ah > paralysis of the urinary bladder.   14

Cystoscopy > sis-**toss**-ko-pee > instrument to look into the urinary bladder.   14

Cystostomy > **sis**-tos-**toe**-me > creating a new opening to allow urine escape.   14

Cytology > sigh-**tol**-oh-gee > study of cells – which includes anatomy (form);
physiology (function); pathology (disease); and chemistry (elements).   3, 9

Cytolysis > sigh-**tol**-ee-sis > breakdown or dissolution of the cell.   3

Cytoplasm > sigh-**tol**-plazm > gel-like environment of the interior cell
(intracellular) environment floating the organelles and other structures.   3

Cytoskeleton > **sigh**-toe-**skel**-eh-ton > support structures of the cell, all proteins:
microfilaments, microtubules, and intermediate filaments. Also referred to as
the centrioles.   3

Cytotoxin > **sigh**-toe-**tok**-sin > identifiable substance, inhibits or destroys the cell.   3

Dacryolith > **dak**-ree-oh-lith > tear duct stone.   8

Debridement > dee-**breed**-ment > removal of nonviable tissue.   4

Decubitus > deh-**Q**-bee-tus > Latin for 'to lay down', these pressure sores occur
due to poor circulation, recurring friction, shearing pressure, and/or the
presence of moisture.   4

Deep > deep > direction: interior, toward the back. The pancreas is deep to the
stomach. It is the opposite of superficial.   2

Defecation > **def**-eh-**kay**-shun > discharge of feces, a bowel movement or
'stooling'.   13

Deltoid > **del**-toyd > Latin for triangular, muscle drapes the shoulder.   6

Delusion > deh-**lew**-shun-al > false or incorrect judgment.   7

Dementia > deh-**men**-she-ah > progressive loss of cognitive intelligence at any
age and several causes.   7

Dendritic > den-**drit**-ik > branching processes reaching out from a cell body
such as nerve endings and melanocytes.   4, 7

Dental > pertaining to the teeth, used primarily to denote anatomy.   13

Unit

Deoxyribonucleic acid > dee-**oks**-ee-**rye**-bo-nu-**kle**-ik > DNA carries the genetic inclusion (chromosomes) making each individual different. 3

Depression > deh-**presh**-un > mood disorder characterized by profound sadness, loss of interests, fatigue, and more. 7

Dermatitis > **dur**-ma-**tie**-tis > inflammation of the skin. 1, 4

Dermatologist > **dur**-ma-**tol**-oh-jist > provider who evaluates and treats skin conditions. 1, 4

Dermatology > **dur**-ma-**tol**-oh-gee > study of skin. 4

Dermatome > **dur**-ma-tohm > instrument to cut or slice the skin. 1, 4

Dermatosis > **dur**-ma-**toe**-sis > abnormal condition of the skin. 1, 4

Dermis > **dur**-mis > active layer of the skin, provides the blood and lymphatic support of the epidermis. 3, 4

Diabetes mellitus > **die**-ah-**bee**-tis **mel**-i-tus > abnormal glucose/carbohydrate metabolism, a disease process. 8, 9

Diagnosis (Dx) > die-ag-**no**-sis > discernment through knowledge, this is the disease or injury the person is believed to have after taking a history and doing a physical exam/laboratory. 1, 2

Diapedesis > **dye**-ah-pee-**dee**-sis > 'feet through', process of WBCs squeezing through blood vessels to combat inflammation. 9

Diaphragm > **die**-ah-fram > large muscle providing the negative pressure motion to pull air into the tubes and alveoli. 5, 12

Diaphysis > die-**af**-ee-sis > shaft of the long and short bones. Dia > through or between. 5

Diarrhea > **die**-ah-**ree**-ah > 'flow through', the passage of watery stool on a regular basis. 13

Diarthrosis > **die**-are-**throw**-sis > freely mobile joint or articulation. *Synonym*: synovial joint. 5

Diastema > **die**-ah-**steh**-mah > space between adjacent teeth. 13

Diastolic > **die**-ah-**stol**-ik > ambient resting pressure *between* heartbeats. 11

Diencephalon > **die**-en-**sef**-a-lon > through + inside the brain > is deep to the cortex of the brain – in the middle. 7

Digest > **die**-jest > to separate, break apart, or dissolve. In the body it is done mechanically and chemically. **Digestion** > die-**jest**-shun. 2, 13

Diphtheria > dif-**thear**-ee-ah > mild to life-threatening respiratory illness, bacterial. 9, 12

Diplopia > dip-**low**-pee-ah > di- is the Greek for two, to see double. 2, 8

Discectomy > disk-**ek**-toe-me > surgical removal of the spinal disc. 5, 7

Dissect > die-**sek**-ted > to be cut apart (become two) or separate the tissues of the body. 2

Distal > **dis**-tal > direction: away from the center, pertaining to a part of the body furthest from the point of origin. 2

Diuresis > die-yur-**ee**-sis > through (dia) urine > recurrent urination with large volumes. 14

Unit

Diuretics > **die**-U-**eh**-tiks > medication class, forces water to 'run through' the kidneys to decrease blood pressure and edema. 11, 14

Diverticula > **die**-ver-**tik**-U-lah > hernias of the mucosa and submucosal layers of the colon. 13

Diverticulosis > **die**-ver-**tik**-U-**low**-sis > abnormal condition of 'turning away'. 13

Dopamine > **doe**-pah-mean > neurotransmitter, mostly inhibitory, regulating mood and motor control. 7, 9

Doppler > **dop**-plur > ultrasound study using microphone technology to hear the quality of the pulse whether over the carotid or another arteries. 11

Dorsal > **door**-sal > direction: pertaining to the back of, referring to the back of the body or the back of the hand. 2

Drug–drug interactions > when medications are taken together, may enhance or negate each other in a negative or dangerous way. 3

Drug–food interactions > undesirable effects between a medication and food. 3

Drug–herb interactions > undesirable effects between a medication and herb. 3

Duodenitis > **dew**-oh-**den**-eye-tis > inflammation of the C-loop of the small intestines. 13

Dura mater > **dur**-ah **ma**-tur > hard, thick, tough connective tissue, part of the inner periosteum of the cranial bones, brain protection. 7

Durables > **dur**-ah-bals > refers to medical items, may be used again such as wheelchairs, crutches, blood pressure cuffs. 5

Dyscrasia > dis-**kray**-zee-ah > 'bad mixing', an abnormal blood condition. 10

Dysesthesia > **dis**-es-**thee**-zee-ah > bad or painful sensations. 6, 7, 8

Dyskinesia > **dis**-key-**knee**-see-ah > difficult or poor movement. 6, 7

Dyslexia > dis-**lek**-see-a > difficulty in reading. 7

Dysmenorrhea > dis-**men**-oh-**ree**-ah > painful or difficult menstrual flow. 15

Dyspnea > dis-**knee**-ah > difficult breathing, an example of the silent 'p' with a consonant in front or the beginning of a word. 1, 12

Dysthymia > dis-**thigh**-me-a > long-term sense of unhappiness, sadness, and hopelessness. 7

Dystonia > dis-**toe**-knee-ah > poor tone or tension, is also seen as **dystonic**. 6

Dystrophin > dis-**trow**-fin > muscle protein, helps prevent sarcomere breakage. 6

Dystrophy > dis-**trow**-fee > difficult or bad development. 6

Dysuria > dis-**yur**-ee-ah > difficult or painful urination associated with UTIs and sexually transmitted disease (STD). 14

Eccentric > ek-**sen**-trik > moving away from the center, abnormal behavior. 1

Ecchymosis > ek-key-**moe**-sis > condition of blood under the skin, usually quite purple and common in elders with slight strike trauma. 4, 10

Eccrine > **ek**-krin > sweat glands – deposit their secretions on surface of the skin. 4

Echocardiography > **ek**-oh-kar-dee-oh-**graf**-ee > uses high-intensity sound waves to review the heart valves and chambers (**ECHO**). 11

Echolalia > **ek**-hoe-la-**lee**-ah > repeating words over and over again. 7

Unit

Ectopic > **ek**-top-ik > something is out of place, a pregnancy or organ.　　1, 15

Ectropion > ek-**trow**-pee-on > when the lid and lashes roll outward.　　8

Eczema > **ek**-zeh-ma > interchangeable term with atopic dermatitis; known for thickening of the skin with pronounced skin lines.　　4

Effacement > ee-**fas**-ment > cervix dilates and flattens as the baby progresses down the cervical canal.　　15

Efferent > **ef**-air-ent > moving outward, away from the center. Moving fluid or impulses away from the center, like the peripheral nerves take impulses from the brain to a muscle or an organ to create an action. The opposite of afferent.　　2, 7, 14

Egophony > ee-**gof**-oh-knee > patient says an 'E' but is heard as an 'A' with consolidation of fluid, pneumonia or mass.　　12

Elastin > ee-**las**-tin > flexible, rebounding mucoprotein – part of connective tissue and cell matrix.　　4

Electrocardiogram > ee-**lek**-tro-**kar**-dee-oh-gram > (**ECG** or **EKG**) > a record of the electrical action of the heart.　　11

Electrocautery > ee-**lek**-tro-**kaw**-tur-ee > procedure: an instrument directing high-frequency current into tissue. Used to destroy tissue (ablation) or stop bleeding.　　3

Electrolysis > ee-lek-**trol**-ee-sis > dissolution or destruction of a salt or compound which conducts electricity. It is also destruction of hair follicles via electricity.　　3

Electrolytes > ee-**lek**-tro-lites > elements or compounds which will conduct electricity. These elements are also known as ions.　　3, 14

Electromyogram (EMG) > ee-**lek**-trow-**my**-oh-gram > record of electrical action of the muscle.　　6

Electronic Health Record (EHR) > e-**lek**-tron-**ik** health **wrek**-ord > methodical collection of the electronic health information produced by visits and events pertaining to a specific individual. Also called Electronic Medical Record (**EMR**).　　1

Electrophoresis > ee-**lek**-tro-for-**ee**-sis > specialized laboratory analysis for separating DNA fragments. DNA samples are placed in a gel and exposed to an electric field.　　3

Embolectomy > **em**-bow-**lek**-toe-me > surgical: removal of a 'plug', an embolism.　　1, 11

Embolus > **em**-bow-lus > clot in motion until it gets stuck.　　10, 11

Embryo > **em**-bree-oh > zygote will implant in the uterine wall. This stage is 8 weeks long.　　15

Emesis > **em**-e-sis > medical term for vomit, the actual product and the action.　　3, 13

Emphysema > **em**-fe-**see**-mah > chronic lung disease that stretches out the alveoli, which cannot rebound for the next breath.　　12

Encephalitis > en-**sef**-ah-lie-tis > inflammation inside the head, used specifically for the brain.　　1, 7

Encephalomalacia > en-**sef**-ah-low-oh-mah-**lay**-she-ah > softening of the brain.　　7

Endocarditis > **en**-doe-kar-**die**-tis > inflammation of the inner lining of the heart.　　1, 11

Endocrine > **en**-doe-krin > body system, specialized tissue secretes hormones into the bloodstream to affect other tissues elsewhere.　　1, 2, 9

Unit

Endocytosis > **en**-doe-**sigh**-toe-sis > condition inside of the cell or cells.   1, 3, 7

Endometriosis > **en**-doe-me-try-**oh**-sis > abnormal condition of the inner lining of the uterus which is out of place.   15

Endometritis > **en**-doe-me-**try**-tis > inflammation of the inner lining of the uterus.   15

Endomyocarditis > **en**-doe-**my**-oh-**kar**-die-tis > inflammation of the inside lining of the heart muscle.   1, 11

Endomysium > **en**-doe-**mis**-ee-um > fine, delicate, connective tissue covering muscle fiber, inside the muscle.   6

Endoneurium > **en**-doe-**nur**-ree-um > fine, delicate but strong wrapping around each axon.   7

Endoplasmic reticulum > **en**-doe-**plaz**-mik re-**tik**-you-lum > network of canals, receives directions via the cell nucleus to produce proteins and other structures to enable cell function. RER is rough endoplasmic reticulum and SER is smooth endoplasmic reticulum.   3

Enkephalins and **endorphins** > en-**kef**-ah-lins; en-door-fins > localized neurotransmitter-like. These are our natural pain killers, they act like opiates covering pain receptors.   7

Enterology > **en**-ter-**ol**-oh-gee > process of studying the small intestines: duodenum, jejunum, and ileum.   1, 13

Enterostomy > **en**-ter-os-**toe**-me > surgical: surgery to create a new opening into the small intestines.   1, 13

Entropion > en-**trow**-pee-on > when the lashes turn inward to the eyeball, which can damage structures.   8

Enuresis > en-yur-**ee**-sis > urinary incontinence, particularly at night. This is also called 'bed wetting'.   14

Eosinophil > **ee**-oh-**sin**-oh-fil > one of the WBC types called granulocytes; they combat parasites in the bloodstream.   4, 10

Eosinophilia > **ee**-oh-sin-oh-**fil**-ee-ah > 'to like pink (the stain)', noted in patients with asthma.   10

Ependymal > eh-**pen**-dee-mal > cells line the central canals of the spine and brain ventricles, producing cerebral spinal fluid (CSF).   3, 7

Epicondylitis > **ep**-ee-kon-dee-**lie**-tis > inflammation of the condyles of the joint epiphysis, such as the elbow or ankle.   5, 6

Epidemiologist > **ep**-ee-dee-me-**ol**-oh-jist > specialist who studies the patterns, causes, and effects of health and disease conditions in defined populations.   1, 9

Epidermis > **ep**-ee-**dur**-miss > top layer of the skin, 30+ layers of epithelial cells, keratinized.   4

Epididymitis > **ep**-ee-**did**-ee-**my**-tis > inflammation of the epididymis.   15

Epididymoorchitis > **ep**-ee-**did**-ee-moe-or-**keye**-tis > inflammation of both the testi and epididymis.   15

Epigastric > **ep**-ee-**gas**-trik > region: above the stomach, this area includes the pylorus of the stomach, head of the pancreas, common bile duct, and the abdominal aorta.   2, 13

Unit

Epiglottitis > **eh**-pee-**glot**-tie-tis > glott/o Greek for opening; epi- > near, above > making this flap of flexible cartilage 'above the opening', acting as a door on a hinge.   12

Epimysium > **ep**-ee-**mis**-ee-um > thick connective tissue, binding muscle fascicles into a muscle.   6

Epinephrine > **ep**-ee-**nef**-rin > neurotransmitter, mostly excitatory to fight or flee.   7, 9

Epineurium > **ep**-i-**nur**-ree-um > thickest wrapping around sets of fascicles – is called a nerve.   7

Epiphysis > eh-**pif**-ee-sis > distal/proximal ends of long bones provide attachment for ligaments and tendons.   5

Episiotomy > ee-**piz**-ee-**ot**-oh-me > to cut into the vulva and proximal perineum to expand space for birthing. Episi/o > perineal area.   15

Epistaxis (**ep**-ee-**stay**-sis) > Greek for nose bleed, for 'dropping'.   12

Epithelial > **ep**-ee-**the**-lee-al > pertaining (-al) to avascular (without blood) cells on the surface of the body structure protecting both outside (skin) and inside (mucosa and serosa).   3, 11, 13

Eponyms > **ep**-oh-nims > names of the people who discovered or described a particular structure or set of symptoms.   1

Ergonomics > **ur**-go-**no**-miks > science of the workplace, tools, and equipment to maximize safety.   6

Erythema > **eh**-ree-**thee**-ma > condition of being red, inflammation description.   4, 12

Erythrocytes (RBC) > eh-**rith**-row-sites > red blood cells; when mature they are anucleic, live 120 days. Carry oxygen to the body cells.   3, 10

Erythropoiesis > eh-rith-row-poe-ee-sis > production of blood cells.   3, 14

Erythropoietin > eh-**rith**-row-**poe**-eh-tin > renal hormone, response to oxygen level; bone responds by producing erythrocytes (RBCs).   5, 9, 14

Eschar > **es**-kar > thick crust made of coagulated blood and debris – forms over thermal burns which can constrict healing.   4

Esophagitis > eh-**sof**-ah-**jie**-tis > inflammation of the esophagus.   1, 13

Esophagogastroanastomosis > eh-**sof**-ah-go-**gas**-tro-ah-nas-toe-**mow**-sis > surgical formation of a connection between the esophagus and stomach.   13

Esophagogastroduodenoscopy (EGD) > eh-**sof**-ah-go-**gas**-tro-**due**-oh-deh-**nos**-ko-pee > procedure: the process of using a scope to look at the esophagus, stomach, and small intestine (duodenum portion), an EGD.   1, 13

Esotropia > **es**-oh-**trow**-pee-ah > condition of one eye turning in.   8

Estrogen > **es**-trow-jen > sexual hormone for women, excreted via the ovary.   5, 9, 15

Ethmoid > **eth**-moyd > complex irregular bone, the anterior floor of the cranium serving support for the nose, eyes, and sinuses.   5

Eustachian > yu-**stay**-she-an > tube or auditory tube, this middle ear structure allows the normal fluid of the area to drain to the pharynx.   8

Eversion > ee-**vur**-zhun > roll-over action; the great toe is outgoing, moving away from the center.   5

Exanthema or **exanthem** > eg-**zan**-thee-ma, eg-**zan**-them > skin eruption secondary to viral or bacterial systemic infection.   4

Unit

Excision > ek-**sizh**-un > procedure: the removal of the tumor with some normal tissue (clean margins). 3

Excitatory > ek-**sigh**-tah-tor-ee > act of increasing the rapidity or intensity. 7

Excoriation > eks-**kor**-ee-a-shun > superficial injury to skin, a scratch. 4

Exocrine > ek-so-krine > gland, secretes to the outside via a duct. 4, 9

Exocytosis > **eks**-oh-sigh-**toe**-sis > pushing a substance, debris, or foreign body out of the cell. 3

Exogenous > eks-**oh**-je-nus > produced or originating from outside the organism or cell. 1

Exotropia > eks-oh-**trow**-pee-ah > condition of one eye turning outward. 8

Exposure > eks-**poe**-zur > contact with an element from the outside, the environment. 1

Extraocular movement > eks-tra-**ock**-U-lar > six muscle sets which move the eyes, **EOMs**. 8

Extrapyramidal symptoms > ek-stra-peer-**am**-ee-dal > abnormal involuntary movements. 6, 7

Facial > **fay**-shal > CN VII gives taste and pain reception to the anterior two-thirds of the tongue and motion to all the facial muscles. 8

Fascia > **fash**-ee-ah > tough connective tissue, can be as thick as a ligament or a spider-web like to wrap muscle fibers. 4, 6

Fascicles > **fas**-ee-kel > band or bundle of muscle or nerve fibers. 6, 7

Fasciculation > fa-**sik**-Q-**lay**-shun > twitching of the muscle fibers. 6, 7

Fasciitis > **fash**-ee-**eye**-tis > inflammation of the connective tissue, fascia. 6

Fatigue > fa-**teeg** > sensation of being tired, less capacity to do normal activities or weariness. 3, 9

Fear > rational reaction to external danger. It usually initiates a flight-or-fight reaction. 7

Feces > **fee**-seez > the expelled waste product of the GI tract. 13

Ferritin > **fair**-i-tin > laboratory: indirect measure of stored iron via the RBCs, it is a complex protein containing about 23% iron. 10

Fetus > **fee**-tus > Latin for offspring; used from the end of week 8 until the moment of birth. 15

Fibrillation > **fib**-ri-**lay**-shun > muscle fibers contract rapidly, irregularly, or randomly. 6, 11

Fibrin > **fie**-breen > elastic-like, thin fibers or threads (protein), it essentially helps tie up the platelets to form the scab or clot. Protein is **fibrinogen** > **fie**-bree-**noh**-jen. 10

Fibroblasts > **fie**-bro-blasts > mature cells, produce (or become) the collagen and elastic fibers giving connective tissue strength and flexibility. 3

Fibrocystic > **fie**-bro-**cis**-tik > pertaining to cystic (bladder-like) lesion, mostly fibrous tissue. 3, 15

Fibromyalgia > **fie**-brow-my-**al**-gee-ah > painful muscle condition without weakness. 6

Unit

Filiform > **fil**-lee-form > tiny papules found on the face, neck, and creases of the body. *Synonym*: milia.   4

Fissures > **fish**-ur > deep furrows in the skin, usually associated with very dry skin or wet, macerated skin.   4, 7

Fluorescein > floor-**es**-eh-cen > stain viewed through a cobalt-blue light.   8

Follicle-stimulating > **fol**-ee-kal **hormone** (**FSH**) > travels to the gonads to stimulate puberty hormones.   9

Folliculitis > foe-**lick**-ule-**eye**-tis > inflammation of the hair follicles.   4

Fovea > **foe**-vee-ah centralis > center of the macula retina; point of most precise vision.   8

Frontal > **fron**-tal > forehead bone, it covers the frontal area of the brain.   5

Fungus (singular) > **fung**-us; **fungi** > **fung**-eye > growth, it grows in irregular masses so the skin lesions are usually papulosquamous. **KOH** is used to visualize the branching hyphae.   4

Furuncle > fir-**un**-kel > large, inflamed hair follicle.   4

Fusiform > **fue**-see-form > muscle belly, bulky when contracted, such as the biceps brachii.   6

Gallop > **gal**-up > addition of a third and/or fourth heart sound (**S3, S4**) because valves are closing off cycle.   11

Gangliocytoma > **gang**-klee-oh-sigh-**toe**-ma > rare tumor of a peripheral neuronal node.   7

Ganglion cyst > **gang**-klee-on sist > usually benign tumor in a hand or foot ganglion.   7

Gas gangrene > **gan**-green > fermentation of bacteria releases gas, which takes up room and destroys muscle and other tissues.   4, 6

Gastrectomy > gas-**trek**-toe-me > surgical: surgery to remove the stomach.   1, 13

Gastric ulcer > peptic ulcers occur in the stomach rarely because the mucosa is designed for acid, BUT a *Helicobacter pylori* infection can make it happen.   13

Gastroduodenostomy > gas-tro-**due**-oh-de-**nos**-toe-me > surgical: surgery to create a new opening between the stomach and duodenum.   1, 13

Gastroenteritis > gas-tro-en-tur-**eye**-tis > inflammation of the stomach and small intestines. Gastroesophageal reflux disease (**GERD**) > when gastric acid is able to splash up on to the esophagus.   13

Gastroenterology > **gas**-tro-**en**-ter-**ol**-oh-gee > inflammation of the stomach and small intestines.   1, 13

Gastrointestinal (GI) > gas-tro-in-**tes**-ti-nal > pertaining to the body system including the stomach and intestines. Acronym is GI system. It is the digestive tract of the body – mouth to anus.   2, 13

Gastromegaly > gas-tro-**meg**-ah-lee > overeating may cause enlargement of the stomach.   13

Gastroparesis > gas-tro-**par**-ee-sis > when the gut stops due to inflammation, injury, medication, or neurologic changes. Churning stops as does peristalsis.   13

Genetics > je-**net**-iks > study of the functional unit of heredity – the DNA/chromosomes.   3, 10, 15

Unit

Gestation > jes-**tay**-shun > to bear, the act of bearing (a child). 9, 15

GFR > glomerular filtration rate > a ratio based on age, sex, race, and creatinine indicates the function of the nephrons. 14

Gingivitis > **jin**-ji-**vie**-tis > inflammation of the gums which can occur with vitamin deficiency and medication side effects. 13

Glaucoma > glaw-**ko**-ma > steadily, progressive optic neuropathy characterized by increased intraocular pressure. 8

Glomeruli > glo-**mar**-U-lie > 'ball of yarn' (Latin). The arteriole (little artery) becomes a capillary cluster within the 'sink' of Bowman's capsule. 14

Glomerulopathy > glo-**mar**-U-**lop**-ah-thee > disease of the glomeruli. 14

Glossitis > **glos**-sigh-tis > inflammation of the tongue. 13

Glossopharyngeal > **glos**-sow-**fair**-in-jee-al > CN IX gives taste, pain reception, muscle action for swallowing, and secretion of saliva. 8

Glossoplasty > **glos**-oh-**plaz**-tea > surgical repair of the tongue is required for deep bites or tears. 8

Glossotrichia > **glos**-oh-**trik**-ee-ah > hairy tongue which occurs due to use of chewing tobacco. 8, 13

Glucagon > glue-**ka**-gon > endocrine hormone secreted by pancreas; increases the level of glucose in the blood from stored energy when food is not available. 9, 13

Gluconeogenesis > glue-**ko**-knee-oh-**jen**-eh-sis > metabolic process converts lipids or proteins to glucose for cell use via the liver. 9, 13

Glucose > **glue**-kose > functional carbohydrate used by all cells for energy production by mitochondria. It requires insulin to move into the cells. 3, 9, 13

Glycosuria > gli-**kos**-ur-ee-ah > glucose in the urine. 3, 9, 14

Goiter > **goy**-tur > specific term for chronic thyromegaly associated with iodine insufficiency. 9

Golgi apparatus > **goal**-gee **app**-are-**rat**-us > packaging department of the cell following the SER; it packages protein for use in the cell (endocytosis) and outside the cell (exocytosis). An eponym. 3

Gomphosis > gom-**foe**-sis > specialized socket in which the teeth sit. 5

Gonadotropin > go-**nad**-oh-**trow**-pin > hormone promoting growth and function of the gonads. 9, 15

Goniometer > **go**-knee-**om**-ee-tur > instrument to measure joint motion precisely in degrees of motion. 5

Gonorrhea > gon-or-**rhee**-ah > bacterial infection which causes severe dysuria in men and is generally asymptomatic in women. 14, 15

Goodpasture's syndrome > loss of reproduction of the epithelial cells, rapidly causing destruction leading to renal failure and death. 14

Gout > gowt > abnormal metabolism of uric acid causes crystallization over joints and skin. 4, 5

Gracilis > **gras**-i-lis > slender, long parallel muscle of the medial thigh. 6

Granulocytes > **gran**-U-low-sites > white blood cells, have a granular appearance: neutrophils, eosinophils, and basophils. 10

Unit

Gravida > **grav**-ee-dah (**G**) > pregnant, to be heavy with (a child).   15

Growth hormone > protein hormone from anterior pituitary; body growth, fat mobilization, and inhibition of glucose utilization.   5, 9

Gynecology > **gi**-neh-**kol**-oh-gee > study of women.   15

Hallucination > hal-**lew**-si-**nah**-shun > perception of a stimulus that does not exist.   7

Hallux > **hal**-lux > proper name for the great toe; it is the 1st finger in anatomical position.   2, 5

Haustra > **haw**s-trah > pouches; the colon has a series of these pouches which push the feces up and around and enable water reabsorption. **Haustrum** is singular.   13

HCG: human chorionic gonadotropin > **kor**-ee-**on**-ik go-**nad**-oh-**trow**-pin > hormone which is checked to determine pregnancy.   15

Hectometers > **hek**-toe-me-ters > 100 meters, a length measure, metric system.   2

Hemangioma > he-**man**-gee-**oh**-ma > congenital anomaly in which over-production of blood vessels leads to a mass effect.   4

Hematemesis > **he**-mah-**tem**-ee-sis > bloody vomit associated with UGI bleeding. It can be bright red or coffee-ground appearance (older blood).   13

Hematochezia > **hem**-ah-toe-**key**-zi-ah > passage of bloody stool, bright red from local mass or hemorrhoids.   13

Hematocrit (Hct) > he-**mat**-**oh**-krit > percentage of the volume of the blood taken up by whole cells.   10

Hematology > he-mah-**tohl**-oh-jee > study of blood, a laboratory science.   10

Hematoma > he-mah-**toe**-ma > collection of blood under the skin. The bleeding is contained or walled-off in a specific location, usually in the soft tissue or even muscle.   4, 10

Hematopoiesis > **hem**-at-toe-**poy**-ee-sis > production of the red blood cells.   10, 14

Hematuria > **hem**-at-**ur**-ee-ah > RBCs in urine.   14

Hemianopia > **hem**-ee-an-**oh**-pee-ah > condition of loss of one half of the visual fields of one or both eyes.   8

Hemiplegia > **hem**-ee-**play**-gee-ah > ipsilateral, both the arm and leg are paralyzed.   2, 6, 7

Hemoccult > **he**-moe-kult > method to check stool for blood, including DNA to check for colon cancer.   13

Hemoglobin (Hgb, Hb) > **he**-moe-**glow**-bin > red respiratory protein within the red blood cells. About 4% heme (iron) and 96% globin (a protein).   3, 10

Hemolysis > hem-**ol**-i-sis > destruction of blood cells.   10

Hemophilia > **he**-moe-**fil**-ee-ah > inherited blood disorder resulting from a deficiency of factor VIII.   10

Hemopoiesis > **he**-mah-poy-**ee**-sis > process or formation of blood cells by bone marrow.   10

Hemoptysis > he-**mop**-ti-sis > coughing up or spitting blood.   12

Hemorrhage > **hem**-or-ahj > flowing blood > vessel has ruptured (like a pipe) or been cut or torn (injury) and blood is escaping into the surrounding tissues.   8, 11

Hemorrhea > **hem**-oh-ree-ah > bloody discharge from the ear, nose, mouth.   8

Unit

Hemorrhoids > **hem**-or-oydz > the varicose (**var**-i-kos) veins of the anus. 13

Hemostasis > **he**-moe-**stay**-sis > stop bleeding. 4, 10

Heparin > **hep**-are-rin > neurotransmitter and medication: released by the basophils and acts as an ANTI-coagulant to stop clots forming. 10

Hepatic > **hep**-**at**-ik > pertaining (-ic) to the liver. 1

Hepatitis > **hep**-ah-**tie**-tis > inflammation of the liver. 13

Hepatoma > **hep**-ah-**toe**-mah > tumor of the liver. 13

Hepatomegaly > **hep**-at-oh-**meg**-ah-lee > enlargement of the liver. 13

Heptachromic > **hep**-ta-**crow**-mik > seeing seven colors: yellow, orange, green, blue, red, indigo, and violet. 2

Herpes simplex (HSV 1 or 2) > **her**-pees **sim**-plex > canker sore or fever blister, this is the painful vesicle on an erythematous base. 4, 15

Histamine > **his**-tah-mean > neurotransmitter, chemically reactive in all cells, usually excitatory. 7, 9

Histology > **his**-**tol**-oh-gee > study of tissues. 3

History (Hx) > **hiss**-tor-ee > systematic medical record of past events, current symptoms, medication, allergies, and more relating to an individual. 1

Homeostasis > **hoe**-me-oh-**stay**-sis > dynamic balance between opposing systems in the body which keeps us alive. It can be as simple as the triceps of the arm relaxing so the biceps can bend the elbow. 2, 9

Hordeolum > hor-**deh**-oh-lum > a stye of the eyelid caused by the same staphylococcal infection at an eyelash. 8

Human genome > **hue**-man **jean**-ome > complete set of chromosomes, mapped to about 100,000 genes or 3 billion DNA base pairs. 3

Human Papilloma Virus (HPV) > **pap**-il-**low**-ma > over 100 HPV: warts: hand, foot, face and body, and genitalia. 4, 15

Human placental lactogen > **lak**-toe-jen (HPL) > stimulates maternal fat and protein actions to provide adequate nutrition to the growing fetus. 15

Hydatiform > **hi**-da-**tid**-oh-form > mole is a polycystic mass; it can mimic pregnancy with elevated HCG numbers. 15

Hydronephrosis > **hi**-drow-**nef**-row-sis > abnormal condition of 'water on the kidney'. 14

Hymen > **high**-men > thin membrane which covers the vaginal opening prior to use of tampons or sexual activity. 15

Hyoid > **hi**-oyd > small bone in anterior neck, no joint, provides attachments for tongue and voice muscles. 5, 12

Hyperacusis > **hi**-purr-ah-**kyu**-sis > hypersensitivity to sounds. 8

Hypercalcemia > **hi**-purr-kal-**see**-me-ah > high blood calcium. 14

Hypercapnia (**hi**-purr-**kap**-knee-ah) > abnormal elevation of CO_2 in the arterial blood. 12

Hypercoagulable > **hi**-purr-ko-**ag**-U-la-bel > any condition increasing the tendency for the blood to clot. 10

Hyperesthesias > hi-**purr**-es-**thee**-zee-ah > oversensitivity to touch. 9

Unit

Hyperglycemia > hi-**purr**-gleye-**see**-me-ah > abnormal elevation of serum glucose. 9, 14

Hyperkalemia > hi-**purr**-ka-**lee**-me-ah > laboratory result: elevated blood potassium, in adults greater than 5.1 mEq/L. 3, 14

Hyperlordosis > **hi**-purr-lor-**doh**-sis > normal anterior curvature of the lumbar spine. It is exacerbated during pregnancy. 5

Hypernatremia > **hi**-purr-nah-**tree**-me-ah > high blood sodium. 14

Hyperopia > **hi**-purr-**oh**-pee-ah > condition of farsightedness; vision is better at a distance because the light meets behind the retina. 8

Hypersensitivity > **hi**-purr-**sen**-i-**tiv**-i-tea > an exaggerated response of the body to a foreign body or antigen. 9

Hyperthyroidism > hi-**purr**-thigh-**royd**-izm > collection of symptoms due to overstimulation of the thyroid gland. 9

Hypertrophy > hi-purr-**trow**-fee > overdevelopment, used to describe muscle enlargement. 6, 14

Hypertropia > **hi**-purr-**trow**-pee-ah > condition of one eye turning upward. 8

Hyperuricemia > hi-**purr**-ur-ee-**see**-me-ah > laboratory result: elevated uric acid, in adult males greater than 7.2 mg/dL. 3

Hypnosis > hip-**no**-sis > 'condition of less knowledge' – a state of awareness, deeply relaxed. 7

Hypocalcemia > hi-poe-kal-**see**-me-ah > low blood calcium. 14

Hypocapnia (**hi**-poe-**kap**-knee-ah) > abnormal decrease in arterial CO_2 associated with hyperventilation. 12

Hypochromic > hi-poe-**krow**-mik > decreased color, used to describe red blood cells. 10

Hypocretin > hi-poe-**crey**-tin > chemically reactive substance, helps manage arousal, wakefulness, and appetite at the limbic system and pineal gland. 7, 9

Hypodermis > hi-poe-**dur**-mis > under the skin, the SQ layer of fat and soft tissues support and anchor the skin. 4

Hypoglossal > hi-poe-**glos**-al > CN XII movement and proprioceptive sense to the tongue. 8

Hypokalemia > hi-**poe**-kay-**lee**-me-ah > laboratory result: low blood potassium, in adults less than 3.5 mEq/L. 3, 14

Hyponatremia > hi-poe-nah-**tree**-me-ah > low blood (serum) sodium. 14

Hypopharynx (hi-poe-**fair**-inks) > below or under the throat is a very short link to the larynx (voice box). 12

Hypothalamus > hi-poe-**thal**-ah-muss > below the thalamus. This area contains several structures which form the floor of the 3rd ventricle of the brain. 7, 9

Hypothyroidism > hi-poe-**thigh**-roid-ism > condition of the thyroid, not producing sufficient thyroid hormone to maintain homeostasis. A collection of symptoms. 1, 9

Hypotropia > hi-poe-**trow**-pee-ah > condition of one eye turning downward. 8

Hypoxia (hi-**pok**-see-ah) > abnormally low levels of oxygen in arterial blood. *Synonym*: hypoxemia. 12, 15

Unit

Hysterectomy > **his**-tur-**ek**-toe-me > removal of the uterus.   15

Hysterocleisis > **his**-tur-oh-**kleye**-sis > surgery to close the uterus.   15

Hysteromyoma > **his**-tur-oh-**my**-oh-mah > muscle tumor of the uterus.   15

Icterus > **ick**-tear-us > collection of bile pigments in the dermis and eye sclera indicating liver malfunction.   4

IgA nephropathy > neh-**frop**-ah-thee > abnormal deposit of the protein IgA in the glomeruli.   14

Ileus > **il**-ee-us > a mechanical or adynamic obstruction of the intestines.   13

Immune > im-**mewn** > protection, protective, exempt from.   2, 9

Immunity > i-**mew**-nee-tea > status or quality (-ity) of being immune. The complex system of the body defending against harmful cells, organisms, and foreign bodies.   2, 9

Immunocyte > im-**mewn**-it-ee > cell capable of producing antibodies.   9

Immunodeficiency > **im**-mew-no-de-**fish**-en-see > decreased or defective immune response.   9

Immunoglobulins > **im**-mew-no-**glob**-u-lins > protective proteins, antibodies: IgA, IgD, IgE, IgG, and IgM.   9

Immunomodulators (**im**-mew-no-**mod**-U-**lay**-tors) > these target specific immunologic protective mechanisms.   12

Immunostaining > i-**mew**-no-stain-ing > biochemistry term used for antibody-based approach to detect specific proteins in a tissue specimen.   3

Immunosuppression > **i**-mew-no-sue-**pres**-shun > knocking down or diminishing the function of hormones which stimulate protection mechanisms to fight infections.   3

Impetigo > **im**-peh-**tie**-go > contagious skin infection due to *Staphylococcus*.   4

Incisal > in-**sigh**-zal > pertaining to the biting edges of the incisor teeth.   13

Incision > in-**si**-zhun > to cut into.   1

Incus > **ing**-kus > anvil, it is one of the bones of the middle ear.   8

Infant > live birth, from the moment of delivery.   15

Infection > in-**fek**-shun > to enter or to corrupt, pathogens causing inflammation.   1, 9

Inferior > in-**fear**-ee-or > direction: a descriptor indicating it is below, under, or directed downward. The ankle is inferior to the knee. It is the opposite of superior.   2

Inflammation > in-flam-**may**-shun > 'in flames'. A set of intricate responses to injury occurring in injured tissue. An essential reaction for the body to recognize and begin repair of the injury characterized by pain, redness, swelling, and heat generation.   2, 9

Influenza > in-**flew**-en-zah > severe lower respiratory infection, viral.   6, 12

Inhibitory > in-**hib**-ee-tor-ee > act of depressing or stopping a function.   7

Injection > in-**jek**-shun > medication delivered via a needle (most common), or a medication pushed into rectum or vagina or taken orally by mouth: 'to push inside'.   1, 4, 10, 14

Insertion > **in**-sir-shun > 'planted in', the most mobile muscle attachment of the muscle to bone, where movement occurs.   6

Insomnia > in-**som**-knee-ah > inability to sleep including difficulty falling or staying asleep. Known to increase stress, trigger depression, and cause chronic illnesses.   7

Insulin > in-**sue**-lin > endocrine hormone secreted by pancreas. It reduces the level of glucose in the blood by enabling glucose to cross the cell walls.   9, 13

Integumentary > in-**teg**-U-**men**-tar-ee > relating to the skin. It is an envelope including the epidermis and dermis, providing protection and temperature control for the whole body.   2, 4

Interferons > in-ter-**fear**-ons > produced by T-lymphocytes; inhibit viral growth and trigger phagocytes into action.   9

Interneurons > in-tur-**nur**-ons > between the neurons. Found only in the spine and brain, these are like quick turn-arounds on the highway for ultrafast reaction.   7

Internist > in-**tur**-nist > specialist who studies and treats diseases of the internal organs.   1

Interphalangeal > in-ter-fa-**lan**-gee-al > between the finger bones, the joints or knuckles of the fingers or toes.   2

Interproximal > between neighboring surfaces of adjacent teeth.   13

Interstitial > in-**tur**-stish-al > 'between tissues', condition of interrupting deep tissue levels in a number of systems: lung, bladder, heart . . .   10, 12

Intestinal > in-**tes**-ti-nal > pertaining (-al) to the intestines of the GI tract. It is the digestive tube beginning at the duodenum (C-loop) and ending at the anus.   2, 13

Intradermal > **in**-tra-**der**-mal > pertaining to within the dermis; injection types include TB skin test, Botox, and allergy testing.   4

Intramuscular (IM) > **in**-tra-**mus**-Q-lar > pertaining to within the muscle, injection types include antibiotics, pain medications, and more.   4

Intraorbital > **in**-tra-**or**-bit-al > inside the orbit of the eye.   1

Intravenous (IV) > **in**-tra-**vee**-nus > pertaining to within the veins, to inject the vein with fluids and medications, or withdraw blood.   4, 11, 14

Intussusception > **in**-tu-sue-**sep**-shun > telescoping of the intestine on itself, causing an obstruction. Currant-like stool (blood + mucus).   13

Inversion > in-**vur**-zhun > roll-over action; the great toe is ingoing, moving more inward to the center.   5

Ionization > **eye**-on-eye-**zay**-shun > dissolution of a compound into the specific ions when an electrolyte is dissolved in water.   3

Ions > **eye**-ons > an atom or group of atoms carrying an electrical charge, these electrolytes are present in our cells and bloodstream.   3

Ipsilateral > **ip**-see-**lat**-er-al > structures on the same side, right hand and right leg for instance.   2

Iridoplegia > **ir**-e-doe-**pleh**-jee-ah > condition of paralysis of the iris.   8

Iritis > eye-**rye**-tis > inflammation of the iris.   8

Irritable bowel syndrome (IBS) > specific to the motility of the colon.   13

Ischemia > is-**key**-me-ah > localized loss of blood due to a mechanical blockage.   11, 13

Unit

Isometric > **eye**-sew-**met**-rik > contraction where the tone increases without changing the length of the muscle.

6

Isotonic > **eye**-sew-**tohn**-ik > contraction where tone stays the same as the length of the muscle changes.

6

Jaundice > **jahn**-dis > collection of bile pigments in the dermis and eye sclera indicating liver malfunction.

4, 13

Jejunoplasty > jeh-**jun**-oh-plaz-tee > repair of the jejunum.

13

Justice > **jus**-tis > giving equal treatment to all patients.

15

Keratin > **care**-a-tin > protein produced by the skin cells (epithelials) to waterproof the epidermis, and it hardens to become nails and hair.

2, 4

Keratinocytes > ca-**rat**-in-oh-sites > cells producing the protein and keratin – waterproofs skin and forms our hair and nails.

4

Keratotomy > **ker**-ah-**tot**-oh-me > a cut into the cornea.

8

Ketoacidosis > **key**-toe-ass-ee-**doe**-sis > high level of acid in the bloodstream associated with starvation or uncontrolled diabetes mellitus (**DM**).

14

Ketonemia > **key**-toe-**knee**-me-ah > ketone bodies in the blood.

14

Ketonuria > **key**-toe-nur-ee-ah > ketones in urine.

14

Kilogram > **kill**-oh-gram > 1,000 grams, a metric weight. 1 kg = 2.2 lb.

2

Kinesalgia > ki-**neh**-sal-gee-ah > painful movement.

6

Kinesis > ki-**knee**-sis > movement.

6

Labia > lay-**bee**-ah > lips, in this case, the outer (majora) and inner (minora) set which protect the vaginal opening.

15

Labiogingival > **lay**-be-oh-**jin**-ji-val > pertaining to the lips and gums.

13

Labioplasty > lay-**bee**-oh-**plaz**-tee > repair of the lips. This is used primarily for dental repair.

15

Lacerations > **las**-ur-a-shuns > jagged or torn skin. FST (full skin thickness) and PST (partial skin thickness).

4

Lacrimal > **lak**-rim-al > tiny bones of the face (2), behind and lateral to nasal bones, help form eye orbit and support the tear ducts.

5, 8

Lacteal > **lak**-teels > specialized lymph tissue – resides in the center of all microvilli. It absorbs chyle (kile) (emulsified fat) from the duodenum.

10, 13

Lamella > lah-**mel**-ah > thin layer or shell or of bone.

5

Laparotomy > **lap**-ar-**ot**-toe-me > surgical: a surgical incision over the abdomen, usually vertically.

1

Laryngismus > **lair**-in-**jiz**-mus > spasm of the vocal cords.

12

Laryngitis > **lair**-in-**jie**-tis > inflammation of the voice box.

12

Lateral > **lat**-er-al > direction: 'on the side' – a lateral view will look at the body or object from the side. It is the furthest away from the center of the body or area.

2

Leiomyoma > **lie**-oh-my-**oh**-ma > neoplasm of the smooth muscle.

3, 6

Leukemia > **lew**-key-**me**-ah > proliferation of white blood cells, a carcinoma.

4, 9

Leukocytes > **lew**-koh-**sites** > type of white blood cells.

4, 10

Leukoplakia > **lew**-ko-**play**-key-ah > condition typified by white patch of oral mucus – cannot be scraped off.

4

Unit

Leukopoiesis > **lew**-ko-poe-**ee**-sis > production of blood cells to counteract this effect to some degree.   3

Leukotrienes > **lew**-ko-**try**-enz > fatty molecules impart slow and steady vascular changes associated with inflammation.   9, 12

Lichenification > **lie**-ken-ee-**fi**-kay-shun > like the lichen on a rock; this type of lesion seems to accentuate the skin lines.   4

Limbic > **lim**-bik > pertaining to the area of the brain most involved with emotions.   7

Lingua > **ling**-gwa > singular; **Linguae** (**ling**-gwee) is the plural > tongue from the Latin.   8, 13

Lingual > **ling**-gwal > pertaining to the tongue.   8, 13

Lipase > **lie**-pace > enzymes, breaks fats down into **monoglycerides** (**mon**-oh-**glis**-er-ides) and two fatty acids.   13

Lipid profile > blood test, reviews the level of circulating lipid proteins.   9, 10, 11, 13

Lobectomy > low-**bek**-toe-me > surgical removal of a lung lobe.   12

Luteinizing > **lew**-tin-i-zing **hormone** (**LH**) > travels to the gonads, testicles, and ovaries.   9, 15

Lymph > limf > fluid of life. Used both for the interstitial fluid and specific WBC.   10

Lymphadenography > lim-**fad**-en-**nog**-raf-ee > process of taking a radiographic picture.   10

Lymphadenopathy > lim-**fad**-en-**nop**-ah-thee > disease of the lymph nodes.   10, 13

Lymphangioma > lim-**fan**-gee-**oh**-ma > tumor of the lymph vessels.   10

Lymphangiophlebitis > lim-**fan**-gee-oh-fle-**by**-tis > inflammation of the lymph vessels and veins.   10

Lymphatic > lim-**fat**-ik > pertaining (-ic) to the lymph system, which is the third vascular system of the body – collects the leftovers of fluids, proteins, dead bacteria, etc. . . . to clean and recycle products and put them back into circulation.   2, 9, 10

Lymphocytes > lim-**foe**-sites > specific type of white blood cell, begins in the bone marrow and matures in the thymus, spleen, or other lymph tissue.   2, 9, 10

Lymphocytic > **lim**-foe-**sit**-ik leukemia > proliferation of lymphoblasts.   10

Lymphocytopenia > **lim**-foe-**sigh**-toe-**pee**-knee-ah > low number of lymphocytes occurs with autoimmune diseases.   10

Lymphocytosis < **lim**-foe-sigh-**toe**-sis > abnormal condition of the lymph cells.   10

Lymphoma > **lim**-foe-mah > tumor begins with infection-fighting lymphocytes, often in the lymph nodes.   1, 10

Lysosomes > **lie**-so-soms > clean-up workers of the cells, they contain **lysozymes** (**lie**-so-zoms) to digest cellular debris, foreign bodies, and invaders.   3, 13

Macrocyte > **mak**-row-sites > 'large cell', either large RBC or WBC. *Synonym*: **macrophage** > **mak**-row-fahj.   9, 12

Macroglossia > **mak**-roe-**glos**-ee-ah > condition of enlarged tongue.   8

Macula > **mak**-U-lah retina > small spot. For the eyes, this site has the maximum number of color receptors.   8

Macular > **mak**-U-lar degeneration > slowly developing loss of the macula of the eye, the point of optimal central vision.   4, 8

Unit

Macule (singular) > **mak**-yule; **maculae** (plural > **mak**-yu-lee > 'Spot' in Latin, flat discoloration of the skin no larger than 2 cm, a freckle. — 4

Malleus > **mal**-ee-us > largest of the three middle ear bones, firmly attached to the backside of the TM. — 8

Malocclusion > **mal**-oh-**klue**-shun > poor alignment of the bite or chewing. — 13

Malpractice > patient is harmed when a provider fails to competently perform their medical duties. — 14

Mammary > **mam**-ah-ree > breast, anterior chest. — 2

Mammogram > **mam**-oh-gram > a record of the breast (tissue). — 15

Mandible > **man**-dee-bel > lower jaw bone, only mobile joint in the cranium. It articulates at the TMJ and holds the gomphosis sockets for the lower 16 teeth. — 5

Mastectomy > mas-**tek**-toe-me > to remove the breast. — 15

Mastication > **mas**-tea-**kay**-shun > process of chewing and grinding food with the teeth. — 13

Mastitis > mas-**tie**-tis > inflammation of the breast, common with early breast feeding. — 15

Mastodynia > **mas**-toe-**die**-knee-ah > pain in the breast. — 15

Maxilla > **max**-il-lah > upper jaw bones (2), forms part of the floor of the eye orbit, part of the roof of the mouth, the maxilla sinuses, and the gomphosis joints of the upper teeth. — 5

Meatoplasty > **me**-ah-**toe**-plaz-tee > repair of the opening is done to repair a hypospadia. — 15

Mechanoreceptors > **mek**-ah-no-reh-**sep**-tours > sensory receptors that respond to mechanical pressure or distortion, e.g. sound waves on the eardrum, pressure on a blood vessel, or a fly landing on the skin. — 8

Meconium > me-**ko**-knee-um > green-yellowish stool, may be expelled prior to birth by the fetus. — 15

Medial > **me**-dee-al > direction: relating to the middle or center of the body or part. — 2

Mediastinum > **me**-dee-ah-**sty**-num > area of the chest midline containing the heart, pulmonary arteries and veins, and great vessels. — 2, 11

Medulla > meh-**due**-lah > the inner area of an organ. In the brain, the medulla oblongata is part of the brain stem. Location of the nephron's convoluted tubules. — 7, 9, 14

Medulla oblongata > meh-**duel**-ah ob-long-**gah**-ta > reflex center for breathing, cardiac rate, blood vessel dilatation/contraction, vomiting (emesis), cough, sneezing, and swallowing. — 7

Megacolon > **meh**-ga-**ko**-lon > an enlarged colon. — 13

Megakaryocytes > **meg**-ah-**kar**-ee-oh-sites > platelet cell, derived from the same myeloid stem cell as the erythrocytes. — 10

Megalomania > **meg**-al-oh-**may**-knee-ah > extravagant self-importance. — 7

Melanin > **mel**-an-in > black or dark color; it provides the dark hue pigments, color of the skin, iris of the eyes, and hair. — 4

Unit

Melanocytes > **mel**-ah-no-sites > mature cells of melanin, these cells produce color for skin protection. 4, 9

Melanocyte-stimulating > **mel**-ah-no-sites **hormone** (**MSH**) > travels to melanocytes of the skin, eyes, and mucous membranes. 9

Melanoma > **mel**-ah-**no**-ma > pigmented lesion with an aggressive malignancy behavior can arise from any melanic cell, be it in the skin or eye or under the nails. 4, 8

Melatonin > mel-ah-**tone**-in > pineal gland hormone is associated with maintaining the sleep cycle. 9

Melena > meh-**leh**-nah > passage of tarry (black) stool indicating bleeding higher up the GI tract. 13

Menarche > men-**ark**-he > first menses. 15

Meningioma > meh-**nin**-jee-**oh**-ma > tumor of the meninges. 7

Meningitis > **men**-in-**ji**-tis > inflammation of the meninges. 7

Meningocele > meh-**ning**-oh-seal > herniation of the meninges. 7

Meniscus, menisci > me-**nis**-kus, men-**is**-keye > the cartilage pad, cup-shaped between the femur and tibia. 5

Menopause > **men**-oh-paws > last menses. 15

Menstruation > **men**-stru-**ah**-shun > cyclic shedding and discharge of vascular fluids and tissues from the uterus. 15

Mental retardation > loss of intellect, inability to adapt readily. 7

Mesentery > **mes**-en-**tear**-ree > middle area of the peritoneum. 11, 13

Mesothelioma > **mez**-oh-**thee**-lee-**oh**-ma > lung cancer associated with exposure to asbestos (as-**bes**-toes). 12

Metabolism > meh-**tab**-oh-lizm > sum of the give and take of anabolism (building) and catabolism (breaking), which maintains the body's homeostasis. 3

Metabolite > meh-**tab**-oh-lite > any intermediate or final waste product associated with metabolism. 3

Metabolomics > **met**-ah-**bol**-oh-miks > study of individual chemical fingerprint of the cellular processes left behind, metabolites. 3

Metacarpal > **met**-ah-**car**-pal > beyond the wrist bones, these are the hand bones. 2, 5

Metastatic > **meh**-tah-**sta**-tik > pertaining to the spread of disease from the original location to a distant location. **Metastasis** > meh-tah-**stay**-sis. 3, 10, 15

Metatarsal > **met**-ah-**tar**-sal > beyond the ankle bones, these are the foot bones. 2, 5

Metrorrhagia > **me**-trow-**ra**-jeh-ah > off-cycle bleeding from the uterus. It is also used for excessive bleeding. 15

Microfilament > **my**-krow-**fil**-a-ments > commonly called centrioles as well, these cell structural supports are made of actin, a protein. A key component of cells and motion. 3

Microglia > my-**krow**-glee-ah > smallest of the neuroglial cells; these act as the leukocytes of the brain. They fight bacteria, viruses, fungi, and other foreign bodies. 3, 7

Microglossia > **mik**-roe-**glos**-ee-al > condition of a small tongue; also called atrophy. 8

Unit

Microscope > mike-**row**-scope > instrument, looks at really small things. — 1

Microtubules > **my**-krow-**tube**-ules > proteins configured in a spiral tube pattern allowing them to move things across the cell like a spring. A cytoskeleton structure. — 3

Microvilli > **my**-krow-**vil**-lie (plural) > minute finger-like projections, line the mucosal lining of the nose and sinuses, intestines, and other structures. *Synonym*: cilia. — 3, 12, 13

Micturition > mik-thur-**ish**-on > pertains to the neurologic feedback loops, causing the internal sphincter to relax so the bladder can be emptied. — 14

Middle ear bones > **mal**-ee-us; **in**-kus; **stay**-pees > Malleus (hammer); Incus (anvil); Stapes (stirrup). — 5

Milliliter > **mil**-ee-**lit**-er > 1/1000th of a liter (10^{-3}), a volume measure, metric system, ml. — 2

Millimeter > **mil**-ee-**me**-ter > 1/1000th of a meter (10^{-3}), a length measure, metric system, mm. — 2

Misadventure > patient is harmed due to inadvertent outcome of an intended action. — 14

Mitochondria > **migh**-toe-**kon**-dree-ah > the energy factory of the cell, an organelle. It produces ATP most efficiently with oxygen (O) and glucose. — 3

Mitral > **my**-tral > valve between left atrium and left ventricle, **bicuspid**. — 11

Monilia candidiasis > moe-**nil**-ee-ah **can**-dee-**die**-ah-sis > yeast or fungal infestation presents with thick, white discharge (cottage-cheese look) and pruritus (prue-**ree**-tus) > itchy. — 15

Monocytes > **mon**-oh-sites > type of WBC which is a phagocytes, also called macrocyte. — 9, 10

Monocytosis > **moan**-oh-**sigh**-toe-sis > abnormal condition of monocytes. — 10

Mononeuralgia > **mon**-oh-**nur**-al-gee-ah > pain in one nerve or one nerve pathway. — 2, 7

Monoplegia > **mon**-oh-**play**-gee-ah > paralysis of one or a single limb. — 2, 7

Morbidity > mor-**bid**-it-ee > disease state, it is used as a ratio of sick or injured people versus well people. It tracks disease, injury, and medical efforts to correct these by CDC and other agencies. — 1

Morbilliform > more-**bill**-ee-form > resembling the rash of measles, soft red exanthem of many viral illnesses. — 4

Morphology > more-**fol**-oh-gee > study of shape and form of structures. — 3

Mortality > mor-**tal**-it-ee > state of being mortal, the ability to die. It is used to track the number of deaths, age, and cause as a report of the CDC and other agencies. — 1

Mucolytics > **mew**-ko-**lit**-iks > break up or helps liquify thick mucus, making it easier to cough and move air. — 12

Mucous > **mew**-kus > pertaining to sticky (the descriptive). — 12, 13

Mucus > **mew**-kus > substance, the noun of sticky fluid. — 12, 13

Multinodular > **mul**-tea-**nod**-u-lar > pertaining to having many nodules: kidneys or ovaries. — 2

Unit

Multisynaptic > **mul**-tea-si-**nap**-tik > pertaining to having many nerve
connections.   2, 7

Murmur > **mer**-mur > sound created by the rush of blood over a valve or
vessel.   11

Muscular > **mus**-Q-lar > pertaining (-ar) to the muscles of the body, the
specialized tissue – can contract to move the body (skeletal); or the blood
via the circulation, cardiac (heart) muscle; or moving food through the GI
tract, smooth muscle.   2, 5, 6

Myasthenia gravis > my-as-**thee**-knee-ah **gra**-vis > an autoimmune disease,
attacks muscle cells leading to loss of tone and strength.   6, 7, 9

Myelitis > my-eh-**lie**-tis > inflammation of the spinal cord.   7

Myelocytic > my-ee-low-**sit**-ik **leukemia** > overproduction of immature
granulocytes.   10

Myelogenesis > mi-eh-low-**jen**-eh-sis > development of bone marrow.   10

Myelosuppression > mi-eh-low-soup-**pres**-hun > reduction of bone marrow's
ability to produce cells.   3, 10

Myocardial infarction > my-oh-**kar**-dee-al in-**fark**-shun > (**MI**) death of
heart muscle, a heart attack.   11

Myoclonus > my-oh-**cloy**-nus > one or a series of muscle contractions.   6, 7

Myofibrils > my-oh-**fie**-brils > tiny muscle fibers group together to become
the muscle fiber or cell.   3, 6

Myoglobin > my-oh-**glow**-bin > oxygen transportation protein is stored in the
muscles giving them their deep red coloration.   6

Myogram > **my**-oh-gram > record of muscle motion. -graphy > process of
recording; -graphy > instrument making the record.   6

Myonecrosis > my-oh-neh-**krow**-sis > abnormal condition of muscle death.   5, 6

Myopia > my-**oh**-pee-ah > condition of nearsightedness; vision is better up
close because the light joins in front of the retina.   8

Myosin > **my**-oh-sin > muscle protein, oar shape grasps the actin of the
sarcomere to pull, developing a muscle contraction.   6

Myositis > my-oh-**sigh**-tis > inflammation of the muscles.   5, 6

Nasal > **nay**-zal > nose bones (2), form the upper part of the nose, the end is
cartilage.   5, 8

Nasal cilia > **sil**-ee-ah > microscopic equivalent of nasal hair. It is part of the
mucus production floating debris up and out.   8

Nasogastric > nay-zo-**gas**-trik > pertaining to the nasal passage to the
stomach.   8, 13

Nasogastric lavage > nay-zo-**gas**-trik la-**vahj** > irrigation of the stomach via a
tube (**NG tube**) placed down the nasopharyngeal route.   13

Nasopharyngeal > nay-zo-fa-**rin**-jeel > pertaining to the nose and throat.
Nas/o is used to designate anatomy.   12

Nasopharynx > nay-zo-**fair**-inks > nose and posterior throat area; this allows
the flow of air into the pharynx.   1, 8, 12

Unit

Nausea > **naw**-zee-ah > sensation of a queazy stomach, the sensation of needing to vomit.   3, 13

Necrosis > **nek**-row-sis > abnormal condition of death, dead tissue.   3, 6, 11

Necrotizing fasciitis > **nek**-row-**tie**-zing **fash**-ee-**eye**-tis > inflammation of the fascia, death of tissue.   4

Neglect > failure to provide adequate care which results in physical illness or injury.   14

Neoplasm > **knee**-oh-plazm > 'new growth', used to indicate the abnormal growth of cells, carcinoma.   3

Nephritis > neh-**fry**-tis > inflammation of the kidneys due to infection, injury, congenital abnormalities, or autoimmune disease.   14

Nephroblastoma > **nef**-row-blast-**oh**-ma > tumor of the cells which build the nephrons. Eponym: Wilms' tumor.   14

Nephrolithiasis > **nef**-row-li-**thigh**-ah-sis > infestation of kidney stones.   14

Nephron > **neh**-fron > functional unit of the kidneys.   14

Nephropathy > neh-**frop**-ah-thee > disease condition of the kidneys.   9, 14

Nephrotic > neh-**fro**-tik syndrome > pertaining to a set of symptoms including edema, proteinuria, and fatty urine casts indicating the glomeruli are leaking larger elements – renal disease.   14

Nervous > **nur**-vus > pertaining (-ous) to the nerves. The nervous system consists of the brain (the hard drive), spinal cord, and all the nerves sensing our environment and then sending signals to respond with an action from movement to hormone secretion.   2, 7

Neurilemma > **nur**-ee-**lem**-ma > cell wall, encloses one or more axons of the peripheral nervous system.   3, 7

Neurofibrils > **nur**-oh-**fie**-brils > cytoskeleton parts of the neuron.   3, 7

Neuroglial > **nur**-oh-**glee**-al > group of four cell types – support, protect, and maintain the neurons of the brain and spine.   3, 7

Neurology > nur-**ol**-oh-gee > study of the nervous system.   7

Neuron > **nur**-on > individual brain cells – make up the nervous system.   2, 3, 7

Neuropathy > **nur**-oh-**nop**-ah-thee > disease of the nerve/neurons.   7

Neurotransmitter > **nur**-oh-**trans**-mit-turs > specific chemical agents of the nervous system, some are active in all cells.   6, 7, 8, 9

Neutropenia > **new**-trow-**pee**-knee-ah > decreased numbers of circulating neutrophils.   3, 10

Neutrophils > **new**-trow-fils > so called due to its 'neutral' dye staining, these are the most abundant leukocytes.   3, 10

Nevus > **knee**-vus; **nevi** > **knee**-vi (plural) > well-defined lesion of the skin, may be epidermal, nerve, vascular, or connective tissue elements. Common colors are brown, black, blue, or pink.   4

Nociceptors > **no**-see-**sep**-tours > generated by injury such as surgery, burn, chemical irritant, pressure, loud sounds, or intense light.   8

Nocturia > nok-**tyur**-ee-ah > night urination, specifically having to rise too often to empty the bladder.   14

Unit

Nodule > **nod**-yule > firm, elevated mass or lesion like a papule but larger (0.5 to 5 cm); 'knot' from the Latin. 4

Noncompliance > **non**-come-**ply**-ants > patient who fails to follow provider advice or directions. 2

Non-durables > non-**dur**-ah-bals > refers to medical items used only once such as needles, syringes, gauge pads, medications, etc. 5

Nonigravida > **no**-knee-**grav**-ee-da > history of nine pregnancies. 2, 15

Nonmaleficence > **non**-mah-**lef**-ee-sens > if a provider cannot do 'good'; at least do no harm. 15

Norepinephrine > nor-**ep**-ee-**nef**-rin > neurotransmitter, similar to epinephrine, vital to fight-or-flight responses. 7, 9

Nucleic acid > **new**-clay-ik > specific molecules found in the nuclear chromosomes and other structures of the cell; part of the DNA and RNA. 3

Nucleoplasm > **new**-klee-oh-plazm > living matter (protoplasm) is gel-like inside the nucleus of all cells. 3

Nucleus (singular); **nuclei** (plural) > **new**-klee-us, **new**-klee-eye > control center of all cells with the exception of red blood cells. 3

Nulligravida > nul-lee-grav-ee-da > woman who has never been pregnant. 2, 15

Nulliparous > nul-**ip**-ah-rus > woman who may have been pregnant but did not deliver a child. 2, 15

Nummular > **num**-yule-ar > pertaining to a skin lesion – looks like a stack of coins usually seen with eczema. 4

Objective > ob-**jek**-tiv > facts which can be seen, touched, heard, or perceived by a provider during an exam. It is the findings of things measured and analyzed such as lab, radiology, and procedure results. The 'O' in the SOAP note. 1, 2

Oblique > oh-**bleek** > direction: at an angle, neither anterior nor lateral. 2, 5, 6

Obstipation > **ob**-sti-**pay**-shun > intestinal obstruction due to severe constipation. 13

Obstruction > ob-**struk**-shun > blockage of any sort from masses, stool impaction, volvulus, or intussusception. 13

Occipital > ock-**sip**-ee-tall > large bone at the base of the skull which covers the occipital brain. 5, 7

Octan > **ock**-tan > fever reoccurrings every eight days. 2

Octuplets > ock-**tup**-lets > eight infants born of a single birth. 2

Oculodynia > ok-**yu**-low-**dine**-ee-ah > eye pain. 8

Oculomotor > ock-**U**-low-**moe**-tur > CN III, motion of lids, cornea, pain sensation of the eye. 8

Odontiasis > o-don-**tea**-ah-sis > teething, multiple eruptions of baby teeth. 13

Olecranon > oh-**lek**-rah-non > elbow, the olecranon process of the proximal ulna fits in the fossa of the distal humerus. 5

Olfactory > ohl-**fak**-tor-ee > to smell, the sense of smelling. 8

Oligodendrocytes > **ol**-ee-go-**den**-dro-sites > 'scant' cells build and apply their fibers to the axons of the neuron, speeding the electrical impulse. They make the myelin sheaths. 3, 7

	Unit
Oligomenorrhea > ol-ee-go-**men**-oh-ree-ah > scant menstrual flow.	15
Oliguria > ol-ee-**gyur**-ee-ah > scant flow of urine with obstructions, BPH, and UTIs.	14
Oncogene > **on**-ko-jean > family of genes – code proteins for cell growth, causing the rapid growth of the cancer.	3
Oncogenesis > **on**-ko-**jen**-ee-sis > production or development of a neoplasm.	3
Oncolysis > ong-**ko**-lie-sis > any process which destroys or reduces the size of a tumor or mass.	3
Onychectomy > **on**-ee-kek-**toe**-mee > removal of the nail.	4
Onychia > oh-**nik**-ee-ah > inflammation of the nail.	4
Onychomalacia > **on**-ee-ko-mah-**lay**-she-a > nail softening.	4
Onychomycosis > **on**-ee-ko-**my**-ko-sis > fungal infection of the nails.	4
Onychorrhexis > **on**-ee-ko-**rek**-is > abnormal nail splitting or brittleness.	4
Oocyte > **oh**-oo-sight > immature egg or ovum under construction.	9, 15
Oogenesis > **oh**-ou-**jen**-ee-sis > process of developing eggs.	15
Oophorectomy > **oh**-ou-for-**ek**-toe-me > removal of an ovary.	15
Oophoropexy > **oh**-ou-for-oh-**pek**-see > to fix the ovary in place.	15
Ophthalmology > of-thal-**mol**-oh-gee > study of the eyes.	8
Ophthalmoscope > of-**thal**-moe-scope > instrument used to look at the eyes.	1, 8
Optic > **op**-tik > CN 2, optic nerve; sole activity is sensing light.	8
Optic neuritis > **op**-tik **nur**-eye-tis > inflammation of the optic nerve.	8
Oral > **or**-al > pertaining to the mouth.	13
Orbicularis > or-**bik**-U-**la**-ris > round, circular muscle fibers – form a sphincter.	6
Orchialgia > or-**key**-al-**jee**-ah > pain of the testicle. **Orchalgia** and **testalgia** are also correct.	15
Orchidopexy > or-**key**-doe-**pek**-see > fixing the testicle in place so it does not sneak back up into the pelvis.	15
Organ systems > **or**-gan sis-tems > organs of the body combine to provide specific needs to the human body like the GI system with its many organs that digest, absorb, and utilize nutrients from food.	2
Organelles > **or**-gah-**nels** > 'small organs', the structures of the internal cell environment.	3
Origin > **or**-ee-jin > source, the least mobile or more stable attachment of muscle to the skeleton.	6
Orolingual > **or**-oh-**ling**-gwal > pertaining to the tongue and mouth.	12
Oropharynx > **or**-oh-**fair**-inks > mouth and posterior throat area.	12
Orthodontist > **or**-tho-**don**-tist > specialist who straightens teeth.	5, 13
Orthognathic > **or**-thog-**nath**-ik > pertaining to the 'straightness' between the maxilla **and** mandible (chin > gnath/o).	13
Orthopedic > **or**-tho-**pee**-dik > concerning being 'straight', a practice taking care of bone and joint disease and injury.	5

Unit

Orthopedist > **or**-tho-**pee**-dist > specialist who studies and treats disease and injury of the bones, including surgery.

1, 5

Orthopnea > or-**thop**-knee-ah > having to sit up straight to breathe is an example of a hard 'p' because of the vowels (e, i, y).

12

Osmoreceptors > **oz**-moe-reh-**sep**-tours > caused by chemical or the shift of fluid balance of the body. This is a function of the hypothalamus to maintain homeostasis.

8

Osteitis > os-tea-**eye**-tis > inflammation of bone.

1, 5

Osteoarthritis > **os**-tea-oh-are-**thri**-tis > inflammation of bones and joints. Usually used as a term describing the wear and tear on joints.

1, 5

Osteoblasts > **os**-tea-oh-blasts > immature cells for the bone, builders.

3, 5, 9

Osteoclasts > **os**-tea-oh-klasts > bone carvers, these bone cells are phagocytes that release bone calcium to the bloodstream.

3, 5, 9

Osteocytes > **os**-tea-oh-sites > bone cells, contain nucleus and organelles of the osteon.

5

Osteodystrophy > **os**-tea-oh-**dis**-trow-fee > defective or abnormal bone formation.

5

Osteogenic > **os**-tea-oh-**jeh**-nik > origin of bone, producing bone.

5

Osteolysis > **os**-tea-**ol**-eye-sis > destruction of bone.

5

Osteomyelitis > **os**-tea-oh-my-eh-**lie**-tis > infection of the bone (bone marrow) leading to tissue death.

5

Osteon > **oz**-tea-on > functional unit of the bone.

5

Osteopath (DO) > **os**-tea-oh-path > specialist on disease of the bones originally, now they may practice a full scope of medicine.

5

Osteopoikilosis > **os**-tea-oh-**poke**-ill-**oh**-sis > mottled or varied bone textures.

5

Osteoporosis > **os**-tea-oh-pore-**oh**-sis > weakening of the bone, -porosis > having pores, pitted, indicates loss of calcium matrix.

5

Osteosclerosis > **os**-tea-oh-sklar-**oh**-sis > abnormal condition of hardening of the bone – too heavy, too hard, too brittle.

5

Osteotome > **os**-tea-oh-tohm > instrument for cutting or slicing bone.

1, 5

Otic > **oh**-tik > pertaining to the ear.

2, 8

Otitis media > oh-**tie**-tis **me**-dee-ah > OM, inflammation of the middle ear.

8

Otodynia > oh-toe-**dine**-ee-ah > earache, ear pain. *Synonym*: **otalgia** > ot-al-**jee**-ah.

8

Otoliths > oh-**toe**-liths > ear stones, tiny crystals sitting on the gel-like membranes of the inner ear.

8

Otology > oh-**tol**-oh-gee > study of the ear.

8

Otomycosis > oh-toe-my-**ko**-sis > abnormal condition of ear fungus.

8

Otosclerosis > oh-toe-skleh-**roe**-sis > hardening of the ossicles.

8

Ovarian follicle > oh-**ver**-ee-an fol-ee-kel > one of the stages of development, a spherical cell accretion in the ovary which contains an oocyte.

15

Oxytocin > **ock**-see-**toe**-sin > hormone, travels to the uterus to begin contractions of birth and the breast to let milk down for the infant.

9, 15

Unit

Pachymeter > **pah**-**kim**-ee-tur > measurement of the thickness of the cornea. 8

Paget's disease > **pah**-jets > disease where both the osteoclasts and osteoblasts are working too hard, creating patches of weakened bone. 5

Palatine > **pal**-ah-tine > small bones (2) forming the hard palate and the floor of the eye orbits. 5

Palatoplasty > **pal**-ah-toe-plaz-tee > repair of the palate is a surgery to treat snoring. 13

Palilalia > **pal**-i-la-**lee**-ah > repeating phrases which others speak over and over again. 7

Palpation > pal-**pay**-shun > process of touching the body to feeling vibrations or discerning pain. 11

Palpebral > **pal**-peh-bral > pertaining to the eyelids. 8

Palpitations > **pal**-pee-**tay**-shuns > sensation of the force of or irregular heartbeat. 11

Pancreatectomy > **pan**-kree-ah-**tek**-toe-me > excision or removal of a part of the pancreas. 9, 13

Pancreatic > **pan**-kree-at-ik cancer > arises in the exocrine glands of the pancreas. 9, 13

Pancreatitis > **pan**-kree-ah-**tie**-tis > inflammation of the pancreas. It is associated with certain medications, alcoholism, tobacco use, and the presence of gallbladder disease. 9, 13

Pancytopenia > **pan**-sigh-toe-**pee**-knee-ah > marked decline in the number of all blood cells: RBCs, WBCs, and platelets. 2, 10

Panic disorder > a severe anxiety reaction with intense apprehension, fear, or terror. 7

Papillary muscles > **pap**-il-lar-ee > sit on the floor of each ventricle; slight contraction pulls on chordae to keep valves closed under pressure. 11

Papilledema > **pap**-il-eh-**dee**-ma > bilateral swelling of the optic discs caused by intracranial pressure from a brain mass. 8

Papule > **pap**-yule > firm, solid elevation of the skin, smaller than 0.5 cm; common with acne. 4

Papulonodular > **pap**-u-low-**nod**-u-lar > the condition of being mixed as papular and nodular (size difference) of solid lesions. 4

Papulosquamous > **pap**-u-low-**sqwa**-mus > condition of being mixed papular and scaly skin lesions. 4

Paracrines > **pear**-ah-krines > 'near secretions', localized hormones affecting local and distant tissue. 9

Parallel > **par**-ah-lel > side to side, equidistant fibers or configuration. 6

Paraplegia > **pair**-ah-**play**-gee-ah > both legs are paralyzed. 6, 7

Parasympathetic > **pear**-ah-**sim**-pah-**thet**-ik > division of the CNS most responsible for slowing the body to rest and recuperate. 7

Parathyroid (PTH) > **pair**-ah-**thigh**-royd > four tiny hormone glands behind the thyroid. They control calcium and phosphate levels in the body via bone building and carving. 5, 9

Unit

Paresis > **pah**-ree-sis > partial paralysis.   9

Paresthesias > pair-es-**thee**-zee-as > uncomfortable or painful sensations.   7, 9

Parietal > pah-**rye**-eh-tal > skull bones (2) cover the top of the brain in connection
with occipital and frontal bones with flat sutures or membrane of the wall.
Also outer layer of bilayer sac around heart, lungs, and abdomen.   2, 5, 11, 13

Parkinsonism (an eponym) > **parh**-kin-**son**-izm > collection of symptoms
associated with a progressive disorder of the nervous system.   1, 7

Paronychia > pair-oh-**knee**-key-ah > inflammation or infection of the nail
fold surrounding the nail bed.   4

Parous > **pahr**-us (**P**) > Latin for to bear, to carry.   15

Patch > pach > larger than 2 cm, flat discoloration of the skin.   4

Pathogen > **path**-oh-jen > any virus, microorganism, or other substance which
can cause disease.   2, 9

Pathologist > pah-**thol**-oh-jist > specialist in the study of disease via visualization
of cell and tissue changes.   3

Pathology > pah-**thol**-oh-gee > study of disease via visualization of cell and tissue
changes with laboratory analysis, gross inspection, and microscopic review.   3, 9

Pectinate > **pek**-tea-nate > comb, comb-like, ridges.   6, 13

Pectoral > **pek**-tor-al > muscle group covering most of the anterior chest,
P. major and P. minor.   2, 6

Pectoriloquy > **pek**-toe-**real**-oh-kwee > whisper is generally not heard until it
passes through a consolidation, a more solid area of the lung indicating
pneumonia or mass-effect.   12

Pelvimetry > pel-**vim**-eh-tree > measurement of the pelvic inlet; used to
determine ability to deliver infant.   5, 15

Pelvis (singular), **pelves** (plural) > **pel**-vis > large, cup-shaped ring of bone
which provides the end-point of the trunk. It holds and protects the pelvic
organs: bladder, reproductive organs, and more.   2

Penetrating > **pen**-ee-**trait**-ing > puncture wounds like ice picks, thorns, nails,
splinters.   4

Pennate > **pen**-nate > muscle fascicles – resemble a feather: uni-, bi-, multi-.   6

Pentad > **pen**-tad > group of 5 elements – related or may signify a syndrome.   2

Percussion > purr-**kus**-shun methods > utilize tapping on the chest wall (anterior
and posteriorly) to discern hollow (air-filled) versus dull (solid consolidation).   12

Pericardial tamponade > **tam**-poe-nad > compression of the heart due to fluid
and/or blood in the pericardial sac.   11

Pericarditis > pear-i-**kar**-die-tis > inflammation of the pericardial sac due to
infection or injury.   11

Pericardium > pear-i-**kar**-dee-um > pertaining to around the heart.   11

Perimysium > pear-ee-**mis**-ee-um > connective tissue binding 10–15 muscle
fibers.   6

Perineurium > pear-ee-**nur**-ree-um > thicker wrapping around sets of axons
called a fascicle.   7

Unit

Periosteitis > **pear**-eh-**os**-tea-**eye**-tis > proper name for 'shin splints', inflammation of the periosteum.   6

Periosteum > **pear**-eh-**os**-tea-um > around the bone, connective tissue, fascia, and bone tissue, allows nerve, vessel, and lymph access to bone.   5

Peripheral neuropathy > **nur**-oh-**nop**-ah-thee > disease of the nerve/neurons at a distance. Common cause diabetes.   8

Peristalsis > **pear**-ee-**stal**-sis > rhythmic squeezing moves food (the bolus) down the alimentary canal. Esophagospasm is the term used when the rhythm is broken.   6, 13

Peritoneocentesis > **pear**-ee-toe-**knee**-oh-sen-**tea**-sis > procedure: to withdraw fluid for the abdominal cavity (peritoneal sac) for evaluation or therapy.   2, 13

Peritoneoclysis > **pear**-ee-toe-knee-**oh**-klie-sis > procedure: to irrigate or flush out the peritoneal sac to remove debris such as blood, pus, or stool.   2, 13

Peritoneum > **pear**-i-toe-**knee**-um > double-layer serous membrane encloses the abdominal cavity and covers most of the organs (viscera) providing cushioning, blood vessels, and nerve supply.   2, 13

Peritonitis > **pear**-i-toe-**nigh**-tis > inflammation of the peritoneal sac or space due to inflammation of another organ, such as appendicitis or enteritis.   13

Pernicious > purr-**nish**-us **anemia** > due to inadequate intake or absorption of vitamin B_{12}.   10

Peroxisomes > pear-**ock**-see-soms > cell janitors, they contain oxidative enzymes to destroy debris in the intracellular environment.   3

PERRLA > pupils equal round and reactive to light and accommodation, physical exam acronym.   8

Pertussis > purr-**tus**-is > bacterial lung infection, also called whooping cough.   9, 12

Petechia > peh-**tea**-key-ah > minute (pin-point) hemorrhage, will not blanch.   10

Peyer's > **pie**-yhers > patches, collections of lymphoid tissue – help protect the small intestines.   10

Phacoemulsification > **fak**-oh-ee-mul-see-fi-**kay**-shun > procedure to emulsify and aspirate the lens of the eye.   8

Phagocytes > **fag**-oh-sites > white blood cells, eat (phag/o) debris and foreign bodies.   3, 9

Phagocytosis > **fag**-oh-sigh-**toe**-sis > white blood cells eating (phag/o) debris and foreign bodies.   9

Phalanges, phalanx > fay-**lan**-geez, **fay**-langks > finger and toe bones, 14 each.   5

Phallodynia > **fal**-oh-**din**-ee-ah > pain in the penis.   15

Phalloplasty > **fal**-oh-**plaz**-tea > repair of the penis.   15

Pharyngitis > **fair**-in-**jie**-tis > inflammation of the pharynx, the back of the throat.   1, 12

Phenylketonuria > **fen**-il-**key**-toe-**nyur**-ee-ah (**PKU**) > an inherited disorder interrupting the breakdown (lysis) of phenylalanine, an amino acid.   14

Pheromones > **fair**-oh-monz > specialized molecules, provide specific odors attracting the opposite sex.   4

Unit

Phlebostasis > fleh-**bos**-tay-sis > abnormally slow motion of blood in the veins.   11

Phlebotomy > fleh-**bot**-oh-me > 'to cut into vein' is the process of drawing blood for laboratory study.   10, 11

Phobic > foe-bik > marked or persistent fear of objects or situations.   7

Photoreceptors > foe-to-reh-**sep**-tours > produced by light only – this is used by the eyes, vision specifically.   8

Physical exam (PE) > **fiz**-zi-kal x-am > set of procedures performed on or with the patient to define the body's status and function for health exam, illness, or injury.   1

Pia mater > **pee**-ah **ma**-tur > tender, delicate matter. It is the fine mesh adhering to every nook and cranny of the cortex of the brain.   7

Pilonidal > **pie**-low-**nigh**-dal > presence of hair in a dermoid cyst.   4

Pineal > **pie**-kneel gland > brain endocrine gland associated with rest and sleep cycles.   9

Pinguecula > ping-**qwek**-U-la > white to yellow accumulation of protein on the bulbar conjunctiva.   8

Piriformis > **peer**-i-**form**-is > wedge- or pear-shaped muscle, deep pelvic area, protects sciatic nerve.   6

Pituitary > pi-**tu**-i-ter-ee **gland** > master gland of the body; it is about the size of a large pea.   7, 9

Placenta > play-**cen**-tah > organ of pregnancy; part of the implantation of the embryo is the formation of the chorionic villi into the fetomaternal connection.   15

Placenta previa > pre-**vee**-ah > placenta is located in the wrong place in the distal uterus.   15

Plantar > **plant**-ar > as a *direction* it pertains to the feet and toes. It is the sole of our foot 'planting' on the ground.   2

Plaque > plak > larger (greater than 1 cm), raised lesion with a flatter top with well-demarcated edges as seen in eczema and psoriasis.   4

Plasma membrane > **plaz**-ma **mem**-brain > cell wall with its flexible outer boundary usually constructed of phospholipids walls.   3

Platelets > **playt**-lets > thrombocytes, the cell fragments which provide blood clotting ability.   10

Platysma > platz > flat, wide muscle, neck and head.   6

Pleura (singular), **pleurae** (plural) > **plur**-ah, **plur**-ree > visceral and parietal membranes wrap and protect the lungs from the hilum.   2, 12

Pleurisy > **plur**-i-see or **pleuritis** (**plur**-eye-tis) > inflammation of the pleura.   12

Pleurodesis > plur-ow-**dee**-sis > artificial production of scar tissue of the pleura to seal a reoccurring pneumothorax or hemothorax.   12

Plexus > **pleks**-us > grouped network of nerves – branch off to specific areas.   7

Pneumatocardia > **new**-mat-toe-**kar**-dee-a > presence of air or gas in the blood of the heart.   12

Pneumoconiosis > **new**-mow-ko-knee-**oh**-sis > black lung resulting from coal dust exposure.   12

Unit

Pneumonia > new-**mow**-knee-ah > inflammation of the lung tissues (alveoli) which tends to consolidate in a specific lobe.   1, 12

Pneumothorax > **new**-moe-**thor**-aks > when the potential space fills with air between the layers, it crushes the tissue as it enlarges.   12

Podiatrist > poe-**die**-ah-trists > specialist who diagnoses, treats, and performs surgery on the foot exclusively.   5

Poliomyelitis > **poy**-lee-oh-my-eh-**lie**-tis > viral illness causing ascending muscle weakness and atrophy.   6, 7

Pollex > **pol**-lex > proper name for the 1st finger, the thumb.   2, 5

Polyarticular > pol-ee-are-**tik**-u-lar > pertaining to multiple joints.   2, 5

Polycystic kidney disease (PKD) > hereditary disease characterized by multiple cysts on both kidneys.   14

Polycystic ovarian disease (PCO) > ovarian cysts form, fill with fluid, and change hormone levels.   15

Polycythemia > **pol**-ee-sigh-**thee**-me-ah > abnormal increase in the number of red blood cells.   2, 10

Polydipsia > pol-ee-**dip**-see-ah > excessive drinking of fluids, often associated with diabetes mellitus.   9, 14

Polymyositis > pol-ee-**my**-oh-**sigh**-tis > inflammation of several voluntary muscles simultaneously.   6

Polyphagia > **pol**-ee-**fay**-see-ah > excessive eating.   9, 13

Polyposis > pol-ee-**poe**-sis > abnormal condition of multiple polyps; these are more likely to be converted to a cancer.   13

Polysynaptic > **pohl**-ee-sin-**ap**-tik > many connections work together in response to complex needs, such as protection from a flame or sharp object.   7

Polyuria > pol-ee-**yur**-ee-ah > many urinations.   9, 14

Posterior > pos-**tier**-ee-or > direction: it denotes the back of the body, our back end. *Synonym* of dorsum and more commonly used. Opposite of anterior.   2

Postictal > post-**ik**-tal > slight confusion or disorientation of the person after the seizure.   7

Postpartum > post-**pahr**-tum > after birth.   15

Potassium > poe-**tass**-ee-um > cation, symbol K^+, intracellular ion.   3, 14

Pregnancy > **preg**-nan-see > female condition of carrying the product of conception until termination of this product.   15

Prepuce > **pre**-pyus > foreskin, loose, folded skin covering the glans penis.   15

Presbycusis > **prez**-bee-**kyu**-sis > 'old hearing'. This term is used of the normal hearing changes of aging.   8

Presbyopia > **prez**-bee-oh-pee-ah > 'old eyes'. It refers to the condition of the loss of accommodation with aging.   8

Prevention > using common sense or activities such as vaccinations to avoid injury or illness: sunscreen, seat belts, driving without a cell phone in your hand . . .   3

Primigravida > **pre**-me-**grav**-ee-dah > first pregnancy.   15

Unit

Progesterone > pro-**jes**-tur-ohn > female hormone, provides the balance of the menstrual cycle or preparation for zygote implantation.

9, 15

Prognosis > prog-**no**-sis > condition of predicting knowledge, a forecast of outcome.

1

Prolactin > pro-**lak**-tin (**PRL**) > brain hormone travels to the breast to stimulate milk production.

9

Pronated > **pro**-nated > direction: placing the body or forearm in a face-down position. When the arm is pronated, the palm is facing down.

2

Proprioception > **pro**-pre-oh-**cep**-shun > knowing where a limb is in space without looking.

6, 7

Prostaglandin > **pros**-tah-**glan**-din > paracrine found in all cells, stimulates inflammation, harm, or contamination.

9

Prostatitis > **pros**-tah-**tie**-tis > inflammation of the prostate.

14, 15

Prosthesis > pros-**thee**-sis > an artificial device or appliance – replaces a missing body part.

5

Proteases > pro-**tee**-ayses > enzymes to break down proteins are secreted by the exocrine functions of the pancreas.

13

Protein > **pro**-teen > combination of amino acids, nitrogen, carbon, hydrogen, and carboxyl group. Vital to all cell activities.

3, 13

Protein-energy malnutrition (PEM) > most serious type of malnutrition due to the lack of calories and protein intake.

6

Proteinuria > **pro**-tee-**nur**-ee-ah > protein in the urine.

14

Proteomics > **pro**-tea-oh-miks > study of how proteins are organized, built, and function in the cells based on DNA instructions.

3

Proximal > **prok**-si-mal > direction: it is nearest to center or point of origin. Opposite of distal. The elbow is proximal of the wrist.

2

Pruritus > pru-**ree**-tus > itching, is from the French; this term is often used in relationship to the intense itchy reaction of allergies.

9

Pseudocyesis > **sue**-doe-sigh-**ee**-sis > false pregnancy.

15

Psoriasis > soar-**eye**-ah-sis > characterized by papulosquamous plaques on red bases, these are well defined.

4

Psychopathy > **sigh**-ko-**pah**-thee > diseases of the emotion or mentation or psyche.

7

Pterygium > tear-**i**-jeh-um > tissue mass encroaching past the limbus onto the cornea.

8

Pubic > **pew**-bik > region: above the pelvic cavity with the urinary bladder, sigmoid colon, rectum, and anus. Prostate in men and uterus in women.

2, 5, 15

Pulmonary > **pul**-moe-nar-ee valve > between the right ventricle and pulmonary arteries (2).

11, 12

Punch biopsy > 1 to 5 mm core biopsy.

15

Purpura > **purr**-purr-ah > hemorrhage under the skin, starts out red, becomes dark purple. Large, deep, flat due to systemic issues.

4, 10

Pustules > **pust**-yule > vesicles, full of the debris of inflammation including leukocytes. Larger lesions: boil, furuncles, carbuncles.

4

Unit

Pyelogram > **pi**-el-oh-gram > X-ray exam of the ureter and renal pelvis. 14

Pyelonephritis > **pi**-e-low-neh-**fri**-tis > inflammation of the renal pelvis and kidneys. 14

Pyloric stenosis > pie-**lor**-ik **sten**-oh-sis > narrowing of the sphincter between the stomach and duodenum. 13

Pyrexia > pie-**rek**-see-a > condition of fever, fire, or heat. 9

Pyuria > pie-**ur**-i-ah > pus in the urine. 14

Quadrant > **kwad**-rant > region: 25% of an area, usually referring to the four quadrants of the abdomen. 2, 13

Quadratus > qwah-**dra**-tus > square-like, there are several muscles with this configuration. 6

Quadriplegia > **qwa**-dree-**play**-gee-ah > all four limbs are paralyzed. 6, 7

Quadruplets > kwad-**rup**-lets > four infants born at one birth. 2

Quintuplets > kwin-**tup**-lets > five infants born at one single birth. 2

Rachiocentesis > **rah**-key-oh-sen-**tea**-sis > lumbar puncture to gather cerebral spinal fluid, CSF. 5, 7

Radiculitis > rah-**dik**-U-**lie**-tis > inflammation of the nerve root. 7

Radiculoneuropathy > rah-**dik**-U-low-nur-**op**-ath-ee > disease of the spinal nerve roots and nerves. 7

Radiology > **ray**-dee-**ol**-oh-gee > study of and treatment with X-rays. 2, 5

Rales > rahls > intermittent bubbling sounds or rattles with inspiration. 12

Rami; ramus > **ray**-my or **ray**-mus > nerve division, branches out for motor control from the ventral root or ganglia. 7

Recumbent > re-**come**-bent > direction: to lie down on one's side, left or right lateral. 2

Regurgitation > ree-**gur**-jeh-**tay**-shun > medical term for vomiting, bringing food up (burping), or back-up of blood. 3, 11, 13

Renal > **ree**-nul > pertaining to the kidneys. The renal system filters our blood for waste products and balances electrolytes while producing urine. 2, 14

Renin > **rey**-nin > specific to the kidneys, it raises the blood pressure (**BP**) in the glomeruli by causing vasoconstriction to force fluid into the tubules. 14

Reproductive > **ree**-pro-**duk**-tiv > only system of the human body not essential to life BUT it is absolutely needed to produce children – the next generation of humans. 2, 15

Respiratory > **res**-peer-a-tor-ee > pertaining to respiration, the fundamental process of life of moving oxygen into the body and expelling carbon dioxide, a waste product. 2, 12

Respire > **res**-pyre > to breathe, to move gases over and over again. 2, 12

Reticular > re-**tik**-U-lar > network of delicate tissue, almost spider-web like – permitting support and free motion of leukocytes and lymphatics. 3, 9, 12

Reticulocytes > re-**tik**-U-low-site > laboratory: actual number or percentage of young erythrocytes. 10

Unit

Retinacula (plural) > **reh**-tea-**nak**-u-lah > retaining band, soft tissue – connective tissues, wrap ankle and wrists.   4, 6

Retinal detachment > **ret**-i-nal > loss of part of the retina from its layers.   8

Retinitis pigmentosa > **ret**-i-nal **pig**-men-**toe**-sah > gradually progressive degeneration of the retina beginning in childhood.   8

Retinoblastoma > **ret**-i-tin-**oh**-blas-**toe**-ma > tumor of the retina produced by overgrowth of the development cells.   8

Retinopathy > **ret**-i-**nop**-ah-thee > disease conditions of the eye's retina.   8, 9

Retroperitoneum > **ret**-row-**pear**-i-toe-**knee**-um > behind the abdominal double-layered membrane covering the abdominal contents. Protects, cushions, and lends stability to kidneys, adrenal glands, duodenum, pancreas, parts of the colon, and great abdominal vessels.   2, 13, 14

Rhabdomyolysis > **rab**-doe-my-**oh**-lie-sis > destruction of skeletal muscle tissues.   6

Rhabdomyosarcoma > **rab**-doe-**my**-oh-sar-**ko**-ma > typically, an aggressive malignant muscle tumor.   6

Rheumatologist > **roo**-mah-**tol**-oh-jist > specialist of inflammatory or auto-immune diseases.   5, 9

Rheumatology > **roo**-mah-**tol**-oh-gee > specialist who studies and treats diseases of the joints.   1, 9

Rhinitis > rye-**nigh**-tis > inflammation of the nose.   1, 8, 12

Rhinoantritis > **rye**-no-an-**try**-tis > inflammation of the nose and one or both maxillary sinuses.   8, 12

Rhinolith > rye-**no**-lith > a nose stone.   12

Rhinoplasty > **rye**-no-plas-tee > surgical: surgery to repair the nose.   1, 12

Rhinorrhea > **rye**-no-**ree**-ya > runny nose, discharge or flow from the nose.   1, 12

Rhinoscopy > rye-**nos**-kop-ee > procedure: the process of using an instrument to look in or at the nose.   1, 12

Rhomboid > **rohm**-boyd > geometric rhomboid-shaped muscle of the upper, medial scapula.   6

Rhonchi > **rong**-ki > similar to a wheeze but deeper tone and can be continuous or intermittent.   12

Ribonucleic acid > **rye**-bow-**new**-klay-ik > macromolecule, carries (messenger) and translates the DNA instruction to build proteins in the endoplasmic reticulum of the cell.   3

Ribosomes > **rye**-bow-soms > workers in the ER produce the proteins according to the directions of the DNA as translated by the RNA. rRNA is the combination of proteins and RNA.   3

Rubella > ruw-**bel**-la > German measles; it presents with a 'dim red' or pink rash.   9

Rubeola > **ruw**-bee-oh-lah > measles; it presents with a 'dim red' or pink rash.   9

Sagittal > **saj**-it-tal > direction: term pertaining to the plane – bisects the body vertically, right to left.   2

Salpingectomy > **sal**-pin-**jek**-toe-me > removal of uterine tube.   15

Salpingopexy > sal-**ping**-go-pek-see > fixing the uterine tube in place.   15

Unit

Salpingoscope > sal-**ping**-go-skop > instrument to look at the uterine tube; done when a patient has difficulty getting pregnant to see if there is a blockage.   15

Sarcoidosis > **sahr**-koy-**doe**-sis > chronic inflammatory disease of unknown origin.   12

Sarcolemma > **sar**-ko-**lem**-ma > cell membrane of the muscle fiber or cell. Special name.   3

Sarcomere > **sar**-ko-meer > functional unit of the skeletal muscle cells.   3, 6

Sarcopenia > **sahr**-ko-**peh**-knee-ah > progressive reduction of the muscle associated with aging.   6

Sarcoplasmic > **sar**-ko-plaz-mik > specific name for the muscle endoplasmic reticulum. Wraps each cell in a network to aid rapid chemical exchange.   3

Sarcopoietic > **sahr**-ko-poy-**et**-ik > forming muscle.   6

Scale > increase in the thickness and dryness of the top layer, the stratum corneum. It appears flakey.   4

Scar > fibrous tissue replacing healthy tissue after an illness or injury. *Synonym*: cicatrix > **sik**-ah-tricks from the Latin.   4

Schizophrenia > **skiz**-oh-**fre**-knee-ah > severe form of psychopathology with deep loss of functioning and withdrawal from reality.   7

Scleritis > **sklar**-eye-tis > inflammation of the sclera, the whites of the eyes.   8

Sclerosis > **sklar**-oh-sis > abnormal condition of hardening.   1, 7, 9, 11, 13

Scoliosis > **sko**-lee-**oh**-sis > abnormal lateral curvature of the spine, S-shaped.   5

Scotoma > sko-**toe**-ma > area in the visual field is blank, empty, or muted. A blind spot.   8

Screening > checking for the presence of early disease in an effort to stop it early, such as with coloscopy or mammogram.   3

Scrotal hydrocele > high-**trow**-seal > trauma or inflammation can cause fluid to fill the scrotum.   15

Scrotal raphe > **skro**-tal **ray**-fee > tendinous connective cord running the length of the scrotum to the anus.   15

Scrotal varicocele > **var**-ee-**ko**-seal > varicose veins of the scrotum.   15

Sebaceous > sey-**bay**-shus > relating to sebum, oily or fatty substance; sebaceous gland lubricates hair and skin.   4

Seborrheic dermatitis > **seb**-or-**rhee**-ik **dur**-mah-**tie**-tis > chronic skin condition presents with oily scaling and/or plaques.   4

Sebum > **see**-bum > pertaining to oily fluid.   4

Semen > **sea**-men > penile ejaculate, a thick, slightly sweet sticky fluid, combines the sperm and other fluids to push the sperm into the cervix of the woman.   15

Semicircular canals > balance side of the inner ear, a bony labyrinth.   8

Semicomatose > **sem**-eye-**ko**-mah-tose, **sem**-ee-**ko**-mah-tose > concerning the loss of consciousness or drowsiness.   2

Sensorineural > **sen**-soar-ee-**nur**-al > pertaining to the nerves' ability to sense.   8

Serology > sair-**ol**-oh-gee > study of the immune response observed in the blood, in the serum, the liquid portion of the blood.   10

Unit

Serotonin > **ser**-oh-**toe**-nin > found primarily in the brain and gastrointestinal tract. In the brain, it is linked to supporting mood balance. ... 7

Serratus > seh-**rate**-us > notched, insertion appearance of the lateral, upper thorax muscle sets. ... 6

Sex > seks > features which distinguish male from female. It is based on gonads, internal and external physical findings, chromosome pattern, and hormones. ... 15

Sextuplets > sex-**tup**-lets > six infants born of a single birth. ... 2

Sexuality > **sek**-shu-**al**-i-tee > sum of person's preferred sexual behaviors and tendencies. ... 15

Sialodochoplasty > **sigh**-ah-low-**do**-ko-**plaz**-tee > repair of the salivary duct. ... 13

Sialolithiasis > **sigh**-ah-low-lee-**thigh**-ah-sis > salivary gland stone infestation. ... 13

Sickle > **sik**-**el** cell > abnormality of hemoglobin S, c-shaped cells. ... 10

Silicosis > **seal**-ee-**ko**-sis > inhalation of sand dust of any type. ... 12

Sinoatrial > **sigh**-no-**ay**-tree-al > (**SA**) node > self-starting electrical tissue, the normal trigger for the heartbeat. ... 11

Sinusitis > **sigh**-nu-**sigh**-tis > inflammation of the paranasal sinuses. ... 8, 12

Sinusotomy > **sigh**-nu-**sot**-oh-me > incision into a sinus. ... 8, 12

Skeletal > **skel**-et-al > bony framework of the human body, from the combining form skelet/o = dried up (bones). ... 2, 5

SLE, Systemic lupus erythematosus > **lew**-pus er-**ith**-ee-mah-**toe**-sus > connective tissue disorder that disrupts glomerular function in the renal system. It also affects skin, eyes, joints, and results in pericarditis or anemia. ... 14

Smegma > **smeg**-mah > cheese-like substance which forms under the foreskin if the glans under the foreskin is not cleaned properly. ... 15

Sodium chloride > so-**dee**-um **klor**-ide > table salt, NaCl. ... 3, 14

Spasticity > spas-**tis**-i-tee > increased muscle tone. ... 6

Spermatocide > **spur**-mat-oh-side > process of killing sperm. Heat, radiation, and some medications can destroy sperm. *Synonym*: spermicide. ... 15

Spermatogenesis > **spur**-mat-oh-**jen**-eh-sis > process of producing sperm. ... 15

Sphenoid > **sfee**-noyd > called the bat-bone because of its configuration, foundation of the cranial floor with the sella turcica. ... 5

Spherocytosis > **sfear**-oh-**sigh**-toe-sis > hereditary hemolytic disorder, the RBCs appear as spheres instead of flexible discs. ... 10

Sphincter > **sfink**-tur > a band, like a purse-string, the GI tract has several rate limiters which open and close depending on hormone, mechanical, and some voluntary controls. ... 13

Sphygmomanometer > **sfig**-mo-mah-**nom**-eh-tur > measures pressure, comes in hand-held kits, wall-assemblies, and any number of computerized configurations. ... 11

Splenectomy > sple-**nek**-toe-me > surgical: surgery to remove the spleen. ... 1, 10

Splenomegaly > **sple**-no-**meg**-ah-lee > enlargement of the spleen. ... 10

Spondylolisthesis > **spon**-di-low-lis-**thee**-sis > slipping, falling of the vertebra, on X-ray, the anterior disk area is compressed a bit. ... 5

Unit

Spondylolysis > **spon**-dee-**low**-lie-sis > degeneration of the vertebrae.   5

Stapedius > stay-**pee**-dee-us > muscle, protects the ear's oval window.   8

Stapes > **stay**-pees > stirrup, it is the last and smallest of the middle ear bones.   8

Staphylococcus > **staff**-ee-low-**kock**-us > bacterial type, common to skin infections:
boils, impetigo (crusts), and cellulitis. Looks like clusters of round grapes.   4, 6, 12

Stasis dermatitis > **stay**-sis **dur**-mah-**tie**-tis > acutely inflamed area usually
found over the legs or foot area due to poor circulation.   4

STDs > chlamydia, gonorrhea, herpes (HSV), and genital warts (HPV).   15

Stenosis > **sten**-oh-sis > condition of narrowing of any structure.   5, 11

Sternocleidomastoid > **ster**-no-**klie**-eh-doe-**mas**-toyd muscles > neck muscles.   6, 12

Stethoscope > **steth**-oh-scope > instrument to listen to body sounds; from the
Greek for chest.   1

Stoma > **stoy**-mah > opening, may refer to the artificial opening of the colon
to the skin level to bypass a portion of the colon.   13

Stomatitis > **stoy**-mah-**tie**-tis > inflammation of the mouth.   12, 13

Stomatodynia > **stoy**-mat-oh-**die**-knee-ah > pain in the mouth.   12

Strabismus > strah-**biz**-mus > one eye is not parallel to the other.   8

Stratum basale > **strat**-um ba-**sah**-leh > active layer of the epidermis,
producing new skin cells which migrate up.   4

Stratum corneum > **strat**-um **kor**-knee-um > top layers of the epidermis –
slough off regularly taking contaminants with them.   4

Streptococcus > **strep**-toe-**kock**-us > bacterial type, twisted round bacteria,
common to skin and respiratory infections.   4, 6, 12

Stridor > **stri**-dur > deep, discordant whistle because the air is struggling to
squeak by.   12

Subconjunctival hemorrhage > sub-**kon**-junk-**tie**-val **hem**-or-ahj > bleeding
under the clear layers overlying the eye sclera.   8

Subcostal > **sub**-kos-tal > pertaining to under the ribs.   5

Subcutaneous > sub-Q-**tay**-knee-us > pertaining to under the skin, layer of fat
and soft tissues; support and anchor the skin.   4

Subjective > sub-**jek**-tiv > concern of the patient, in their own words, with
their own descriptions of events related to illness or injury. It is the given
history.   1, 2

Sublingual > sub-**ling**-gwal > under the tongue, used typically for medication
delivery.   13

Subluxation > sub-**luks**-ay-shun > slight dislocation of the joint articulation,
common at the rib heads.   5

Subungual > sub-**ung**-wal > under the nail.   4

Sudoriferous > **su**-door-**if**-ur-us > specialized sweat gland known from their odor.
Synonym: apocrine.   4

Sulci; sulcus > **sul**-sigh or **sul**-kus > shallow fissure or hollow.   7

Superficial > **sue**-pur-**fish**-al > direction: toward the surface; scratches are
superficial. It is the opposite of deep.   2

Unit

Superior > sue-**peer**-ee-or > direction: denotes a structure above or directed upward. The shoulder is superior to the elbow. It is the opposite of inferior. — 2, 5

Supinated > **sue**-pi-nat-ed > direction: term or act of lying face up or turning your hand, palm up. An easy way to remember is hold soup in your hand. — 2

Surfactant > sir-**fak**-tant > lipoprotein acting as a wetting agent to the internal alveoli. — 12

Surgical > **sur**-gee-cal > pertaining to surgery. — 3

Sympathetic > **sim**-pah-**thet**-ik > division of the CNS most responsible for maintaining or speeding up body reactions. — 7

Symptoms > **simp**-tom > collection of feelings, or a departure from normal as perceived by the patient. — 3

Synapsis > si-**nap**-sis > functional membrane to membrane contact between nerve cells. — 7

Synarthrosis > **sin**-are-**throw**-sis > tight joint, immobile such as the skull sutures. — 5

Syncytium > sin-**sish**-ee-um > individual cells working in unison for near simultaneous action. — 6, 11, 12

Synergist > **sin**-er-jist > muscles working together, assisting each other. — 6

Syphilis > **sif**-i-lus > systemic disease caused by *Treponema pallidum*. It has three stages which can be found with a blood test, **RPR**, Rapid Plasma Reagin or other immunoassays. — 3, 10, 15

Systolic > sis-**tol**-ik > contraction of the heart, the squeezing increases the pressure throughout the arterial system. — 11

Tachycardia > **tak**-ee-**kar**-dee-ah > fast heart rate, greater than 100 bpm. — 11

Tachypnea > **tac**-key-**pee**-knee-ah > fast breathing. — 12

Tactile cells > **tak**-till sells or **tak**-tile > nerve ending type, picks up touch; quite abundant in fingertips. — 4

Tamponade > **tam**-poe-nod > compression of the heart by an accumulation of fluid in the pericardial sac. Emergency. — 11

Telangiectasia > tel-**an**-gee-ek-**taz**-ee-ah > dilation of a tiny vessel previously not seen on the surface of the skin. — 4

Temporal > **tem**-pore-al > skull bones (2) cover the sides of the brain, provide support for ear canal, TMJ (jaw), connecting with parietal, occipital, and sphenoid bones. — 5, 7

Tendinoplasty > **ten**-din-oh-plaz-tee > surgical repair of the tendon. *Synonym*: tendoplasty (**ten**-do-plaz-tee). — 5, 6

Tendolysis > **ten**-**doh**-lie-sis > release of a tendon (lysis > destruction). — 5, 6

Tendonitis > **ten**-doe-**nigh**-tis > inflammation of the tendon. — 5, 6

Tenosynovitis > **ten**-oh-sin-oh-**vie**-tis > inflammation of the synovium (of the joint) and tendon. — 5, 6

Tensor tympani > **tim**-pah-knee > muscle, protects the eardrum from excessive motion, attaches to the handle of the malleus. — 8

Teres > **tear**-ez > rounded, smooth, muscle on the posterior chest. — 6

Unit

Terminology > **tur**-min-ol-**oh**-gee > process of studying the vocabulary or words of a specific language. 1

Testosterone > tes-**tos**-tur-ohn > male hormone, stimulates sperm formation; the smallest cell of the body, at about 5 micrometers. 9, 15

Tetanus > **tet**-ah-nus > muscle in prolonged contract. Also infectious disease which causes muscle paralysis and death. A vaccination. 6, 9

Tetany > **tet**-ah-knee > sustained muscle contraction. 6

Tetradactyl > **tet**-rah-**dak**-teal > presence of four toes on one foot or hand. 2

Tetralogy of Fallot > **tet**-ral-**oh**-gee of **Fa**-low > eponym: named for the nineteenth-century French physician Étienne-Louis Arthur Fallot who described the four congenital heart defects. 2

Thalamotomy > **thal**-ah-**mot**-oh-me > to cut into the thalamus. 7

Thalassemia > **thal**-ah-**see**-me-ah > genetic condition, thalassemia major is associated with severe anemia. 10

Thermoreceptors > **ther**-moe-reh-**sep**-tours > sparked via changes in temperature – this is touch, smell, and taste. 8

Thoracic > thor-**as**-ik > related to the thorax, the chest cavity which contains the heart, lungs, esophagus, great vessels, and lymph glands. 2, 5, 10, 12

Thorax > **tho**-raks > chest, protected by the rib cage and thoracic spine. 2, 5, 11

Thrill > vibration of a heart or vessel felt on palpation. 11

Thrombocytes > **thrawm**-bow-sights > laboratory: Platelets, the cells cause blood to clot. 10

Thrombus > throhm-bus > clot, usually associated with blood or the mixed atherosclerotic plaque. 10, 11

Thymosin > **thigh**-moe-zin > hormone, secreted by thymus gland to trigger T-cell function. 9, 10

Thymus > **thigh**-mus > endocrine in the mediastinal area. Large at birth, it shrinks but is vital to maturation of the T-lymphocytes. 9

Thyroid > **thigh**-royd > endocrine gland at the base of the anterior neck. Vital to overall metabolic functions. 9

Thyroiditis > **thigh**-royd-**eye**-tis > inflammation of the thyroid. 9

Tics > tiks > habitual contractions of a specific muscle. 6

Tinea corporis > **tin**-ee-ah **kor**-pore-sis > commonly called ringworm, it is a fungal infection typified by red, raised, itchy rings. 4

Tinea cruris > **tin**-ee-ah **krew**-is > jock itch, red, itchy rash over the genitalia. 4

Tinea pedis > **tin**-ee-ah **ped**-is > athlete's foot, a fungal infection distinguished by redness, peeling skin, itching, and blisters. 4

Tinnitus > **tin**-knee-tus > noise in the ears: ringing, wind noise, booming, buzzing, clicking, or whistling. 8

Tissue > **tis**-shoe > grouping or aggregation of similar cells, together perform an identifiable function. Bone, connective, epithelium, and nerve tissues are the four large categories of tissue. 2, 3, 4

Tomogram > **toe**-moe-gram > imaging: A radiographic procedure, takes a series of X-rays in slices or cuts. 1

Unit

Tonicity > toe-**nis**-i-tea > quality of having muscle tone or resistance. 6

Tonography > **ton**-oh-**graf**-ee > records intraocular pressure. 8

Tonsillitis > **tohn**-si-**lie**-tis > inflammation of the tonsils, lymphatic tissue found at the back of the throat. 1, 10, 12

Torsion testicle > **tor**-shun **tes**-tik-ce > when the testicle rotates around the spermatic cord, blocking blood supply. 15

Torticollis > **tor**-tea-**kol**-lis > contraction of neck muscles. 6

Trabecular > tra-**bek**-U-lar > spongy bone of the bone, inner arches, location of red blood marrow. 5

Tracheobronchitis > **tray**-key-oh-brong-**keye**-tis > inflammation of the trachea and bronchi is seen with the childhood disease. 12

Tracheoscopy > **tray**-key-**os**-kop-ee > process of looking into the windpipe. 12

Tracheostomy > **tray**-key-**os**-toe-me > creation of a new opening of the windpipe. 12

Tracheotomy > **trake**-ee-**ot**-oh-me > surgical: surgery to cut into the trachea (windpipe). 1, 12

Transcriptome > trans-**grip**-tohm > study of how the transcription of RNA makes errors in metabolism. 3

Trapezius > tra-**pee**-zee-us > muscle shaped like a trapezoid. 6

Treatment (Tx) > **treet**-ment > medical, surgical, dental, or psychiatric management of a patient's illness or injury. It can also include preventive medicine to avoid illness and injury. It is part of the plan in the acronym SOAP. 1, 2

Trephination > **tref**-i-**na**-shun > alternate term for craniotomy, which is used when fluid/blood is evacuated via a drill or burr hole. 7

Triad > **try**-ad > group of three elements having things in common or may be associated with a syndrome. 2

Trichoepithelioma > **trik**-oh-**ep**-ee-**thee**-lee-**oh**-ma > abundant small benign nodules of the hair roots. 4

Trichomoniasis > **trik**-oh-moe-**nigh**-ah-sis > infestation of malodorous, green-yellow, thin discharge with colpodynia. 15

Trichomycosis > **trik**-oh-**my**-ko-sis > disease of the hair caused by fungi. 4

Trichorrhexis > **trik**-oh-**rek**-sis > disorder in which the hairs tend to break or split. 4

Tricuspid > try-**kus**-pid > having three cusps used to describe and name the heart valve between the right atrium and right ventricle; has three leaflets held by 4–6 chordae tendineae. 11

Trigeminal > try-**gem**-in-al > three pathways. Used for the Trigeminal nerve (CN 5) with three branches of the face. Trigeminal pulse is heartbeats in a pattern of three. 2, 11

Triglyceride > tri-**glis**-er-ide > most abundant fat of the body made up of a glycerol and three fatty acids. 13

Trochlear > tro-**klee**-ar **>** CN IV, nerve moves the eye in (nasally) and up. 8

Tropomyosin > **trow**-poe-**my**-oh-sin > muscle protein. 6

Unit

Troponin > **trow**-poe-nin > (**Tn-I** or **Tn-L**) > muscle protein of troponin I and troponin T increase with cardiac damage. 6, 11

Tuberculosis > two-**bur**-Q-**low**-sis > infectious disease caused by the bacterium *Mycobacterium tuberculosis* (**MTB**); generally affects the lungs but can affect all tissues. 12

Tumor > **too**-mur > swelling, used as a neoplasm, an abnormal growth. 4

Turbinate > **tur**-bi-nate > Latin for 'shaped like a top'; three turbinates filter and warm the air on the way to the lungs. An alternate term for turbinate is **concha** (**kong**-ka) > shell-shape. 5, 8

Turbinectomy > **tur**-bi-**nek**-toe-me > surgical removal of the turbinate bone. 8

Turbinotomy > **tur**-bi-**not**-oh-me > surgical incision into the turbinate bone. 8

Tympanocentesis > **tim**-pah-no-sen-**tea**-sis > surgical puncture of the TM with a needle to aspirate fluid. 8

Tympanogram > **tim**-pan-**oh**-gram > record of the movement of the TM. 8

Tympanometry > **tim**-pah-**nom**-ee-tree > specific measurement of the compliance of the drum. 8

Ulcer > **ul**-sir > loss of the epidermis and portion of the dermis; it is associated with poor circulation. 4

Ulcerative colitis > **ul**-sir-ah-tiv ko-**lie**-tis (**UC**) > inflammatory bowel disease (**IBD**). 9, 13

Umami > **u**-mah-me > Japanese for savory taste. 8

Umbilical > um-**bill**-ee-kal > region: the middle square with the umbilicus (belly button) – includes most of the small intestines (jejunum), abdominal aorta, inferior vena cava. 2

Ungual > **ung**-wal > pertaining to the nail. 4

Unilateral > **u**-knee-**lat**-er-al > occurring on one side of the body. 2

Ureterectasia > yur-ee-tur-ek-**tay**-zee-ah > dilating the ureter > done when disease or injury narrows the tube (stenosis). 14

Ureterolith > yur-**ee**-tur-**oh**-lith > stone in the ureter; painful contractions by the ureter tries to clear the stone. 14

Ureteropyeloplasty > yur-**ee**-tur-oh-**pie**-eh-low-**plaz**-tee > surgical repair or reconstruction of a ureter from the renal pelvis. 14

Ureteropyosis > yur-**ee**-tur-oh-**pie**-oh-sis > accumulation of pus in the ureter. 14

Urethritis > **yur**-ee-**thri**-tis > inflammation of the urethra. 14

Urethrocystometry > **yur**-ee-throw-sis-**toe**-meh-tree > procedure, measures the pressure during the release of urine at the urethral and urinary bladder levels. 14

Urinalysis > **yur**-in-**al**-i-sis > laboratory: analysis of urine specimen for electrolytes and cells. 3, 14

Urinary > **your**-in-air-ee > pertaining to urine. The urinary tract begins in the renal pelvis of the kidneys, flows down the ureters, to the urinary bladder, and finally out of the urethra. 2, 14

Urine > **your**-in > waste product of the kidneys: ammonia, creatinine, and urea. 2, 14

Unit

Urobilinogen > **yur**-oh-bi-**lin**-oh-jen > liver waste product bilirubin is found in the urine. 13, 14

Urticaria > **ur**-tea-**kare**-ee-ah > eruption of itchy wheals usually associated with allergies, cold, or heat. *Synonym*: hives. 4, 9

Uterine atony > **U**-tur-ine **at**-oh-knee > failure of the myometrium (muscle layers of the uterus) to contract. 15

Uterosalpingography > **U**-tur-oh-**sal**-ping-**goh**-graf-ee > process of recording the uterine tube and uterus for open passageway. 15

Vaginal atrophy > **at**-row-fee > loss of hydration and hormone stimulation causes the mucosal layer to be dry and friable. 15

Vaginitis > **vaj**-ee-**nigh**-tis > inflammation of the vagina. 15

Vaginosis > **vaj**-ee-**knee**-oh-sis > abnormal condition of the vagina. 15

Vagus > **vay**-gus > CN X is the only CN to leave the cranium and is active with the heart, pharynx, larynx, and the GI tract. 8

Varicella zoster (VZV) > **vair**-ee-**sell**-ah **zos**-tur > shingles, painful, plaque of vesicles and bullae on red bases following the nerve root across the dermatome. 4, 7

Variolation or Inoculation> **vair**-ee-oh-**lay**-shun or **in**-oc-**U**-**lay**-shun > use of a two-prong needle set – connects with the epithelial line. Used for Smallpox vaccination. 4

Vasculitis > **vaz**-Q-**lie**-tis > inflammation of the blood vessels. *Synonym*: angiitis. 4, 9

Vasectomy > vas-**ek**-toe-me > to cut out or remove the vas deferens. 15

Vasoactive > **vay**-so-**ak**-tiv > influencing the size and tone of the vessels. 11

Vasodilation > **vay**-so-die-**lay**-shun > increase in the diameter or caliber of the vessel. 11

Vasovasostomy > **vah**-so-vah-**sos**-toe-me > repair of a vasectomy, a new opening is created by joining the two cut ends together. This is also called an anastomosis. 15

Vegetations > **vej**-eh-ta-shuns > growing or functioning improperly on structures such as the leaflets of the cardiac valves. 11

Veins > vain > smaller than arteries, weaker, less muscle, low pressure, carry deoxygenated blood. 10, 11

Venipuncture > **ven**-i-**punkt**-shur > to puncture the vein to withdraw blood. 11

Ventral > **ven**-tral > front of, anterior, used primarily to describe internal organs which are more anterior. 2

Ventricle > **ven**-tree-kel > cavity, chamber of the heart or brain. 7, 11

Ventricular fibrillation (VF or VFib) > life-threatening arrhythmia where the normal impulses triggering an ordered contraction of the heart muscle become disorganized to the point that the heart is quivering. 11

Verruca plana > **vair**-u-kah **play**-nah > dome-shaped lesion, gets flattened and deeper into the skin on the feet. *Synonym*: plantar warts. 4

Verruca vulgaris > **vair**-u-kah vul-**gah**-ris > waxy lesion on the skin, wart, HPV. 4

Unit

Vertebra, **Vertebrae** > **vur**-teh-brah; **vur**-teh-breh > stack of 33 bones is a segmented curved rod with three distinct curves. Cervical > 7, Thoracic > 12, Lumbar > 5, Sacrum > 5 fused, and Coccyx > 4 fused. *Synonym*: Rachi/o and Spondyl/o.   5, 7

Vertebral > **vur**-teh-bral > pertaining to the vertebra (singular), vertebrae (plural), the bones of the spinal column.   2

Vertigo > **vur**-tea-go > extreme dizziness, spinning sensation associated with inner ear malfunction.   8

Vesicles > **ves**-ee-kels > small container or bladder. Tiny carriers found in most cells. Any small sac such as the gallbladder or urinary bladder.   3, 14

Vesicoclysis > **ves**-i-**kok**-lie-sis > washing out the bladder or irrigation.   14

Vesicotomy > **ves**-i-**kot**-oh-me > to cut into the bladder.   14

Vesicouterine > **ves**-i-ko-**U**-tur-ine **fistula** > abnormal opening between the bladder and uterus.   14

Vestibulotomy > ves-**tib**-U-**lot**-oh-me > to cut into the vestibule of the ear.   8

Vibrissae > vie-**bris**-ay (plural) > nose hairs which are visible; these are designed to capture larger particles of dust, sawdust, and dirt. **Vibrissa** > singular.   8, 12

Visceral > **vis**-ur-al > pertaining to the membrane; will cling to or touch the organs it protects.   2, 11, 12, 13

Vitreous > **vit**-ree-us **floaters** > tiny collagen fibers of the stroma, have been dislodged.   8

Voiding cystourethrogram (VCUG) > **voy**-ding **sis**-to-yur-ee-**throw**-gram > X-ray image made as a patient voids (urinates) a bladder full of X-ray dye.   14

Voiding or **Urination** > **yur**-i-**nay**-shun > evacuating urine.   14

Volvulus > **vol**-vyu-lus > twisting of the intestines causing an obstruction.   13

Vomer > **voe**-mur > single, small bone forms the bottom and back of the nasal septum.   5

Vomit > **vom**-it > ejection of stomach contents via the mouth. *Synonym*: emesis.   3, 13

Vulva > **vul**-vah > general term describing the area including the clitoris, labia, hymen, and vaginal opening.   15

Vulvitis > **vul**-vie-tis > inflammation of the vulva, associated with yeast infections or similar.   15

Wheals > wheels > raised papules or plaques, represent capillary swelling or permeability (weeping). *Synonym*: welts.   4

Wheezing > **we**-zing > musical and tends to be a higher pitch. Occurs with obstruction such as asthma. Occurs with both inspiration and expiration.   12

Withdrawal syndrome > with the cessation of an addictive substance, a specific set of symptoms occurring which can be uncomfortable or even deadly.   7

Xanthelasma > **zan**-the-**laz**-ma > yellow-appearing nodules around the eyes, associated with elevated cholesterol.   4

Xenograft > **zen**-oh-graft > graft from one species used on another species.   4

Unit

Xiphoid > **zeye**-foyd > distal bone of the breast bone; sword-tip in Latin.   2, 5, 11

Yersinia pestis > yur-**sin**-knee-ah **pest**-is > bacterium causing bubonic plague.
Causes ulcers.   4

Zygomatic > **zi**-go-**mat**-ik > cheekbones (2), helps form the eye socket
(laterally and bottom).   5

Zygote > **zeye**-goat > fertilization of an oocyte by a sperm, joining chromosomes.   9, 15

Appendix A

Singular and plural suffix list

These all pertain to NOUNS, a thing or place. They are used as the SUBJECT of the following sentences: 'The *axilla* is an area of lymphadenopathy associated with breast cancer'. 'The *foramina* of the skull number 20'. 'Dr. Henry reviewed several *diagnoses* to explain Mrs. Rey's symptoms'. It is not an action such as 'explain' or 'confined' or a descriptive such as 'cyanotic (skin)' or 'tachycardic (heart)'.

While there is a proper plural for these nouns, some are seldom seen because injury or illness involve the singular more often. Example: 'The *pleura* of the lungs confine the lung tissue'. Technically, it should be '*pleurae*' because there are two lungs. It is an example of 'convention', everyone uses it this way.

(-a) at the end of the word, make it a singular NOUN. The plural is most commonly (-ae)

- Ameba   Amebae   Single-cell organism
- Axilla   Axillae   Underarm area
- Bulla   Bullae   Larger blister
- Bursa   Bursae   Closed sac cushions joint actions
- Conjunctiva   Conjunctivae   Mucous membrane anterior eye, exterior
- Cornea   Corneae   Transparent, anterior portion of the eye sclera
- Fimbria   Fimbriae   Fringe or finger-like trumpet surrounding ovary
- Fossa   Fossae   Depression on a bone or surface area
- Fovea   Foveae   Depression on the surface: bone, skin, eye
- Gingiva   Gingivae   Dense tissue, helps anchor the teeth
- Hypha   Hyphae   Branching, tubular cell appearance of mold (fungus)
- Lacuna   Lacunae   A small space, cavity, or depression (bone)
- Larva   Larvae   Developmental stage of insects
- Macula   Maculae   A small spot, different color than surroundings
- Palpebra   Palpebrae   Eyelids

- Patella   Patellae   Kneecap
- Pleura   Pleurae   Serous membrane enveloping the lungs
- Ruga   Rugae   Wrinkle or fold
- Scapula   Scapulae   Large, triangular bone, shoulder blade
- Stria   Striae   Stripe, band, streak, or line
- Trachea   Tracheae   Windpipe, cartilaginous tube
- Tunica   Tunicae   Coat or layers, commonly used for blood vessels
- Uvula   Uvulae   The appendix structure of the upper palatine region
- Vagina   Vaginae   Genital canal of women
- Vertebra   Vertebrae   Bone segment of the spine
- Vulva   Vulvae   External genitalia of women

(–is) at the end of the word, make it a singular NOUN. The plural is most commonly (-es)

- Anastomosis   Anastomoses   Connection surgically joining two structures
- Crisis   Crises   Time of intense difficulty or trouble
- Diagnosis   Diagnoses   Through knowledge, identify the nature of an illness
- Epiphysis   Epiphyses   The end part of the long bones, growth plate
- Genesis   Geneses   The origin or beginning of formation
- Metastasis   Metastases   Spread of a cancer from primary site to distant areas
- Prognosis   Prognoses   With knowledge, prediction of outcome
- Prosthesis   Prostheses   An artificial body part: hand, leg, heart valve
- Pubis   Pubes   Most anterior set of bones in the pelvis, forms 1st arch
- Synapsis   Synapses   Connection or junction between structures
- Synopsis   Synopses   Findings on a specific subject or reading
- Testis   Testes   Male gonad gland housed in the scrotum

(–ex, –ix, or –yx) at the end of the word, make it a singular NOUN. The plural most commonly becomes (–ices)

- Apex   Apices   The tip, point, or vertex of a structure
- Appendix   Appendices   A process or projection in anatomy
- Calix   Calices   Cup-like, the shape of collection areas in kidneys
- Cervix   Cervices   Any neck-like part
- Coccyx   Coccyges   Our tail end, the end of the spinal column
- Cortex   Cortices   Outer region of an organ or structure
- Fornix   Fornices   Arching fibrous formations in the brain
- Helix   Helices   A spiral as in the shape of the ear, DNA, cochlea
- Index   Indices   Alphabetical listing or the finger we point with

• Matrix	Matrices	A formative structure like the nail bed
• Suffix	Suffices	(Suffixes is also correct) affix to the end of a word
• Thorax	Thoraces	Chest cavity as a whole
• Varix	Varices	Abnormal dilation and lengthening of a vein
• Vertex	Vertices	Top or crown of the head

(–um) at the end of the word, make it a singular NOUN. The plural most commonly becomes (–a)

• Agendum	Agenda	A list, plan, or outline to be discussed or reviewed
• Bacterium	Bacteria	One-cell organism: spiral, rod-shaped, or round
• Brachium	Brachia	The upper arm, from shoulder to the elbow
• Cilium	Cilia	Tiny, finger-like projects to move and filter
• Diverticulum	Diverticula	Tiny blind pocket of the lumen of the intestines
• Filum	Fila	A filament, a thin thread-like structure
• Frenulum	Frenula	A tether or bridle, a structure to attach
• Hilum	Hila	Medial aspect where vessels/nerves emerge
• Ilium	Ilia	Broad, upper part of the pelvis
• Inoculum	Inocula	The substance inside the syringe, usually a vaccine
• Labium	Labia	A lip or lip shape
• Millennium	Millennia	A period of 1,000 years
• Ovum	Ova	Female reproductive cell or egg or gamete
• Sacrum	Sacra	Five-fused vertebra forms posterior wall of pelvis
• Scrotum	Scrota	The pouch of skin containing the male testes
• Serum	Sera	Clear, pale-yellow liquid separates clotted blood

(–itis) at the end of the word, make it a singular NOUN. The plural most commonly becomes (–ides). Technically, any word ending in (–itis), meaning inflammation is made plural by (–ides); by convention, it is seldom seen.

• Arteritis	Arteritides	Inflammation of the arteries
• Arthritis	Arthritides	Inflammation of the joints
• Glottitis	Glottides	Inflammation of the epiglottis (closure over trachea)
• Hepatitis	Hepatitides	Inflammation or infection of the liver
• Iris	Irides	Inflammation of the iris (eye)
• Myelitis	Myelitides	Inflammation of the bone marrow or spinal cord
• Otitis	Otitides	Inflammation of the ears
• Phlebitis	Phlebitides	Inflammation of the veins
• Rhinitis	Rhinitides	Inflammation of the nose

(-on) at the end of the word, make it a singular NOUN. The plural most commonly becomes (-a)

- Criterion   Criteria
- Ganglion   Ganglia
- Mitochondrion   Mitochondria
- Protozoon   Protozoa
- Spermatozoon   Spermatozoa

There are many (-on) words which become plural with an (-s)

- Addiction   Addictions
- Capitation   Capitations
- Classification   Classifications
- Condition   Conditions
- Neuron   Neurons
- And many more, when in doubt, look it up!

(-us) at the end of the word, make it a singular NOUN. The plural most commonly becomes (-i)

- Alveolus   Alveoli   Functional unit of the lungs
- Bacillus   Bacilli   One-cell organism, treated with antibiotics
- Bronchus   Bronchi   Two subdivisions of the trachea, airways
- Calcaneus   Calcanei   Heel bone
- Calculus   Calculi   Stones: renal, gallbladder, salivary
- Canthus   Canthi   Corner of the eye, medial or lateral
- Carpus   Carpi   Wrist bone
- Cubitus   Cubiti   Elbow, originally a measure, finger to elbow = cubit
- Embolus   Emboli   A plug or blockage: blood, air, cholesterol plaque
- Esophagus   Esophagi   Transit tube mouth to stomach
- Limbus   Limbi   Border or edge, reference to corneal/sclera edge
- Locum   Loci   Location or place, used in reference to genetics
- Malleolus   Malleoli   Rounded prominence at medial and lateral ankle
- Meniscus   Menisci   Crescent-shaped, knee fibrocartilage cushion
- Nucleus   Nuclei   Center or core of the cells in this case
- Oculus   Oculi   Eye, eyeball
- Ramus   Rami   Linked branching of nerves or vessels
- Sacculus   Sacculi   Tiny sac, part of the vestibule of the inner ear
- Syllabus   Syllabi   Short summary
- Thrombus   Thrombi   Clot, obstruction: blood, air, cholesterol plaque
- Villus   Villi   Fingerlike or hairlike projections

Exceptions always occur:

- Plexus   Plexus or plexuses   A network of spinal nerves
- Sinus   Sinuses   Air filled cavities of the face
- Virus   Viruses   Tiny infectious agent, not an organism

(-nx) at the end of the word, make it a singular NOUN. The plural most commonly becomes (-ges)

- Larynx   Larynges   Voice box
- Meninx   Meninges   Coverings of the brain and spinal cord
- Nasopharynx   Nasopharynges   Area behind the nose, connecting to the pharynx
- Phalanx   Phalanges   Digits, fingers and/or toes
- Pharynx   Pharynges   Extension of the GI tract between the mouth and esophagus
- Salpinx   Salpinges   Tubes, uterine tubes between ovary and uterus
- Syrinx   Syringes   Instrument to inject or remove fluids

(-en) at the end of the word, make it a singular NOUN. The plural most commonly becomes (-ina)

- Foramen   Foramina   Opening, aperture to cross
- Lumen   Lumina   Inside, opening of a tubular structure, such as the GI tract
- Putamen   Putamina   A specific area of the mid-brain, branching

(-y) at the end of the word, make it a singular NOUN. The plural most commonly becomes (-ies) like most other non-medical words.

- Anomaly   Anomalies   Irregular, birth defect defined by structural changes
- Biopsy   Biopsies   Process of removing cells or tissues for investigation

(-oma, -ma) at the end of the word, make it a singular NOUN. The plural most commonly becomes (-mata). These are correct, however you will see the second choice as well.

- Carcinoma   Carcinomata   Carcinomas   Malignant (spreading) neoplasm
- Condyloma   Condylomata   A wart-like skin lesion
- Fibroma   Fibromata   Fibromas   Generally considered a benign neoplasm
- Leiomyoma   Leiomyomata   Leiomyomas   Smooth muscle tumor, usually benign
- Meningioma   Meningiomata   Tumor of the covering of the brain
- Neuroma   Neuromata   Neuromas   Tumor of the neurons or neuroglia
- Osteoma   Osteomata   Osteomas   Neoplasm of the bone
- Sarcoma   Sarcomata   Sarcomas   Connective tissue neoplasm
- Stigma   Stigmata   Stigmas   Visual, visible evidence of disease or change

Appendix B

The likes, the opposites, and the very close! Sounds and spelled alike yet different

- Corne/o > horny layer > describes the look of the tissue, it is used for the layer of epidermis producing new skin cells AND the cornea of the eye, the clear window of the sclera.

- Cyan/o > blue color OR compound containing cyanide.

- Myel/o > bone marrow OR spinal cord, medulla oblongata > the tissue seemed similar to the early anatomist.

- Neur/o > nerve, neuron > is the word root for brain cells and some of their organelles. Neur/o > also means 'sinew' (Greek), the tough connective tissue sheets binding muscle to muscle or muscle to bone.

- Pariet/o > wall; the outermost wall of the pleural sac of the lungs or abdominal cavity. It is also a cranial bone, a lobe of the brain, and the name of the cells of the stomach producing hydrochloric acid.

- Phren/o > diaphragm > the muscle contracts to create air pressure, filling the lung. Phren/o > also means mind, the heart sits on the diaphragm, the heart is the seat of emotions.

- Salping/o > tubes; the external auditory canal may be referred to by this word root. It is commonly used to refer to the uterine tubes of the female reproductive system.

- Sarc/o > flesh; specialize cell names for muscle; common name for members of the Sarcoptidae, a family of mites.

- Trich/o > hair as on our body or head OR the hair-like tails of parasitic protozoan flagellates.

The likes

These word parts have two or more terms which may be used.

- **Word roots with linking vowel**
  - Air: aer/o; pneum/o; pneumat/o
  - Black: melan/o; negr/o
  - Bone: oste/o; osse/o; ossi/o
  - Brain: cephal/o; encephal/o
  - Breathing: pneum/o; spir/o
  - Cell: cyt/o; kary/o (kary/o is seen as the nucleus, center)
  - Cornea: of the eye or the hard surface of skin, meaning 'scaly or horny': corne/o; kerat/o; or squam/o > scale, used for tissue designation
  - Death: mort/o; necr/o; thanat/o
  - Ear: aur/o; auricul/o; ot/o
  - Eardrum: myring/o; tympan/o
  - Egg, ovum: o/o; ov/o; ov/i; ovul/o
  - Fat: adip/o; lip/o; steat/o
  - Feces: corp/o; scat/o; sterc/o
  - Glucose/sugar: gluc/o; glyc/o; glycos/o; sacchar/o
  - Granular: mito-; chondr/o
  - Hair: trich/o; pil/o
  - Hearing: audi/o; acous/o
  - Lungs: pneum/o; pheumat/o; pulmon/o
  - Movement: kine/o; kinesi/o
  - Muscles: muscul/o; my/o; myos/o
  - Nail: onych/o; ungu/o
  - Nerve root: radic/o; radicul/o; rhiz/o
  - Nucleus: nucle/o; kary/o (kary/o may be used as cell but it is not seen often)
  - Oily: seb/o; sebace/o
  - Ovary: ovari/o; oophor/o
  - Skin: derm/o; dermat/o; cutane/o; cut/i
  - Spinal bone: vertebr/o; rachi/o; spondyl/o
  - Tendons: ten/o; tendin/o; tend/o
  - Testicle: test/i; orchid/o; orchi/o; testicul/o
  - Thread or fiber: fibr/o; fila-; mito-; coll/a
  - Tympanic membrane (TM): tympan/o; myring/o
  - Uterus: hyster/o; uter/o; men/o; metri/o
  - Yellow: xanth/o is the yellow discoloration of fatty plaques; jaundice is the yellow of liver dysfunction, staining the skin and mucous membranes; icterus also means

yellow, used to describe the color produced by dysfunctional liver or RBC destruction.

- **Prefixes**
  - Abnormal, poor, bad: dys-; mal-; dis- (removal, separation)
  - Above, on top, on, upon: supra-, epi-
  - After, behind: post-; retro-; meta- (after or beyond a point)
  - Against: contra-; anti-; counter-
  - Around, near: para-; peri-; circum- (circle)
  - Before, forward, in front of: pre-; pro-; ante-
  - Below, under: infra-; under-; sub-
  - Beyond, extreme: ultra-; meta-
  - Down, reduce, down from, less than: de-; down-; hypo-
  - First, primary: primi-; proto- (prototype protoplasm)
  - Half: hemi-; semi-
  - In, inner, inside, within, internal: in-; en-, endo-, intra- (**LIKE ALERT!** in- can mean 'no' as well)
  - Increased, more, elevated, above normal: hyper-; up-; super-; supra-
  - Many, more, increased: hyper-; multi-; poly-
  - No, not, absent, lack of: a-; an-; ig- (before gn, ignore); il- (before l, illegal); im- (before b, m, or p, immobile, imbalance); in- (before other letters, incomplete, infirm); ir- (before r, irregular); un- (not); and under- (not enough); de- (dehydration); no-; non-; nulli-
  - Out, outside, external, outer most: ec-; ecto-; ex-; exo-; extra- (outside)
  - Through: per-, dia-, di-
  - Together, with: co-; sym- (before b, p, ph, or m); syn-
  - Two, twice: bi-; di-

- **Suffixes**
  - Breaking: -clasis; -clast; -clasia; -ase
  - Building, development, beginning: -genesis; -blasts; -genic; -trophy; -tropic
  - Condition of (noun): -ia; -ism; -osis; -sis; -y; -iasis
  - Eating, devour: -phage; -phagia; -phagy
  - Pain: -algesia; -algia; -dynia
  - Pertaining to (adjectives): -al; -ar; -ary; -ic; -ac; -ile; -ory; -ous; -oid; -ive; -ine
  - Stone: -lith, -lithiasis, petrosis
  - Vision: -opia; -opsia

- **The opposites**
  - ab-　　　　　　　　　　Away from the center, not normal
  - ad-　　　　　　　　　　Toward the middle, additive

– hyper-	Increased, more than, higher, excessive
– hypo-	Decreased, less than, lower, deficient
– macro-	Large, bigger
– micro-	Smaller, smallest, tiny
– in-, intra-, en-, endo-	In, within, inner, internal, within
– ec-, ecto-, ex-, exo-	Out, outer, external, outer most
– brady-	Slow
– tachy-	Fast
– epi-, supra-	Above, on, upon, on top of
– sub-, under-	Under, below, less than, downward
– ante-, pre-	Before, forward, a head of
– post-, retro-	After, behind
– eu-	Good, normal
– dys-, mal-	Bad, difficult, painful, abnormal
– ana-	Up, toward, apart
– cata-	Down, break

Sound or spell alike potential

Dye > staining color and Die > death

Hidr/o > Sweat and Hydr/o > Water

Humerus > arm bone and humorous > funny

Malleus > a small bone in the middle ear and Malleolus > a bony protuberance at the ankle

Onch/o > tumor and Onych/o > nail

Myel/o > bone marrow or spinal cord and my/o > muscle and myl/o > tooth molar

Ilium > bone of the pelvis and Ileum > last segment of the small intestines

Prostate > part of male urinary system and Prostrate > to lay down prone

Ureter > tube from the kidney to the bladder and Urethra > tube from the bladder to the outside

Trapezius > a muscle in the back and Trapezium > a bone in the wrist

Sore > skin lesion or pain and soar > to fly

Digestive: breakdown of food by mechanical or chemical means carries down the GI tract and Gestation: to carry or bear a pregnancy

Ictal: term used to describe symptoms that occur after a stroke or seizure (Latin > stroke) and Icteric or icterus: yellow coloration of the skin or mucous membranes (Greek > yellowish)

American versus British spelling

Anemia	Anaemia	Etiology	Aetiology
Anesthetic	Anaesthetic	Fetus	Foetus
Celiac	Coeliac	Fiber	Fibre
Centimeter	Centimetre	Gynecology	Gynaecology
Cesarean	Caesarean	Hemoglobin	Haemoglobin
Color	Colour	Hemorrhage	Haemorrhage
Defecation	Defaecation	Ischemic	Ischaemic
Defense	Defence	Labor	Labour
Diarrhea	Diarrhoea	Leukemia	Leukaemia
Dyslipidemia	Dyslipidaemia	Leukocyte	Leucocyte
Dyspnea	Dyspnoea	Liter	Litre
Edema	Oedema	Orthopedic	Orthopaedic
Esophagus	Oesophagus	Paralyze	Paralyse
Estrogen	Oestrogen	Tumor	Tumour

Index of word parts

WORD ROOT WITH LINKING FORM

PREFIXES

SUFFIXES

General index